Dietary Reference Intake Values for Energy for Active Individuals*
Food and Nutrition Board, Institute of Medicine, National Academies

Life-Stage Group	Criterion	Active Pal Eer (kcal/day)†	
		Male	Female
Infants			
0-6 mo	Energy expenditure + Energy deposition	570	520 (3 mo)
7-12 mo	Energy expenditure + Energy deposition	743	676 (9 mo)
Children			
1-2 yr	Energy expenditure + Energy deposition	1046	992 (24 mo)
3-8 yr	Energy expenditure + Energy deposition	1742	1642 (6 yr)
9-13 yr	Energy expenditure + Energy deposition	2279	2071 (11 yr)
14-18 yr	Energy expenditure + Energy deposition	3152	2368 (16 yr)
Adults			
>18 yr	Energy expenditure	3067‡	2403‡ (19 yr)
Pregnant Women			
14-18 yr	Adolescent female EER + Change in TEE + Pregnancy energy deposition		
First trimester			2368 (16 yr)
Second trimester			2708 (16 yr)
Third trimester			2820 (16 yr)
19-50 yr	Adult female EER + Change in TEE + Pregnancy energy deposition		
First trimester			2403‡ (19 yr)
Second trimester			2743‡ (19 yr)
Third trimester			2855‡ (19 yr)
Lactating Women			
14-18 yr	Adolescent female EER + Milk energy output—Weight loss		
First 6 mo			2698 (16 yr)
Second 6 mo			2768 (16 yr)
19-50 yr	Adult female EER + Milk energy output—Weight loss		
First 6 mo			2733‡ (19 yr)
Second 6 mo			2803‡ (19 yr)

om Institute of Medicine of The National Academies: Dietary reference intakes for energy, carbohydrate, fiber, fat, fatty acids, cholesterol, protein, and amino acids. Washington, DC: The National Academies Press, 2002.
or healthy active Americans and Canadians at the reference height and weight.
PAL, Physical activity level; *EER*, estimated energy requirement; *TEE*, total energy expenditure.
Subtract 10 kcal/day for men and 7 kcal/day for women for each year of age above 19 years.

Dietary Reference Intakes (DRIs): Recommended Intakes for Individuals, Macronutrients
Food and Nutrition Board, Institute of Medicine, National Academies

Life-Stage Group	Protein RDA/AI g/day[a]	Protein AMDR[b]	Carbohydrate RDA/AI g/day	Carbohydrate AMDR	Fiber RDA/AI g/day	Fiber AMDR	Fat RDA/AI g/day	Fat AMDR	n-6 Polyunsaturated Fatty Acids (Linoleic Acid) RDA/AI g/day	n-6 AMDR	n-3 Polyunsaturated Fatty Acids (α-Linoleic Acid) RDA/AI g/day	n-3 AMDR[d]	Saturated and Trans Fatty Acids and Cholesterol RDA/AI g/day	S&T AMDR
Infants														
0-6 mo	9.1	ND[c]	60	ND	ND		31		4.4	ND	0.5	ND		
7-12 mo	13.5	ND	95	ND	ND		30		4.6	ND	0.5	ND		
Children														
1-3 yr	13	5-20	130	45-65	19			30-40	7	5-10	0.7	0.6-1.2		
4-8 yr	19	10-30	130	45-65	25			25-35	10	5-10	0.9	0.6-1.2		
Males														
9-13 yr	34	10-30	130	45-65	31			25-35	12	5-10	1.2	0.6-1.2		
14-18 yr	52	10-30	130	45-65	38			25-35	16	5-10	1.6	0.6-1.2		
19-30 yr	56	10-35	130	45-65	38			20-35	17	5-10	1.6	0.6-1.2		
31-50 yr	56	10-35	130	45-65	38			20-35	17	5-10	1.6	0.6-1.2		
50-70 yr	56	10-35	130	45-65	30			20-35	14	5-10	1.6	0.6-1.2		
>70 yr	56	10-35	130	45-65	30			20-35	14	5-10	1.6	0.6-1.2		
Females														
9-13 yr	34	10-30	130	45-65	26			25-35	10	5-10	1.0	0.6-1.2		
14-18 yr	46	10-30	130	45-65	26			25-35	11	5-10	1.1	0.6-1.2		
19-30 yr	46	10-35	130	45-65	25			20-35	12	5-10	1.1	0.6-1.2		
31-50 yr	46	10-35	130	45-65	25			20-35	12	5-10	1.1	0.6-1.2		
50-70 yr	46	10-35	130	45-65	21			20-35	11	5-10	1.1	0.6-1.2		
>70 yr	46	10-35	130	45-65	21			20-35	11	5-10	1.1	0.6-1.2		
Pregnant														
≤18 yr	71	10-35	175	45-65	28			20-35	13	5-10	1.4	0.6-1.2		
19-30 yr	71	10-35	175	45-65	28			20-35	13	5-10	1.4	0.6-1.2		
31-50 yr	71	10-35		45-65	28			20-35	13	5-10	1.4	0.6-1.2		
Lactating														
≤18 yr	71	10-35	210	45-65	29			20-35	13	5-10	1.3	0.6-1.2		
19-30 yr	71	10-35	210	45-65	29			20-35	13	5-10	1.3	0.6-1.2		
31-50 yr	71	10-35	210	45-65	29			20-35	13	5-10	1.3	0.6-1.2		

ata from Dietary reference intakes for energy, carbohydrate, fiber, fat, fatty acids, cholesterol, protein, and amino acids. Washington, DC: The National Academies Press, 2002.
OTE: This table represents Recommended Dietary Allowances (RDAs) in **bold type** and Adequate Intakes (AIs) in ordinary type. RDAs and AIs may both be used as goals for individual intake. RDAs are set to meet the needs of almost all (97%-98%) indi-duals in a group. For healthy breastfed infants, the AI is the mean intake. The AI for other life-stage and gender groups is believed to cover the needs of all individuals in the group, but lack of data prevents being able to specify with confidence the per-entage of individuals covered by this intake.
ased on 1.5 g/kg/day for infants, 1.1 g/kg/day for 1-3 yr, 0.95 g/kg/day for 4-13 yr, 0.85 g/kg/day for 14-18 yr, 0.8 g/kg/day for adults, and 1.1 g/kg/day for pregnant (using prepregnancy weight) and lactating women.
cceptable Macronutrient Distribution Range (AMDR) is the range of intake for a particular energy source that is associated with reduced risk of chronic disease while providing intakes of essential nutrients. If an individual has consumed in excess of e AMDR, there is a potential of increasing the risk of chronic diseases and insufficient intakes of essential nutrients.
ND 5 Not determinable due to lack of data of adverse effects in this age group and concern with regard to lack of ability to handle excess amounts. Source of intake should be from food only to prevent high levels of intake.
pproximately 10% of the total can come from longer-chain, n-3 fatty acids.

Dietary Reference Intakes (DRIs): Recommended Intakes for Individuals, Vitamins
Food and Nutrition Board, Institute of Medicine, National Academies

Life-Stage Group	Vitamin A (µg/d)[a]	Vitamin C (mg/d)	Vitamin D (µg/d)[b,c]	Vitamin E (mg/d)[d]	Vitamin K (µg/d)	Thiamin (mg/d)	Riboflavin (mg/d)	Niacin (mg/d)[e]	Vitamin B_6 (mg/d)	Folate (µg/d)[f]	Vitamin B_{12} (µg/d)	Pantothenic Acid (mg/d)	Biotin (µg/d)	Choline (mg/d)[g]
Infants														
0-6 mo	400*	40*	5*	4*	2.0*	0.2*	0.3*	2*	0.1*	65*	0.4*	1.7*	5*	125*
7-12 mo	500*	50*	5*	5*	2.5*	0.3*	0.4*	4*	0.3*	80*	0.5*	1.8*	6*	150*
Children														
1-3 yr	**300**	**15**	5*	**6**	30*	**0.5**	**0.5**	**6**	**0.5**	**150**	**0.9**	2*	8*	200*
4-8 yr	**400**	**25**	5*	**7**	55*	**0.6**	**0.6**	**8**	**0.6**	**200**	**1.2**	3*	12*	250*
Males														
9-13 yr	**600**	**45**	5*	**11**	60*	**0.9**	**0.9**	**12**	**1.0**	**300**	**1.8**	4*	20*	375*
14-18 yr	**900**	**75**	5*	**15**	75*	**1.2**	**1.3**	**16**	**1.3**	**400**	**2.4**	5*	25*	550*
19-30 yr	**900**	**90**	5*	**15**	120*	**1.2**	**1.3**	**16**	**1.3**	**400**	**2.4**	5*	30*	550*
31-50 yr	**900**	**90**	5*	**15**	120*	**1.2**	**1.3**	**16**	**1.3**	**400**	**2.4**	5*	30*	550*
51-70 yr	**900**	**90**	10*	**15**	120*	**1.2**	**1.3**	**16**	**1.7**	**400**	**2.4**[h]	5*	30*	550*
> 70 yr	**900**	**90**	15*	**15**	120*	**1.2**	**1.3**	**16**	**1.7**	**400**	**2.4**[h]	5*	30*	550*
Females														
9-13 yr	**600**	**45**	5*	**11**	60*	**0.9**	**0.9**	**12**	**1.0**	**300**	**1.8**	4*	20*	375*
14-18 yr	**700**	**65**	5*	**15**	75*	**1.0**	**1.0**	**14**	**1.2**	**400**[i]	**2.4**	5*	25*	400*
19-30 yr	**700**	**75**	5*	**15**	90*	**1.1**	**1.1**	**14**	**1.3**	**400**[i]	**2.4**	5*	30*	425*
31-50 yr	**700**	**75**	5*	**15**	90*	**1.1**	**1.1**	**14**	**1.3**	**400**[i]	**2.4**	5*	30*	425*
51-70 yr	**700**	**75**	10*	**15**	90*	**1.1**	**1.1**	**14**	**1.5**	**400**	**2.4**[h]	5*	30*	425*
> 70 yr	**700**	**75**	15*	**15**	90*	**1.1**	**1.1**	**14**	**1.5**	**400**	**2.4**[h]	5*	30*	425*
Pregnancy														
≤18 yr	**750**	**80**	5*	**15**	75*	**1.4**	**1.4**	**18**	**1.9**	**600**[j]	**2.6**	6*	30*	450*
19-30 yr	**770**	**85**	5*	**15**	90*	**1.4**	**1.4**	**18**	**1.9**	**600**[j]	**2.6**	6*	30*	450*
31-50 yr	**770**	**85**	5*	**15**	90*	**1.4**	**1.4**	**18**	**1.9**	**600**[j]	**2.6**	6*	30*	450*
Lactation														
≤18 yr	**1200**	**115**	5*	**19**	75*	**1.4**	**1.6**	**17**	**2.0**	**500**	**2.8**	7*	35*	550*
19-30 yr	**1300**	**120**	5*	**19**	90*	**1.4**	**1.6**	**17**	**2.0**	**500**	**2.8**	7*	35*	550*
31-50 yr	**1300**	**120**	5*	**19**	90*	**1.4**	**1.6**	**17**	**2.0**	**500**	**2.8**	7*	35*	550*

SOURCES: Dietary Reference Intakes for Calcium, Phosphorous, Magnesium, Vitamin D, and Fluoride (1997); Dietary Reference Intakes for Thiamin, Riboflavin, Niacin, Vitamin B_6, Folate, Vitamin B_{12}, Pantothenic Acid, Biotin, and Choline (1998); Dietary Reference Intakes for Vitamin C, Vitamin E, Selenium, and Carotenoids (2000); and Dietary Reference Intakes for Vitamin A, Vitamin K, Arsenic, Boron, Chromium, Copper, Iodine, Iron, Manganese, Molybdenum, Nickel, Silicon, Vanadium, and Zinc (2001). These reports may be accessed via www.nap.edu. Copyright 2001 by the National Academy of Sciences. All rights reserved.

NOTE: This table (taken from the DRI reports, see www.nap.edu) presents Recommended Dietary Allowances (RDAs) in **bold type** and Adequate Intakes (AIs) in ordinary type followed by an asterisk (*). RDAs and AIs may both be used as goals for individual intake. RDAs are set to meet the needs of almost all (97%-98%) individuals in a group. For healthy breastfed infants, the AI is the mean intake. The AI for other life-stage and gender groups is believed to cover needs of all individuals in the group, but lack of data or uncertainty in the data prevent being able to specify with confidence the percentage of individuals covered by this intake.

[a] As retinol activity equivalents (RAEs). 1 RAE = 1 µg retinol, 12 µg β-carotene, 24 µg α-carotene, or 24 µg β-cryptoxanthin. To calculate RAEs from REs of provitamin A carotenoids in foods, divide the REs by 2. For preformed vitamin A in foods or supplements and for provitamin A carotenoids in supplements, 1 RE = 1 RAE.

[b] Calciferol. 1 µg calciferol = 40 IU vitamin D.

[c] In the absence of adequate exposure to sunlight.

[d] As α-tocopherol. α-Tocopherol includes RRR- α-tocopherol, the only form of α-tocopherol that occurs naturally in foods, and the 2R-stereoisometric forms of α-tocopherol (RRR-, RSR-, RRS-, and RSS-α-tocopherol) that occur in fortified foods and supplements. It does not include the 2S-stereoisometric forms of α-tocopherol (SRR-, SSR-, SR-, and SSS-α-tocopherol), also found in fortified foods and supplements.

[e] As niacin equivalents (NE). 1 mg of niacin = 60 mg of tryptophan; 0-6 months = preformed niacin (not NE).

[f] As dietary folate equivalents (DFE). 1 DFE = 1 µg food folate = 0.6 µg of folic acid from fortified food or as a supplement consumed with food = 0.5 µg of a supplement taken on an empty stomach.

[g] Although AIs have been set for choline, few data assess whether a dietary supply of choline is needed at all stages of the life cycle, and it may be that the choline requirement can be met by endogenous synthesis at some of these stages.

[h] Because 10 to 30 percent of older people may malabsorb food-bound B_{12}, it is advisable for those older than 50 years to meet their RDA mainly by consuming foods fortified with B_{12} or a supplement containing B_{12}.

[i] In view of evidence linking folate intake with neural tube defects in the fetus, it is recommended that all women capable of becoming pregnant consume 400 µg from supplements or fortified foods in addition to intake of food folate from a varied diet.

[j] It is assumed that women will continue consuming 400 µg from supplements or fortified food until their pregnancy is confirmed and they enter prenatal care, which ordinarily occurs after the end of the periconceptional period—the critical time for formation of the neural tube.

Dietary Reference Intakes (DRIs): Tolerable Upper Intake Levels (UL[a]), Vitamins
Food and Nutrition Board, Institute of Medicine, National Academies

Life-Stage Group	Vitamin A (µg/d)[b]	Vitamin C (mg/d)	Vitamin D (µg/d)	Vitamin E (mg/d)[c,d]	Vitamin K	Thiamin	Riboflavin	Niacin (mg/d)[d]	Vitamin B_6 (mg/d)[d]	Folate (µg/d)[d]	Vitamin B_{12}	Pantothenic Acid	Biotin	Choline (g/d)	Carotenoids[e]
Infants															
0-6 mo	600	ND[f]	25	ND	ND	ND	ND	ND	ND	ND	ND	ND	ND	ND	ND
7-12 mo	600	ND	25	ND	ND	ND	ND	ND	ND	ND	ND	ND	ND	ND	ND
Children															
1-3 yr	600	400	50	200	ND	ND	ND	10	30	300	ND	ND	ND	1.0	ND
4-8 yr	900	650	50	300	ND	ND	ND	15	40	400	ND	ND	ND	1.0	ND
Males, Females															
9-13 yr	1700	1200	50	600	ND	ND	ND	20	60	600	ND	ND	ND	2.0	ND
14-18 yr	2800	1800	50	800	ND	ND	ND	30	80	800	ND	ND	ND	3.0	ND
19-70 yr	3000	2000	50	1000	ND	ND	ND	35	100	1000	ND	ND	ND	3.5	ND
>70 yr	3000	2000	50	1000	ND	ND	ND	35	100	1000	ND	ND	ND	3.5	ND
Pregnancy															
≤18 yr	2800	1800	50	800	ND	ND	ND	30	80	800	ND	ND	ND	3.0	ND
19-50 yr	3000	2000	50	1000	ND	ND	ND	35	100	1000	ND	ND	ND	3.5	ND
Lactation															
18 yr	2800	1800	50	800	ND	ND	ND	30	80	800	ND	ND	ND	3.0	ND
19-50 yr	3000	2000	50	1000	ND	ND	ND	35	100	1000	ND	ND	ND	3.5	ND

SOURCES: Dietary Reference Intakes for Calcium, Phosphorous, Magnesium, Vitamin D, and Fluoride (1997); Dietary Reference Intakes for Thiamin, Riboflavin, Niacin, Vitamin B_6, Folate, Vitamin B_{12}, Pantothenic Acid, Biotin, and Choline (1998); Dietary Reference Intakes for Vitamin C, Vitamin E, Selenium, and Carotenoids (2000); and Dietary Reference Intakes for Vitamin A, Vitamin K, Arsenic, Boron, Chromium, Copper, Iodine, Iron, Manganese, Molybdenum, Nickel, Silicon, Vanadium, and Zinc (2001). These reports may be accessed via www.nap.edu. Copyright 2001 by the National Academy of Sciences. All rights reserved.

[a] UL = The maximum level of daily nutrient intake that is likely to pose no risk of adverse effects. Unless otherwise specified, the UL represents total intake from food, water, and supplements. Due to lack of suitable data, ULs could not be established for vitamin K, thiamin, riboflavin, vitamin B_{12}, pantothenic acid, biotin, or carotenoids. In the absence of ULs, extra caution may be warranted in consuming levels above recommended intakes.

[b] As preformed vitamin A only.

[c] As α-tocopherol; applies to any form of supplemental α-tocopherol.

[d] The ULs for vitamin E, niacin, and folate apply to synthetic forms obtained from supplements, fortified foods, or a combination of the two.

[e] β-Carotene supplements are advised only to serve as a provitamin A source for individuals at risk of vitamin A deficiency.

[f] ND = Not determinable due to lack of data of adverse effects in this age group and concern with regard to lack of ability to handle excess amounts. Source of intake should be from food only to prevent high levels of intake.

Dietary Reference Intakes (DRIs): Recommended Intakes for Individuals, Minerals
Food and Nutrition Board, Institute of Medicine, National Academies

Life-Stage Group	Calcium (mg/d)	Chromium (µg/d)	Copper (µg/d)	Fluoride (mg/d)	Iodine (µg/d)	Iron (mg/d)	Magnesium (mg/d)	Manganese (mg/d)	Molybdenum (µg/d)	Phosphorus (mg/d)	Potassium (mg/d)	Selenium (µg/d)	Sodium (mg/d)	Zinc (mg/d)
Infants														
0-6 mo	210*	0.2*	200*	0.01*	110*	0.27*	30*	0.003*	2*	100*	400*	15*	120*	2*
7-12 mo	270*	5.5*	220*	0.5*	130*	11	75*	0.6*	3*	275*	700*	20*	370*	3
Children														
1-3 yr	500*	11*	340	0.7*	90	7	80	1.2*	17	460	3000*	20	1000*	3
4-8 yr	800*	15*	440	1*	90	10	130	1.5*	22	500	3800*	30	1200*	5
Males														
9-13 yr	1300*	25*	700	2*	120	8	240	1.9*	34	1250	4500*	40	1500*	8
14-18 yr	1300*	35*	890	3*	150	11	410	2.2*	43	1250	4700*	55	1500*	11
19-30 yr	1000*	35*	900	4*	150	8	400	2.3*	45	700	4700*	55	1500*	11
31-50 yr	1000*	35*	900	4*	150	8	420	2.3*	45	700	4700*	55	1500*	11
51-70 yr	1200*	30*	900	4*	150	8	420	2.3*	45	700	4700*	55	1300*	11
>70 yr	1200*	30*	900	4*	150	8	420	2.3*	45	700	4700*	55	1200*	11
Females														
9-13 yr	1300*	21*	700	2*	120	8	240	1.6*	34	1250	4500*	40	1500*	8
14-18 yr	1300*	24*	890	3*	150	15	360	1.6*	43	1250	4700*	55	1500*	9
19-30 yr	1000*	25*	900	3*	150	18	310	1.8*	45	700	4700*	55	1500*	8
31-50 yr	1000*	25*	900	3*	150	18	320	1.8*	45	700	4700*	55	1500*	8
51-70 yr	1200*	20*	900	3*	150	8	320	1.8*	45	700	4700*	55	1300*	8
>70 yr	1200*	20*	900	3*	150	8	320	1.8*	45	700	4700*	55	1200*	8
Pregnancy														
≤18 yr	1300*	29*	1000	3*	220	27	400	2.0*	50	1250	4700*	60	1500*	13
19-30 yr	1000*	30*	1000	3*	220	27	350	2.0*	50	700	4700*	60	1500*	11
31-50 yr	1000*	30*	1000	3*	220	27	360	2.0*	50	700	4700*	60	1500*	11
Lactation														
≤18 yr	1300*	44*	1300	3*	290	10	360	2.6*	50	1250	5100*	70	1500*	14
19-30 yr	1000*	45*	1300	3*	290	9	310	2.6*	50	700	5100*	70	1500*	12
31-50 yr	1000*	45*	1300	3*	290	9	320	2.6*	50	700	5100*	70	1500*	12

SOURCES: Dietary reference intakes for calcium, phosphorus, magnesium, vitamin D, and fluoride (1997); Dietary reference intakes for thiamin, riboflavin, niacin, vitamin B6, folate, vitamin B12, pantothenic acid, biotin, and choline (1998); Dietary reference intakes for vitamin C, vitamin E, selenium, and carotenoids (2000); Dietary reference intakes for vitamin A, vitamin K, arsenic, boron, chromium, copper, iodine, iron, manganese, molybdenum, nickel, silicon, vanadium, and zinc (2001); and Dietary reference intakes for water, potassium, sodium, chloride, and sulphate (2004). Copyright 2001 by the National Academy of Sciences. All rights reserved.

NOTE: This table presents Recommended Dietary Allowances (RDAs) in **bold type** and Adequate Intakes (AIs) in ordinary type followed by an asterisk (*). RDAs and AIs may both be used as goals for individual intake. RDAs are set to meet the needs of almost all (97%–98%) individuals in a group. For healthy breastfed infants, the AI is the mean intake. The AI for other life-stage and gender groups is believed to cover needs of all individuals in the group, but lack of data or uncertainty in the data prevent being able to specify with confidence the percentage of individuals covered by this intake.

Dietary Reference Intakes (DRIs): Tolerable Upper Intake Levels (UL[a]), Minerals
Food and Nutrition Board, Institute of Medicine, National Academies

Life-Stage Group	Arsenic[b]	Boron (mg/d)	Calcium (mg/d)	Chromium	Copper (µg/d)	Fluoride (mg/d)	Iodine (µg/d)	Iron (mg/d)	Magnesium (mg/d)[c]	Manganese (mg/d)	Molybdenum (µg/d)	Nickel (mg/d)	Phosphorus (g/d)	Selenium (µg/d)	Silicon[d]	Vanadium (mg/d)[e]	Zinc (mg/d)
Infants																	
0-6 mo	ND[f]	ND	ND	ND	ND	0.7	ND	40	ND	ND	ND	ND	ND	45	ND	ND	4
7-12 mo	ND	ND	ND	ND	ND	0.9	ND	40	ND	ND	ND	ND	ND	60	ND	ND	5
Children																	
1-3 yr	ND	3	2.5	ND	1000	1.3	200	40	65	2	300	0.2	3	90	ND	ND	7
4-8 yr	ND	6	2.5	ND	3000	2.2	300	40	110	3	600	0.3	3	150	ND	ND	12
Males, Females																	
9-13 yr	ND	11	2.5	ND	5000	10	600	40	350	6	1100	0.6	4	280	ND	ND	23
14-18 yr	ND	17	2.5	ND	8000	10	900	45	350	9	1700	1.0	4	400	ND	ND	34
19-70 yr	ND	20	2.5	ND	10,000	10	1100	45	350	11	2000	1.0	4	400	ND	1.8	40
>70 yr	ND	20	2.5	ND	10,000	10	1100	45	350	11	2000	1.0	3	400	ND	1.8	40
Pregnancy																	
≤18 yr	ND	17	2.5	ND	8000	10	900	45	350	9	1700	1.0	3.5	400	ND	ND	34
19-50 yr	ND	20	2.5	ND	10,000	10	1100	45	350	11	2000	1.0	3.5	400	ND	ND	40
Lactation																	
≤18 yr	ND	17	2.5	ND	8000	10	900	45	350	9	1700	1.0	4	400	ND	ND	34
19-50 yr	ND	20	2.5	ND	10,000	10	1100	45	350	11	2000	1.0	4	400	ND	ND	40

SOURCES: Dietary reference intakes for calcium, phosphorous, magnesium, vitamin D, and fluoride (1997); Dietary reference intakes for thiamin, riboflavin, niacin, vitamin B6, folate, vitamin B12, pantothenic acid, biotin, and choline (1998); Dietary reference intakes for vitamin C, vitamin E, selenium, and carotenoids (2000); and Dietary reference intakes for vitamin A, vitamin K, arsenic, boron, chromium, copper, iodine, iron, manganese, molybdenum, nickel, silicon, vanadium, and zinc (2001). These reports may be accessed via www.nap.edu. Copyright 2001 by the National Academy of Sciences. All rights reserved.

a. The maximum level of daily nutrient intake that is likely to pose no risk of adverse effects. Unless otherwise specified, the UL represents total intake from food, water, and supplements. Due to lack of suitable data, ULs could not be established for arsenic, chromium, and silicon. In the absence of ULs, extra caution may be warranted in consuming levels above recommended intakes.
b. Although the UL was not determined for arsenic, there is no justification for adding arsenic to food or supplements.
c. The ULs for magnesium represent intake from a pharmacologic agent only and do not include intake from food and water.
d. Although silicon has not been shown to cause adverse effects in humans, there is no justification for adding silicon to supplements.
e. Although vanadium in food has not been shown to cause adverse effects in humans, there is no justification for adding vanadium to food, and vanadium supplements should be used with caution. The UL is based on adverse effects in laboratory animals, and this data could be used to set a UL for adults but not children and adolescents.
f. ND = Not determinable due to lack of data of adverse effects in this age group and concern with regard to lack of ability to handle excess amounts. Source of intake should be from food only to prevent high levels of intake.

Determining BMI

Find the height in the left column. Move across the row to the best indicator of weight. The number at the top of the row that corresponds will indicate the BMI. BMI is not applicable to children, adolescents, frail elderly, pregna and lactating women, and highly muscular individuals.

BMI	19	20	21	22	23	24	25	26	27	28	29	30	31	32	33	34	35
Height								Weight (in pounds)									
4'10" (58")	91	96	100	105	110	115	119	124	129	134	138	143	148	153	158	162	167
4'11" (59")	94	99	104	109	114	119	124	128	133	138	143	148	153	158	163	168	173
5' (60")	97	102	107	112	118	123	128	133	138	143	148	153	158	163	168	174	179
5'1" (61")	100	106	111	116	122	127	132	137	143	148	153	158	164	169	174	180	185
5'2" (62")	104	109	115	120	126	131	136	142	147	153	158	164	169	175	180	186	191
5'3" (63")	107	113	118	124	130	135	141	146	152	158	163	169	175	180	186	191	197
5'4" (64")	110	116	122	128	134	140	145	151	157	163	169	174	180	186	192	197	204
5'5" (65")	114	120	126	132	138	144	150	156	162	168	174	180	186	192	198	204	210
5'6" (66")	118	124	130	136	142	148	155	161	167	173	179	186	192	198	204	210	216
5'7" (67")	121	127	134	140	146	153	159	166	172	178	185	191	198	204	211	217	223
5'8" (68")	125	131	138	144	151	158	164	171	177	184	190	197	203	210	216	223	230
5'9" (69")	128	135	142	149	155	162	169	176	182	189	196	203	209	216	223	230	236
5'10" (70")	132	139	146	153	160	167	174	181	188	195	202	209	216	222	229	236	243
5'11" (71")	136	143	150	157	165	172	179	186	193	200	208	215	222	229	236	243	250
6' (72")	140	147	154	162	169	177	184	191	199	206	213	221	228	235	242	250	258
6'1" (73")	144	151	159	166	174	182	189	197	204	212	219	227	235	242	250	257	265
6'2" (74")	148	155	163	171	179	186	194	202	210	218	225	233	241	249	256	264	272
6'3" (75")	152	160	168	176	184	192	200	208	216	224	232	240	248	256	264	272	279

Classification of Weight

Classification	BMI
Underweight	<18.5
Normal	18.5-24.9
Overweight	25.0-29.9
Obesity	30.3-34.9
Extreme Obesity	>40.0

Source: *National Institutes of Health, 1998*

Data from NIH / National Heart, Lung, and Blood Institute (NHLBI). Evidence report of clinical guidelines on the identification, evaluation, and treatment of overweight and obesity in adults. Bethesda, MD: NIH / NHLBI, 1998.
19-24, Minimal health risk; *25-26*, low heaslth risk; *27-29*, moderate health risk; *30-34*, high health risk; *35-39*, very high health risk; *40+*, extremely high health risk.

The Dental Hygienist's Guide to

Nutritional Care

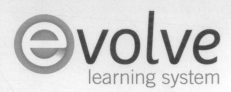

learning system

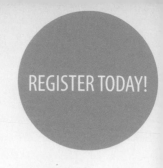

REGISTER TODAY!

To access your Student Resources, visit:

http://evolve.elsevier.com/Stegeman/ nutritional/

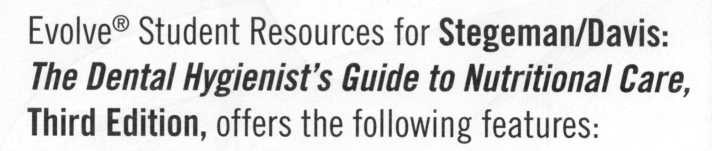

Evolve® Student Resources for **Stegeman/Davis:**
The Dental Hygienist's Guide to Nutritional Care,
Third Edition, offers the following features:

- **Illustrated Case Studies.** 10 written scenarios with accompanying photographs and follow-up questions present situations that may be encountered in practice. An excellent review source for the National Board Dental Hygiene Examination.

- **Food Pyramids and Guides from Around the World.** Food pyramids and guides from a variety of different countries including Mexico, Puerto Rico, the Philippines, Korea, China, Great Britain, Germany, Australia, Portugal, and Sweden. Also included are the Native American Food Pyramid and the Mediterranean Diet Pyramid.

- **Food Diary and Food Analysis Forms.** Printable versions of the forms needed to complete the Personal Assessment Project.

- **Weblinks.** A variety of weblinks provide additional means of study and research.

- **Printable Appendices.** Printable versions of the appendices allow for inclusion in class notebooks and easy transport from class to class.

ELSEVIER

THIRD EDITION

The Dental Hygienist's Guide to

Nutritional Care

Cynthia A. Stegeman, RDH, MEd, RD, LD, CDE
Associate Professor
Dental Hygiene Program
Raymond Walters College
University of Cincinnati
Cincinnati, Ohio

Judi Ratliff Davis, MS, RD
Texas Department of Health
Quality Assurance Nutrition Consultant for Women, Infants, and Children (WIC)
Austin, Texas

with

Linda D. Boyd, RDH, RD, LD, EdD
Professor
Director, Division of Graduate Studies
Department of Dental Hygiene
Idaho State University
Boise, Idaho

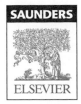

SAUNDERS

ELSEVIER

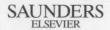

11830 Westline Industrial Drive
St. Louis, Missouri 63146

THE DENTAL HYGIENIST'S GUIDE TO NUTRITIONAL CARE,
THIRD EDITION   ISBN: 978-1-4160-6398-8
Copyright © 2010, 2005, 1998 by Saunders, an imprint of Elsevier Inc.

Notice

Knowledge and best practice in this field are constantly changing. As new research and experience broaden our knowledge, changes in practice, treatment and drug therapy may become necessary or appropriate. Readers are advised to check the most current information provided (i) on procedures featured or (ii) by the manufacturer of each product to be administered, to verify the recommended dose or formula, the method and duration of administration, and contraindications. It is the responsibility of the practitioner, relying on their own experience and knowledge of the patient, to make diagnoses, to determine dosages and the best treatment for each individual patient, and to take all appropriate safety precautions. To the fullest extent of the law, neither the Publisher nor the Editors assumes any liability for any injury and/or damage to persons or property arising out or related to any use of the material contained in this book.

Library of Congress Cataloging in Publication Data

Stegeman, Cynthia A.
   The dental hygienist's guide to nutritional care / Cynthia A. Stegeman, Judi Ratliff Davis, with Linda D. Boyd.—3rd ed.
     p. ; cm.
   Includes bibliographical references and index.
   ISBN 978-1-4160-6398-8 (pbk. : alk. paper)
   1. Nutrition and dental health.   2. Dental hygienists.   I. Davis, Judi Ratliff.   II. Boyd, Linda D.
III. Title.   IV. Title: Guide to nutritional care.
   [DNLM: 1. Oral Health.   2. Dental Hygienists.   3. Nutritional Requirements. WU 113 S817d 2010]
   RK281.S74 2010
   617.6'01—dc22

                                                    2009003940

Vice President and Publisher: Linda Duncan
Senior Editor: John Dolan
Senior Developmental Editor: Courtney Sprehe
Associate Development Editor: Joslyn Dumas
Publishing Services Manager: Patricia Tannian
Senior Project Manager: John Casey
Design Direction: Kim Denando

Printed in Canada
Last digit is the print number: 9 8 7 6 5 4 3 2

The study of nutrition is an interesting and rewarding subject for dental hygiene students, not only as it relates to patient education, but also for how it can affect the hygienist's own health. *The Dental Hygienist's Guide to Nutritional Care* is designed to show both dental hygiene students and practicing dental hygienists how to apply sound nutrition principles when assessing, diagnosing, planning, implementing, and evaluating the total care of patients, as well as to help them contribute to the nutritional well-being of patients. *The American Dietetic Association* recognizes nutrition as an integral component of oral health. The dental hygienist should be able to assess the oral cavity in relation to the patient's nutrition, dietary habits, and overall health status. A holistic approach to dietary management of a disease by all members of the healthcare team is especially appropriate to coordinate managed health care.

Since the subject of nutrition, especially obesity, is a top priority in today's society, the public faces the challenge of understanding a wide range of nutritional information that can often be confusing and overwhelming. As the health professional that patients may see most often, the dental hygienist should be able to knowledgeably and authoritatively discuss nutritional practices with his or her patients.

NEW TO THIS EDITION

In this expertly revised, **full color** edition you will find information on the most recent developments in the field including:

- *2005 Dietary Guidelines for Americans* and MyPyramid
- Pros and cons of popular high protein diets
- Ways to maintain brain health
- Recent research surrounding vitamin D, a vitamin deficiency prevalent in the United States
- Nutritional value of bottled water, energy drinks, and sports drinks
- Symptoms of menopause and how they can be decreased through diet
- Genomics and diet-disease relationships

Also included with the new edition is the addition of more **Evolve** resources. A complete listing of the material available on Evolve can be found on the *About Evolve* page following the preface.

ORGANIZATION

Nutrition information in this book is organized clearly and concisely to provide an understanding of the therapeutic value of foods in a normal diet.

Part I, Orientation to Basic Nutrition, deals with basic principles of nutrition. A basic understanding of fundamental nutrition facts enables the dental hygienist to make wise judgments about eating habits, counsel patients about needed dietary changes, and evaluate the flood of new information available. Nutrient deficiencies and excesses are addressed in sections entitled *Hyper-States* and *Hypo-States,* terms that

are more congruent with real-life occurrences. Chapters addressing vitamins and minerals are arranged separately to cover the specific nutrients involved in oral calcified structures or oral soft tissues.

Part II, Considerations of Clinical Nutrition, addresses problems specifically involved in the application of basic nutrition principles through the lifespan and within ethnic groups. This helps the dental hygienist to recognize that food choices different from his or her own food patterns may actually be very good. By approaching any necessary modifications with sensitivity and respect, patients are more likely to make suggested changes. Alterations in nutritional requirements and eating patterns affected by various stages of life, specifically females, infants and children, and older adults, are discussed.

Part III, Nutritional Aspects of Oral Health, looks at factors involved in oral problems and the nutritional treatment of these problems. In these chapters, Dental Hygiene Considerations boxes provide specific information to consider during an assessment by the dental hygienist including: (1) note *physical* status and *dietary* habits; (2) address *interventions*, or factors that need to be considered when caring for the patient; and (3) *evaluation* concerns the patient's ability or motivation to make changes based on what he or she has learned during the appointment with the dental hygienist. Educational information the dental hygienist can discuss with the patient during the counseling is provided in the Nutritional Directions boxes. A nutritional assessment is a basic essential for the nutritional well-being of all patients and this involves performing a physical assessment, evaluating dietary intake/history, and counseling patients about recommended changes in food choices. Many conditions or their outcome are improved by encouraging patients to eat well or to make minor changes in food choices to improve their health.

The **Appendices** contain a variety of reference material, including a glossary of the key terms. Since food composition tables are not included, the authors encourage instructors to make arrangements to have nutritional software available for students or to have computer access to USDA Home and Garden Bulletin No. 72 available at http://www.nal.usda.gov/fnic/foodcomp/ for student reference and to analyze food intake using the governmental free website http://www.usda.gov/cnpp/healthyeating.html. Frequently updated nutrition software usually has nutritional values of many processed foods, fast foods, and the newest products available. The Appendices also include a list of resources, including organizations, governmental agencies, reliable journals and newsletters, and websites. The latest Centers for Disease Control and Prevention growth charts for children are included in Appendix B.

A variety of features throughout the text help to enhance the learning experience:

- **Learning Objectives**: A list of objectives provide a guide to the important information to acquire from the chapter.

- **Key Terms**: A list of unfamiliar terms at the beginning of each chapter; terms are **bolded** in the text where they are defined and are also compiled in the **Glossary** for easy reference.
- **Test Your NQ** (nutrition quotient): An initial true-false pretest used to stimulate interest in the reading assignment; answers are conveniently located in Appendix F and on Evolve.
- **Dental Hygiene Considerations**: Practical information that can affect the patient's care or nutritional status.
- **Nutritional Directions:** Information the patient should know or be taught to improve oral health and overall health status.
- **Health Applications:** Information presented in Chapters 1 through 15 covers current "hot topics" in nutrition including the ways a vegetarian can obtain an adequate balance of nutrients, causes and treatment of obesity, and use of vitamin and mineral supplements.
- **Case Application**: Potential patient situations describing a clinical situation and providing the five-step care plan to help "pull it all together."

- **Student Readiness:** Questions at the end of each chapter help students determine their comprehension of the subject.
- **Case Studies:** Practice case studies help students test their ability to make sound judgments when faced with real-life patient scenarios.

NOTE FROM THE AUTHORS

With a better understanding of the importance of food choices, the members of an entire healthcare team can complement each other and provide optimal care for the patient. Even though specific amounts of nutrients are mentioned, the intent of this text is not for prescriptive use. Instead, its purpose is to provide dental hygiene students and practicing dental hygienists with a relative idea of the amounts of various nutrients needed so viable food sources can be recommended.

Cynthia A. Stegeman
Judi Ratliff Davis

The expanded Evolve website offers a variety of additional learning tools that greatly enhances the text for both students and instructors. Spearheading the expansion of the Evolve material is Professor Linda Boyd of Idaho State University (see the next section for a complete listing of her affiliations), an expert in educational coursework and the clinical aspects of the curriculum, and Mary E. Bossart, RDH, BSDH, MSDH Student and Graduate Teaching Assistant at Idaho State University.

FOR THE STUDENT

Evolve Student Resources offers the following:

- **Illustrated Case Studies.** 10 written scenarios with accompanying photographs and follow-up questions present situations that may be encountered in practice. An excellent review source for the National Board Dental Hygiene Examination.
- **Food Pyramids and Guides from Around the World.** Food pyramids and guides from a variety of countries including Mexico, Puerto Rico, the Philippines, Korea, China, Great Britain, Germany, Australia, Portugal, and Sweden. Also included are the Native American Food Pyramid and the Mediterranean Diet Pyramid.
- **Food Diary and Food Analysis Forms.** Printable versions of the forms needed to complete the Personal Assessment Project. Also included are printable versions of the Carbohydrate Intake Analysis Worksheet and Menu Planning Record.
- **Weblinks.** A variety of weblinks provide additional means of study and research.

- **Printable Appendices.** Printable versions of the appendices allow for inclusion in class notebooks and easy transport from class to class.
- **MNA Mini Nutritional Assessment.** A validated nutrition screening tool that can assess for malnutrition in patients 65 years and older.

FOR THE INSTRUCTOR

Evolve Instructor Resources offers the following:

- **Image Collection.** An image collection that includes all of the illustrations from the book, making it easy to incorporate a photo or drawing into a lecture or quiz.
- **PowerPoint Presentations.** Presentations that provide ready-made lectures compliant with the content found in the text.
- **Testbank.** An extensive testbank makes the creation of quizzes and exams much easier.
- **Personal Assessment Project.** A classroom learning activity designed to help students objectively assess their own personal dietary patterns, practice the process of recording and analyzing food intake for its nutritive and cariogenic value, and use nutritional and dental knowledge to contribute to better general and oral health for self and clients.
- **Classroom Learning Activities.** A variety of interactive learning activities that can be incorporated into class to stimulate discussion and teamwork.

ACKNOWLEDGMENTS

Because of the diversity of subjects presented in a general nutrition textbook, a compilation of the work of many people, whether direct or indirect, is necessary to present up-to-date information. Whether the aid was in the area of a research study or was verbal or written communications, each person's help and support is truly appreciated.

Our sincere thanks to Barbara Altshuler, Assistant Professor Emeritus, Caruth School of Dental Hygiene, Baylor College of Dentistry, who "birthed" this nutrition textbook for dental hygienists and took this baby to W.B. Saunders to develop a resource for dental hygienists to assess the nutritional status of their patients. While your "early retirement" is a true loss to the dental hygiene profession, we hope you are enjoying your family time.

Special thanks to the dental hygiene faculty, staff, and students at Raymond Walters College, University of Cincinnati, for their encouragement, expertise, provision of research, and use of many clinical forms. Their consistent support and praise make the incredible task of creating a textbook easier and rewarding.

A special thanks to the librarians at the Texas Department of State Health Services, Carolyn Medina and David McLellan, who were superb at locating scientific references for "dramatic findings" publicized by the press. In addition to those listed, there are countless other friends and relatives to whom we wish to express our gratitude for their encouragement and support.

Objective critiques from reviewers are invaluable to a good publication. We appreciate the insight, perspective, words of encouragement, and valuable ideas of the following reviewers: Lisa F. Harper Mallonee, BSDH, MPH, RD/LD, Baylor College of Dentistry, Dallas, Texas, and Tina Banning, MS, RD, LD, Capital Health Services, Inc., Dayton, Ohio.

We also wish to thank the many staff at Elsevier who worked so tirelessly in the various phases of planning and producing this book. We are especially grateful to John Dolan, Senior Editor, for his helpful ideas and for seeing us through this project. We also appreciate the invaluable input, assistance, and encouragement of Courtney Sprehe, Senior Developmental Editor, who has been an invaluable resource and advocate in this revision.

Cynthia A. Stegeman
Judi Ratliff Davis

Cynthia A. Stegeman, RDH, MEd, RD, LD, CDE is an Associate Professor in the Dental Hygiene Program at the University of Cincinnati, Raymond Walters College and has taught Nutrition and Health Education for almost 20 years. Cyndee has been a dental hygienist for 30 years and a long-time member of the American Dental Hygienists' Association. She is also a Certified Diabetes Educator and practiced in clinical dietetics with emphasis in cardiac rehabilitation, diabetes education, disordered eating, and sports nutrition. In addition, she speaks to numerous community and professional groups and has written several publications on nutrition and dentistry. She plays a very active leadership role in the local, state, and national American Dietetic Association. She is currently completing a doctorate degree with a dissertation emphasis on dentistry, diabetes, and nutrition.

Judi Ratliff Davis, MS, RD is currently employed in Austin, Texas, at the State Department of State Health Services as a Quality Assurance Nutrition Consultant for the Women, Infants and Children (WIC) program. She has been an active member of the American Dietetic Association for 40 years. She has had a variety of experiences in the field of nutrition, including teaching, clinical dietitian, and consultant. She has taught various nutrition and food service courses at Tarrant County Junior College in Fort Worth, Texas. Her roles as a clinical dietitian include Home-Based Community Support, Tarrant County Mental Health Mental Retardation; Rehabilitation Hospital of North Texas, Arlington, Texas; Fort Worth State School, Fort Worth, Texas; Rex Hospital in Raleigh, North Carolina; and Baptist Memorial Hospital in San Antonio, Texas. She has also worked as a nutrition consultant for nursing homes and mental health facilities in western Virginia, San Antonio, and the Dallas-Fort Worth area, for the Greenhouse, a health spa in Arlington, Texas, and the Sugar Association. She is also the author of the book *Applied Nutrition and Diet Therapy for Nurses*.

Linda Boyd, RDH, RD, LD, EdD is a Professor and Director of the Master of Science Degree in Dental Hygiene in the Department of Dental Hygiene at Idaho State University. Linda has over 30 years of experience in dental hygiene practice in both general and periodontal offices. She has been a dental and dental hygiene educator for 11 years specializing in teaching prevention, periodontology, special needs, clinical dental hygiene, and educational theory and methodology. In addition, she has been involved in educational and clinical research addressing diabetes, complementary and alternative medicine (CAM) and periodontal disease, and critical thinking. Dr. Boyd is actively involved in the American Dental Hygienists' Association as a member of the Council of Research and an ADHA nominee for Curriculum Consultant to the Commission on Dental Accreditation. She is a member of the American Dietetic Association and has served as content advisor for the association's position paper on Oral Health and Nutrition and is currently serving as Chair, Evidence Analysis Library Work Group on Fluoride. In addition, Linda serves in many leadership roles in the American Dental Education Association, including being an officer for the Dental Hygiene Graduate Program Directors and Biochemistry, Nutrition and Microbiology Section. She has published widely in textbooks and journals on the topic of nutrition and oral health as well as on the development of critical thinking in dental students. She presents continuing education courses nationwide to state and local dental and dental hygiene professionals.

CONTENTS

PART I

Orientation to Basic Nutrition

Chapter 1

Overview of Healthy Eating Habits

LEARNING OBJECTIVES

Upon completion of this chapter, the student will be able to achieve the following objectives:
- List the general physiological functions of the six nutrient classifications of foods.
- Identify factors that influence food habits.
- Name the food groups in MyPyramid.
- State the amounts needed from each of the food groups in MyPyramid for a well-balanced 2000 kilocalorie diet.
- Identify significant nutrient contributions of each food group, and assess their implications for oral health.

- State the *Dietary Guidelines for Americans* and their purpose.
- Assess dietary intake of a patient, using the *Dietary Guidelines for Americans* and *MyPyramid Food Guidance System*.
- Explain the different purposes of dietary reference intakes (DRIs), MyPyramid, and reference daily intakes (RDIs).
- Apply basic nutritional concepts to help patients with nutrition-related problems.

KEY TERMS

Acceptable macronutrient distribution ranges
  (AMDRs)
Adequate intake (AI)
Bariatric surgery
Body mass index (BMI)
Calorie
Cruciferous
Daily reference value (DRV)
Daily value (DV)
Dietary reference intakes (DRIs)
Energy
Enrichment
Estimated average requirement (EAR)
Estimated energy requirement (EER)
Fortification
Ghrelin
Health claims

Hypertension
Kilocalorie (kcal)
Macronutrients
Micronutrients
Nutrient density
Nutrients
Nutrient content claims
Nutrition
Nutritionist
Obesity
Overweight
Precursor
Recommended dietary allowances (RDAs)
Reference daily intake (RDI)
Registered dietitian
Satiety
Tolerable upper intake level (UL)

Test Your NQ

1. **T/F** Milk is a perfect food for everyone.
2. **T/F** According to the *Dietary Guidelines for Americans,* consumption of all sugars should be reduced.
3. **T/F** Water is the most important nutrient.
4. **T/F** DRIs are required daily intakes essential for all patients to be healthy.
5. **T/F** Good nutrition is possible regardless of a patient's cultural habits.
6. **T/F** Based on MyPyramid, two to four servings daily are needed from the fruit and vegetable group.

7. **T/F** The *Dietary Guidelines for Americans* were written for healthy people to help reduce their risk of developing chronic diseases.
8. **T/F** Sugar is the leading cause of chronic health problems.
9. **T/F** The goal of the *MyPyramid Food Guidance System* is to convey the importance of variety, moderation, and proportion.
10. **T/F** The only nutrients that provide energy are carbohydrates, fats, and vitamins.

The dental hygiene profession continues to grow and rapidly move into the forefront of health care. To function as valuable members of today's healthcare team, the dental hygienist must be knowledgeable in various aspects of health care. Because of the lifelong synergistic bidirectional relationship between oral health and nutritional status, dental hygienists and **registered dietitians** and **nutritionists** need to be competent in assessing and providing basic education to patients, and provide referral to each other to effect comprehensive patient care.

All registered dietitians and some nutritionists are considered experts in the field, but their training prepares them for slightly different areas. A nutritionist has at least a 4-year degree in foods and nutrition and usually works in a public health setting assisting people in the community, such as pregnant teenagers or older individuals, with diet-related health issues. In many states, a nutritionist is legally defined and is licensed or certified. Nutritionists work in local or

state health departments and in the extension service of a land-grant university. A registered dietitian (RD) has completed a minimum of a bachelor's degree in foods and nutrition with training in normal and clinical nutrition, food science, and food service management, and advanced training in medical nutrition therapy. A registered dietitian must pass a national registration examination and receive continuing education. Registered dietitians work in hospitals, long-term care facilities, healthcare providers' offices, pharmaceutical companies, schools, community and research settings, wellness and fitness centers, and many other settings.

Dental professionals typically see patients on a more regular basis than other healthcare professionals; this allows observation of many physical signs, particularly oral signs, of a nutrient deficiency or medical condition that affects nutritional status before it is diagnosed. Recognition of abnormal conditions and early referral to an appropriate healthcare professional can lead to positive health outcomes for patients. Assessment of dietary information obtained from a patient can also uncover habits detrimental to oral health that can be addressed in the dental office. Additionally, compromised oral health may affect food choices. For example, patients who lose their teeth may avoid foods that are hard to chew and reduce the quality and variety of their diets.

Finally, dental hygienists can follow up on the goals established by patients to evaluate their understanding and compliance. Overall, the dental hygienist is committed to prevention of oral disease along with promotion of health and wellness. All healthcare professionals must work together to enhance patient care. The purpose of this textbook is to provide the dental hygienist with the nutrition information that can realistically be applied to and practiced with patients in the dental setting.

BASIC NUTRITION

Nutrition is the process by which living things use food to obtain nutrients for energy, growth and development, and maintenance. **Energy** is the ability or power to do work. **Nutrients** are biochemical substances that can be supplied only in adequate amounts from an outside source, normally from food. One aspect of nutrition is the integration of physiological and biochemical reactions within the body: (1) digesting food to make nutrients available, (2) absorbing and delivering nutrients to the cells where they are used, and (3) eliminating waste products.

Nutrition is a relatively new science and still an evolving discipline. People want science to be definitive; they become confused and concerned when scientific research challenges what the public assumes to be factual. In nutrition, something that is considered to be true today may be disrupted by future research refuting established beliefs. In many cases, the media exacerbates this situation by highlighting findings from a new research study that cannot be reproduced in further research. The pace of research has quickened; this text is based on current, well-established, and evidence-based nutrition advice. Everyone in the healthcare field must continue to stay abreast of ongoing research to be able to respond to questions from patients.

Psychological and social factors that enter into frequent decisions concerning food choices are also important aspects of nutrition. Freedom of choice and variety in consumption are important components of an individual's personal and social life. Tastes, budget, environment, and cultural attitudes influence food choices. The systemic and environmental effects of nutrients, which are determined by these food choices, affect dental health.

PHYSIOLOGICAL FUNCTIONS OF NUTRIENTS

Physiologically, foods eaten are used for energy, tissue building maintenance and replacement or repair, and obtaining or producing numerous regulatory substances. The classes of macronutrients and micronutrients obtained from foods are the following:

1. Water
2. Proteins
3. Carbohydrates
4. Fats
5. Alcohol
6. Minerals
7. Vitamins

Of the above-listed nutrients, only proteins, carbohydrates, fats, and alcohol provide energy. The potential energy value of foods within the body is expressed in terms of the **kilocalorie (kcal)**, more frequently referred to as the **calorie**. A kilocalorie is a measure of heat equivalent to 1000 calories.

Nutrients work together and interact in complex metabolic reactions. Proteins, carbohydrates, fats, and alcohol provide energy that the body needs for metabolic processes. However, the body cannot use the energy from these energy-containing components of food without adequate amounts of vitamins and minerals. Vitamins and minerals, along with protein and water, are essential for the body to build and maintain body tissues and to regulate essential body processes.

BASIC CONCEPTS OF NUTRITION

Foods differ in the amount of nutrients they furnish. Any individual food can be compatible with good nutrition but should be evaluated in the context of the patient's physiological needs, the food's nutrient content, and other food choices. The premise of nutritional care is that, in any cultural or environmental circumstance or for any personal taste or preference, good nutrition is possible.

Increasing the variety of foods consumed reduces the probability of developing isolated nutrient deficiencies, nutrient excesses, and toxicities resulting from non-nutritive components or contaminants in any particular food. A dietary change to eliminate or increase intake of one specific food component or nutrient usually alters the intake of other nutrients. For instance, because red meats are an excellent source of iron and zinc, decreasing cholesterol intake by limiting these meats can reduce dietary iron and zinc intake.

Essential nutrients are needed throughout life on a regular basis; only the amounts of nutrients needed change. The patient's use of foods eaten, stage of growth and development, sex, body size, weight, physical activity, and state of health influence nutrient requirements.

Some nutrients can be converted by the body to meet its physiological needs. Nonessential nutrients can be used by the body, but either are not required or can be synthesized from dietary precursors. **Precursors** are substances from which an active substance is formed. An example is carotene, found in fruits and vegetables, which the liver can convert into an active form of vitamin A.

Water is the most important nutrient. After water, the nutrients of highest priority are those that provide energy, which must be supplied from foods or can be supplied from quantities stored in the body. The human body has adaptive mechanisms that allow toleration of modest ranges in nutrient intakes. For instance, the metabolic rate usually decreases as a result of decreased caloric intake.

Dental Hygiene Considerations

- Because nutrients work interdependently, a lack or excess of one can interfere with or prevent use of another. Asking the patient to record food and beverage intake for the past 24 hours allows assessment of nutrient intake.
- Evaluation of the patient's intake of macronutrients and micronutrients can help determine whether intake is adequate or excessive.

Nutritional Directions

- No single food contains all the essential nutrients in amounts needed for optimal health.
- Nutritional intake can either improve or adversely affect health.

GOVERNMENT NUTRITION CONCERNS

Before 1977, nutritional efforts focused on ensuring that the U.S. food supply provided adequate nutrients to prevent deficiency diseases. The U.S. government recognized nutritional problems related to food choices in 1977 with the *United States Dietary Goals,* which addressed excessive consumption of some nutrients. In 1988, the Surgeon General issued a report confirming that 5 of the 10 leading causes of death (coronary heart disease [CHD], certain types of cancer, stroke, diabetes mellitus, and atherosclerosis) were associated with dietary intake.

HEALTHY PEOPLE NUTRITION OBJECTIVES

The *Healthy People 2000* report, issued in 1990 by the U.S. Department of Health and Human Services (USDHHS), identified public health goals to improve the overall health of the United States. It promoted health and disease prevention and addressed disparities in health status and health outcomes between diverse population groups. To help meet these goals within 10 years, specific objectives involving nutrition were identified in 21 different priority areas. The goals for *Healthy People 2010*[1] focus on (1) increasing the quality and years of healthy life, and (2) eliminating health disparities among racial and ethnic groups. The report emphasizes that public and private organizations must share responsibility for improving Americans' health. *Healthy People 2010* targets many objectives related to nutrition, weight, and oral health (Box 1-1).

Box 1-1   *Healthy People 2010*: Nutri Priority Areas

- Reduce the proportion of children, adolescents, and adults who are overweight or obese.
- Increase the proportion of adults who are at a healthy weight.
- Reduce growth retardation among low-income children younger than age 5 years.
- Increase the proportion of all individuals who consume desirable levels of fruits, vegetables (at least one serving of dark green or orange), and grain products (at least six daily servings including three whole grain).
- Increase the proportion of individuals older than age 2 years who consume less than 10% of kilocalories from saturated fat and no more than 30% of kilocalories from total fat.
- Increase the proportion of individuals 2 years and older who consume 2400 mg or less of sodium.
- Increase the proportion of individuals 2 years and older who meet dietary recommendations for calcium.
- Reduce iron deficiency among young children, women of childbearing age, and pregnant women.
- Increase the proportion of children and adolescents whose intakes from meals and snacks at school contribute proportionally to overall dietary quality.
- Increase the number of worksites that offer nutrition or weight management classes or counseling.
- Increase the number of physician office visits that include counseling or education related to diet and nutrition for patients with cardiovascular disease, diabetes, and hyperlipidemia.
- Achieve food security and reduce hunger in U.S. households.
- Increase the number of mothers who breastfeed their infants.
- Reduce the number of low-birth-weight and very-low-birth-weight infants.
- Increase the proportion of mothers who achieve a recommended weight gain during their pregnancy.
- Increase the proportion of pregnancies that begin with an optimum folic acid level.
- Reduce the proportion of children and adolescents who have dental caries in their primary or permanent teeth.
- Increase the numbers of community water systems containing optimal amounts of fluoride.

Adapted from U.S. Department of Health and Human Services: Healthy People 2010: understanding and improving health. Washington, DC: U.S. Government Printing Office, 2000. Available at http://www.health.gov/healthypeople/.

By 2004, some objectives showed positive results, whereas several objectives showed negative results. In particular, negative outcomes included decreasing numbers of people with a healthy weight, increasing prevalence of overweight people (adults, children, and adolescents), and children with dental caries and untreated dental decay.[2]

NUTRIENT RECOMMENDATIONS: DIETARY REFERENCE INTAKES

Recommendations for the amounts of required nutrients have undergone significant changes in recent years, and the revised sets of nutrient-based reference values is collectively called the **dietary reference intakes (DRIs)** (see inside front cover and pp. i-iii). In 1993, the Food and Nutrition Board of the Institute of Medicine (IOM) undertook this major project, which was completed in 2004. The government publishes the DRIs that are established by an expert group of scientists and registered dietitians from the United States and Canada. These groups of experts base their recommendations on available scientific evidence from different types of studies on the nutrients and their application to individual requirements.

Previous **recommended dietary allowances (RDAs)** focused on amounts of nutrients necessary to prevent deficiency diseases. The current DRIs additionally attempt to (1) estimate amounts of required nutrients to improve the long-term health and well-being of people by reducing the risk of chronic diseases, such as heart disease, osteoporosis, and cancer, affected by nutrition, and to (2) establish maximum safe levels of tolerance. The four categories of nutrient-based reference values are relevant for various stages of life.

The DRIs were intended for planning and assessing diets of healthy Americans and Canadians. The DRIs are inappropriate for malnourished individuals or patients whose requirements are affected by a disease state.

ESTIMATED AVERAGE REQUIREMENT

The **estimated average requirement (EAR)** is the amount of a nutrient that is estimated to meet the needs of half of the healthy individuals in a specific age and gender group. This set of values is useful in assessing nutrient adequacy or planning intakes of population groups, not individuals.

RECOMMENDED DIETARY ALLOWANCE

The new RDA is generally higher than the EAR and provides a sufficient amount of a nutrient to meet the requirements of nearly all (97% to 98%) healthy individuals. These recommendations provide a generous margin of safety and are intended as a goal for achieving adequate intakes. No health benefits are established for consuming intakes greater than the RDA.

ADEQUATE INTAKES

If sufficient scientific evidence was unavailable to determine an EAR or RDA, an **adequate intake (AI)** was established, based on scientific judgments. An AI, which is derived from mean nutrient intakes by groups of healthy people, is the average amount of a nutrient that seems to maintain a defined nutritional state. An AI is expected to exceed average requirements of virtually all members of a life stage/gender group, but is more tentative than an RDA. AI values were established for various life stages for calcium, vitamin D, and fluoride because of uncertainties about the scientific data to determine EAR and RDA values that would reduce the risk of chronic disease.

TOLERABLE UPPER INTAKE LEVEL

A **tolerable upper intake level (UL)** is the maximum daily level of nutrient intake that probably would not cause adverse

health effects or toxic effects for most individuals in the general population. The potential risk of adverse effects increases as intake exceeds the UL. The term *tolerable intake* was selected to avoid the implication that these higher levels would result in beneficial effects. These values are especially helpful because of increased consumption of nutrients in the form of dietary supplements or from enrichment and fortification. This recommendation pertains to habitual daily use and is based on the combined intake of food, water, dietary supplements, and fortified foods.

Acceptable Macronutrient Distribution Ranges

Acceptable macronutrient distribution ranges (AMDRs) were established for the macronutrients, fat, carbohydrate, protein, and two polyunsaturated fatty acids, to ensure sufficient intakes of essential nutrients, while reducing risk of chronic disease. **Macronutrients** are the energy-providing nutrients needed in larger amounts than **micronutrients**, such as vitamins and minerals. As shown in Table 1-1, the AMDR is a range of intakes for food components that provide kilocalories; these are expressed as a percentage of total energy intake because the intake of each depends on intake of the others or of the total energy requirement of the individual. Increasing or decreasing one energy source while consuming a set amount of kilocalories affects the intake of the other sources of energy. For instance, if an individual who routinely consumes 2000 kcal decides to reduce the amount of fat, either the protein or carbohydrate intake would need to increase to provide the 2000 kcal. CHD may occur from diets very low in fat with very high intakes of carbohydrates as well as from diets that are very high in fat. Consuming amounts outside of the ranges increases risk of insufficient intake of essential nutrients. The recommended ranges for carbohydrates, fats, and proteins allow for more

Table 1-1	Acceptable Macronutrient Distribution Range		
	Range (Percent of Energy)		
Macronutrient	*Children, 1-3 years*	*Children, 4-18 years*	*Adults*
Fat	30-40	25-35	20-35
n-6 polyunsaturated fatty acids* (linoleic acid)	5-10	5-10	5-10
n-3 polyunsaturated fatty acids* (α-linolenic acid)	0.6-1.2	0.6-1.2	0.6-1.2
Carbohydrate	45-65	45-65	45-65
Protein	5-20	10-30	10-35

Data from the Institute of Medicine (IOM) of the National Academies: Dietary Reference Intakes for Energy, Carbohydrate, Fiber, Fat, Fatty Acids, Cholesterol, Protein, and Amino Acids. Washington, DC, The National Academies Press, 2002.
*Approximately 10% of the total can come from longer chain n-3 or n-6 fatty acids.

flexibility in dietary planning for healthy individuals and development of eating plans to meet an individual's preferences.

ESTIMATED ENERGY REQUIREMENT

The **estimated energy requirement (EER)** is defined as the dietary energy intake that is predicted to maintain energy balance in healthy, normal-weight individuals of a defined age, gender, weight, height, and physical activity level consistent with good health (see p. i). The EER is similar to the EAR, and no RDA was established because consuming more kilocalories than are needed would result in weight gain. Since energy requirement depends on activity level, four different activity levels are presented.

SUMMARY OF DIETARY REFERENCE INTAKES

Because nutrient requirements are influenced by age and sexual development, the DRIs are listed for 16 groups, separating gender groups after 10 years of age. Separate levels are established for three categories of pregnant and lactating women. Also, two age groups for the older American population were added.

No definitive guidelines exist for establishing the point at which diets become inadequate. These guidelines apply to average daily intakes. Meeting the recommendations for every nutrient on a daily basis is very difficult and unnecessary. These nutrient goals are intended to be met by consuming a variety of foods whenever possible.

Dental Hygiene Considerations

- Use of DRIs as an assessment guide is for healthy patients only.
- An individual's exact requirement for a specific nutrient is not known for certain.
- The ULs may be used to warn patients that excessive intake of nutrients from nutritional supplements could lead to adverse effects if taken on a regular basis.

Nutritional Directions

- The DRIs are general guidelines for good health, rather than specific requirements.
- Generally, specific foods or food groups, rather than nutrients, should be discussed with patients.
- If an individual's food consumption is below the RDA for a nutrient over several days, more food choices containing that particular nutrient should be encouraged.

FOOD GUIDANCE SYSTEMS FOR AMERICANS

The identification of nutrients and knowledge of their physiological function were significant developments. However,

patients eat and think in terms of food, not nutrients. Nutrient requirements and information must be interpreted into the "food" language patients understand. In 2005, the USDHHS and the U.S. Department of Agriculture (USDA) released the sixth edition of the *Dietary Guidelines for Americans*. These guidelines, based on scientific knowledge to promote health and reduce risk for major chronic disease through diet, physical activity, and food safety, are the basis for federal nutrition policies and education. They are designed to help Americans choose foods meeting nutrient requirements, promote health, support active lives, and reduce risks of chronic disease. The USDHHS and the USDA have appointed a new advisory committee responsible for establishing 2010 dietary guidelines.

The *Dietary Guidelines for Americans* is the foundation for the *MyPyramid Food Guidance System*, also released in 2005, which assists consumers to become healthier by applying nutrition science to their own lives.

Another helpful tool is the food label, which helps consumers determine what kind of food to eat and how much of a particular food to eat. Nutrition labeling, required for most packaged foods, provides information on certain nutrients. The Nutrition Facts panel provides information on nutrient content of food and the number of servings in the package. Knowing how to interpret label facts enables consumers to accurately apply key Dietary Guidelines messages that correspond to the nutrients and other information on the Nutrition Facts panel.

DIETARY GUIDELINES FOR AMERICANS

Because of new scientific information related to nutrient requirements, the Dietary Guidelines are revised every 5 years to promote health and reduce chronic diseases. The Dietary Guidelines address diet, physical activity, and other issues related to food intake and energy expenditure. They reflect the preponderance of scientific evidence and summarize information regarding individual nutrients and food components into recommendations for eating patterns that can be adopted by the public (Fig. 1-1). Government nutrition programs use the Dietary Guidelines to determine funding for research, nutrition labeling, and to develop nutrition education information for the public. The Dietary Guidelines contain technical information involved in key issues, such as energy balance. They are primarily oriented toward policymakers, nutrition educators, nutritionists, and healthcare providers, rather than the general public. The Dietary Guidelines are translated into a consumer-friendly form through the *MyPyramid Food Guidance System* to implement the Dietary Guidelines recommendations. MyPyramid replaced the 12-year-old Food Guide Pyramid.

The Dietary Guidelines for 2005 include nine focus areas with 23 key recommendations. In general, the message is simple: monitor portion size, be more active, and eat a variety of foods. The guidelines support healthy eating habits to improve health and quality of life, as shown in the sample menu in Figure 1-2. Unique nutrient needs of

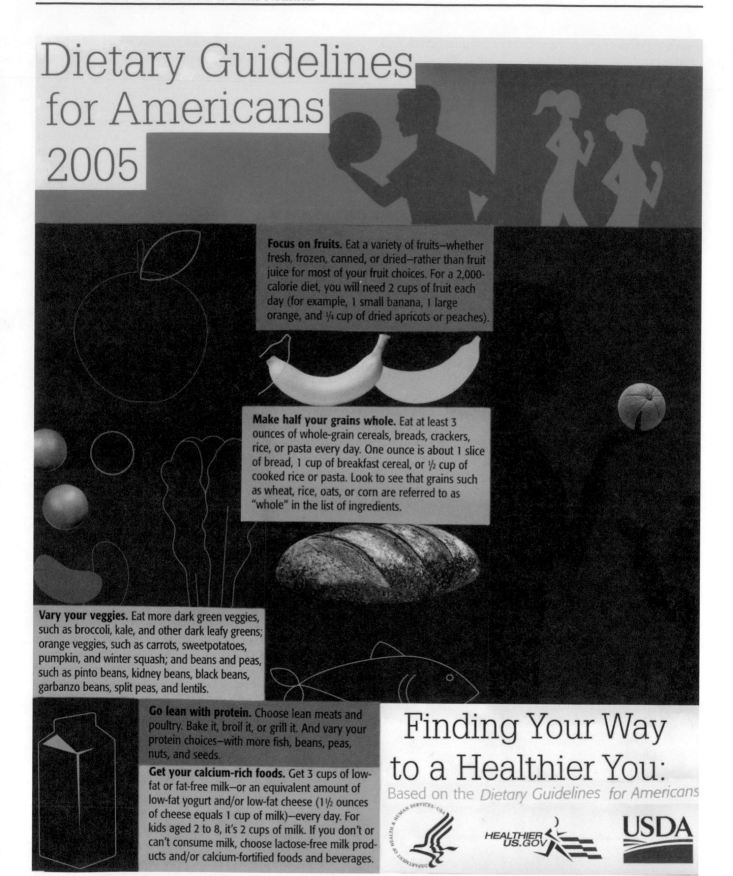

FIGURE I-I *Dietary Guidelines for Americans 2005.* (From the U.S. Department of Health and Human Services and U.S. Department of Agriculture. Available at www.healthierus.gov/dietaryguidelines.)

specific population groups, such as people older than age 50, pregnant women, and children and adolescents, are addressed in Key Recommendations for Specific Population Groups; these are addressed in relevant chapters in this text.

ADEQUATE NUTRIENTS WITHIN KILOCALORIE NEEDS

Many Americans consume excessive kilocalories but inadequate amounts of some nutrients. Meeting nutrient recommendations must be balanced with keeping caloric levels under control. In other words, food choices need to change when caloric levels are decreased to include foods containing more nutrients.

Dietary intake data and evidence of public health problems indicate that adults consume inadequate amounts of calcium, potassium, dietary fiber, magnesium, and vitamins A, C, and E. In addition, older men, women, and adolescent girls fail to consume adequate amounts of zinc, and older women are not getting enough vitamin B_6 from their diets.[3]

The Dietary Guidelines promote the use of foods to meet physiological nutrient needs. In addition to the array of nutrients provided by food, hundreds of other naturally occurring substances present may protect against chronic health conditions. In some cases, fortified foods are advisable sources of nutrients that otherwise might be consumed in less than recommended amounts (e.g., folic acid). Supplements, recommended if a specific nutrient cannot or is not otherwise being met by food intake, cannot replace a healthful diet. A high-quality diet that does not provide excess kilocalories, in addition to physical activity, should enhance the health of most Americans.

In addition to consuming the number of servings recommended from each of the food groups, consumers should choose a variety of foods within each group, with emphasis on choosing nutrient-dense foods. Nutrient-dense foods provide substantial amounts of vitamins and minerals, but relatively few kilocalories. When more foods or beverages are chosen that are low in **nutrient density** (having a high fat, alcohol, or sugar content), consuming enough nutrients without gaining weight is more difficult.

Key Recommendations
- Consume a variety of nutrient-dense foods and beverages within and among the basic food groups, while choosing foods that limit the intake of saturated and *trans* fats, cholesterol, added sugars, salt, and alcohol.
- Meet recommended intakes with energy needs by adopting a balanced eating pattern, such as MyPyramid or the DASH (Dietary Approaches to Stop Hypertension) Eating Plan (discussed in Health Application 11).

WEIGHT MANAGEMENT

Weight management is difficult for a number of Americans because of the abundance of food and lack of physical activity. Body weight should be evaluated in relation to a person's height using the body mass index (BMI) to determine health risks that increase at higher levels of overweight and obesity (see p. iv). **Body mass index (BMI)** is the current preferred method of defining healthy weight because it correlates more closely with actual body fat than height and weight tables. BMI can be determined by using the table on p. iv, or it can be determined by dividing weight (in lbs) by the height (in inches), dividing that number by the height (in inches) again, then multiplying the answer by 703. A BMI of less than 25 is generally considered the upper limit of healthy weight, since chronic disease risk increases in most people who are above this level. A BMI of 25 or greater is considered **overweight;** a BMI of 30 or greater is identified as **obesity.** BMI is not appropriate for infants and children younger than 2. Special tables are available for determining BMI for children.

Overweight and obesity have increased significantly among adults and children during the last 2 decades in the United States. Although most Americans are consuming more kilocalories than they expend, intake is only one side of the energy balance equation. To reverse this obesity trend, most Americans need to eat more fruits and vegetables, engage in more physical activity, and reduce the consumption of high-calorie foods and sugar-sweetened beverages.

Because weight loss is a challenge requiring changes in many behaviors and patterns, prevention of weight gain is ideal. Even small decreases in caloric intake can help avoid weight gain. It is much easier to reduce caloric intake by 100 kcal per day to prevent gradual weight gain than to reduce intake by 500 kcal to lose weight.

Portion sizes require special attention. Studies show that controlling portion sizes helps limit energy intake, especially when eating high-kilocalorie foods. In general, the best choice for weight loss involves a change in lifestyle, both in diet and in physical activity. Kilocalories are the key factor to controlling body weight—not the proportions of fat, carbohydrates, and protein, but balancing caloric intake with expenditure.

Key Recommendations
- To maintain body weight in a healthy range, balance kilocalories from foods and beverages with kilocalories expended.
- To prevent gradual weight gain over time, make small decreases in kilocalories from foods and beverages, and increase physical activity.

PHYSICAL ACTIVITY

For all age groups, regular physical activity and physical fitness are important factors for an individual's health, sense of well-being, and maintenance of a healthy body weight. However, Americans are relatively inactive. Physical activity is defined as any body movement produced by skeletal muscles resulting in energy expenditure. Physical activity is not the same as physical fitness, which is related to the ability to perform physical activity. People with high levels of physical fitness are at lower risk of developing chronic diseases, whereas a sedentary lifestyle increases risk for

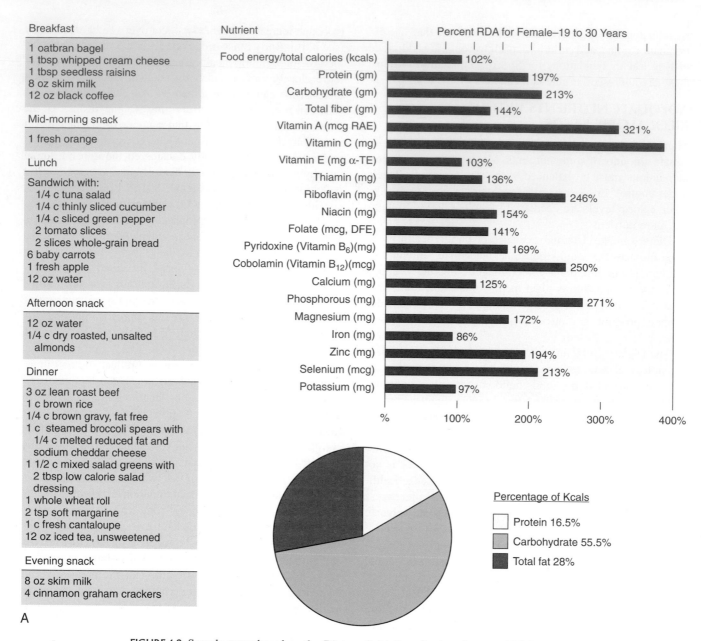

FIGURE I-2 Sample menu based on the *Dietary Guidelines for Americans* and MyPyramid.

overweight, obesity, and many chronic diseases. Additionally, physical activity can aid in managing mild to moderate depression and anxiety.

Different intensities and types of exercise yield distinct benefits. Vigorous activity improves physical fitness more than moderate physical activity and burns more kilocalories per unit of time. Resistance exercise increases muscular strength and endurance and maintains or increases muscle mass. Weight-bearing exercise may reduce the risk of osteoporosis by increasing peak bone mass during growth, maintaining peak bone mass during adulthood, and reducing the rate of bone loss during aging. Also, regular exercise can help prevent falls in older adults.

Physical activity may be accomplished in short bouts (10-minute periods) of moderate-intensity activity three to six times during a day; it is the accumulated total that results

in improved health status and increased caloric expenditure. The higher an individual's physical activity level, the more kilocalories can be consumed without gaining weight. This makes it easier to plan a daily food intake pattern that meets recommended nutrient requirements.

In the fall of 2008, the USDHHS issued physical activity guidelines for Americans to complement the *Dietary Guidelines for Americans.** These comprehensive guidelines indicate that additional health benefits occur as the amount of physical activity increases through higher intensity, greater frequency, and/or longer duration of moderate intensity physical activity, such as brisk walking. Regular physical

*U. S. Department of Health and Human Services: 2008 Physical Activity Guidelines for Americans. Available online: www.health.gov/paguidelines. Accessed January 10, 2009.

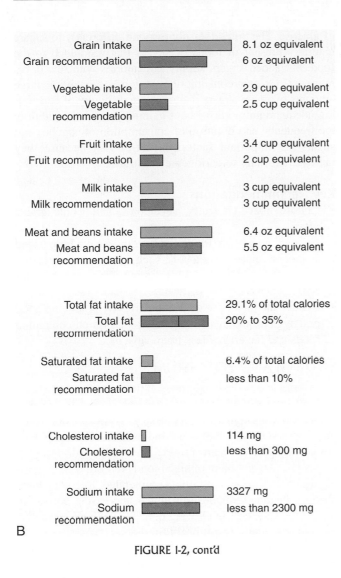

Grain intake		8.1 oz equivalent
Grain recommendation		6 oz equivalent
Vegetable intake		2.9 cup equivalent
Vegetable recommendation		2.5 cup equivalent
Fruit intake		3.4 cup equivalent
Fruit recommendation		2 cup equivalent
Milk intake		3 cup equivalent
Milk recommendation		3 cup equivalent
Meat and beans intake		6.4 oz equivalent
Meat and beans recommendation		5.5 oz equivalent
Total fat intake		29.1% of total calories
Total fat recommendation		20% to 35%
Saturated fat intake		6.4% of total calories
Saturated fat recommendation		less than 10%
Cholesterol intake		114 mg
Cholesterol recommendation		less than 300 mg
Sodium intake		3327 mg
Sodium recommendation		less than 2300 mg

B

FIGURE 1-2, cont'd

activity reduces the risk in adults of early death, coronary heart disease, stroke, hypertension, type 2 diabetes, colon and breast cancer, and depression. These guidelines will most likely replace the current physical activity guidelines from the 2005 *Dietary Guidelines for Americans* when it is updated.

Key Recommendations
- Engage in regular physical activity and reduce sedentary activities to promote health, psychological well-being, and a healthy body weight.
- Achieve physical fitness by including cardiovascular conditioning, stretching exercises for flexibility, and resistance exercises or calisthenics for muscle strength and endurance.

NEW PHYSICAL ACTIVITY GUIDELINES FOR ADULTS
- All adults should avoid inactivity. Some physical activity is better than none, and adults who participate in any amount of physical activity gain some health benefits.

- For substantial health benefits, adults should do at least 150 minutes (2½ hrs) a week of moderate-intensity, or 75 minutes (1¼ hrs) weekly of vigorous-intensity aerobic physical activity, or an equivalent combination of moderate- and vigorous-intensity aerobic activity. Aerobic activity should be performed in episodes of at least 10 minutes, and preferably, it should be spread throughout the week.
- For additional and more extensive health benefits, adults should increase their aerobic physical activity to 300 minutes (5 hours) a week of moderate-intensity, or (2½ hrs) a week of vigorous-intensity aerobic physical activity, or an equivalent combination of moderate- and vigorous-intensity activity. Additional health benefits are gained by engaging in physical activity beyond this amount.
- Adults should also do muscle-strengthening activities that are moderate or high intensity and involve all major muscle groups on 2 or more days a week, as these activities provide additional health benefits.

FOOD GROUPS TO ENCOURAGE
Protein-containing foods are important, but most Americans consume adequate amounts, so an increase is not recommended. Adding more fruits, vegetables, whole grains, and fat-free or low-fat milk and milk products may have beneficial health effects. These food groups provide good sources of the nutrients frequently lacking in American diets. (Good sources of various nutrients are listed in the specific chapters where the nutrient is discussed.) When adding these beneficial foods, a decrease of less nutrient-dense foods is recommended to control kilocalorie intake.

People who consume more fruits and vegetables have a reduced risk of chronic diseases, including stroke and other cardiovascular diseases, type 2 diabetes, and certain cancers (oral cavity and pharynx, larynx, lung, esophagus, stomach, and colorectal). High-fiber diets from foods such as fruits, vegetables, and whole grains may reduce the risk of CHD.

Despite the initiation of the 5-A-Day campaign by the Centers for Disease Control and Prevention (CDC) in 1991 to increase fruit and vegetable consumption to five servings daily, Americans' fruit and vegetable consumption did not increase between 1988-1994 and 1999-2002. Vegetable consumption decreased with only 11% of consumers meeting the dietary recommendations.[4] Later, the CDC replaced its fruits and vegetables website to reflect the Fruits & Veggies—More Matters campaign (see Relevant Websites listed on the Evolve site).

Key Recommendations
- Consume a sufficient amount of fruits and vegetables while staying within energy needs. Two cups of fruit and 2½ cups of vegetables per day are recommended for a reference 2000-kcal intake, with higher or lower amounts depending on the kilocalorie level.
- Choose a variety of fruits and vegetables each day. In particular, select from all five vegetable subgroups (dark

green, orange, legumes, starchy vegetables, and other vegetables) several times a week.
- Consume 3 or more ounce-equivalents of whole-grain products per day, with the rest of the recommended grains coming from enriched or whole-grain products. In general, at least half the grains should come from whole grains.
- Consume 3 cups per day of fat-free or low-fat milk or equivalent milk products.

FATS

Although fats and oils are important in a healthful diet, heart health is affected by the type and total amount of fat. Too much saturated fats, *trans* fats, and cholesterol increase the risk of elevated blood lipid levels, which may increase the risk of CHD. Usually, high fat intake (more than 35% of kilocalories) is associated with a higher saturated fat intake and consumption of excess kilocalories. If fat intake is less than 20% of kilocalories, there is a risk of inadequate intakes of vitamin E and essential fatty acids that may lead to unfavorable changes in high-density lipoproteins (HDL) ("good" type of cholesterol) and triglycerides in the blood.

Key Recommendations
- Consume less than 10% of kilocalories from saturated fatty acids, and keep *trans* fatty acid consumption as low as possible.
- Keep total fat intake between 20% and 35% of kilocalories, with most fats coming from sources of polyunsaturated and monounsaturated fatty acids, such as fish, nuts, and vegetable oils.
- When selecting and preparing meat, poultry, dry beans, and milk or milk products, make choices that are lean, low-fat, or fat-free.
- Limit intake of fats and oils high in saturated or *trans* fatty acids, and choose products low in such fats and oils.

CARBOHYDRATES

Carbohydrates are the principal source for dietary fiber, which is composed of nondigestible carbohydrates and lignin in plants. Carbohydrates are essential for a healthful diet. Dietary fiber has numerous beneficial effects on health, including decreased risk of CHD and decreased constipation. A fiber-rich diet may also lower the risk of type 2 diabetes. Because fruit juices contain little or no fiber, most fruit servings should be eaten in the form of whole fruit (fresh, frozen, canned, or dried). Legumes, or dry beans and peas, should be consumed several times weekly because of their high-fiber content. At least half the recommended grain servings should be whole-grain foods to meet the fiber recommendation. Consuming at least 3 ounce-equivalents of whole grains daily can reduce the risk of CHD, may help with weight maintenance, and may reduce risk for other chronic diseases.

Sugars and starches, whether they are naturally present or added to food, supply physiological energy in the form of glucose. The body does not respond differently to sugars naturally present in foods or sugars that are added to the food, but added sugars supply kilocalories with few or no nutrients. Greater consumption of foods containing large amounts of added sugars increases the difficulty of consuming adequate nutrients without gaining weight. In addition, the frequency and duration of consumption of starches and sugars are important factors in caries risk because they increase exposure to cariogenic substrates.

Key Recommendations
- Choose fiber-rich fruits, vegetables, and whole grains often.
- Choose and prepare foods and beverages with little added sugars or caloric sweeteners, such as amounts suggested by MyPyramid and DASH Eating Plan (see Chapter 11).
- Reduce the incidence of dental caries by practicing good oral hygiene and consuming sugar- and starch-containing foods and beverages less frequently.

SODIUM AND POTASSIUM

Most Americans consume more salt than they need; decreasing salt intake is advisable. In general, high salt intake is associated with higher blood pressure. **Hypertension** (high blood pressure) increases an individual's risk of CHD, stroke, congestive heart failure, and kidney disease. To prevent the development of high blood pressure with increasing age, lifestyle changes are recommended. Recommended changes include reducing salt intake, increasing potassium intake, losing excess body weight, increasing physical activity, and eating an overall healthful diet.

The natural salt content of food accounts for only about 10% of total intake. Discretionary salt (salt added at the table or in cooking) provides another 5% to 10% of total intake. Approximately 75% is added to prepared foods by manufacturers and food establishments. Because most of the salt consumed is from processed foods, the goal should concentrate primarily on reducing the salt added during food processing, and on changing food selections to more fresh foods and fewer processed items.

Key Recommendations
- Consume less than 2300 mg (approximately 1 tsp of salt) of sodium per day.
- Choose and prepare foods with less salt. At the same time, consume potassium-rich foods, such as fruits and vegetables.

ALCOHOLIC BEVERAGES

Alcohol consumption can have beneficial or harmful effects depending on the amount consumed, age and other characteristics of the individuals consuming the alcohol, and specifics of the situation. Fewer Americans consume alcohol today compared with 50 to 100 years ago.

The risks of heavy alcohol consumption include increased potential for liver cirrhosis, hypertension, cancers of the upper gastrointestinal tract, injury, violence, and death. Because alcoholic beverages supply kilocalories with few nutrients, adequate nutrient intake without weight gain is difficult with excessive alcohol consumption. Some individuals are more susceptible to the harmful effects of alcohol and should abstain—children and adolescents; women who may become pregnant or who are pregnant; individuals who cannot limit their drinking to moderate levels; and individuals who plan to drive, operate machinery, or take part in other activities that require attention, skill, or coordination or are taking medications that can interact with alcohol.

In moderation, alcohol may have beneficial effects for middle-aged and older adults, but not for young people. Adults who consume one to two alcoholic beverages a day seem to have a lower risk of CHD. Alcohol use among young adults is associated with a higher risk of traumatic injury and death. A distinct disadvantage of alcohol consumption (even one drink per day) is a significantly increased risk for oral and pharyngeal cancers.[5]

An alcoholic beverage is defined as 12 oz of regular beer, 5 oz of wine, or 1.5 oz of distilled spirits (80 proof). Moderation is not intended as an average over several days, but rather as the amount consumed on any single day. Because of the adverse effects of alcohol consumption for many individuals, other factors that reduce the risk of heart disease (e.g., healthy diet, physical activity, avoidance of smoking, and maintenance of a healthy weight) are more advisable than recommending alcohol intake.

Key Recommendations
- Individuals who choose to drink alcoholic beverages should do so sensibly and in moderation—defined as the consumption of up to one drink per day for women and up to two drinks per day for men.
- Alcoholic beverages should not be consumed by some individuals, including individuals who cannot restrict their alcohol intake, women of childbearing age who may become pregnant, pregnant and lactating women, children and adolescents, individuals taking medications that can interact with alcohol, and individuals with specific medical conditions.
- Alcoholic beverages should be avoided by individuals engaging in activities that require attention, skill, or coordination, such as driving or operating machinery.

FOOD SAFETY

The food safety guideline is designed to reduce the risks from foods that are contaminated with harmful bacteria, viruses, parasites, toxins, and chemical and physical contaminants. Healthful eating requires a safe food supply provided by farmers, food producers, markets, food service establishments, and other food handlers. The guideline addresses simple food-handling principles to practice when preparing, serving, and storing food to minimize the risk of foodborne illness. This topic is addressed further in Chapter 15.

Key Recommendations
- Do the following to avoid microbial foodborne illness:
  - Clean hands, food contact surfaces, and fruits and vegetables. Meat and poultry should not be washed or rinsed.
  - Separate raw, cooked, and ready-to-eat foods while shopping, preparing, or storing foods.
  - Cook foods to a safe temperature to kill microorganisms.
  - Chill (refrigerate) perishable food promptly, and defrost foods properly.
- Avoid raw (unpasteurized) milk or any products made from unpasteurized milk, raw or partially cooked eggs or foods containing raw eggs, raw or undercooked meat and poultry, unpasteurized juices, and raw sprouts.

Dental Hygiene Considerations
- These guidelines do not apply to patients with conditions that interfere with normal nutrition or for children younger than 2 years of age.
- These guidelines may be inappropriate if the patient has been told to follow a special diet or is ill or immunocompromised.
- Nutrient-dense foods provide substantial amounts of vitamins and minerals and relatively few kilocalories. Foods that can be suggested to patients are noted in Table 1-2.
- Fats provide energy and essential fatty acids and are important for absorption of fat-soluble vitamins A, D, E, and K and carotenoids.
- Processed foods and oils provide approximately 80% of trans fats, with the remainder coming from animal sources.
- The recommended dietary fiber intake is 14 g per 1000 kcal consumed.
- Provide the patient with a definition or example of moderation (e.g., $\frac{1}{4}$ tsp salt per day or 5 oz glass of wine for a woman per day).

Nutritional Directions
- Nutritional advice should recommend diets that follow national nutrition guidelines and provide all the nutrients needed for growth and health.
- Encourage patients to consume more dark green and orange vegetables, legumes, fruits, whole grains, and low-fat milk and milk products.
- Encourage patients to consume less refined grains, total fats (especially saturated and trans fats), added sugars, and kilocalories.
- A patient needing 2000 kcal daily should limit saturated fat intake to 20 g or less.
- Carbohydrate-containing foods—fruits, vegetables, grains, and milk—are important sources of many nutrients, but carbohydrate selections should be chosen wisely, within the context of a calorie-controlled diet.
- Dental caries can be minimized by reducing the frequency and duration of oral exposure to fermentable carbohydrate intake, and optimizing oral hygiene practices, such as drinking fluoridated water and brushing and flossing teeth.

Table 1-2   Frequency of Use of Foods for Implementing Dietary Guidelines

Food Groups	Choose More Often	Choose Less Often	Major Contributions
Fats	Corn, cottonseed, olive, sesame, soybean, safflower, sunflower, peanut, canola oils Mayonnaise or salad dressing (made from the above oils) Avocado Olives	Butter, lard Margarine made from hydrogenated or saturated fats Coconut or palm oil Hydrogenated vegetable shortening Bacon Meat fat/drippings, gravy, sauces	Vitamin A, kilocalories, essential fatty acids
Soups	Lightly salted soups with fat skimmed Cream-style soups (with low-fat milk)	Commercially prepared soups and mixes	Fluid, kilocalories (may contain a variety of vitamins, minerals, and protein, depending on type)
Sweets and desserts	Desserts that have been sweetened lightly or contain only moderate fat, such as puddings made from skim milk, angel food cake, fruit-based desserts	Desserts high in sugar or fats, candy, pastries, cakes, pies, whole-milk puddings, cookies	Kilocalories (fats, carbohydrates)
Beverages	Water Unsweetened soft drinks Decaffeinated drinks	Sweetened beverages Caffeine-containing beverages Alcoholic beverages	Fluid, kilocalories (unless sugar-free)
Milk and milk products	Low-fat or skim milk Low-fat cheese Low-fat yogurt	Whole milk Whole-milk cheeses Whole-milk yogurt Ice cream	Kilocalories, calcium, protein, phosphorus, vitamins A and D, riboflavin
Vegetables, including starchy vegetables	Fresh, frozen, or canned; potatoes—baked or boiled Include one dark green or deep orange vegetable daily	Deep-fried vegetables, chips Pickled vegetables Highly salted vegetables or juices	Kilocalories, vitamins A and C, dietary fiber, potassium, zinc, cobalt, folic acid
Fruits	Unsweetened fruits or juices Include one citrus fruit/juice or one tomato juice daily	Sweetened fruits or juices Coconut Avocado	Kilocalories, dietary fiber, vitamins A and C
Breads, starches, and cereals	Whole-grain breads or cereals Muffins, bagels, tortillas Enriched pasta, rice, grits or noodles	Snack chips or crackers Sweetened cereals Pancakes, doughnuts, and biscuits	Kilocalories, B-complex vitamins, magnesium, copper, iron, dietary fiber
Meats or substitutes	Lean meats, fish, shellfish, poultry without skin Low-fat cheese (e.g., cottage cheese and part skim mozzarella) Peanut butter Soybeans, tofu Dry beans and peas	Fried or fatty meats/fish Fried poultry or poultry with skin High-fat cheeses (e.g., cheddar and processed cheese) Eggs Nuts	Kilocalories, protein, iron, zinc, copper, B-complex vitamins
Miscellaneous	Herbs, spices, flavorings	Salt and salt/spice combinations	Sodium

From Peckenpaugh NJ: Nutrition Essentials and Diet Therapy, 10th ed. Philadelphia: Saunders, 2007.

- A person's preference for salt is not fixed; the desire for salty foods tends to decrease after consuming foods lower in salt for a period of time.
- Residual moisture on produce may promote survival and growth of microbes. Drying the food is crucial if the item is not going to be eaten or cooked immediately.
- Dietetic, sugar-free, or reduced-fat products may not be low in kilocalories; this depends on other ingredients in the food.

MYPYRAMID FOOD GUIDANCE SYSTEM

The *MyPyramid Food Guidance System* provides assistance in implementing the recommendations of the Dietary Guide-lines and the DRI from the IOM. MyPyramid is a system that includes interactive websites and educational modules. The key tool of this guidance system is the website, www.mypyramid.gov. MyPyramid, the new food guidance system, is revolutionary for numerous reasons. The new pyramid is part of a system designed to be an interactive nutrition education tool to help consumers apply personalized dietary guidance to achieve a healthful lifestyle. Implementation of these guidelines is shown in the sample menu outlined in Figure 1-2. This menu was analyzed by the MyPyramid website to determine the nutrient content of food intake and evaluate the healthfulness of food choices.

MyPyramid (shown on the inside front cover) provides a wide array of patterns, or energy levels, to cover the span of energy needs in the population and the associated nutrient requirements. MyPyramid continues with the principles embodied in the previous Food Guide Pyramid, but is more specific in certain areas, reflecting evolving knowledge about diet and health.

The tools, particularly the graphics, are designed to help Americans make food choices that are adequate for meeting nutritional standards yet are moderate in energy level (kilocalories) and in food components or nutrients often consumed in excess (fats and sodium). Foods providing similar kinds of nutrients are grouped together, and as a rule, foods in one group cannot replace those in another (Table 1-3). The website is designed to make dietary advice relevant and attainable by personalizing it based on age, gender, and level of physical activity. As with the previous Food Guide Pyramid, MyPyramid is intended to be used as food guidance for the U.S. general public and not a therapeutic diet for any specific health condition. MyPyramid does not address adequate intake of water.

The biggest drawback of this interactive website is the dependency on access to a computer and an Internet connection. Many people in need of this information may not have access to computers. However, Nielsen Net Ratings reported that in 2004 nearly 75% of Americans have access to the Internet at home.[6] The MyPyramid website has recorded more than 3.6 billion "hits." MyPyramid: Steps to a Healthier You (see figure on inside front cover of textbook) illustrates options to establish smarter eating habits and physical activities. It is designed to convey the same message of balance, variety, moderation, and adequate nutrients. MyPyramid is individualized to help consumers personalize their food intake to achieve a healthier lifestyle through better eating and increased physical activity. MyPyramid shows six vertical color bands, each representing one of the five familiar food groups and varying proportions of the pyramid.

Each food group is in the shape of a pyramid, depicting that there are healthier choices among the foods in each group and reinforcing the concept of moderation. The vertical bands are different colors and different widths because each group represents proportions, or how much food to choose from each group. The largest groups are the grain and vegetable groups, meaning plenty of the foods in these groups should be chosen, whereas the oils in the narrowest band should be limited. The wider base in each group represents foods with little or no fats and no added sugars. For instance, whole-grain breads would be at the bottom of the grain groups and donuts at the top, indicating one should choose whole-grain breads more frequently than donuts.

By clicking on each colored vertical band inside MyPyramid, in-depth information is available for every food group: (1) what foods are included in each group and subgroup for specific types of foods, such as whole grains and refined grains, and dark green vegetables, orange vegetables, and starchy vegetables; (2) how much of each group is needed daily for various stages of life; (3) what counts as an equivalent serving; (4) the importance of eating foods from each group, presenting the health benefits and nutrients provided; and (5) tips to help you eat foods from each group. Replacing the old reference to "servings," MyPyramid uses cups, ounces, and other common household measurements to indicate the daily recommendation. Serving sizes, in relation to items patients can relate to, are shown in Box 1-2.

Physical activity, represented by the person climbing the pyramid steps, is an integral part of the nutrition graphic. Linking nutrition and fitness is essential for a healthier you, whether the goal is to maintain weight, prevent the development of diabetes, or increase energy. The physical activity component is a reminder that if less kilocalories are burned than consumed, the excess ends up as weight gain.

By entering age, gender, and level of physical activity, a pyramid designed for individual needs is immediately

Table 1-3 Principal Nutrient Contributions of Each Food Group

Nutrients	Vegetable	Fruit	Meat	Milk	Grain
Protein			X	X	X
Vitamin A	X	X			
Vitamin D				X*	
Vitamin E	X				
Vitamin C	X	X			
Thiamin			X		X
Riboflavin				X	X†
Niacin			X		X
Vitamin B6			X	X	
Folate/folic acid	X	X			X†
Vitamin B12			X‡	X‡	
Calcium				X	
Phosphorus			X	X	X
Magnesium	X			X	X§
Iron			X		X†
Zinc			X	X	X
Fiber	X	X			X§

*If fortified.
†If enriched.
‡Only animal products.
§Whole grains.

Box 1-2 What Counts as a Serving?

3 oz meat—deck of cards or the size of your palm
2 oz meat—small chicken drumstick or thigh
1 oz meat—about 3 tbsp
1 cup vegetables—size of a fist
Medium apple, orange, peach—size of a tennis ball
¼ cup dried fruit—golf ball
½ cup fruit or vegetable—half of a baseball
1 cup broccoli—light bulb
Medium potato—computer mouse
½ cup cooked pasta—ice cream scoop or half a baseball
1 bagel—diameter of a compact disc (CD)
1 oz cheese—2 dominos or 2 dice
2 Tbsp peanut butter—ping-pong ball
1 tsp butter or margarine—tip of thumb

available. The 12 intake levels, ranging from 1000 to 3200 kcal per day, are designed to help individuals find the caloric balance that will help them achieve a healthier weight. MyPyramid Plan can be printed, which includes the recommended amounts per day from each food group and an allotment of discretionary kilocalories from fat, sugar, and alcohol. This personalized plan, based on an individual's age, gender, and activity level, indicates an appropriate kilocalorie level. MyPyramid is not intended to be a weight loss tool, but is geared to individuals wishing to maintain their weight. However, MyPyramid Tracker tool on MyPyramid. com can be used for gradual weight loss because energy intake is the basis for the 12 food patterns (different energy levels). Numerous online tips are available on how to translate the recommendations into practical everyday eating patterns.

The Calculate Healthy Eating History option allows individuals to follow their average food group and nutrient intake for 1 week, 1 month, 3 months, 6 months, or 1 year. Information presented in a bar graph and a table is helpful because intake over time is more important than what is consumed on any single day.

A link to another website, MyPyramidtracker.gov, offers a database of 8000 foods and 600 types of physical activity. Individuals can keep a record of 1 year's worth of food intake and physical activity on the website. It evaluates physical activity status and provides related energy expenditure information and educational messages.

Calculate Dietary Guidelines Comparison provides a quick visual check of how food intake compares with recommendations from the Dietary Guidelines with text along with smiling, neutral, or frowning faces. Based on an individual's energy needs, the information is compared with the recommended amounts from the grain, vegetable, fruit, milk, and meat and beans food groups. It also displays a comparison of intake with Dietary Guidelines recommendations for total fat, saturated fat, cholesterol, sodium, and oils. Another option, Calculate MyPyramid Stats, takes individuals to a bar graph and table showing their food group intakes relative to recommendations and based on the energy needs of the individual.

MyPyramid Menu Planner is an interactive multimedia tool to help individuals plan meals based on the *Dietary Guidelines for Americans*. After inputting the individual's information (age, height, weight, and physical activity), foods and amounts for each food are selected. As each item is added, the screen displays a comparison to the goals and limits on kilocalories, saturated fats, added sugars, and alcohol.

For Professionals provides many tips, such as background information on MyPyramid, downloadable resources, and relevant links for further information, to help a consumer implement any necessary changes.

Of benefit to consumers, several food industry groups have elected to partner with the USDA to promote MyPyramid.[7] By doing this, they reinforce the government's nutrition education program in supermarket aisles. Educating consumers when they are purchasing food is an effective way to ensure that they make more healthful food choices.

GRAINS GROUP (ORANGE VERTICAL BAND)

Five to 8 oz of grains are recommended daily with a goal of choosing at least half of the total recommended servings from whole grains. A variety of whole-grain products should be selected, including wheat, rice, oats, and corn. All whole-grain, refined and enriched, and fortified-grain products are included in this group.

Most Americans believe they are consuming adequate amounts of whole grains, but the difficulty in identifying them is a major barrier. There is no universally accepted definition of whole-grain foods, and labels may be deceiving. Labels such as "wheat bread," "stone-ground," and "seven-grain bread" do not guarantee that the food contains whole grain. Color is a poor indicator of whole grains because molasses or caramel food coloring may be added. Based on U.S. Food and Drug Administration (FDA) draft guidelines, whole grain is defined as "cereal grains that consist of the intact, ground, cracked or flaked fruit of the grains whose principal components—the starchy endosperm, germ and bran—are present in the same relative proportions as they exist in the initial grain."[8]

Since the release of the Dietary Guidelines, food manufacturers have introduced more processed foods with higher whole-grain content. Whole-grain bread purchases increased nearly 12%, whole-grain rice (brown rice) purchases increased by almost 19%, and whole-grain ready-to-eat cereal purchases increased by 16%.[9]

Enrichment is the process of restoring the iron, thiamin, riboflavin, folic acid, and niacin that are removed from food during processing to approximately their original levels. This process is federally controlled by the FDA, which establishes the quantity of nutrients that can be added. The outer layer of whole grains naturally contains bran (the outer layer) and germ (the internal embryo). When the bran is removed during the refining process, important disease-preventing nutrients are lost. Whole-grain products contribute more fiber, magnesium, phosphorus, and zinc than do enriched products (Table 1-4).

Fortification is the process of adding nutrients not present in the natural product or increasing the amount above that in the original product. Most processed breakfast cereals undergo fortification to achieve nutrient levels higher than those occurring naturally in the grain. Folic acid was the most recent addition for fortification. Most breakfast cereals and some grain products have added folic acid to reduce the risk of serious birth defects that may occur during early pregnancy if adequate amounts are unavailable.

VEGETABLE GROUP (GREEN VERTICAL BAND)

Two to 3 cups of vegetables are recommended daily, to include a weekly amount of 2 to 3 cups of dark green vegetables, $1\frac{1}{2}$ to 2 cups of orange vegetables, $2\frac{1}{2}$ cups of dry beans and peas, 3 to 6 cups of starchy vegetables, and $5\frac{1}{2}$ to 7 cups of other vegetables. Vegetables are primary sources

Table 1-4 Comparison of Nutrient Values of Selected Whole-Grain and Enriched Products

Types of Bread	Protein (g)	Total Dietary Fiber (g)	Thiamin (mg)	Riboflavin (mg)	Niacin (mg)	Vitamin B$_6$ (mg)	Total Folate (µg)	Pantothenic Acid (µg)	Iron (mg)	Zinc (mg)	Calcium (mg)	Phosphorus (mg)	Magnesium (mg)
Enriched white	1.91	0.6	0.114	0.083	1.096	0.021	28	0.051	0.94	0.18	38	25	0.119
Whole wheat	3.63	1.9	0.099	0.060	1.320	0.059	14	0.192	0.68	0.50	30	57	0.598
Whole grain	3.47	1.9	0.073	0.034	1.051	0.063	20	0.087	0.65	0.44	27	59	20
Rye	2.72	1.9	0.139	0.107	1.218	0.024	35	0.141	0.91	0.36	23	40	13

Nutrient data from U.S. Department of Agriculture, Agriculture Research Service. USDA National nutrient database for standard reference, Release 20. Available at http://www.nal.usda.gov/fnic/foodcom. Accessed July 7, 2008.

Table 1-5	Contributions of Selected Fruits and Vegetables			
Fruit/Vegetable	Vitamin A	Vitamin C*	Fiber	Cruciferous Vegetable
Acorn squash	X			
Apple		X		
Avocado		X		
Banana		X		
Bell pepper	X	XX		
Broccoli	X	XX	X	X
Brussels sprouts		XX	X	X
Cabbage		X	X	X
Cantaloupe	X	XX	X	
Carrot	X		X	
Cauliflower		X	X	X
Celery			X	
Collard greens	X	X		
Grapefruit		X	X	
Iceberg lettuce			X	
Kale	X	X		
Kiwi		X	X	
Kohlrabi				X
Mango	X	X		
Orange		XX	X	
Papaya	X	X	X	
Pear			X	
Prune			X	
Romaine lettuce	X	X	X	
Spinach	X		X	
Strawberry		XX	X	
Sweet potato	X		X	
Swiss chard	X			X
Tomato		X	X	

*X, good source of vitamin C; XX, excellent source of vitamin C.

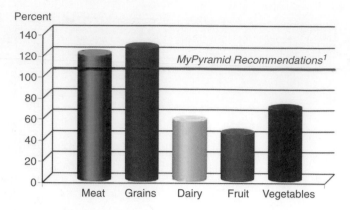

Note: Food availability data serve as proxies for actual food consumption.
[1]2006 data based on a 2,000-calorie diet.

FIGURE 1-3 American diets are out of balance with dietary recommendations. (From the U.S. Department of Agriculture and Economic Research Center. Available at http://www.ers.usda.gov/Briefing/DietQuality/Availability.htm. Accessed August 26, 2008.)

of the required nutrients dietary fiber, vitamin A (carotenoids), vitamin C, folic acid, and potassium (Table 1-5). Most vegetables are low in fat in their natural state and are cholesterol-free. Because of high water and high fiber content, most vegetables are relatively low in kilocalories. Dark green vegetables also contribute calcium, iron, magnesium, and riboflavin. **Cruciferous** vegetables, or vegetables from the mustard family are especially encouraged because of their healthful potent anticancer properties. Beans are unusual because they are in two groups, the vegetable group and meat group. Beans contain protein, fiber, calcium, folic acid, and potassium.

FRUIT GROUP (RED VERTICAL BAND)

The daily recommendation for fruit is 1½ to 2 cups. Any fruit or 100% fruit juice counts as part of the fruit group. Fruits are naturally low in fat, sodium, and kilocalories, and do not contain cholesterol. In addition, they are important sources of potassium, dietary fiber, vitamin C, and folate. Because of their fiber content, fresh, frozen, canned, or dried

fruits are recommended, suggesting that fruit juice be minimized. This food group is the most poorly implemented by consumers, as shown in Figure 1-3.

MILK, YOGURT, AND CHEESE GROUP (BLUE VERTICAL BAND)

The recommendation for this group is 3 cups for all age groups except children younger than 8 years of age. Milk products provide calcium and potassium, and may be a good source of vitamin D. Fortified milk products are important sources of vitamin D; however, many milk substitutes (cheese, yogurt, and ice cream) are not fortified with vitamin D (unless made with fortified milk). Whole milk and many cheeses are high in saturated fat and can have negative health implications. Low-fat or fat-free milk products provide little or no fat and should be chosen most often to avoid consuming more kilocalories than are needed. Although whole milk consumption has decreased, intake of reduced-fat milk has remained stable, which indicates overall milk consumption is declining. The dairy group does not include high-fat products, such as butter and cream, because they are not high in calcium, riboflavin, and protein.

The consumption of milk and milk products can promote achievement of peak bone mass in children and adolescents, and reduce the risk of low bone mass and osteoporosis. In terms of oral health, two studies have indicated that higher dairy product consumption is associated with decreased prevalence and severity of periodontal disease.[10,11]

MEATS, POULTRY, FISH, DRY BEANS AND PEAS, EGGS, AND NUTS GROUP (PURPLE VERTICAL BAND)

This group includes all foods containing predominantly meat, poultry, fish, dry beans or peas, eggs, nuts, and seeds. Lean or low-fat meat and poultry selections are recom-

Table 1-6	Outstanding Contributions of Various Protein Foods
Protein Food	**Nutrient**
Lean red meats	Iron
	B vitamins
	Zinc
Pork	Thiamin
	Zinc
Poultry	Potassium
	Niacin
Liver and egg yolks	Vitamin A
	Iron
	Zinc
Dry peas and beans, soybeans, and nuts	Magnesium
	Fiber
	Zinc

mended. Fish, nuts, and seeds contain a healthy type of fat, so these are recommended more frequently than meat or poultry. Dry beans and peas are included in this group as well as in the vegetable group.

The daily recommendation is for 5 to 6½ oz. The foods in this group are important sources of protein, B vitamins (niacin, thiamin, riboflavin, and B_6), vitamin E, iron, zinc, and magnesium. A variety of foods from this group should be included because each food has distinct nutritional advantages (Table 1-6). By varying choices and including fish, nuts, beans, and seeds, the intake of healthful fats, such as monounsaturated fatty acids and polyunsaturated fatty acids, is increased. Current scientific evidence indicates protein intake is not a public health concern for adults and children older than 4 years of age.

Dry beans and peas, such as kidney beans, pinto beans, lima beans, black-eyed peas, and lentils, can be counted as a vegetable (dry beans and peas subgroup) or in the meat, poultry, fish, dry beans, eggs, and nuts group. They are excellent sources of plant protein and dietary fiber, and contribute other nutrients similar to meats, poultry, and fish. Whether they are counted as a vegetable or a meat, frequent consumption—several cups a week—is recommended. Vegetarians can choose eggs, beans, nuts, nut butters, peas, and soy products to obtain adequate amounts of protein.

Most Americans consume approximately twice as much protein as they need. Although this may not be harmful, high-fat meats may be an undesirable source of kilocalories, cholesterol, and saturated fatty acids. Protein supplements promoted to increase muscle mass do not contain other nutrients important for health that foods provide. These supplements should be used only after consulting a healthcare provider or registered dietitian.

OILS GROUP (YELLOW VERTICAL BAND)

Fats that are liquid at room temperature are called oils. They are extracted from different plants, fish, and seeds and nuts. The daily recommendation for oils depends on age, sex, and level of physical activity, but generally 5 to 7 tsp of oils is

sufficient to provide the e
amount is limited to balance to
contain about 120 kcal per Tbsp.

DISCRETIONARY KILOCALORIES

Kilocalories are necessary to provide energy
activities and other body functions. The amount
tionary kilocalories is based on estimated caloric nee
age, sex, and activity level. Physical activity increase
caloric needs, so physically active individuals need more
total kilocalories and have a larger discretionary caloric
allowance.

For adults, the total number of kilocalories needed minus the number of kilocalories consumed by the required food groups would yield the amount of discretionary kilocalories allowable without weight gain. For example:

Total kcal – kcal from required food groups
= discretionary kcal

Therefore, whole milk is 120 kcal – 90 kcal for skim milk
= 30 discretionary kcal

The daily estimated discretionary kilocalorie allowance ranges from 154 kcals for young children, whose energy requirement is 1000 kcals, to 334 kcal for adults, whose energy requirement is 3000 kcals. Discretionary kilocalorie allowance is greater for those who are physically active.

Foods included in discretionary kilocalories include solid fats (e.g., stick margarine; shortening; and beef, chicken, and pork fat), added sugars (regular soft drinks, candy, cakes, cookies, pies, donuts, and sweet rolls as well as sugar, corn syrup, and high fructose corn syrup), and alcoholic beverages. All of the kilocalories in candy, sodas, alcoholic beverages, and solid fats are discretionary kilocalories. Many foods such as regular meats, many cheeses, well-marbled cuts of meats, biscuits, and French fries may be counted as servings from another food group, but their estimated discretionary kilocalories must be counted against the total caloric allowance.

Discretionary kilocalories include (1) additional foods from any food group more than MyPyramid recommends; (2) higher caloric foods containing larger amounts of fat or sugar, such as whole milk, cheese, biscuits, and sweetened yogurt; (3) fats or sweeteners added to foods, such as sauces and salad dressings; and (4) foods that are principally fats, caloric sweeteners, or alcohol, such as candy, soda, and beer. By choosing foods that are lower in fats, such as skim milk rather than whole milk, individuals could consume more of these "luxury" items without exceeding their total caloric allowance.

Most individuals should use these foods sparingly, especially if their physical activity is minimal. In some instances, these items contribute to palatability and make some nutritious foods more desirable (e.g., some patients may dislike milk but enjoy pudding or custard). In addition to providing a prolonged feeling of **satiety** (fullness), some fats and oils are good sources of vitamins A and E and are considered

... of healthy
... otivation to
... questions or
... d food group
... wledgeable to
... le grains, types
... essential fatty acids needed. The
... al caloric intake because oils

... ient adequacy or
... ninates fruits and
... s may develop; if
... ated, calcium defi-

GROUP
for physical
... of discre-
... s by

- Ensure th... number and size of
  servings recomme... group daily to obtain
  adequate nutrients.
- Although consumers are getting the message that they need
  to make positive dietary and lifestyle changes, putting that
  advice into practice is challenging and confusing for many,
  and there is still a wide gap between the Dietary Guidelines
  and actual eating patterns (see Fig. 1-3).
- Encourage small practical changes in food choices to help
  patients gradually make significant improvement toward the
  Dietary Guidelines.
- Less than one-third of American adults meet the recommendations to consume five or more servings of fruits and vegetables daily.[14]
- A large proportion of Americans, regardless of their weight,
  are malnourished in terms of vitamins and mineral intake.
  However, they should not be told to eat less food, but to
  choose more nutrient-dense foods.

Nutritional Directions

- Within each food group, individual foods can vary widely
  in the number of kilocalories furnished; knowledge about
  serving sizes is important.
- Consumers should understand that the caloric level is much
  higher if foods with higher fat or added sugar are chosen
  from a food group (e.g., choosing high-fat ice cream rather
  than skim milk).
- If only nutrient-dense foods are selected from each food
  group in the amounts recommended, a small amount of discretionary kilocalories can be consumed as added fats or
  sugars, alcohol, or other foods.
- Dairy products are poor sources of iron and vitamin C, but
  they are good sources of protein, calcium, and riboflavin.
- Caloric consumption can be decreased by substituting low-
  fat or skim milk for whole milk. The nutrient content is the
  same for whole milk and low-fat milk except for the amount
  of fat and kilocalories. Low-fat or skim milk is recommended for healthy Americans older than age 2 years.
- Foods in the grains group are economical and nutritious;
  they may be staple items for people in lower socioeconomic
  groups. However, whole-grain products may be more expensive, so patients need to be encouraged to increase these
  food choices as much as possible.
- Cholesterol occurs naturally in all foods of animal origin.
- Elimination or reduction of one or more food groups reduces
  the variety of food intake, reducing the number or amount
  of nutrients consumed.
- Adults watching their weight should choose the minimal
  amounts of servings recommended from all groups, choose
  foods from the lower part of the band, and limit portion
  sizes.

healthy fats. Based on the *National Health and Nutrition
Examination Survey* (NHANES), sweets, desserts, soft
drinks, and alcoholic beverages account for almost 30% of
all kilocalories consumed by Americans.[12]

OTHER FOOD GUIDES

Not all healthcare professionals agree that MyPyramid is the
ideal method to promote health and wellness. However, the
recommendations in MyPyramid are remarkably consistent
with other population-based recommendations designed to
control obesity, diabetes, heart disease and stroke, hypertension, cancer, and osteoporosis. Although different guides
were derived from different types of nutrition research and
for different purposes, they share consistent messages: eat
more fruits, vegetables, legumes, and whole grains; eat less
added sugar and saturated fat; and emphasize plant oils.
Primary differences are in the types of recommended vegetables and protein sources, and the amount of recommended
dairy products and total oil. Overall nutrient values are also
similar for most nutrients except for vitamins A and E and
calcium.

As shown in Table 1-7, the recommendations in MyPyramid are similar to the recommendations of the DASH Eating
Plan (discussed in Chapter 11), the American Heart Association (discussed in Chapter 5), and the American Cancer
Society. In addition, calculated nutrient intakes associated

with following the guide are generally within the ranges of
nutrient recommendations from the *Clinical Guidelines on
Overweight and Obesity,* the American Diabetes Association
(discussed in Chapter 6), the National Cholesterol Education
Program, the National Committee on High Blood Pressure,
and the American Institute for Cancer Research.

HEALTHY EATING PYRAMID

One alternative food guide is the Healthy Eating Pyramid
created by the nutrition faculty at Harvard School of Public
Health (Fig. 1-4). The goal of this pyramid is staying healthy,
which depends on an individual's daily exercise and weight
control. More food from the bottom part of the pyramid
(vegetables and whole grains) should be consumed and less
from the top (red meat and refined grains). Tips for following the Healthy Eating Pyramid include: (1) Start with exercise to keep kilocalories in balance and weight in check. (2)
Focus on food, not grams, to guide how you should eat. (3)
Go with plant sources, including plenty of vegetables, fruits,
whole grains, and healthy fats, such as olive and canola oil.
(4) Cut back on American staples such as red meat, refined
grains, potatoes, sugary drinks, and salty snacks. (5) Take a
multivitamin with nutrients not exceeding the RDAs as a
nutrition insurance policy, and maybe have a drink, which
is beneficial for many people.

Table 1-7 Comparison of Authoritative Groups' Nutrient and Other Recommendations to Address Chronic Diseases and Conditions with Calculated Nutrient Content of MyPyramid 2000-kcal Pattern

Dietary Component		Recommending Body					
	MyPyramid*	Clinical Guidelines on Overweight and Obesity in Adults	American Diabetes Association	National Cholesterol Education Program	American Heart Association	National Committee on High Blood Pressure	American Institute for Cancer Research
Protein	18% of energy	≈15% of energy	15%-20% of energy	≈15% of energy		Follow Dietary Approaches to Stop Hypertension Eating Plan‡	
Total fat	29% of energy	≤30% of energy		25%-35% of energy			Select foods low in fat
Saturated fat	7.8% of energy	8%-10% of energy	≤10% of energy; £7% for those with low-density lipoprotein cholesterol ≥2.6 mmol/L (≥100 mg/dL)†	<7% of energy	Limit how much saturated fat, *trans* fat, and cholesterol you eat		
Monounsaturated fat	10.7% of energy	≤15% of energy	See carbohydrate	≤20% of energy			
Polyunsaturated fat	8.9% of energy	≤10% of energy	≈10% of energy	≤10% of energy			
Trans fatty acids	Estimate unavailable	Not mentioned	Minimize		Limit how much saturated fat, *trans* fat, and cholesterol you eat		
Cholesterol	230 mg/d	<300 mg/d	<300 mg/d; <200 mg/d for those with low-density lipoprotein cholesterol ≥2.6 mmol/L (≥100 mg/dL)†	<200 mg/d	<300 mg/d		Choose diet rich in plant-based foods and eat plenty of fruits and vegetables
Carbohydrate	55% of energy	≥55% of energy	60%-70% of total energy when combined with monounsaturated fat	50%-60% of energy			
Fiber	31 g/d	20-30 g/d	20-30 g/d	20-30 g/d	≈25 g/d		
Sodium	1779 mg/d	≤2400 mg/d	≤2400 mg/d	≤2400 mg/d	<2300 mg/d: African Americans, middle-aged and older adults, and people with high blood pressure need <1500 mg/d	≤2400 mg/d	Low
Energy	1987 kcal/d	500-1000 kcal/d below usual intake	Balance energy intake and expenditure to maintain weight		Use as many kilocalories as you take in every day		
Alcohol	Estimate not provided‡	Provides unneeded energy and displaces more nutritious foods	Limit to 1 drink/d for women and 2 drinks/d for men	Limit to 1 drink/d for women and 2 drinks/d for men	Limit to 1 drink/d per day for women and 2 drinks/d for men	Limit to 1 drink/ d for women and 2 drinks/d for men	In moderation

From Krebs-Smith SM, Kris-Etherton P: How does MyPyramid compare to other population-based recommendations for controlling chronic disease? J Am Diet Assoc 2007 May; 107(5):830.

*Values represent estimated levels assuming typical choices.

†To convert mg/dL cholesterol to mmol/L, multiply mg/dL by 0.026. To convert mmol/L cholesterol to mg/dL, multiply mmol/L by 38.6. Cholesterol of 100 mg/dL = 2.6 mmol/L.

‡Alcohol would be counted as discretionary calories. No specific advice given in MyPyramid.

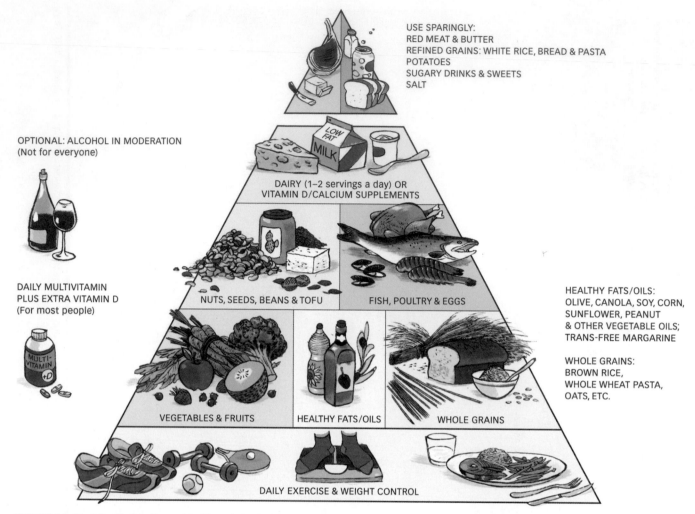

USE SPARINGLY:
RED MEAT & BUTTER
REFINED GRAINS: WHITE RICE, BREAD & PASTA
POTATOES
SUGARY DRINKS & SWEETS
SALT

OPTIONAL: ALCOHOL IN MODERATION
(Not for everyone)

DAIRY (1–2 servings a day) OR
VITAMIN D/CALCIUM SUPPLEMENTS

DAILY MULTIVITAMIN
PLUS EXTRA VITAMIN D
(For most people)

NUTS, SEEDS, BEANS & TOFU

FISH, POULTRY & EGGS

HEALTHY FATS/OILS:
OLIVE, CANOLA, SOY, CORN,
SUNFLOWER, PEANUT
& OTHER VEGETABLE OILS;
TRANS-FREE MARGARINE

WHOLE GRAINS:
BROWN RICE,
WHOLE WHEAT PASTA,
OATS, ETC.

VEGETABLES & FRUITS

HEALTHY FATS/OILS

WHOLE GRAINS

DAILY EXERCISE & WEIGHT CONTROL

FIGURE 1-4 Healthy Eating Pyramid. (Copyright © 2008 Harvard University. For more information about The Healthy Eating Pyramid, please see The Nutrition Source, Department of Nutrition, Harvard School of Public Health, www.thenutritionsource.org, and Eat, Drink, and Be Healthy, by Walter C. Willett, MD, and Patrick J. Skerrett (2005), Free Press/Simon & Schuster, Inc.)

CANADA'S FOOD GUIDE

Canada has also developed a pictorial food guide to assist Canadians to choose food wisely (Fig. 1-5). The Food Guide rainbow encourages consumers to find their own healthy lifestyle—a pot of gold. The website, www.hc-sc.gc.ca/fn-an/food-guide-aliment/index_e.html, allows consumers to personalize the food guide, providing recipes, tips for healthy eating and physical activity, and other educational materials.

NUTRITION LABELING

NUTRITION FACTS LABEL

Two categories of claims currently can be used on foods in the United States—nutrient content claims and health claims. **Nutrient content claims** describe the percentage of a nutrient in a product relative to the daily value. **Health claims** describe a relationship between a food or food component and reducing risk of a disease or health-related condition.

These claims are based on a very high standard of scientific evidence and significant scientific agreement.

In a concerted effort by the USDA and the FDA to improve the health and well-being of the American people by enhancing nutritional knowledge, the Nutrition Facts label was established as a graphic tool to inform consumers about nutrient content of foods available in the supermarket (Fig. 1-6). Nutrition labels on product packaging help health educators and consumers know what nutrients are in a food to be able to compare nutritional values of various products. These labels provide nutrition information regarding general recommendations for most adults. Approximately 52% of consumers indicate they frequently refer to the Nutrition Facts panel when making decisions about purchasing or consuming a food or beverage.[15]

The labeling policy requires approximately 90% of all foods, including some fresh produce, meat, and fish, provide nutritional information based on the nutrients provided in a single serving. For foods that are not packaged, the information must be displayed at the point of purchase (e.g., in a counter card, sign, or booklet).

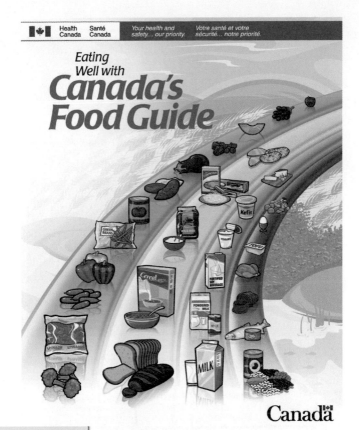

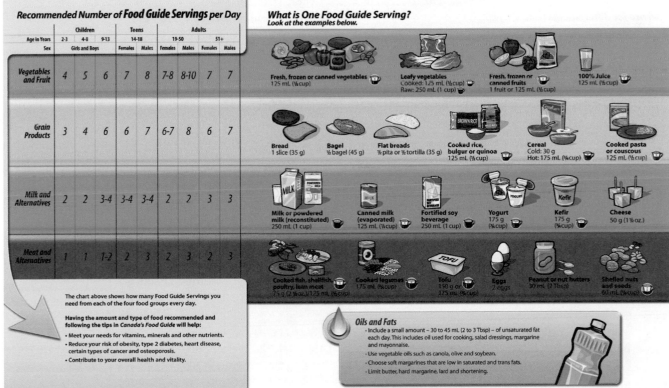

FIGURE 1-5 Eating well with Canada's food guide. (From Eating Well with Canada's Food Guide (2007), Health Canada. Reproduced with permission of the Minister of Public Works and Government Services Canada, 2009. Available at www.hc-sc.gc.ca/fn-an/food-guide-aliment. Accessed January 25, 2008.)

Make each Food Guide Serving count...
wherever you are – at home, at school, at work or when eating out!

▶ **Eat at least one dark green and one orange vegetable each day.**
  Go for dark green vegetables such as broccoli, romaine lettuce and spinach.
  Go for orange vegetables such as carrots, sweet potatoes and winter squash.

▶ **Choose vegetables and fruit prepared with little or no added fat, sugar or salt.**
  Enjoy vegetables steamed, baked or stir-fried instead of deep-fried.

▶ **Have vegetables and fruit more often than juice.**

▶ **Make at least half of your grain products whole grain each day.**
  Eat a variety of whole grains such as barley, brown rice, oats, quinoa and wild rice.
  Enjoy whole grain breads, oatmeal or whole wheat pasta.

▶ **Choose grain products that are lower in fat, sugar or salt.**
  Compare the Nutrition Facts table on labels to make wise choices.
  Enjoy the true taste of grain products. When adding sauces or spreads, use small amounts.

▶ **Drink skim, 1%, or 2% milk each day.**
  Have 500 mL (2 cups) of milk every day for adequate vitamin D.
  Drink fortified soy beverages if you do not drink milk.

▶ **Select lower fat milk alternatives.**
  Compare the Nutrition Facts table on yogurts or cheeses to make wise choices.

▶ **Have meat alternatives such as beans, lentils and tofu often.**

▶ **Eat at least two Food Guide Servings of fish each week.***
  Choose fish such as char, herring, mackerel, salmon, sardines and trout.

▶ **Select lean meat and alternatives prepared with little or no added fat or salt.**
  Trim the visible fat from meats. Remove the skin on poultry.
  Use cooking methods such as roasting, baking or poaching that require little or no added fat.
  If you eat luncheon meats, sausages or prepackaged meats, choose those lower in salt (sodium) and fat.

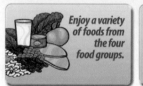
Enjoy a variety of foods from the four food groups.

Satisfy your thirst with water!
Drink water regularly. It's a calorie-free way to quench your thirst. Drink more water in hot weather or when you are very active.

* Health Canada provides advice for limiting exposure to mercury from certain types of fish. Refer to www.healthcanada.gc.ca for the latest information.

Advice for different ages and stages...

Children

Following *Canada's Food Guide* helps children grow and thrive.

Young children have small appetites and need calories for growth and development.

- Serve small nutritious meals and snacks each day.
- Do not restrict nutritious foods because of their fat content. Offer a variety of foods from the four food groups.
- Most of all... be a good role model.

Women of childbearing age

All women who could become pregnant and those who are pregnant or breastfeeding need a multivitamin containing *folic acid* every day. Pregnant women need to ensure that their multivitamin also contains *iron*. A health care professional can help you find the multivitamin that's right for you.

Pregnant and breastfeeding women need more calories. Include an extra 2 to 3 Food Guide Servings each day.

Here are two examples:
- Have fruit and yogurt for a snack, or
- Have an extra slice of toast at breakfast and an extra glass of milk at supper.

Men and women over 50

The need for *vitamin D* increases after the age of 50.

In addition to following *Canada's Food Guide*, everyone over the age of 50 should take a daily vitamin D supplement of 10 µg (400 IU).

Eat well and be active today and every day!

The benefits of eating well and being active include:
- Better overall health.   - Feeling and looking better.
- Lower risk of disease.   - More energy.
- A healthy body weight.   - Stronger muscles and bones.

Be active

To be active every day is a step towards better health and a healthy body weight.

Canada's Physical Activity Guide recommends building 30 to 60 minutes of moderate physical activity into daily life for adults and at least 90 minutes a day for children and youth. You don't have to do it all at once. Add it up in periods of at least 10 minutes at a time for adults and five minutes at a time for children and youth.

Start slowly and build up.

Eat well

Another important step towards better health and a healthy body weight is to follow *Canada's Food Guide* by:

- Eating the recommended amount and type of food each day.
- Limiting foods and beverages high in calories, fat, sugar or salt (sodium) such as cakes and pastries, chocolate and candies, cookies and granola bars, doughnuts and muffins, ice cream and frozen desserts, french fries, potato chips, nachos and other salty snacks, alcohol, fruit flavoured drinks, soft drinks, sports and energy drinks, and sweetened hot or cold drinks.

Read the label

- Compare the Nutrition Facts table on food labels to choose products that contain less fat, saturated fat, trans fat, sugar and sodium.
- Keep in mind that the calories and nutrients listed are for the amount of food found at the top of the Nutrition Facts table.

Limit trans fat

When a Nutrition Facts table is not available, ask for nutrition information to choose foods lower in trans and saturated fats.

Nutrition Facts		
Per 0 mL (0 g)		
Amount		**% Daily Value**
Calories 0		
Fat 0 g		0 %
Saturates 0 g		0 %
+ Trans 0 g		
Cholesterol 0 mg		
Sodium 0 mg		0 %
Carbohydrate 0 g		0 %
Fibre 0 g		0 %
Sugars 0 g		
Protein 0 g		
Vitamin A 0 %	Vitamin C	0 %
Calcium 0 %	Iron	0 %

Take a step today...

✓ Have breakfast every day. It may help control your hunger later in the day.
✓ Walk wherever you can – get off the bus early, use the stairs.
✓ Benefit from eating vegetables and fruit at all meals and as snacks.
✓ Spend less time being inactive such as watching TV or playing computer games.
✓ Request nutrition information about menu items when eating out to help you make healthier choices.
✓ Enjoy eating with family and friends!
✓ Take time to eat and savour every bite!

For more information, interactive tools, or additional copies visit Canada's Food Guide on-line at:
www.healthcanada.gc.ca/foodguide

or contact:
Publications
Health Canada
Ottawa, Ontario K1A 0K9
E-Mail: publications@hc-sc.gc.ca
Tel.: 1-866-225-0709
Fax: (613) 941-5366
TTY: 1-800-267-1245

Également disponible en français sous le titre :
Bien manger avec le Guide alimentaire canadien

This publication can be made available on request on diskette, large print, audio-cassette and braille.

How do I count Food Guide Servings in a meal?

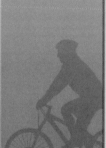

Here is an example:

Vegetable and beef stir-fry with rice, a glass of milk and an apple for dessert		
250 mL (1 cup) mixed broccoli, carrot and sweet red pepper	=	**2 Vegetables and Fruit** Food Guide Servings
75 g (2½ oz.) lean beef	=	**1 Meat and Alternatives** Food Guide Serving
250 mL (1 cup) brown rice	=	**2 Grain Products** Food Guide Servings
5 mL (1 tsp) canola oil	=	part of your **Oils and Fats** intake for the day
250 mL (1 cup) 1% milk	=	**1 Milk and Alternatives** Food Guide Serving
1 apple	=	**1 Vegetables and Fruit** Food Guide Serving

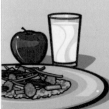

FIGURE 1-5, cont'd

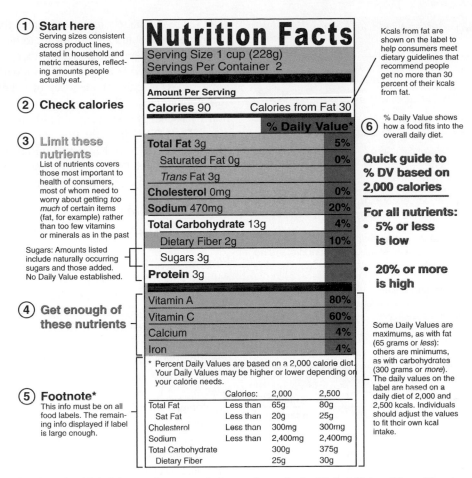

① **Start here**
Serving sizes consistent across product lines, stated in household and metric measures, reflecting amounts people actually eat.

② **Check calories**

③ **Limit these nutrients**
List of nutrients covers those most important to health of consumers, most of whom need to worry about getting *too much* of certain items (fat, for example) rather than too few vitamins or minerals as in the past

Sugars: Amounts listed include naturally occurring sugars and those added. No Daily Value established.

④ **Get enough of these nutrients**

⑤ **Footnote***
This info must be on all food labels. The remaining info displayed if label is large enough.

Nutrition Facts
Serving Size 1 cup (228g)
Servings Per Container 2

Amount Per Serving

Calories 90   Calories from Fat 30

                                                % Daily Value*

Total Fat 3g	**5%**
Saturated Fat 0g	**0%**
Trans Fat 3g	
Cholesterol 0mg	**0%**
Sodium 470mg	**20%**
Total Carbohydrate 13g	**4%**
Dietary Fiber 2g	**10%**
Sugars 3g	
Protein 3g	

Vitamin A	**80%**
Vitamin C	**60%**
Calcium	**4%**
Iron	**4%**

* Percent Daily Values are based on a 2,000 calorie diet. Your Daily Values may be higher or lower depending on your calorie needs.

		Calories:	2,000	2,500
Total Fat	Less than		65g	80g
Sat Fat	Less than		20g	25g
Cholesterol	Less than		300mg	300mg
Sodium	Less than		2,400mg	2,400mg
Total Carbohydrate			300g	375g
Dietary Fiber			25g	30g

Kcals from fat are shown on the label to help consumers meet dietary guidelines that recommend people get no more than 30 percent of their kcals from fat.

⑥ % Daily Value shows how a food fits into the overall daily diet.

Quick guide to % DV based on 2,000 calories

For all nutrients:
• **5% or less is low**

• **20% or more is high**

Some Daily Values are maximums, as with fat (65 grams or *less*): others are minimums, as with carbohydrates (300 grams or *more*). The daily values on the label are based on a daily diet of 2,000 and 2,500 kcals. Individuals should adjust the values to fit their own kcal intake.

FIGURE 1-6 An example of the food label format that currently is mandatory in the United States. (From How to understand and use the nutrition facts label. Department of Health and Human Services, Food and Drug Administration, June 2000; updated July 2003 and November 2004. Available at www.cfsan.fda.gov/~dms/foodlab.html. Accessed August 26, 2008.)

The FDA established standardized serving portions based on a reference amount for food labels in an effort to educate and provide the consumer with information about how foods fit into a healthy diet. The number of servings in a container is expressed to the nearest whole number. One of the main issues with nutrition labeling is that rules for labeling portions can be confusing for consumers and are complicated further by the fact that Americans usually eat larger portions. For example, a 12-oz can of soda has 140 kcal and is legally considered a single serving, but a 20-oz bottle lists 100 kcal per serving because a single serving in a larger container is 8 oz. Per FDA regulations, a serving of bagel is about 2 oz, which is one-fourth the size of most bagels. Misleading serving sizes may be a reason consumers are eating far more kilocalories than they think.

The requirement to label products has caused food manufacturers to reformulate foods. From January 2005 through September 2007, manufacturers introduced more than 5000 products with labels touting low or zero *trans* fat content.[16] A survey by the Grocery Manufacturers Association indicated that 92% of food manufacturing firms are reformulating foods or planning to introduce new products that contain less fat or sugar or both. In the past 5 years, manufacturers

have introduced more than 10,000 products that were nutritionally improved.[17]

Nutrients provided on the nutrition label include total kilocalories; total kilocalories from fats; total fat and saturated fat (g); *trans* fat (g); cholesterol (g); total carbohydrates, complex carbohydrates, and sugars (g); dietary fiber (g); protein (g); sodium (mg); and vitamins and minerals (%). **Daily reference values (DRVs)** are the levels of nutrients considered desirable for health for total fat, saturated fat, protein, cholesterol, carbohydrate, fiber, and sodium. A product's nutrient profile is based on the percentage of DRVs (Table 1-8), but the term **daily value (DV)** is used on the label. The DV for most vitamins and minerals is based on the highest value in the 1968 RDAs. DVs for protein, fat, fatty acids, cholesterol, sodium and potassium, total carbohydrate, and dietary fiber are based on various scientific documents written between 1987 and 1991, extracting recommended intakes to establish a basis for DVs for nutrients without RDAs.

For ease of standardizing the label, 2000 kcal is the reference amount for calculating the percentage of the DV provided in a serving. The vitamin and mineral content of a product is listed only in terms of percent DV (%DV). This

Table 1-8 Daily Reference Values (DRVs)*

Food Component	DRV
Protein	50 g†
Carbohydrate	300 g
Total fat	<65 g
Saturated fat	<20 g
Cholesterol	<300 mg
Sodium	<2400 mg
Potassium	>3500 mg
Fiber	25 g

From Kurtzweil P: "Daily values" encourage healthy diet. In FDA Consumer: Focus on Food Labeling. Washington, DC, Department of Health and Human Services, 1993.
*Daily reference values (DRVs) do not appear on the nutrient label. The term *daily value* appears on the label for ease of understanding and reflects the DRV and the DRI standards to encourage a healthy diet.
†Protein amount is for adults and children older than age 4 years only. The RDI for protein has been established for certain groups: children 1-4 years, 16 mg; infants <1 year, 14 g; pregnant women, 60 g; nursing mothers, 65 g.

Table 1-9 Reference Daily Intakes

Nutrient	Amount
Vitamin A	5000 IU
Vitamin C	60 mg
Thiamin	1.5 mg
Riboflavin	1.7 mg
Niacin	20 mg
Calcium	1 g
Iron	18 mg
Vitamin D	400 IU
Vitamin E	30 IU
Vitamin B_6	2 mg
Folic acid	400 µg
Vitamin B_{12}	6 µg
Phosphorus	1 g
Iodine	150 µg
Magnesium	400 mg
Zinc	15 mg
Copper	2 mg
Biotin	0.3 mg
Pantothenic acid	10 mg

rough guide indicates whether the food contains a small or large amount of a nutrient and is useful in comparing the nutrient content of various products. Foods that provide 20% or more of the DV are considered high in a nutrient. Although nutrient label information uses the term *daily value,* the amounts for the nutrients are based on the **reference daily intake (RDI)**, which is usually larger than the RDA for a specific age/gender group (Table 1-9). No %DV has been established for *trans* fats, sugars, and protein. Information regarding sugars and *trans* fats can be used to limit their intake.

DVs are not the recommended intake for an individual or population group and are not meant to be used for planning diets. They are merely reference numbers to compare various foods and to provide a perspective on daily nutrient needs, not to assess nutritional adequacy of a diet.

Although 67% of consumers report that using the Nutrition Fact label is easy, about one-third find the label difficult.[18] The FDA is investigating new ways of labeling food to provide more useful information about fat, calorie, and carbohydrate content, and to encourage healthier food choices to help fight the obesity epidemic.

HEALTH CLAIMS

A label cannot include an explicit or implied nutrient content claim unless it uses terms that have been defined by the FDA, such as "free," "low," "more," or "reduced." Box 1-3 defines some of the established terms and definitions used on food labels. No definition has been established by the FDA for carbohydrate claims. The FDA is expected to establish definitions regarding carbohydrate content of foods in the near future so that consumers can make informed choices based on their own preferences and goals.

Only health claims that have been approved and authorized by the FDA can be used on food products and dietary supplements. Health claims allowed by the FDA include statements dealing with the relationship between a specific nutrient and its ability to reduce the risk of disease or health-related conditions, as listed in Box 1-4. If a food is labeled with such a claim, it must meet specific criteria regarding the amount of that specific nutrient and sometimes other nutrients in the product. Products making a claim are required to use the FDA's exact wording.

The FDA established interim procedures beginning in spring 2004 allowing qualified health claims. Unqualified health claims have been permitted since 1990. Qualified health claims are graded based on the quality and strength of the scientific evidence supporting the claim. The four grading levels, A through D, help consumers evaluate the validity of the claims.[19] The highest level claims (A) are all unqualified health claims that meet the standards established by the FDA indicating a consensus of scientific agreement regarding the claim. Consumers can feel confident about the validity of an "A" claim. Second-level claims (B) have this disclaimer: "Although there is some scientific evidence supporting the claim, the evidence is not conclusive." Third-level claims (C) indicate "some scientific evidence suggests" the claim and carry the statement: "However FDA has determined that this evidence is limited and inconclusive." At the lowest end of the scale (D), to claim a health benefit, the product is required to state that "FDA concludes that there is little scientific evidence supporting this claim."

This grading system can be helpful because consumers have become more responsible for their own healthcare decisions. This changing and flexible grading system can reflect advances made in scientific research. The first qualified claim allowed by the FDA was the association between nuts and heart disease. The required claim statement must

Box 1-3   Food Label Terminology

Calories
- *Calorie free*: Fewer than 5 calories per serving
- *Low calorie*: 40 calories or less per serving, or per 50 g of the food
- *Reduced or fewer calories*: At least 25% fewer calories per serving than reference food

Fat
- *Fat-free*: Less than 0.5 g of fat per serving
- *Saturated fat–free*: Less than 0.5 g per serving, and the level of *trans* fatty acids does not exceed 1% of total fat
- *Low fat*: 3 g or less per serving, or per 50 g of the food
- *Low saturated fat*: 1 g or less per serving and not more than 15% of calories from saturated fatty acids
- *Reduced or less fat*: At least 25% less per serving than reference food
- *Reduced or less saturated fat*: At least 25% less per serving than reference food

Cholesterol
- *Cholesterol-free*: Less than 2 mg of cholesterol and 2 g or less of saturated fat per serving
- *Low cholesterol*: 20 mg or less or 2 g or less of saturated fat per serving, or per 50 g of the food
- *Reduced or less cholesterol*: At least 25% less and 2 g or less of saturated fat per serving than reference food

Sodium
- *Sodium-free*: Less than 5 mg per serving
- *Low sodium*: 140 mg or less per serving, or per 50 g of the food
- *Very low sodium*: 35 mg or less per serving, or per 50 g of the food
- *Reduced or less sodium*: At least 50% less per serving than reference food

Fiber
- *High fiber*: 5 g or more per serving (foods with high-fiber claims must meet the definition for low fat, or the level of total fat must appear next to the high-fiber claim)

- *Good source of fiber*: 2.5 to 4.9 g per serving
- *More or added fiber*: At least 2.5 g more per serving than reference food

Sugar
- *Sugar free*: Less than 0.5 g per serving
- *No added sugar, without added sugar,* or *no sugar added*:
  ○ No sugars are added during processing or packaging, including ingredients that contain sugars (e.g., fruit juices, applesauce, or dried fruit)
  ○ Processing does not increase the sugar content to an amount higher than is naturally present in the ingredients (a functionally insignificant increase in sugars is acceptable from processes used for purposes other than increasing sugar content)
  ○ The food that resembles it and for which it substitutes normally contains added sugars
  ○ If it does not meet the requirements for a low- or reduced-calorie food, that product bears a statement that the food is not low calorie or reduced calorie, and directs consumers' attention to the nutritional panel for additional information on sugars and calorie content
- *Reduced sugar*: At least 25% less sugar per serving than reference food

Healthy
Products using the term "healthy" in the product name or as a claim on the label must contain, per serving, no more than 3 g of fat, 1 g of saturated fat, 350 mg of sodium, or 60 mg of cholesterol. They must supply at least 10% of the daily value for at least one of six nutrients: vitamins A and C, calcium, iron, protein, and fiber. Raw meat, poultry, and fish can be labeled "healthy" if they contain, per serving, no more than 5 g of fat, 2 g of saturated fat, and 95 mg of cholesterol.

Modified from Stehlin D: A little "lite" reading. In FDA Consumer: Focus on Food Labeling. Washington, DC, Department of Health and Human Services, 1993, and Federal Register 59(24219), May 10, 1994; 59(27143), May 25, 1994.

Box 1-4   Claims Authorized by the U.S. Food and Drug Administration

- Calcium and reduced risk of osteoporosis
- Sodium and reduced risk of hypertension
- Dietary fat and increased risk of cancer
- Saturated fat and cholesterol and increased risk of heart disease
- Fiber-containing grain products, fruits, and vegetables and reduced risk of cancer
- Fruits, vegetables, and grain products that contain fiber, particularly soluble fiber, and reduced risk of heart disease
- Fruits and vegetables and reduced risk of cancer
- Folic acid and reduced risk of neural tube defects during pregnancy
- Noncariogenic carbohydrate sweeteners and reduced risk of dental caries

- Soluble fiber from certain foods and reduced risk of heart disease
- Soy protein and reduced risk of heart disease
- Plant sterol/stanol esters and risk of heart disease
- Whole-grain foods and reduced risk of heart disease and certain cancers
- Potassium and reduced risk of hypertension and stroke
- Fluoride and decreased risk of dental caries
- Saturated fat, cholesterol, and *trans* fats and increased risk of heart disease
- Substitute of saturated fat with unsaturated fatty acids and decreased risk of heart disease

read:[20] "Scientific evidence suggests but does not prove 1.5 ounces per day of most nuts such as (insert name of specific nut) as part of a diet low in saturated fat and cholesterol may reduce the risk of heart disease."

ADDITIONAL NUTRITION LABELS

Many consumers are confused by the Nutrition Facts panel and prefer information in a quicker and easier to read format. Food manufacturers, supermarket chains, trade associations, and health organizations began developing independent nutrition symbol systems. These groups have individually and independently implemented food scoring programs to make it easier to choose foods wisely.

These programs include icons on the front of packages, markers on store shelves, and online programs in which foods are scored according to their healthfulness. In these scoring systems, foods are rated according to their nutritional profiles for healthy ingredients (fiber and whole grains) and less healthy ones (saturated and *trans* fats). These ratings allow consumers to compare different types of the same food within a category.

Since 1985, the American Heart Association has tried to make heart-healthy grocery shopping easier with its heart check symbol. A food has to meet certain criteria to qualify to use this symbol. A group of food distributors and manufacturers along with health and nutrition advocates have introduced a universal ranking system to identify healthy food choices. This system, known as the Smart Choice program, provides easy-to-understand, at-a-glance guidance for consumers. The Whole Grain Council has different stamps indicating two different levels of whole grain in a serving. These food rating programs can help individuals make better food choices, but the Nutrition Facts panel still needs to be reviewed along with consideration of the food within the context of the whole diet to make wise decisions.

Dental Hygiene Considerations

- The dental hygienist must ensure the appropriate RDIs are used for the patient's age or grouping (e.g., when talking to a pregnant patient, the RDI for pregnancy should be used).
- To prevent confusion, the acronyms RDI and DRV are not used on labels; however, dental hygienists need to be aware of the basis for the information presented.
- The number of teaspoons of sugar in a food product can be determined from the label (see Fig. 1-6). Four grams of sugar is equivalent to 1 level teaspoon of sugar. A product containing 16 g of sugar has 4 tsp of sugar. Measuring the number of teaspoons of sugar in a product is a valuable visual aid for patients.

- To determine the percentage of sugar in a serving of a food, (1) multiply the number of grams of sugar in a product by 4 (kcal/g), (2) divide this number by the total number of kilocalories per serving, and (3) multiply by 100 to establish the percentage of calories as sugar. Using the example of the label shown in Fig. 1-5:

$$5\,g\;sugar \times 4\,kcal/g = 20\,kcal\;from\;sugar$$

$$20\,kcal\;sugar \div 250\,kcal/serving = 0.08 \times 100\% = 8\%$$

Nutritional Directions

- Read labels carefully. Ingredients are listed in order of quantity (by weight). Choose products that have less fat or oils or in which fats are listed last.
- Food labels are a useful tool to compare nutrient values of foods and learn valuable sources of nutrients. Review a label together with the patient and family. Ask the patient to bring in several labels of commonly used foods in the household for you to discuss with the patient.
- Fortified foods and supplements should not be purchased in an attempt to meet 100% of the RDIs because this may result in greater nutrient consumption than is needed, especially for young children. Concerns should be addressed to a healthcare provider or dietitian.
- Because portion sizes between products can vary, remind patients to compare these when comparing products.

- On a label, point out the DVs that indicate kilocalories (carbohydrate, fat, and protein), those indicating they should be limited (fat, saturated and *trans* fat, cholesterol, and sodium), and how to determine whether a product contains a small or large amount of a nutrient (see Fig. 1-6).
- Unsweetened juices and milk contain significant amounts of sugars because of the natural content of simple carbohydrates. This may be confusing for some patients because both are encouraged in appropriate amounts. Looking at "sugars" on the label may be misleading, whereas the total carbohydrate in the product more closely reflects actual carbohydrate content. Soluble fiber is included in the total carbohydrate kilocalories, but not insoluble fiber.

The goals of the U.S. Public Health Services' *Healthy People 2010* nutritional objectives include increasing the proportion of adults who are at a healthy weight to 60% compared with the current level of 42% in 1988-1994, and reducing the proportion of adults who are obese to 15% compared with 32.7% adults who are overweight, 34.4% obese, and 5.9% extremely obese in 2005-2006. The goal is about half the current level of obesity.[21] In 2007, 26% of the U.S. population was obese, increased nearly 2% from 2005. Not one state had reached the obesity prevalence goal of 15% established by *Healthy People 2010*. More men (26.4%) than women (24.8%) were found to be obese.[22] During the past 20 years, the heaviest body mass index (BMI) groups have been increasing at the fastest rates.[23] More depressing is a study that found that if the trend of the past 3 decades continues, possibly every American adult will be overweight 40 years from now.[24] The 2010 goals related to the objectives to attain a healthy weight include increasing the proportion of adults who (1) engage in moderate physical activity for at least 30 minutes per day and (2) perform physical activities that enhance and maintain muscular strength and endurance.

Maintaining a healthy weight is a major goal to reduce the burden of illness and its consequent reduction in quality of life and life expectancy. Obesity and overweight in adulthood go hand-in-hand with chronic diseases, notably hypertension, osteoarthritis, elevated blood cholesterol or triglyceride levels, heart disease, diabetes, gallbladder disease, sleep apnea and respiratory problems, and many cancers.[25] These conditions are associated with significant decreases in life expectancy. Overweight and obesity are the leading cause of cancer, second only to tobacco as a risk factor for cancer in Americans. The risk for cancer increases even with modest weight gains.[26] Because overweight and obesity seem to contribute to other health problems, their economic impact on the healthcare system is immense. Direct medical costs, which include prevalence, diagnosis, and treatment services, constitute $93 billion, or 9% of the total national medical bill.[27]

The terms *overweight* and *obesity* are used interchangeably, but have different meanings, as defined earlier in this chapter (p. 10). If an individual is very muscular with little fat, a BMI greater than 25 may be acceptable. However, some individuals who are normal or below normal in weight have excess amounts of fat stores. Athletes are usually overweight because of their increased muscle mass, not excess fat. Being overweight is not the same as being fat or obese. Additional muscle tissue aids body functions, but excessive fat interferes with normal body metabolism. A desirable weight depends on the amount and location of body fat and other weight-related medical problems.

Weight distribution is also a factor in predicting health risk. Excess fat in the abdominal area (the "apple-shaped" body), known as android obesity, is characteristic of men, but some women also tend to accumulate more fat around the waist, especially after menopause. Accumulation of fat in the hips or thighs (the "pear-shaped body"), called gynecoid obesity, is typical of women. Any amount of upper body obesity or increased abdominal fat increases health risks. In contrast, lower body or gynecoid obesity is relatively benign and may even be protective. However, patients with this pattern of obesity have more difficulty losing weight and maintaining a healthy weight.

Larger waist measurements indicate accumulating fat stores and are associated with increased health risks. Even normal-weight women face significantly elevated risk of premature death from heart disease, stroke, or cancer with abdominal obesity.[28] Having a proportionately large waist is associated with an accumulation of fat around the heart, liver, and other internal organs. Women greater than 5 feet in height whose waist measurement is more than 35 inches have more health risks, and for men, risk increases at 37 inches with serious concerns with more than 40 inches.[29,30] If the BMI is greater than 35, waist circumference standards may not apply. Waist-to-height ratio seems to be a good indicator of overall health risks. The waist measurement should be less than half of the person's height.

Obesity is the result of consistent caloric overconsumption in excess of energy expenditure. The CDC estimates that average daily energy intake increased almost 7% for men and about 22% for women between 1971-2000. American men consume an average of 2600 kcal, and women consume approximately 1850 kcal.[31] This increased intake reflects a consumption level that is conducive for weight gain in inactive individuals. Genetic influence is a significant factor contributing to obesity.[32] Body weight is affected by genes, metabolism, hormones, food choices, behavior, environment, culture, and socioeconomic status. Although genetics and the environment may increase the risk of weight gain, the foods an individual chooses significantly affect body weight. Many factors in American culture have made food more accessible—fast food restaurants, prepackaged food, and soft drinks. Portion sizes also have increased, and more people are eating less often at home. When eating in a restaurant, people tend to consume slightly more than 100 kcal per meal.[33] The problem results in different characteristics and warrants differing treatments.

In some cases, understanding physiological benefits of weight loss can be motivating for some patients. Weight loss is highly desirable in individuals with certain risk factors and advisable for others. A 10% weight loss is associated with a decrease in serum glucose, cholesterol, systolic blood pressure, and uric acid. Other physical symptoms that can be expected to improve with weight loss include shortness of breath, easy fatigability, fluid retention, gastric disorders, headaches, decreased energy level, decreased sexual interest, joint pains, muscle cramps, elevated pulse rate, sleeping disorders, urinary infection, and varicose veins.

Treatment of obesity has a high level of noncompliance and failure. Weight management is very difficult for most individuals. It is a lifelong commitment to change one's lifestyle—exercise regularly, make wise food choices, and modify behaviors. Weight loss should be motivated by internal rather than external reasons ("I am doing this for myself," rather than "I will lose weight for my son's wedding"). Any treatment for weight loss should always be a serious undertaking with a high level of motivation and long-term commitment. This approach increases chances that the plan will be followed until weight is lost, and that weight loss will be maintained.

One pound of fat equals 3500 kcal. Losing weight can be accomplished by eating fewer kilocalories, increasing activity, or a combination of both. A ½- to 2-lb per week weight loss is recommended to lose body fat while minimizing muscle loss. To accomplish this goal, food intake must be 500 kcal less than needed per day, which results in loss of 1 lb per week. An additional energy expenditure of 500 kcal per day is recommended for the other 1 lb of weight loss. When weight loss is achieved slowly, it is usually more effective and is maintained for a longer period.

Numerous strategies have been implemented to treat overweight and obesity. No one treatment is best for everyone; each modality varies in effectiveness, risk, and cost. Millions of obese individuals have chosen **bariatric surgery** (surgical procedure on the stomach or small intestine or both for weight reduction), which is very effective for weight loss, but affects the absorption of many nutrients. Drugs and surgical procedures currently being used for weight loss are beyond the scope of this text. A realistic goal regarding the rate and amount of weight loss must be established for each individual trying to reduce weight.

Popular weight reduction diets devised for weight loss are abundant (see Appendix E and Evolve site). Although many different plans "guarantee" weight loss, no guaranteed easy cure exists for maintaining a healthy weight. A weight reduction diet needs to be followed for an extended time; it must be appealing and flexible as well as affordable for the individual trying to lose weight. It can be balanced in terms of nutrients, yet hypocaloric. Reducing caloric intake to less than 1200 kcal for women and less than 1400 kcal for men is not recommended because adequate amounts of nutrients are not provided.

Some registered dietitians and scientists believe the low-fat era created an obesity epidemic. The lack of flavor in low-fat foods may have resulted in eating more food and increased caloric intake. This simplistic message to minimize fat intake has some problems. Some types of fat have healthy physiological effects. A certain amount of fat helps individuals feel satisfied longer because fat digestion is slower than carbohydrate or protein. Healthy fats need to be included in a regimen to improve the taste of food and to help increase satiety in addition to their physiological benefits.

Popular diets vary in their nutritional adequacy and consistency with guidelines for risk reduction. Renewed popularity of the low-carbohydrate, high-protein diet resulted in numerous controlled studies to determine effects of various types of diets. The results of several of these studies indicating that low-carbohydrate, high-protein diets are more effective in promoting weight loss and reducing blood lipid levels perplexed the scientific community. However, the long-term effects of this type of diet on health and weight control are unknown. More long-term studies indicate weight is regained when the individual stops following the diet. Some high-fat regimens seem to be unhealthy because of the emphasis on high animal fats and minimal carbohydrates, which include whole-grain products, fruits, and many healthy vegetables. A dietary regimen that stresses meat and high-fat foods but eliminates sugar and most carbohydrates is more successful at

helping people lose weight because high-protein foods provide greater satiety.

Evidence is emerging that higher protein diets, even without weight loss, may be beneficial for health.[34] Proteins seem to suppress **ghrelin** (an appetite-stimulating hormone) better than carbohydrates and lipids.[35] Diets that are considered high fat may cause undesirable cholesterol levels to increase, but weight loss itself usually improves blood lipid levels regardless of the dietary regimen.[36] Another negative side effect of high-protein diets is dehydration. Information about various popular diets is available from the American Dietetic Association at http://www.eatright.org/Public/NutritionInformation/92_11722.cfm or from Consumer Guide at http://www.cg-diet-reviews.com/

Different diets work for different people. A reduction diet should include foods from all food groups to provide necessary nutrients. A diet that totally eliminates one category (fat or carbohydrate) or a specific group of foods (fruits or meats) is inadvisable. Indispensable to any weight loss program is a preplanned food allotment with specified times for eating throughout the day to lessen feelings of deprivation and to eliminate excessive food intake. The total amount of food should be divided into at least three feedings. Eating only once or twice a day has been associated with consuming more kilocalories,[33] impulsive snacking, and increased adipose tissue and serum cholesterol. Some "free" foods or beverages (foods containing less than 20 kcal per serving) may be available for snack periods, but regular mealtimes are important. A diet that requires the least amount of change in usual dietary patterns has better long-term success. A 1200- to 1500-kcal diet is relatively safe; when accompanied by an exercise program, the rate of weight loss is augmented, and muscle mass is maintained.

A weight reduction diet should satisfy the following criteria: (1) meets all nutrient needs except energy, (2) suits tastes and habits, (3) minimizes hunger and fatigue, (4) is accessible and socially acceptable, (5) encourages a change in eating pattern, and (6) favors improvement in overall health. Box 1-5 provides some questions to help determine the validity of a weight reduction diet. Individuals have indicated several reasons for discontinuing a weight loss regimen: (1) trouble controlling food choices, (2) difficulty motivating oneself to eat appropriately, and (3) using food as a reward.[37]

Treatment of obesity is improved when increased energy expenditure occurs along with decreased caloric intake. Exercise alone has a modest effect on weight loss; it positively affects energy metabolism. The initiation of an exercise regimen may lead to weight gain in the form of muscle mass, but the health benefits are significant, including improved cardiovascular fitness, improved plasma lipoprotein profile, improved carbohydrate metabolism, increased energy expenditure, and enhanced psychological well-being.

Behavior modification for weight control refers to getting in touch with the reality of which foods are being consumed and in what quantity, and when and why eating occurs. One of the most important components of an effective weight control program is learning new ways of

HEALTH APPLICATION   Obesity—cont'd

dealing with old habits. Comprehensive behavior-modification programs include diet and exercise programs individually tailored for patients. A team approach including a healthcare provider, a psychologist, a registered dietitian, and the family is more effective in helping the patient make necessary long-lasting changes in food choices and lifestyle behaviors. A food diary for recording amounts and types of food eaten, emotional status, and environmental factors helps to provide new insights to devise strategies for dealing with eating habits.

Although behavior-modification approaches to weight control are helpful, maintaining weight loss remains a major problem. Studies indicate that programs need to be approximately 20 to 24 weeks long and more comprehensive, including relapse prevention training and use of social support systems.

CASE APPLICATION FOR THE DENTAL HYGIENIST

A young healthy mother who has a 3-year-old son at home comes to the dental office for a 6-month recall appointment. She expresses concern about foods she should be eating and feeding her husband and son to improve and maintain their overall health for optimal growth and development of the child. She has learned a little about the food groups, the *Dietary Guidelines for Americans,* and nutrition labels from the press, but does not know how to implement them.

Nutritional Assessment
- Willingness to seek nutritional information
- Desire for increased control of nutritional health habits
- Knowledge of community resources
- Cultural or religious influences
- Knowledge regarding the *Dietary Guidelines for Americans,* food labels, and MyPyramid
- Definition of optimal nutrition

Nutritional Diagnosis
Health-seeking behaviors related to lack of knowledge concerning optimal nutrition and current standards.

Nutritional Goals
The patient verbalizes correct information concerning the Dietary Guidelines and food labels, and can name the food groups, the number of servings needed, and portion sizes from each group of MyPyramid.

Nutritional Implementation
Intervention: Ask the patient to write down everything she ate yesterday from the time she got up yesterday until this morning when she got up.

Rationale: This will help you tailor the information you provide to the patient's needs.

Intervention: Encourage variety of food intake, using MyPyramid. Review the number of servings needed and serving size.

Rationale: The total balance of food intake matters, and the best balance incorporates variety to promote optimal nutrition. Providing the minimal number of servings prevents nutritional deficiencies in healthy individuals.

Intervention: (1) Suggest that the mother and her husband have their blood lipid profiles checked if not recently done; (2) emphasize a decreased intake of fats, saturated and *trans* fats, and cholesterol by trimming excess fat and eating smaller servings of meat (about the size of a fist or a deck of cards).

Rationale: Decreasing fats, saturated and *trans* fats, and cholesterol helps reduce the risk of heart disease.

Intervention: (1) Stress the importance of eating vegetables, fruits, and grains, and (2) explain that complex carbohydrates are not fattening.

Rationale: Dietary fiber is important for healthy bowel functioning and can reduce symptoms of chronic constipation, diverticular disease, and hemorrhoids, and decrease the risk of developing obesity, cancer, and diabetes.

Intervention: (1) Explain how to read labels for sugar. The name of most sugars end in "-ose." (2) Emphasize moderation of sugar intake. (3) Explain that "dietetic" and "sugar-free" do not mean that the product is low in kilocalories. (4) Explain the relationship between sugar and tooth decay, and emphasize the importance of proper oral hygiene after sugar consumption.

Rationale: Refined sugar contains kilocalories and no other nutrients, but is acceptable when used in items that contain appreciable amounts of other nutrients (e.g., a pudding would provide more nutrients than a gelatin dessert or carbonated beverages).

Intervention: (1) Stress using sodium and salt in moderation; (2) emphasize that "no salt added" does not mean that the product is low in sodium.

Rationale: Good habits that do not foster a high level of salt preference are recommended.

Intervention: Emphasize that any alcohol intake should be in moderation (one drink a day for women and two drinks a day for men), if at all.

Rationale: Alcohol is high in kilocalories and contains few, if any, nutrients.

Intervention: (1) Review an entire label with the mother to help her understand how to interpret it. (2) Determine a serving size. (3) Explain the types of carbohydrates. (4) Determine the percentage of fat in a product by multiplying the grams of fat by 9, and compare this number with the total kilocalories; if the amount is more than 30%, do not consume that product every day. (5) Look at cholesterol levels. (6) Emphasize that "no cholesterol" does not indicate that the product contains no saturated or *trans* fat. (7) Point out the sodium level, and if it is greater than 400 mg, encourage its use in moderation.

Rationale: Knowledge increases compliance and allows informed choices regarding food choice.

Intervention: Refer the patient to county extension agencies or to a registered dietitian.

Rationale: These agencies and nutritional professionals provide practical guidelines via newsletters, workshops, and written materials for healthy patients wanting to improve health.

CASE APPLICATION FOR THE DENTAL HYGIENIST—cont'd

Evaluation

To determine effectiveness of care, the patient reads labels and chooses the best buy for the nutrient content. The patient states the basic guidelines for nutrition; the hygienist explains to her that serving sizes for her son are different than the standard serving size indicated on MyPyramid. Additionally, the patient should be able to plan a menu using recommended foods, and to state how to obtain and use community information/support. The patient should be able to indicate how changes in food choices would not only improve overall health, but also maintain health of the oral cavity and ensure optimal growth of her son with minimal or no problems in the oral cavity.

Box 1-5   Evaluating Weight Loss Diets or Programs

The program should evaluate the individual's BMI, and whether the weight is principally from increased fat stores or increased muscle mass and possible contributing factors.

The cost of the program should be realistic and reasonable.

The program should be adaptable for various lifestyles and something an individual can continue indefinitely.

Tips for Evaluating Safety and Effectiveness of Reduction Diets

1. Stay current with scientific research. Nutrition is a relatively new science, and new developments are still evolving to increase our knowledge base.
2. Evaluate diet trends and claims for effects on overall health.
3. Compare recommendations with known nutrition science and recommendations such as MyPyramid and *Dietary Guidelines for Americans*.
4. Calculate nutritional requirements of the individual considering the diet, and determine what nutrients would be lacking.
5. Evaluate diets using the following principles:
   • What is the weight loss recommendation?
   • What is the success rate of the program?
   • What is the basis for advertisements and endorsements?

• Has any scientific research been done to evaluate the safety and effectiveness of the diet?
• What is the cost of the program? Are special foods or nutrient supplements required, and what do they cost? Are there other additional fees?
• Is the program medically supervised?
• Are any major food groups excluded?
• Are the foods appealing to the individual? Does the program allow occasional consumption of favorite foods?
• Is it permissible to eat in restaurants and other people's homes at least occasionally?
• Are certain foods avoided because they cause specific problems?
• Are certain foods used to "cure"?
• Are dramatic statements made that contradict well-established nutrition principles or reputable scientific organizations?
• Are exercise and behavior modification included?
• Can an individual live on the program for a lifetime?
• Is there a maintenance plan?
• Does it promote good food habits?

STUDENT READINESS

1. A patient asks you the difference between food and nutrition. What would you say?
2. Locate an advertisement in a popular magazine or newspaper for a weight reduction product or program, and list the merits of the product or program stated in the ad. Then list information about the product or program that might have been omitted or should be questioned. Evaluate the product or program using information from Box 1-5.
3. Discuss popular weight reduction diets (Appendix E) and how they may have adverse effects.
4. Distinguish between nutrient recommendations and requirements.
5. Keep a record of all the foods you eat for 24 hours. Was your intake adequate as evaluated by MyPyramid? In what areas did you do well? Where can you improve? Provide specific recommendations for making changes.
6. Collect nutrition labels for three similar products. Compare the nutrient values to determine which is a better source of nutrients. Which is a better buy for the amount of nutrients it contains?
7. List the *Dietary Guidelines for Americans*. In which areas do you do well? In which areas would you like to improve your choices? Do you believe you have enough information to make knowledgeable changes?
8. Discuss the pros and cons of allowing nutritional claims on products.
9. If a food label indicates that one serving of the product has 23 g of carbohydrate and 15 g of sugar with 140 kcal (total), how many teaspoons of sugar does the product contain? What percentage of carbohydrate does this product contain?

For relevant website, see the Evolve site.

References

1. U.S. Department of Health and Human Services: Healthy People 2010: understanding and improving health. Washington, DC: U.S. Government Printing Office, 2000. Available at http://www.health.gov/healthypeople/.
2. Department of Health & Human Services. Progress toward Healthy People 2010 targets. Available at http://www.healthypeople.gov/Data/midcourse/html/focusareas. Accessed January 25, 2008.
3. Moshfegh A, Goldman J, Cleveland L: What we eat in America, NHANES 2001-2002: Usual nutrient intakes from

food compared to dietary reference intakes. USDA, Agricultural Research Service. Available at www.ars.usda.gov/foodsurvey. Accessed January 20, 2008.

4. Casagrande SS, et al: Have Americans increased their fruit and vegetable intake? The trends between 1988 and 2002. Am J Prev Med 2007 Apr; 32(4):257-263.

5. Tarvainen L, et al: Cancer of the mouth and pharynx, occupation and exposure to chemical agents in Finland 1971-95. Int J Cancer 2008; 123(3):653-659.

6. Grace K: Three out of four Americans have access to the internet, according to Nielsen//Netratings. Available at http://www.nielsen-netratings.com/pr/pr_040318.pdf. Accessed January 12, 2008.

7. Food industry groups team with USDA on MyPyramid. Progressive Grocer (serial online). Available at www.progressivegrocer.com/progressivegrocer/content_display/features/health-wellness/e3i95a8c8893ac9738a83e4b791ebdb0886. Accessed July 5, 2008.

8. U.S. Food and Drug Administration: FDA provides guidance on "whole grain" for manufacturers. FDA News 2006 Feb 15. Available at www.fda.gov/bbs/topics/news/2006/NEW01317.html. Accessed August 25, 2008.

9. Special report. One year later: Lessons from New Guidelines and Pyramid. Tufts University Health & Nutrition Letter 2006 February; 24(12): 4-5.

10. Shimazaki Y, et al: Intake of dairy products and periodontal disease: the Hisayama study. J Periodontol 2008 Jan; 79(1):131-137.

11. Al-Zahrani MS: Increased intake of dairy products is related to lower periodontitis prevalence. J Periodontol 2006 Feb; 77(2):289-294.

12. Block G: Foods contributing to energy intake in the United States: data from NHANES III and NHANES 1999-2000. J Food Composit Anal 2004; 17(3-4):439-447.

13. Britten P, Haven J, Davis C: Consumer research for development of educational messages for MyPyramid Food Guidance System. J Nutr Educ Behav 2006; Nov-Dec:38(6 Suppl):S108-S123.

14. National Center for Health Statistics, CDC: Third Report on Nutrition Monitoring in the United States. Available at http://www.cdc.gov/nchs/products/pubs/pubd/other/miscpub/nutflyer.htm. Assessed January 13, 2008

15. Todd, JE, Variyam JN: The decline in consumer use of food nutrition labels, 1995-2006. ERR-63, USDA, Economic Research Service, August 2008.

16. Golan E, Kuchlet F, Krissoff B: Do food labels make a difference? Sometimes. Amber Waves (serial online). Available at http://www.ers.usda.gov/AmberWaves/scripts/print.asp?page=November07/Features/Food Labels.htm. Accessed January 12, 2008.

17. McNally A: Industry is taking healthy eating seriously, pool finds. Food USA Navigator.com. Available at http://www.foodnavigator-usa.com/news/ng.asp?id-82626. Accessed January 18, 2008.

18. Keeping up with the changing food label. Food Insight January/February 2006; 1-2:6.

19. U.S. Food and Drug Administration (FDA): Interim procedures for qualified health claims in the labeling of conventional human food and human dietary supplements. 2003 Jul 10. Available at www.cfsan.fda.gov/~dms/hclmgui3.html. Accessed August 26, 2008.

20. U.S. Food and Drug Administration (FDA): Qualified health claims: letter of enforcement discretion—nuts and coronary heart disease. 2003 Jul 14. Available at www.cfsan.fda.gov/~dms/qhcnuts2.html. Accessed August 26, 2008.

21. National Center for Health Statistics, CDC: Prevalence of overweight, obesity and extreme obesity among adults: United States, trends 1976-80 through 2005-2006. December 2008. Available at: http://www.cdc.gov/nchs/products/pubs/pubd/hestats/overweight/overweight_adult.htm. Accessed on January 16, 2009.

22. CDC: State-specific prevalence of obesity among adults—United States, 2007. MMWR Morb Mortal Wkly Rep 2008 Jul 18; 57(28):765-768. Available at www.cdc.gov/mmwr/preview/mmwrhtml/mm5728a1.htm. Accessed July 20, 2008.

23. Sturm R: Increases in morbid obesity in the USA: 2000-2005. Public Health 2007 Jul; 121(7):492-496.

24. Wang Y, et al: Will all Americans become overweight or obese? Estimating the progression and cost of the US obesity epidemic. Obesity (Silver Spring) 2008 Jul 24 [Epub ahead of print].

25. Centers for Disease Control and Prevention: Overweight and obesity, health consequences. Available at http://www.cdc.gov/nccdphp/dnpa/obesity/consequences.htm. Accessed January 21, 2008.

26. American Institute for Cancer Research and the World Cancer Research Fund: Food, nutrition, physical activity and the prevention of cancer: A global perspective, 2007. Available at www.dietandcancerreport.org. Accessed January 25, 2008.

27. Herper M: Obesity's huge hidden costs. Forbes. 2006 Jul 20. Available at www.forbes.com/2006/07/19/obesity-fat-costs_cx_mh_0720obesity.html. Accessed July 25, 2006.

28. Zhang C, et al: Abdominal obesity and the risk of all-cause, cardiovascular, and cancer mortality. Circulation 2008 Apr 1; 117(13):1658-1667.

29. Gut-check time: why belly fat poses extra risks. Tufts Univ Health & Nutrition Letter 2008 Jul; 26(5):6.

30. Mitka M: Obesity's role in heart disease requires apples and pears comparison. JAMA 2005 Aug 6; 294(24):3071-3072.

31. Moshfegh A, Goldman J, Cleveland L: What we eat in America. USDA, Agricultural Research Service. Available at www.ars.usda.gov/ba/bhnrc/fsrg. Accessed January 26, 2008.

32. Wardle J, et al: Evidence for a strong genetic influence on childhood adiposity despite the force of the obesogenic environment. Am J Clin Nutr 2008 Feb; 87(2):398-404.

33. Mancino L, Kinsey J: Is dietary knowledge enough? Hunger, stress, and other roadblocks to healthy eating. ERS Report Summary. ERS/USDA ERR-62. August 2008. Available at www.ers.usda.gov/publications/err62. Accessed August 26, 2008.

34. Souza RJ, et al: Alternatives for macronutrient intake and chronic disease: A comparison of the OmniHeart diets with popular diets and with dietary recommendations. Am J Clin Nutr 2008 Jul; 88(7):1-11.

35. Foster-Schubert K, et al: Acyl and total ghrelin are suppressed strongly by ingested proteins, weakly by lipids and biphasically by carbohydrates. J Clin Endocrinol Metab 2008 May; 93(5):1971-1979.

36. Miller M: High-fat Atkins diet damages blood vessels: study. Presented at the American Heart Association in Orlando, Florida, November 2007.

37. Burke LE, et al: A descriptive study of past experiences with weight-loss treatment. J Am Diet Assoc 2008 Apr; 108(4):640-647.

Chapter 2

The Alimentary Canal: Digestion and Absorption

LEARNING OBJECTIVES

Upon completion of this chapter, the student will be able to achieve the following objectives:
- Discuss factors that influence food intake.
- Describe general functions of each digestive organ.
- Identify chemical secretions necessary for digestion of energy-containing nutrients and in what parts of the gastrointestinal tract they are secreted.
- Name the nutrients that require digestion and the digested products that can be absorbed.
- Explain the role of gastrointestinal motility in the digestion and absorption process.
- Use the information from the points in Nutritional Directions for a dental patient.
- Describe how the digestion and absorption processes may affect nutritional status and oral health.

KEY TERMS

Accessory organs
Alimentary canal
Alveolar process
Anorexia
Anosmia
Bile
Bolus
Cancellous bone

Cortical bone
Demineralization
Dysgeusia
Emulsification
Enteric
Enzymes
Gustatory
Hydrolysis

Hypergeusia	Prebiotics
Hypogeusia	Probiotics
Iatrogenic	Proteolytic enzymes
Large intestine	Remineralization
Lower esophageal sphincter (LES)	Residue
Masticatory efficiency	Small intestine
Microflora	Sphincter muscles
Microvilli	Systemic condition
Olfactory nerves	Synbiotics
Osmosis	Taste buds
Pancreatic enzymes	Trabecular bone
Pathogenic	Valves
Peristalsis	Xerostomia
Phantom taste	

Test Your NQ

1. **T/F** The alimentary tract is about 30 feet long.
2. **T/F** The hydrolysis of carbohydrate yields fatty acid and glycerol.
3. **T/F** Most absorption occurs in the stomach.
4. **T/F** Fat-soluble nutrients always enter the portal circulation.
5. **T/F** Taste disorders are often the result of problems in smell rather than taste.
6. **T/F** Lactose is the name of an enzyme.
7. **T/F** The digestive process begins in the oral cavity.
8. **T/F** Villi are located in the large intestine.
9. **T/F** Missing, decayed, or poorly restored teeth can affect food intake.
10. **T/F** Saliva aids in the oral clearance of food.

Foods are composed of large chemical molecules that cannot be used unless they are broken down to an absorbable form. The digestive system is designed to (1) ingest foods; (2) digest or break down complex molecules into simple, soluble materials that can be absorbed; and (3) eliminate unused residues. Only the energy-providing macronutrients (carbohydrate, protein, and fat) must be digested for absorption. Most vitamins, minerals, alcohol, and water can be absorbed as eaten.

The gastrointestinal tract can also be used to deliver complex chemical substances, such as oral medications. Medications frequently affect or can be affected by foods, modifying absorption, metabolism, or excretion of either the food or the drug. They also may affect nutritional status as a result of changes in taste or salivary flow; both of these conditions influence the amount and types of foods consumed. Dental hygienists need to become familiar with normal gastrointestinal processes because disturbances in the gastrointestinal tract may affect the nutritional status of patients and their oral health.

PHYSIOLOGY OF THE GASTROINTESTINAL TRACT

The digestive system includes the alimentary canal and several accessory organs (Fig. 2-1). The **alimentary canal** comprises all the body parts through which food passes,

extending from the mouth to the anus. The alimentary canal is a tubular structure about 30 feet long (five times the height of an average man). It includes the oral cavity, pharynx, esophagus, stomach, small intestine, and large intestine. The **small intestine** includes the duodenum, jejunum, and ileum; the **large intestine** includes the cecum, colon, and rectum. **Accessory organs**—the salivary glands, liver, gallbladder, and pancreas—provide secretions essential for the digestive process. Digestion involves two basic types of action on food: (1) mechanical activities and (2) chemical activities. Mechanical actions include chewing and peristalsis, which break up and mix foods, permitting better blending with the chemicals. Chemical actions involve salivary enzymes and digestive juices that reduce foodstuffs to absorbable molecules.

CHEMICAL ACTION

A large molecule can be split into smaller ones that are water-soluble and can be used by cells; this process is called **hydrolysis**. The hydrolysis of energy nutrients requires water. The following are basic hydrolysis reactions in food digestion:

$$Protein + H_2O \rightarrow amino\ acids$$

$$Fat + H_2O \rightarrow fatty\ acids + glycerol$$

$$Carbohydrate + H_2O \rightarrow monosaccharides$$

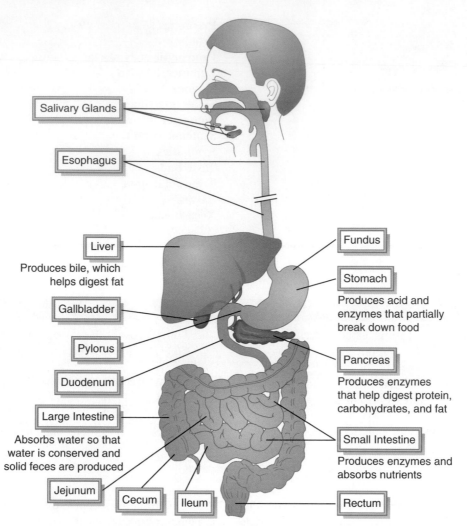

FIGURE 2-1 The digestive process. (From Peckenpaugh NJ: Nutrition Essentials and Diet Therapy, 10th ed. Philadelphia: Saunders, 2007.)

These reactions depend on enzymes. **Enzymes** are complex proteins that enable metabolic reactions to proceed at a faster rate without being exhausted themselves. In protein hydrolysis, the substrate for the enzyme is protein, and amino acids are the basic end product. The enzyme forms a temporary chemical compound with the substrate. When the reaction is completed, the complex separates, releasing new chemical compounds and the enzyme.

Because the enzyme is reused, only small amounts are needed. Enzymes function similar to keys: they are very specific and function on only one substrate, similar to a key fitting a particular lock (Fig. 2-2). The name for some enzymes is derived from the name of the substrate, with the suffix *-ase* (e.g., lactase is the enzyme produced to catalyze the breakdown of lactose).

MECHANICAL ACTION

The wall of the gastrointestinal tract is similar from the esophagus to the rectum (Fig. 2-3). A layer of muscles encircles the tube, allowing the diameter of the tube to expand and contract. Food particles are broken up and mixed by the churning action. The outer fibers of the muscular coat (longitudinal muscle) run lengthwise and are responsible for **peristalsis,** the involuntary rhythmic waves of contraction traveling the whole length of the alimentary tract.

Doorlike mechanisms between the digestive segments, called **valves** or **sphincter muscles,** are designed to (1) retain food in each segment until the work of the mechanical actions and digestive juices has been completed, (2) allow measured amounts of food to pass into the next segment, and (3) prevent food from "backing up" into the preceding area. The regulation of these valves is complex, involving muscular function and different pressures on each side of the valve.

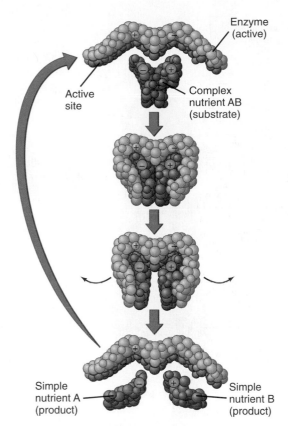

FIGURE 2-2 Model of enzyme action. Enzymes are proteins that allow the substrate to fit into the active sites of the enzyme; notice how the active site of the enzyme chemically fits the substrate in a lock-and-key type of biochemical interaction, and how the enzyme molecule alters its shape to perform its function. The substrate (in this case, molecule *AB*) is broken into simpler smaller molecules (*A* and *B*). After the reaction, the products separate, and the unchanged enzyme is available to catalyze production of additional products. (Adapted from Thibodeau GA, Patton KT: Anatomy and Physiology, 6th ed. St Louis: Mosby, 2007.)

Dental Hygiene Considerations

- Gurgling sounds, caused by air and fluid in the normal abdomen, indicate peristalsis is occurring.
- If the alimentary tract is not functioning properly, adequate amounts of nutrients may not be provided to the body as a result of alterations in digestion and absorption. The patient may be prone to nutrient deficiencies, poor healing, or fecal impactions.
- Loss of motility in the stomach and small intestine results in impaired gastric and intestinal emptying. This allows excessive growth of bacteria, which may injure the surface of the intestine, cause diarrhea, and interfere with nutrient absorption. Patients who are immobile (because of injury, trauma, or debilitating illness) or patients with uncontrolled diabetes are more prone to these disorders.
- Food-drug interactions have the potential to cause nutritional problems or erratic drug responses. Knowledge of the drugs taken, including over-the-counter medications, herbals, and supplements, and how they interact with food is important. For example, consuming milk or milk products while taking tetracycline decreases the amount of tetracycline and calcium available to the body.

Nutritional Directions

Taking over-the-counter enzyme tablets may not be beneficial because the enzymes are digested before they can be used. Prescription pancreatic enzymes have a special **enteric** coating preventing the enzyme from exposure to gastric juices. Lactase, a nonprescription enzyme, is effective for lactose-intolerant individuals because it is either added to or taken with lactose-containing foods, allowing the conversion of lactose into glucose and galactose before the gastric juices can affect the enzyme (see Health Application 2). Patients reporting gastrointestinal problems should be assessed for adequate nutrient intake using national nutrition guidelines. If intake is inadequate, the patient should be referred to his or her primary care provider or a registered dietitian.

ORAL CAVITY

TASTE AND SMELL

Generally, food choices are influenced by the three sensory perceptions: sight, smell, and taste. **Gustatory** (taste) sensations evoke pronounced feelings of pleasure or aversion; in the United States, taste is the primary determinant of food choices. The presentation of food, its color and aroma, may be the basis for acceptance or rejection. Food flavors are prompted from characteristics of substances ingested, including taste, aroma, texture, temperature, and irritating properties. Approximately 75% of flavor is derived from odors.

The mouth, or oral cavity, plays an important role in the digestive system. It is the "port of entry" where receptors for the sense of taste, or **taste buds**, are located. A taste bud consists of 30 to 100 cells embedded in the surrounding epithelium, termed *papillae*. Taste papillae appear on the tongue as little red dots, or raised bumps, and are most numerous on the dorsal epithelium. These cells replace themselves every 3 to 10 days; disease, drugs, nutritional status, radiation, and age can affect them. As food is chewed, gustatory receptors come into contact with chemicals dissolved in the saliva.

Nerve cells carry messages to the brain, which interprets the flavor as sweet, sour, salty, or bitter. These four basic tastes reflect specific constituents of food. Taste buds for all four sensations are located throughout the mouth, but specific kinds of buds are concentrated in certain (but overlapping) areas. Taste buds also are found on the soft palate, epiglottis, larynx, and posterior wall of the pharynx (Fig. 2-4). Taste and smell are essential for maintaining intake to meet physiological needs.

Food stimulates taste buds, and aromas stimulate **olfactory nerves**, the receptors for smell. In contrast to gustatory sensations, an almost unlimited number of unique odors can be detected. No tactile sensation indicates the origin of odor sensations. Food-related aromas may be confused with taste sensations, and taste disorders are often the result of problems in smell rather than taste. The prevalence of olfactory

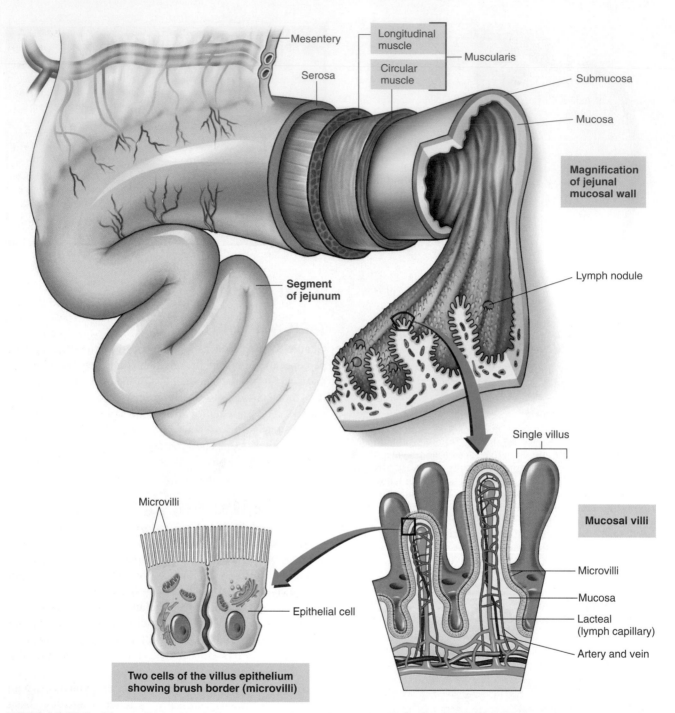

FIGURE 2-3 Wall of the small intestine. **A,** Layers composing the intestinal wall. **B,** The villi covering the mucosa that absorb nutrients. **C,** Further enlargement shows the brush border or microvilli enzymes that are available to hydrolyze nutrients further for absorption. (From Williams P [ed]: Gray's Anatomy: The Anatomical Basis of Medicine and Surgery, 38th ed. London: Churchill Livingstone, 1999.)

impairment is high in older adults, and the problem increases with age. This is most likely the reason an elderly patient will state that food "just doesn't taste good."

Loss of smell, or **anosmia**, results in limited capacity to detect the flavor of food and beverages. Ability to smell food being prepared and eaten influences food selection. Foods are sometimes judged to be harmful or spoiled because of their odors, so the sense of smell is also a protective mecha-

nism. Upper respiratory infections, nasal or sinus problems, neurological disorders, endocrine abnormalities, aging, or head trauma may cause anosmia. Individuals with a cold usually lose their appetite because of a decreased sense of smell, which affects the ability to "taste" and enjoy food. The rate of the continuous renewal process undergone by olfactory receptor cells is depressed in malnutrition and by some antibiotics. Some of these disorders are self-limited;

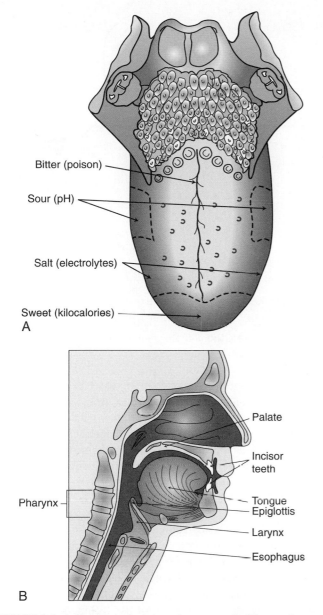

Bitter (poison)

Sour (pH)

Salt (electrolytes)

Sweet (kilocalories)

A

Palate

Incisor teeth

Pharynx

Tongue
Epiglottis

Larynx

Esophagus

B

FIGURE 2-4 **A,** Regions of taste on the tongue. **B,** The oropharyngeal cavity showing the regions that contain taste buds, which include the epiglottis, soft palate, laryngeal pharynx, and oral pharynx.

however, chemosensory losses from chemotherapy, infection, and aging may be irreversible.[1]

Dysgeusia is the persistent, abnormal distortion of taste, including sweet, sour, bitter, salty, or metallic tastes. Dysgeusia without identifiable taste stimuli is called **phantom taste**. Dysgeusia may be caused by a previous viral upper respiratory infection, head trauma, a neurological or psychiatric disorder, a **systemic condition** (a disease or disorder that affects the whole body), **xerostomia** (dry mouth from inadequate salivary secretion), severe nutritional deficiencies, invasive dental procedures resulting in nerve damage, oral bacterial and fungal infections, and burning mouth syndrome,[2] or it may have an iatrogenic causation. **Iatrogenic** refers to an adverse condition resulting from medical treat-

ment (medications, irradiation, surgery). These conditions may also cause **hypogeusia,** or loss of taste, and **hypergeusia,** or heightened taste acuity. Dysgeusia may also result from breathing through the mouth. The dental hygienist is frequently the first healthcare provider to detect a patient's taste disorder. Hyperkeratinization of the epithelium may be observed during an oral examination causing blockage of taste buds, which may affect dietary intake.

Gustatory and olfactory disorders, whether caused by disease states or drugs, are not mere inconveniences or neurotic symptoms. They affect food choices and dietary habits. A poor appetite, also called **anorexia**, may occur when medications cause loss of taste acuity. Taste stimulants affect salivary and pancreatic secretions, gastric contractions, and intestinal motility; gustatory disorders also can affect digestion.

Because gustatory and olfactory disorders can result in deterioration of a patient's general condition or nutritional status, these abnormalities must always be considered in dental and nutritional care. Potentially adverse compensatory habits may develop (e.g., decreased sweetness or saltiness perceptions may result in excessive usage of sweets or salts, which may be potentially harmful, especially for patients with diabetes or hypertension). Also, the addition of sugar can lead to higher incidence of caries. Persistent taste distortions can lead to inadequate caloric intake, resulting in unintentional weight loss or malnutrition.

SALIVA

Adequate saliva flow is essential for oral health and maintenance of soft tissues in the oral cavity, including the taste buds. Saliva, secreted by the salivary glands, is essential in taste sensations, functioning to (1) lubricate oral tissues to assist in chewing, swallowing, and digestion; (2) remove debris from teeth; (3) provide antibacterial action; (4) neutralize, dilute, and buffer bacterial acids; (5) aid in **remineralization** (the restoration or return of calcium, phosphates, and other minerals into areas that have been damaged, as by incipient caries, abrasion, or erosion); (6) affect the rate of plaque accumulation; (7) influence taste; and (8) allow for ease in talking. This complex fluid helps maintain the integrity of the teeth against physical, chemical, and microbial insults. Saliva is supersaturated with calcium phosphates that allow demineralized areas of the hydroxyapatite in enamel to be remineralized. **Demineralization** occurs as a result of the removal or loss of calcium, phosphate, and other minerals from tooth enamel, causing tooth enamel to dissolve.

Acidic, sour, or bitter tastes stimulate saliva flow. Saliva production is also increased with consumption of tasty foods and gum chewing. An increase in oral clearance rate decreases risk of caries formation (for more information, see Chapter 17). Saliva blended with food particles moistens foods so that they are more easily manipulated and prepared for swallowing.

Some chemical action or hydrolysis of nutrients begins in the mouth. The functions of the different constituents in

Table 2-1	Digestive Functions of Saliva	
Saliva Component	**Classification**	**Function**
Mucin	Glycoprotein	Lubricates food for easier passage and protects lining of the gastrointestinal tract
Ptyalin (amylase)	Enzyme	Initiates hydrolysis of complex carbohydrates to simple sugars
Lysozyme (antibody)	Enzyme	Breaks down cell walls of some ingested bacteria

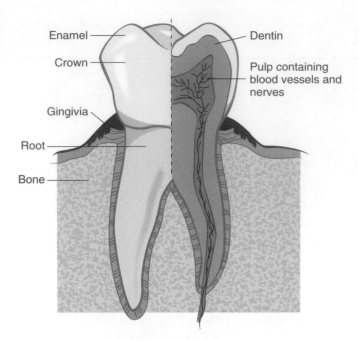

FIGURE 2-5 Diagram of a tooth.

saliva are shown in Table 2-1. Because food is normally in the mouth briefly, ptyalin, or salivary amylase, initiates starch digestion. If a carbohydrate food, such as a cracker, is chewed and held in the mouth for a few seconds, it will begin to taste sweet, denoting the fact that some starch is being hydrolyzed to dextrin and maltose.

Dry mouth from inadequate salivary secretion, also called xerostomia, leads to diminished gustatory function (see Chapter 19 for additional details). Xerostomia may result in frequent oral ulcerations, increased sensitivity of the tongue to spices and flavors, and increased risk of dental caries. Many drugs, including diuretics, cause xerostomia. Diuretics, prescribed to help the body eliminate fluids, also cause a decrease in salivary flow. Increasing fluid intake to 8 to 10 cups daily is important to compensate for these losses.

TEETH

Another important role of the mouth in food digestion is the mechanical action of teeth. In contrast to bone, neither the tooth enamel nor dentin can be repaired or replaced by any natural process other than simple remineralization of small areas and deposition of secondary dentin around the pulp chamber (Fig. 2-5). Mineral deposition and resorption influence the supporting bone structure. Alveolar bone is primarily **trabecular bone** (bony spikes forming a meshwork of spaces in cancellous bone) and **cancellous bone** (internal bone that appears spongy with little hollows that contain bone marrow). When negative calcium balance occurs, the **alveolar process** (crest of the maxilla and mandible serving as the bony investment for the teeth) is more susceptible to resorption than other **cortical bones** (compact external part of the skeleton that surrounds the bone marrow).[3] The maxilla and mandible to some extent depend on the presence of teeth and occlusal forces associated with chewing to prevent calcium resorption. Chewing firm foods helps maintain proper balance between alveolar bone resorption and new bone formation. Teeth and supporting bone structures are affected by intake of adequate nutrients, adequate digestive function, and hormonal balance.

Chewing reduces food particle size. Inability to masticate food adequately may result in larger chunks of food being swallowed. Larger pieces of food increase the potential for food obstruction in the airway. Food asphyxiation, which may result in sudden death, occurs in many individuals with defective, incomplete, or poorly fitting dentures. The loss of even one permanent molar may decrease **masticatory efficiency**, or how well the patient prepares the food for swallowing. Even after patients become fully adjusted to well-fitted dentures, masticatory efficiency is reduced compared with patients with their natural teeth.

Digestion of food is facilitated by increasing its surface area. Whether or not particle size affects its digestibility is uncertain. However, when elderly patients have digestive problems, masticatory efficiency is usually a factor. Frequently, when masticatory efficiency declines, people choose foods that require less chewing or use techniques to soften foods, such as stewing meats, steaming vegetables, or dunking cookies or toast in fluids. In many circumstances, hypersensitive, poorly restored, decayed, abscessed, or periodontally involved teeth affect food choices and limit the variety of foods consumed.

ESOPHAGUS

The swallowing reflex moves a **bolus**, or the mass of food that is swallowed, into the esophagus, where it is transported to the stomach by peristalsis and gravity. The esophagus is a continuous tube about 10 inches long and connects the mouth with the stomach. It penetrates the diaphragm through an opening called the *esophageal hiatus*. The **lower esophageal sphincter (LES)** comprises a group of very strong circular muscle fibers located just above the stomach. The LES relaxes to permit food into the stomach, but contracts tightly to prevent the regurgitation or "backwashing" of the stomach contents.

Dental Hygiene Considerations

- Assess the nutritional status of patients with gustatory or olfactory disorders for changes in dietary habits and appetite that may lead to a dietary deficiency, increased use of spices (especially salt and sugar), food textures, and development of food cravings or dislikes.[4]
- Patients commonly complain about the "taste" or "flavor" of food when olfactory as well as gustatory sensations are impaired.
- Assess patients for possible dietary deficiencies (niacin, vitamins B_{12} and A, zinc, copper, nickel) because these can be a factor in gustatory abnormalities.
- Xerostomia may compound nutritional intake problems related to taste loss. Patients may experience difficulty chewing and swallowing food.
- Patients who have difficulty chewing are likely to develop decreased taste acuity; monitor food intake.
- Edentulous patients or patients with ill-fitting dentures should be monitored because quality and quantity of food intake may be compromised.
- Subjective alterations in taste perception in denture wearers theoretically could be due to altered masticatory efficiency or shielding of palatal taste buds by the prosthesis. Patients with complete dentures exhibit poorer taste and texture tolerance compared with patients with partial dentures or with compromised natural dentition.
- Carefully assess a patient's mandibular bone density, which can result in early diagnosis or detection of osteoporosis. Postmenopausal women with low dental bone mass may have decreased levels of total bone mass.
- Chewing sugar-free gum containing xylitol has many potential benefits, including preventing tooth decay, reducing plaque, and freshening breath. It aids appetite control when used as a substitute for high-calorie snacks. Chewing sugar-free gum containing xylitol improves alertness and concentration, and helps relieve stress.
- Although food intake often decreases when patients receive a set of dentures, after an initial adjustment period, food intake usually increases with improved ability to chew.
- Carefully evaluate anecdotal reports or studies involving limited numbers of patients supporting a beneficial effect of vitamins or minerals on dysgeusia.
- Refer patients with persistent gustatory, masticatory, or swallowing difficulties to a healthcare provider or registered dietitian to determine types of foods needed to obtain adequate nutrients.

Nutritional Directions

- Natural teeth are more efficient for chewing and biting than any prosthesis.
- Tooth losses are not inevitable; most people can maintain their natural dentition throughout life if preventive dental measures are practiced routinely.
- If salivary flow is diminished, increase fluid intake with meals to assist in oral clearance. Nutrient-dense foods in a liquid or semiliquid form are beneficial.
- No proven intervention either enhances taste acuity or ameliorates dysgeusia. Encourage experimentation with texture, spiciness, temperature, and enhanced visual presentation of food in a calm, relaxing environment.
- To improve nutrient intake when mastication is less efficient, special cooking techniques (e.g., stewing meats), chewing longer, and choosing soft foods are preferable to pureeing foods. For example, cream-style corn can replace corn on the cob, and applesauce can replace raw apples.
- Particularly for new denture wearers, herbs and spices and contrasting food taste combinations (e.g., sweet and sour) can be used to enhance taste perception.
- New denture wearers may slow the rate of alveolar resorption by taking calcium and vitamin D supplements. Refer the patient to a healthcare provider or registered dietitian for a nutritional assessment.

GASTRIC DIGESTION

A bolus entering the stomach is mixed with gastric secretions by peristaltic contractions, producing chyme, a semifluid paste. Gastric secretions include mucus, hydrochloric acid (HCl), enzymes, and a component called *intrinsic factor*.

The low pH of the stomach contents (about 1.5 to 3.0) is beneficial for several reasons: (1) it kills or inhibits the growth of most food bacteria, (2) it denatures proteins and makes them more easily hydrolyzed to amino acids, (3) it activates gastric enzymes, (4) it hydrolyzes some of the carbohydrates, and (5) it increases solubility and absorption of calcium and iron.

Two major enzymes are found in gastric juice: pepsin and lipase. Pepsin is capable of hydrolyzing large protein molecules to smaller fragments. Gastric lipase is involved in digestion of short- and medium-chain triglycerides (e.g., the triglycerides found in butterfat). Mucus forms an alkaline coating on the lining of the stomach for protection against digestion of the stomach by pepsin. Intrinsic factor secreted in the stomach is essential for absorption of vitamin B_{12} in the small intestine.

Normal gastric secretion is regulated by nerve and hormonal stimuli. Visual, olfactory, and gustatory senses stimulate gastric secretions. Fear, sadness, pain, and depression are generally accompanied by decreased secretions; anger, stress, and hostility may increase secretions.

The adult stomach functions as a reservoir to hold an average meal for 3 to 4 hours. The stomach empties at different rates depending on its size and the composition of the chyme. The rate of passage through the stomach (fastest to slowest) is liquids, carbohydrates, proteins, and fats. When a mixture of foods is presented, this pattern is not as well defined. The smaller the stomach capacity, the more rapidly the stomach empties. (This is exemplified in infants, who must be fed frequently until the stomach size expands.) Fats remain in the stomach longer, increasing satiety for a longer time than proteins or carbohydrates. Small amounts of chyme are released from the stomach through the pyloric sphincter to allow for adequate digestion and absorption in the small intestine.

Very little absorption occurs in the stomach because few foods are completely hydrolyzed to nutrients the body can use at this stage. Nutrients that can be absorbed from the stomach include some water, alcohol, and a few water-soluble substances (e.g., amino acids and glucose).

Dental Hygiene Considerations

- Dietary constituents that increase HCl and pepsin secretions are proteins, calcium, caffeine, coffee, and alcohol. These may need to be limited in patients with ulcers or certain gastrointestinal tract disorders.
- Because gravity facilitates movement of food down the esophagus, patients who are in a supine position may have some difficulty swallowing and may reflux gastric contents, especially after eating. Aspiration of acid reflux into the lungs is possible. To prevent an emergency situation, place the patient in a semisupine position for treatment. If possible, schedule the appointment 3 hours after a meal to minimize reflux.

Nutritional Directions

- Vomiting is one of the body's methods of eliminating toxins from contaminated foods. Vomiting also can be stimulated by rapid changes in body motion or by drugs.
- Heartburn is a result of regurgitation (reflux) of the stomach contents into the esophagus. Acidic gastric secretions produce discomfort or pain, which may be relieved if the patient remains in an upright position after eating.
- Eating in a calm, relaxing atmosphere helps reduce gastric secretions.
- Over an extended period, chronic problems with vomiting or reflux can result in sensitive teeth and superficial or deep tooth erosion, especially on lingual and occlusal surfaces.

SMALL INTESTINE

Within the small intestine, most of the energy-providing nutrients are completely hydrolyzed and absorbed. Most vitamins and minerals are also absorbed in the small intestine. The small intestine is specially designed to perform these tasks with juices secreted by the accessory organs and its complex luminal wall (Fig. 2-6). The small intestine is approximately 15 feet long, and foods are retained therein for 3 to 10 hours.

DIGESTION

Throughout the walls of the small intestine are villi, finger-like projections rising out of the mucosa into the intestinal lumen (see Fig. 2-3). These villi increase the surface area of the alimentary tract to about 3000 square feet. Each villus is also covered with a layer of epithelial cells containing microvilli, which collectively form the brush border cells. **Microvilli** are minute cylindrical processes located on the surface of the intestinal cells, greatly increasing their absorp-

tive surface area. The pH change and motility in the small intestine inhibit bacterial growth.

Acidic chyme entering the intestine stimulates hormones to release pancreatic juices into the duodenum. Cholecystokinin, a hormone released in response to the presence of fat in chyme, stimulates the gallbladder to contract and release bile. **Bile** is produced and secreted by the liver and is stored in the gallbladder. The action of bile salts allows insoluble molecules to be divided into smaller particles, a process called **emulsification**. This process allows greater exposure of the fats to intestinal and pancreatic lipases. Peristalsis also facilitates the mixing and emulsification process by bile.

Pancreatic enzymes enter the duodenum through the pancreatic duct and function best in the neutralized chyme. Pancreatic enzymes hydrolyze carbohydrates, proteins, and fats. The **proteolytic enzymes** are produced and stored in the pancreas in an inactive form. Proteolytic enzymes function to hydrolyze proteins.

Specific digestive enzymes lining the brush border of the microvilli are responsible for completing the hydrolysis of carbohydrates, proteins, and fats. Not everything in foods can be completely digested; for example, the human body lacks enzymes that can digest cellulose, a carbohydrate found in plants. Other factors affecting digestion and absorption are as important to nutritional status as adequate intake, such as (1) the amount of the nutrient consumed; (2) the physiological need; (3) the condition of the digestive tract, such as the amount of secretions, motility, and absorptive surface; (4) the level of circulating hormones; (5) the presence of other nutrients or drugs ingested at the same time that enhance or interfere with absorption; and (6) the presence of adequate amounts of digestive enzymes.

ABSORPTION OF NUTRIENTS

The small intestine is the principal site for nutrient absorption (see Fig. 2-6). Only after the nutrient is absorbed into the intestinal mucosa is it considered to be "in" the body. Generally, absorption of nutrients occurs by passive diffusion or active transport mechanisms. Passive diffusion is the passage of a permeable substance from more concentrated solution to an area of lower concentration. Active transport occurs when absorption is from a region of low concentration to one of a higher concentration and requires a carrier and cellular energy. Approximately 80% to 90% of fluid intake is absorbed in the small intestine by osmosis. **Osmosis** is the passage of water through a semipermeable membrane to equalize osmotic pressure exerted by ions in solutions. Water moves freely in both directions across the intestinal mucosa. Absorbable nutrients pass through the microvilli and enter the portal circulation if they are water-soluble and the lymphatic circulation if they are fat-soluble.

ABSORPTION INTO PORTAL CIRCULATION

Monosaccharides, amino acids, glycerol, water-soluble vitamins, minerals, and short- and medium-chain fatty acids

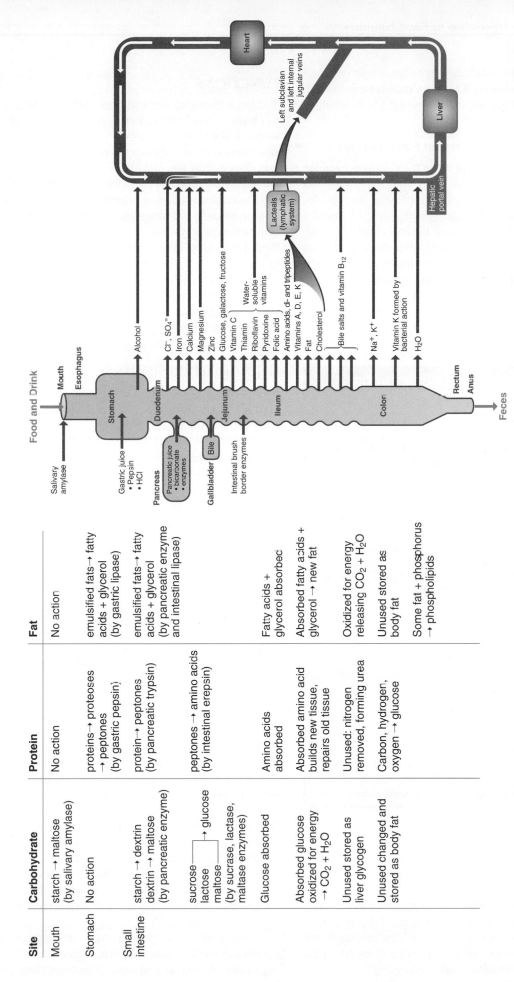

FIGURE 2-6 Digestive process of carbohydrate, protein, and fat. Cl⁻, chloride; CO₂, carbon dioxide; HCl, hydrochloric acid; H₂O, water; K⁺⁺, potassium; Na⁺⁺, sodium; SO₄, sulfate. (From Peckenpaugh NJ: Nutrition Essentials and Diet Therapy, 10th ed. Philadelphia: Saunders, 2008. Modified from Mahan LK, Escott-Stump S: Krause's Food, Nutrition, and Diet Therapy, 12th ed. Philadelphia: Saunders, 2008.)

are absorbed from the small intestine through the mucosa into the portal circulation. They are transported through the portal vein directly to the liver, where metabolism begins.

ABSORPTION OF FAT-SOLUBLE NUTRIENTS

The absorption process for long-chain fatty acids is complex because the molecules are large and insoluble. Long-chain fatty acids are broken apart to allow passage through the intestinal wall into the lymphatic system, which transports them to the left subclavian and internal jugular veins. Absorption of the four fat-soluble vitamins—A, D, E, and K—is not as complex. Bile salts and lipases increase their water solubility so that these vitamins are absorbed along with other fats in the lymphatic system.

Dental Hygiene Considerations

- An enzymatic deficiency in the gastrointestinal tract results in some nutrients not being digested; they cannot be absorbed. The most prevalent enzyme deficiency is lactase deficiency, which is discussed in Health Application 2. Unless preventive care is taken, patients with large portions of the gastrointestinal tract removed, as in bariatric surgery, may develop nutritional deficiency symptoms because digestive secretions or absorptive areas are removed (see Fig. 2-6).
- If motility is increased, such as in diarrhea, nutrients are not exposed to digestive secretions and absorptive surfaces long enough for maximum absorption. Severe or prolonged diarrhea may result in numerous deficiencies, the most rapid being a fluid deficit or dehydration.

Nutritional Directions

- The digestive process may be affected by how well the food is broken apart by the teeth.
- Dietary fat should not be eliminated entirely because it increases satiety, provides transportation for fat-soluble vitamins, and frequently contains fat-soluble vitamins.
- Routine use of mineral oil as a laxative is not advisable because it reduces absorption of fat-soluble vitamins.

LARGE INTESTINE

Small amounts of chyme remaining in the ileum are released through the ileocecal valve into the cecum. Only about 5% of the ingested foods and digestive secretions arrives in the large intestine. For most adults, it takes 16 to 24 hours for foodstuffs to travel the full length of the gut.

FUNCTIONS

The large intestine, so named because of its large diameter, has little or no digestive function. Its main functions are to reabsorb water and electrolytes (mainly sodium and potassium) and to form and store the **residue** (feces) until defecation. Residue in the intestinal tract is defined as the total amount of fecal solids, including undigested or unabsorbed food, and metabolic (bile pigments) and bacterial products. Chyme entering the large intestine with 500 to 1000 mL of water is excreted as feces containing only 100 to 200 mL of fluid. Essentially, all absorption occurs in the proximal half of the colon.

The inner lining of the large intestine is smooth, lacking the numerous villi found in the small intestine. The only important secretion is mucus, which protects the intestinal wall, aids in holding particles of fecal matter together, and helps to control the pH of the large intestine.

UNDIGESTED RESIDUES

Fiber, obtained from fruits and vegetables and whole-grain products, results in increased residue and has a water-holding capacity, contributing to bulkier feces. Dietary fiber is not digestible and works as a laxative. Some foods may contain other substances that increase fecal output. One example is prune juice, which yields no residue on chemical digestion, but is classified as a high-residue food because it contains a laxative that indirectly increases the volume of the stool. Residue has a beneficial side effect of stimulating peristalsis, resulting in better muscle tone.

MICROFLORA

Because of decreased peristalsis and the neutral pH, more than a trillion harmless bacteria thrive in the colon. About 400 different species of microorganisms living in the large intestine are called **microflora**. Microflora have several important roles: They (1) break down substances that human enzymes are unable to digest; (2) synthesize vitamins needed by humans (vitamin K, vitamin B_{12}, biotin, thiamin, and riboflavin); (3) boost the immune system to protect against infection better; and (4) inhibit **pathogenic** (harmful) bacteria. The types of food and medications ingested influence the type, activity, and relative numbers of bacteria. Bacterial activity produces various gases contributing to flatus in the colon. Fecal odor is a result of the compounds produced by these bacteria.

Probiotics are live microorganisms (usually bacteria) that aid in restoring and maintaining good health when adequate amounts are consumed. Currently, there is no legal definition for "probiotic," but this term is being used to market products even though minimum scientific criteria are not established. Each probiotic strain is unique, and the properties and the effects of each strain must be assessed individually (Table 2-2).

Probiotic studies in the scientific literature have reported the following effects: regulation of immune function (including enhanced immune response to disease-promoting organ-

Table 2-2 Probiotics and Prebiotics

Class/Component	Source*	Potential Benefit
Probiotics		
Certain species and strains of *Lactobacillus, Bifidobacterium,* yeast	Certain yogurts, other cultured dairy products, and nondairy applications	May improve gastrointestinal health and systemic immunity
Prebiotics		
Inulin, fructo-oligosaccharides, polydextrose, arabinogalactan, polyols—lactulose, lactitol	Whole grains, onions, bananas, garlic, honey, leeks, artichokes, fortified foods and beverages, dietary supplements, and other food applications	May improve gastrointestinal health; may improve calcium absorption

Adapted from International Food Information Council Foundation: Media Guide on Food Safety and Nutrition: 2004-2006. Available at http://www.ific.org/publications/factsheets/preprobioticsfs.cfm, Accessed January 25, 2008.
*Examples are not all-inclusive.

isms and inflammatory responses), shortening the duration of infectious diarrhea in infants, enhanced gastrointestinal tolerance to antibiotic therapy, and control of symptoms associated with lactose intolerance.[5] *Lactobacillus acidophilus* and *Bifidobacterium bifidus,* found in certain yogurts and other fermented dairy products, have been shown to help prevent pathogenic bacteria from proliferating and healthy bacteria from becoming toxic. Certain types of microorganisms have been shown to improve the ability of lactose-intolerant individuals to digest lactose, improving their tolerance to dairy products, whereas other probiotics decrease the incidence or duration of gastrointestinal infections, such as diarrhea.

Probiotics are found in fermented dairy products, such as kefir, yogurt, and cheeses. Commercial products are generally safe with few side effects, relatively inexpensive, and readily available. These products do not usually disclose the levels or strain designations of added bacteria, so consumers do not know if the product has been shown to be efficacious for specific effects. Not all products on the market claiming to be probiotic meet the minimum criteria established for a probiotic.

Prebiotics are nondigestible food ingredients that have beneficial effects on the host by selectively stimulating the growth or activity, or both, of beneficial microorganisms in the colon. Fiber, particularly fermentable fiber, is crucial for good health. Prebiotics are specialized ingredients targeted to influencing specific bacteria, their fermentation end products, and possible health effects on the host.[5] In other words, prebiotics are food for probiotics. Prebiotics increase mineral absorption (especially calcium and magnesium) from the foods containing them.[6]

Probiotics together with prebiotics that support their growth are called **synbiotics** because they work together to promote probiotic benefits more efficiently. The benefits associated with probiotics and prebiotics are strain- (probiotics) and substance-specific (prebiotics).

PERISTALSIS

The purpose of peristalsis in the large intestine is to force the feces into the rectum. These large waves occur only two to three times daily.

Dental Hygiene Considerations

- Bowel habits, stress, exercise, and nutritional intake (especially the amount of fiber and fluid intake) affect the gastrointestinal transit rate.
- Lengthy retention of feces in the large intestine allows more reabsorption of water, causing the feces to become hard and dry and leading to constipation.
- For most patients, microbes in probiotics are beneficial. However, patients who have a poor immune response should consult a healthcare provider before using probiotics.
- Probiotics are being used to treat traveler's diarrhea, prevent and treat urinary tract infections and irritable bowel disease, and prevent and manage atopic dermatitis in children.
- Many patients may have symptoms of a chronic digestive problem, such as heartburn, abdominal pain, constipation, diarrhea, and gastroesophageal reflux disease. Many of these problems can be addressed with dietary or lifestyle changes.
- Antibiotic therapy normally kills the bacteria in the colon and inhibits bacterial production of vitamins. Patients on long-term antibiotic therapy may develop vitamin K, vitamin B$_{12}$, and biotin deficiencies.

Nutritional Directions

- Constipation can be treated by increasing fluid intake or by gradually increasing nondigestible materials (fiber) in the diet, or both.
- Activity also affects gastrointestinal mobility. Active individuals who routinely choose high-fiber foods and drink adequate amounts of liquids are less likely to become constipated than their sedentary counterparts.
- The frequency of bowel movements varies from after each meal to once every 2 days.
- Probiotics as a dietary supplement are beneficial in providing high levels of bacteria easily, if the products are responsibly formulated and stored properly. These products should be purchased only from reputable companies and should contain the United States Pharmacopeia (USP) or the National Formulary (NF) symbol on their packaging.
- The presence of higher levels of bifidobacteria in the intestines of breastfed infants may be a reason why these infants are generally healthier than formula-fed infants.
- A probiotic should be able to survive and establish itself in the intestinal environment.

HEALTH APPLICATION 2 Lactose Intolerance

Some patients are unable to digest specific carbohydrates because of insufficient amounts of disaccharide enzymes. When those carbohydrates are eaten, the disaccharide is fermented by intestinal bacteria rather than being broken down into simple sugars. This results in malabsorption of the disaccharide, accompanied by diarrhea, abdominal cramps, flatulence, and halitosis. A meta-analysis suggests lactose is not a major cause of the symptoms that many lactose maldigesters attribute to lactose intolerance.[7] Lactase, an intestinal enzyme responsible for lactose digestion, is the only disaccharidase whose activity is reduced in a significant proportion of older children and adults.

Lactose intolerance primarily affects African Americans (75%), Hispanics (50%), Native Americans (100%), and Asians (100%).[8] Lactase deficiency may be an inherited problem with gradual decreases in lactase activity throughout the life span, or a temporary condition caused by gastrointestinal diseases or intestinal mucosa damage. Occasionally, an infant has a lactase deficiency at birth because of an inborn error of metabolism. Lactose intolerance can be diagnosed based on results of a blood, breath, or stool test ordered by a healthcare provider.

Nutritional Care

Treatment of lactase deficiency is simple: reduce lactose-containing foods. Because milk provides significant amounts of calcium, vitamin D, phosphorus, riboflavin, and sometimes protein, elimination is not advisable. The ability to digest lactose is not an all-or-nothing phenomenon; most patients with lactose intolerance can tolerate some lactose. The amount of dairy products is reduced to a patient's tolerance level (Box 2-1). Milk is tolerated better when taken with a meal and limited to 8 oz at a time. Whole milk is tolerated better than skim milk.

Studies indicate an increased frequency of osteoporosis in patients with lactose intolerance because of reduced calcium intake. When adolescent girls restrict dairy products because of perceived milk intolerance, lower spinal bone mineral content results, which may result in osteoporosis.[9] Patients should be taught the approximate calcium composition of the milk products they tolerate (see Table 8-2) so that they can try to consume adequate amounts of calcium.

Fermented dairy products—especially yogurt, buttermilk, aged cheese, and sour cream—are often better tolerated by lactase-deficient individuals. Yogurt made with the organisms *Lactobacillus bulgaricus* or *Streptococcus thermophilus* is better tolerated than nonfermented dairy products because it contains active lactase and less lactose. Most commercially available unflavored yogurt can be beneficial to lactose-intolerant patients. Pasteurization of frozen yogurts decreases the lactase activity and kills lactose-producing bacteria, so most frozen yogurts are not well tolerated by lactose-intolerant patients.

Commercially available lactase in tablet or liquid form can be beneficial. Lactase tablets, taken with a lactose-containing food, are effective in the stomach's acidic environment for approximately 45 minutes. Liquid lactase is effective in a neutral pH, and when added to milk, the lactose is hydrolyzed before ingestion. Specialized lactose-reduced products are also commercially available.

Box 2-1 Suggestions for Lactose-Intolerant Patients

- Adequate amounts of calcium need to be provided when milk and milk products are avoided. Because of different tolerance levels, each patient needs to experiment to determine which method is most effective for providing necessary nutrients without discomfort. Consume small amounts of lactose-containing foods with meals several times a day.
- Consume fermented dairy products—yogurt,* kefir,† and buttermilk—that contain probiotics (live bacteria).
- Choose aged cheeses (Swiss, Colby, Longhorn) that naturally contain less lactose.
- Try small amounts of whole-milk dairy products.
- Buy lactose-reduced or lactose-free products.
- Read ingredient labels for "hidden" lactose (whey, milk by-products, nonfat dry milk powder, malted milk, buttermilk, and dry milk solids). Also check for lactose in prescription and over-the-counter drugs.

- Drink or eat calcium-fortified foods, such as orange juice, soymilk, and cereals.
- Use over-the-counter lactase enzymes available in tablet/liquid form to hydrolyze the lactose in milk products or lactose-hydrolyzed commercially available milk.
- Increase consumption of other calcium-containing foods, such as salmon and sardines canned with bones, spinach, kale, broccoli, turnip and beet greens, molasses, tofu, almonds, orange, eggs, and shrimp.
- Consider commercially available nutrition supplements, such as Ensure (Abbott Nutrition), Resource (Novartis/Sandoz Nutrition), and Sustacal (Mead Johnson Nutritionals).
- If the previous suggestions are not feasible to maintain an adequate intake of 800 mg of calcium, consult a healthcare provider or dietitian for calcium supplements that are well absorbed. These supplements may also need to include vitamin D.

*Unflavored yogurt is usually the best tolerated.
†Kefir is a fermented milk beverage that contains different bacteria than yogurt.

CASE APPLICATION FOR THE DENTAL HYGIENIST

Mr. A complains that he can hardly talk because his mouth is dry and sticky. Sores in his mouth make his dentures very uncomfortable. He states he does not leave his home often because he is unable to find liquids easily to prevent his tongue from sticking to the sides and the roof of his mouth. He also complains that eating is difficult. Mr. A reports his healthcare provider prescribed a diuretic for his hypertension.

Nutritional Assessment
- Recent change in weight
- Dietary intake
- Preferred fluids, frequency of intake
- Food preparation techniques
- Medications taken
- Oral examination to determine the condition of the underlying tissues
- Fit of dentures
- Willingness to learn and to change habits

Nutritional Diagnosis
Knowledge deficit of the effects of diuretics on hydration of the body related to lack of information and understanding.

Nutritional Goals
The patient will continue taking the diuretic. His nutrient intake will improve to prevent further weight loss, and his fluid intake will increase to 8 to 10 glasses of fluid a day.

Nutritional Implementation
Intervention: Discuss the importance of adequate salivary flow for maintenance of soft tissues, taste functions, and teeth. If indicated and desired, suggest use of products designed to relieve xerostomia to provide temporary comfort as needed.
Rationale: Xerostomia has severe deleterious effects on a patient's ability to talk and on the integrity of the oral tissues.
Intervention: Review the importance of meticulous oral hygiene and removal of dentures for periods of time.

Rationale: Xerostomia promotes plaque formation, which can lead to further gingival irritations and caries. Removal of dentures allows the underlying tissue to become healthy again.
Intervention: Discuss that although diuretics may cause this condition, the diuretic is important for his health.
Rationale: To prevent other health problems, Mr. A must continue the medication as prescribed by his healthcare provider.
Intervention: Discuss ways he can increase his fluid intake to 8 to 10 glasses daily: (1) drink more fluid with meals; (2) carry fluids with him in a large covered thermal container.
Rationale: To replace fluids excreted because of the diuretic, adequate fluid intake is essential.
Intervention: Encourage increased intake of nutrient-dense liquid or semiliquid foods, such as milkshakes, cream soups, gravies, and sauces.
Rationale: These foods contain larger proportions of nutrients, which will help Mr. A to consume adequate amounts of nutrients and will prevent weight loss.
Intervention: Recommend tips to relieve the dryness in his mouth, such as sugar-free mints and gum containing xylitol or ice chips.
Rationale: The patient's comfort will be enhanced if his mouth is moist; oral complications associated with xerostomia will be minimized. The use of chewing gum or mints containing xylitol will stimulate salivary flow, reduce caries-causing bacteria, and assist with remineralization of any early carious lesions.

Evaluation
If the patient continues to take the prescribed diuretic, consumes a well-balanced diet, increases fluid intake, uses correct oral hygiene practices, maintains body weight, and can state why he was having all these problems, dental hygiene care was effective.

STUDENT READINESS

1. Make a chart or diagram showing the gastrointestinal secretions, where they are produced, and their digestive actions on the nutrients present in milk. Homogenized milk contains the following: lactose (a disaccharide), proteins, emulsified fats, calcium, riboflavin, and vitamins A and D. Where are the end products absorbed?
2. Define *alimentary canal, hydrolysis, enzyme,* and *residue.*
3. A patient has problems secreting too much HCl. What types of food would you tell a patient to avoid?
4. Cut a small hole (1 mm in diameter) in a piece of paper. Place the tip of your tongue through the hole. Looking in the mirror, count the number of taste buds. Compare your findings with other classmates of varying ages. Observe the number of taste buds on adolescent and older patients.
5. If caloric intake were equal, which of the following breakfasts would probably delay the feeling of hunger the longest? Explain your reason.

   a. Dry cereal with skim milk, toast with jelly, and coffee with sugar.
   b. Egg with ham, toast with butter, and coffee with cream.
6. What are the absorbable products resulting from digestion of carbohydrates, proteins, and fats?
7. Within what section of the alimentary canal does most digestion and absorption take place?
8. Considering the secretions and the functions of the gastrointestinal tract, discuss the fallacy of diets that claim only one type of food (e.g., fruits) should be eaten at a given time.
9. Could constipation be called a nutrient deficiency? Defend your answer.
10. What types of problems might be encountered when a patient does not chew his or her food well? Discuss the dental issues that can lead to decreased ability to masticate food.

CASE STUDY

A 22-year-old Asian woman reports a history of lactose intolerance. She is concerned about her calcium intake because she has eliminated all dairy products from her diet.

1. What should be included in the dietary recommendations made by the dental hygienist?
2. Can this patient consume dairy products?
3. Which dairy products are best tolerated by lactose-deficient individuals?
4. When should lactase tablets be taken?
5. What symptoms may the patient report that are associated with lactose intake?
6. Why should she include dairy products?

References

1. Hutton JL, Baracos VE, Wismer WV: Chemosensory dysfunction is a primary factor in the evolution of declining nutritional status and quality of life in patients with advanced cancer. J Pain Symptom Manage 2007 Feb; 33(2):156-165.
2. Klasser GD, Utsman R, Epstein JB: Taste change associated with a dental procedure: case report and review of the literature. J Can Dent Assoc 2008 Jun; 74(5):455-461.
3. DePaola DP, et al: Nutrition in relation to dental medicine. In Shils ME, et al (eds): Modern Nutrition in Health and Disease, 9th ed. Philadelphia: Lea & Febiger, 1999, pp 1099-1134.
4. Mattes RD, Cowart BJ: Dietary assessment of patients with chemosensory disorders. J Am Diet Assoc 1994 Jan; 94(1):50-56.
5. Douglas LC, Sanders ME: Probiotics and prebiotics in dietetics practice. J Am Diet Assoc 2008 Mar; 108(3):510-521.
6. Adolfsson O: Yogurt and gut function. Am J Clin Nutr 2004 Aug; 80(2):245-256.
7. Savaiano DA, Boushey CJ, McCabe GP: Lactose intolerance symptoms assessed by meta-analysis: a grain of truth that leads to exaggeration. J Nutr 2006 Apr; 136(4):1107-1113.
8. Jackson KA, Savaiano DA: Lactose maldigestion, calcium intake and osteoporosis in African-, Asian-, and Hispanic-Americans. J Am Coll Nutr 2001 Apr; 20(2 Suppl):198S-207S.
9. Matlik L, et al: Perceived milk intolerance is related to bone mineral content in 10- to 13-year-old female adolescents. Pediatrics 2007 Sep; 120(3):e69-e77.

Chapter 3

Carbohydrate: The Efficient Fuel

LEARNING OBJECTIVES

Upon completion of this chapter, the student will be able to achieve the following objectives:
- Identify major carbohydrates in foods and in the body.
- List ways glucose can be used by the body.
- State the functions of dietary carbohydrate.
- State why carbohydrates should be included in the diet.
- Identify dietary sources of lactose, other sugars, and starches.
- State the role and sources of dietary fiber.
- State the number of kilocalories provided per gram of carbohydrate.
- Describe the role of carbohydrate in the caries process.
- Make recommendations concerning carbohydrate consumption when counseling patients to reduce risk for dental caries.

KEY TERMS

Anticariogenic
Cariogenic
Cariostatic
Complex carbohydrates
Dextrins
Dietary fiber
Disaccharides

Fermentable carbohydrate
Functional fiber
Glycogen
Hyperglycemia
Hypoglycemia
Ketones
Lipogenesis

KEY TERMS—cont'd

Monosaccharides
Nondigestible
Nonessential amino acids
Phenylketonuria
Photosynthesis
Plaque biofilm
Polysaccharides
Resistant starch

Streptococcus mutans
Sugar alcohols
Synergistic
Total fiber
Viscous fiber
Xylitol

Test Your NQ

1. **T/F** Raw sugar is nutritionally superior to white sugar.
2. **T/F** Fructose is the principal carbohydrate in honey.
3. **T/F** All caloric sugars can be metabolized by plaque biofilm.
4. **T/F** The desire for sweetness in the diet is an acquired taste.
5. **T/F** Fiber tends to regulate the rate of foods passing through the gastrointestinal tract.
6. **T/F** Carbohydrates are absorbed as monosaccharides.
7. **T/F** Excessive consumption of carbohydrates is the main cause of obesity.
8. **T/F** Glucose is the same as table sugar.
9. **T/F** Eliminating sucrose from the diet prevents the development of dental caries.
10. **T/F** Natural sugars in foods can be just as cariogenic as added sugars.

Carbohydrates have been the major source of energy for people since the dawn of history. Worldwide, carbohydrates are the most important source of energy. The popular belief that carbohydrates have some mysterious "fattening" power is unfounded. Carbohydrates furnish 80% to 90% of the kilocalories for some African and Asian nations. They add variety and palatability to the diet and are the most economical form of energy.

Carbohydrates are made by all plants from carbon, hydrogen, and oxygen in the process of **photosynthesis** (the formation of chemical compounds when chlorophyll-containing plant tissues are exposed to light), when the carbon is combined with a molecule of water, as in C-H$_2$O:

$$6\,CO_2 + 6\,H_2O \rightarrow C_6H_{12}O_6 + 6\,O_2$$
$$\text{(air)} \quad \text{(water)} \quad \text{(glucose)} \text{(oxygen)}$$

It has been stated that a hydrated carbon is a carbohydrate. During the 1950s, carbohydrates acquired a bad reputation in the United States. Statements made in best-selling books indicated we are the victims of "carbohydrate poisoning." Naturally, these unscientific statements affect food consumption patterns. In 1977, the U.S. government began advising Americans of the reduced risk of various chronic diseases from eating foods containing more complex carbohydrates (fruits, vegetables, legumes, and whole-grain cereals and breads). Since then, dietary patterns have been changing. As can be seen in Figure 3-1, carbohydrate intake has fluctuated more than any other macronutrient.

Food supply data for 2005 indicate Americans consuming 2000 kcal per day averaged slightly more than eight servings of grain products.[1] Resurgence of the popular low-carbohydrate, high-protein weight reduction diets caused the pendulum to swing again away from choosing carbohydrate foods by many people. Many of these diets are not balanced nutritionally and may not provide adequate amounts of some nutrients that protect against several chronic diseases. Most food and drink manufacturers have introduced reduced-carbohydrate foods and are actively investing in research and development of new low-carbohydrate products.

Even if people are consuming an adequate number of servings from the bread, cereal, rice, and pasta group, the types of foods chosen need adjustment to increase fiber and decrease added sugars. Because most high-carbohydrate food choices are cakes, cookies, pastries, pies, and regular sodas, intake of fat and sugar is detrimentally affected. Most Americans currently consume less than one serving of whole grains daily.[1] As shown in Figure 3-2, the average intake of caloric sweeteners was stable between 1970-1974, but between 1974-2005, intake increased by 19%.[2] Sugar consumption (sucrose and high fructose corn syrup, and other sweeteners) decreased and stabilized at about 139 lb per capita in 2006.[3]

Misconceptions surrounding the intake of sugars are that (1) sugar is the cause of tooth decay, (2) food with a high sugar concentration is more dangerous to the teeth, and (3) avoidance of sticky sweets prevents tooth decay. The incidence of caries has decreased in industrialized countries with water fluoridation despite increased sugar consumption. Approximately 90% of all snack foods contain **fermentable carbohydrate** (i.e., carbohydrates that can be metabolized by bacteria in plaque biofilm, including all sugars and cooked or processed starches). Dental hygienists

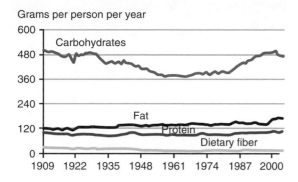

FIGURE 3-1 Carbohydrate intake has fluctuated over time. (From the USDA, Center for Nutrition Policy and Promotion, Nutrient Availability data, 1909-2004. Available at http://www.ers.usda.gov/Briefing/DietQuality/Availability.htm.)

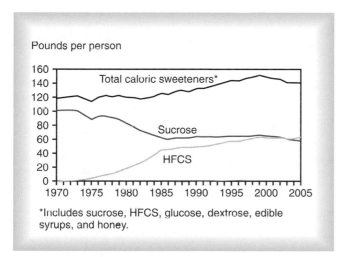

*Includes sucrose, HFCS, glucose, dextrose, edible syrups, and honey.

FIGURE 3-2 Added sugars in the food supply, 1970-2005. (From the ERS Food Availability data. In Wells HF, Buzby JC: High-fructose corn syrup usage may be leveling off. Amber Waves, February 2008, the Economic Research Service, U.S. Department of Agriculture. Available at http://www.ers.usda.gov/AmberWaves/February08/Findings/HighFructose.htm.)

must be knowledgeable about the effect of carbohydrates on soft and hard tissues in the oral cavity as well as chronic health problems caused by low-carbohydrate, high-fat intake. Dental hygienists need to be able to counsel patients about ways to modify carbohydrate consumption and intake patterns that are consistent with overall good health.

CLASSIFICATION

Generally, the chemical components of carbohydrate are in these proportions: $C_n(H_2O)_n$. Empirical formulas such as $C_6H_{12}O_6$ or $C_{12}H_{22}O_{11}$ can readily be identified as a carbohydrate. The number of carbon atoms in the molecule is used to classify carbohydrates. **Monosaccharides** are simple sugars containing two to six carbon atoms. **Disaccharides**

HEXOSES

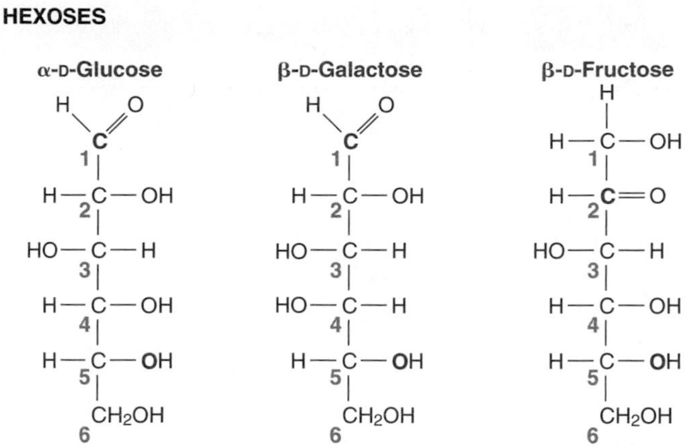

FIGURE 3-3 Chemical structure of monosaccharides. Monosaccharides, or hexoses, are represented as straight chains called *stick formulas*. The chemical formula is the same, but the atoms are arranged differently, as shown by the enriched grouping, resulting in differences in chemical behavior, taste, and sweetness. (Adapted from Mahan LK, Escott-Stump S: Krause's Food, Nutrition and Diet Therapy, 12th ed. Philadelphia: Saunders, 2008.)

are composed of two simple sugars joined together containing 12 carbon atoms. **Polysaccharides** are **complex carbohydrates** containing a minimum of 10 units of various simple sugars.

Monosaccharides and disaccharides contribute to the palatability of a food because of their sweetness. Temperature, pH, and presence of other substances influence the sweetness of a food. Relative sweetness of sugars is measured by subjective sensory tasting; sucrose is used as the standard of comparison (Table 3-1).

MONOSACCHARIDES

The simplest carbohydrates, monosaccharides, are absorbed without further digestion. The monosaccharides of greatest significance in foods and body metabolism are glucose, fructose, and galactose. Figure 3-3 identifies slight differences between three of the six-carbon sugars compared with glucose. A fermentable carbohydrate that can reduce salivary pH to less than 5.5 is referred to as being **cariogenic**.

Glucose

Also called *dextrose* or *corn sugar,* glucose is naturally abundant in many fruits, such as grapes, oranges, and dates, and in some vegetables, including fresh corn. It is prepared commercially as corn syrup or by special processing of starch. Glucose is the principal product formed by the digestion of disaccharides and polysaccharides. It provides energy for cells via the bloodstream. Glucose is the only sugar transported through the bloodstream to help nourish all cells in the body.

Fructose

Fructose, also known as *levulose,* is found naturally in honey and fruits. It is the sweetest of the monosaccharides and is

Table 3-1 Sugars and Sweeteners: Caloric Value, Relative Sweetness, and Cariogenicity

Sugar or Sweetener	Kilocalories/g	Relative Sweetness*	Relative Cariogenicity*
Sugars and Sweeteners			
Fructose	4	173	80-100
Honey (fructose and glucose)	3	130	100
Sucrose	4	100	100
Molasses (sucrose and invert sugar)	2.4	100	100
Brown sugar (sugar and molasses)	3.8	100	100
Dextrose/glucose (corn syrup)	4	74	†
Galactose	4	60	†
Maltose	4	50	†
Lactose	4	16	40-60
Reduced-Calorie Sweeteners‡			
Tagatose	1.5	100	0
Xylitol	2.4	100	§
Maltitol	2.1	90	0
Hydrogenated starch hydrolysates	<3	40-90	0
Erythritol	0.2	60-70	0
Sorbitol	2.6	60	0
Mannitol	1.6	50	0
Trehalose	4	45	Reduced
Isomalt	2	45-65	0
Lactitol	2	40	0
Non-nutritive Sweeteners‡			
Neotame	0	7000-13,000	0
Thaumatin (Talin)¶	0	2000-3000	Unknown
Dihydrochalcones¶	0	1500	Unknown
Sucralose	0	600	0
RebaudiosideA (Truvia)¶	0	300	0
Saccharin	0	300	0
Acesulfame K	0	200	0
Aspartame	0	200	0
Glycyrrhizin**	0	50-100	Unknown
Cyclamate¶	0	30	0

*Relative to sucrose (=100).
†Information not available.
‡Data from Calorie Control Council, Copyright © 2007 Calorie Control Council. Available at http://www.caloriecontrol.org.
§Reduces new caries formation.
¶Not approved by FDA for use in the United States.
¶Approved by FDA for use as a sweetener in December 2008.
**Approved by FDA for use as a flavor and flavor enhancer.

a product of the digestion of sucrose. Fructose can be manufactured from glucose.

Galactose

Glucose, another six-carbon sugar, is a product of lactose digestion (milk sugar). Galactose is rarely found free in nature. Physiologically, it is a constituent of nerve tissue and is produced from glucose during lactation.

Sugar Alcohols

Sugar alcohols, also called *polyols,* are formed from or converted to sugar. Sugar alcohols, such as sorbitol, may appear naturally in foods or be added by a manufacturer. Polyols most frequently used or found naturally in the body include sorbitol, xylitol, and mannitol.

For a given quantity, a sugar alcohol adds about the same amount of sweetness as glucose; it also furnishes the same amount of kilocalories. Incomplete absorption of all the sugar alcohols produces a laxative effect—soft stools or diarrhea—by causing an osmotic transfer of water into the gastrointestinal tract. The advantages of sugar alcohols are that they do not cause sudden increases in blood glucose levels, they do not contribute to tooth decay, and some may contribute to remineralization of enamel.[4,5]

The benefit of sorbitol is that it is absorbed and metabolized more slowly than sucrose. Sorbitol, the most commonly used sugar alcohol, is the least expensive. Mannose is a six-carbon sugar found in some legumes. Mannitol, derived from mannose, is found in foods. **Xylitol** is a sweetener with approximately the same perceived sweetness and 40% less calories than sugar. It is found in fruits and vegetables (lettuce, carrots, and strawberries). As a food additive, it is more expensive than other sugar alcohols, but has no aftertaste. Xylitol shows passive and active anticaries effects along with antimicrobial properties.[6]

DISACCHARIDES

Intact disaccharides cannot be metabolized by the body, but they contribute to body functions after they have been digested. All are hydrolyzed during digestion to their constituent monosaccharides for absorption as shown:

$$Sucrose = glucose + fructose$$

$$Lactose = glucose + galactose$$

$$Maltose = glucose + glucose$$

Sucrose

Granulated table sugar is the most common form of sucrose. Commercially, sucrose is produced from sugar cane or sugar beets (not to be confused with red beets). It is also found in molasses, maple syrup, and maple sugar. Some fruits (apricots, peaches, plums, raspberries, honeydew, cantaloupe) and vegetables (beets, carrots, parsnips, winter squash, peas, corn, and sweet potatoes) naturally contain varying amounts of sucrose.

Lactose

The sugar found in milk is lactose. Lactose is unique to mammalian milk. In the fermentation of milk, some of the lactose is converted to lactic acid, giving buttermilk and yogurt their characteristic flavors.

Maltose

Also called *malt sugar,* maltose does not occur naturally. It is created in bread making and brewing beer and is present in some processed cereals and baby foods.

POLYSACCHARIDES OR COMPLEX CARBOHYDRATES

Complex carbohydrates, also called polysaccharides, contain more than 10 monosaccharides. Some polysaccharides have a role in energy storage and are digestible. Dietary fiber is largely indigestible by human intestinal enzymes.

Starch

Starches are composed of many glucose units that may be in long chains or branched. Most food sources of complex carbohydrates are in the form of starch from cereal grains, roots, vegetables, and legumes. The amount of starch present in a vegetable increases with its maturity. For example, corn tastes much sweeter immediately after it is picked than it does several days later because its simple sugars have not developed into starch. In contrast, the amount of starch in fruit decreases as it ripens—that is, complex carbohydrates are broken down in the ripening process into simple sugars.

The presence of the cell wall, or cellulose, surrounding the starch granule is the reason starches are insoluble in cold water. Cellulose is composed of long straight chains of glucose units bound together in a very strong bonding to provide great mechanical strength with limited flexibility (Fig. 3-4). Cooking facilitates the digestive process by causing the granules to swell, rupturing the cell wall so that digestive enzymes have access to the starch inside the cell. In cooking, this swelling is referred to as thickening, as occurs in making gravy. Industrially, food starch is modified by chemicals to produce a better thickening agent.

Glucose Polymers

Industrially produced carbohydrate supplements are composed of glucose, maltose, and dextrins. **Dextrins** are long glucose chains split into shorter ones or intermediate products of the digestive enzymes on the starch molecules. In the process of toasting bread, dextrins are produced. Consistent with other carbohydrate products, glucose provides 4 kcal/g.

Glycogen

Glycogen is the carbohydrate storage form of energy in humans. Stored in the muscle and liver, glycogen is readily available as a source of glucose and energy. Carbohydrates are frequently consumed in excess of immediate energy needs. Excess glucose is converted to glycogen until the limited glycogen storage capacity is filled; simultaneously, glucose is converted into fats and stored as adipose tissue. The total amount of glycogen stores is relatively small, only enough to meet energy demands for less than a day.

Dietary Fiber

Fiber refers to nondigestible components of food. **Nondigestible** means enzymes in the human gastrointestinal tract cannot digest and absorb the substance; plant cells remain largely intact through the gastrointestinal digestive process. Fiber has demonstrable health effects. Foods contain soluble or insoluble fiber based on whether they become viscous in water. Insoluble fiber and soluble fiber have different physiologic functions in the body. Many naturally occurring com-

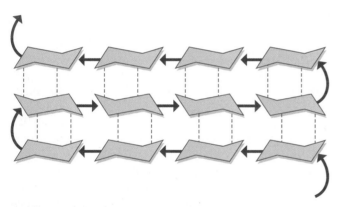

FIGURE 3-4 The ribbon-like structure of cellulose. Note the cross-links between adjacent molecules. (From Mahan LK, Escott-Stump S: Krause's Food, Nutrition and Diet Therapy, 11th ed. Philadelphia: Saunders, 2004.)

ponents in food are classified as dietary fiber. During food processing, many compounds are added that have the same physiological effect as naturally occurring fiber.

Dietary fiber consists of several different types of nondigestible carbohydrates and lignin that occur naturally in plants. Dietary fiber includes polysaccharides, lignin, and associated substances in plants such as whole grains, legumes, vegetables, fruits, seeds, and nuts (Table 3-2). Sources of dietary fiber usually contain other macronutrients, such as digestible carbohydrate and protein normally found in foods.

Resistant starch is a form of dietary fiber that delivers some of the health benefits of soluble and insoluble fibers. Resistant starches are not digested, so they contribute to health by providing fatty acids for bacteria in the colon.[7] Resistant starches trap water and add bulk to the stool, helping with regularity. Small amounts of resistant starches occur naturally in underripe bananas, navy beans, lentils, barley, and whole-grain breads.

Fiber added during the manufacturing process is called **functional fiber**. Functional fiber consists of isolated, nondigestible carbohydrates that have beneficial physiological effects in humans. Functional fibers may be modified from the natural state or commercially produced, as long as scientific research has shown beneficial physiological effects. Manufacturers have isolated various types of fiber from carbohydrate sources to add to foods because of their functional properties, such as thickening or emulsifying. Many of these substances, including carrageenan and guar gum, are commonly used as food additives. **Total fiber** is the sum of dietary fiber and functional (added) fiber. Many fibers can be classified either as dietary fiber or functional fiber, depending on whether they are a natural component of the food or added to the food during processing. Plant-based foods are a good source of dietary fiber, but commercially developed functional fibers for use in processed foods also have a beneficial role in health. Various types of fibers have distinct properties resulting in different physiological effects.

Table 3-2 Synopsis of Total Fibers				
			Physiological Response	
Type of Fiber	**Dietary Fiber Sources**	**Laxation**	**Normalization of Blood Lipid Concentration**	**Attenuation of Blood Glucose Response**
Cellulose	Whole-wheat flour, whole rye, bran, cabbage family, peas/beans, apples, root vegetables, fresh tomatoes	Yes	Neutral	Neutral
Gums and mucilages	Oats, dried beans, legumes	Neutral	Yes	Yes
Hemicellulose	Bran, cereals, whole grains	Yes	Unknown	Unknown
Liginin (noncarbohydrate)	Fruits and edible seeds such as strawberries, mature vegetables, whole grains	Yes	Unknown	Unknown
Pectin	Apples, citrus fruits, berries (especially strawberries), carrots	Somewhat	Yes	Yes

Data from Institute of Medicine of the National Academies: Dietary Reference Intakes: Energy, Carbohydrate, Fiber, Fat, Fatty Acids, Cholesterol, Protein, and Amino Acids. Washington, DC: National Academies Press, 2002.

PHYSIOLOGICAL ROLES

ENERGY

The principal role of absorbed sugars is to provide a source of energy for body functions and activity and heat to maintain body temperature. Glucose is the preferred source of energy for the brain and central nervous system, red blood cells, and lens of the eye. Although many organs can use fats for energy, glucose is the preferred fuel. Carbohydrate, whether it was originally from a sugar or a starch, provides 4 kcal/g. Because of incomplete absorption, sugar alcohols contribute varying amounts of kilocalories (Table 3-3). Glycogen stores are a readily available source of glucose for the tissues.

FAT STORAGE

Sugars in the blood ensure replenishing of glycogen stores; however, excessive intake of energy from any source results in converting glucose to fats in a process known as **lipogenesis**. When carbohydrates are eaten in excess of needs, lipogenesis results in increased fat stores.

CONVERSION TO OTHER CARBOHYDRATES

Monosaccharides are important constituents of many compounds that regulate metabolism. Examples include heparin, which prevents blood clotting; galactolipins, which are constituents of nervous tissue; and dermatan sulfate, which is present in tissues rich in collagen (especially the skin).

CONVERSION TO AMINO ACIDS

The liver can use part of the carbon framework from the sugar molecule and part of the protein molecule contributed by the breakdown of an amino acid to produce **nonessential amino acids**. These are essential to the body, but are not required in the diet.

NORMAL FAT METABOLISM

Oxidation of fats requires the presence of some carbohydrates. When carbohydrate intake is low, the body relies on energy from fat intake or stores. Fats are metabolized faster than the body can oxidize them; the resulting intermediate products are called ketone bodies. **Ketones** are normal products of lipid metabolism in the liver; muscles can use them for energy only if adequate amounts of glucose are available. An accumulation of ketones, or incompletely oxidized fatty products, results in ketosis.

PROTEIN-SPARERS

Carbohydrates, by furnishing energy in the diet, are said to be protein-sparing. Energy is an essential physiological requirement. With insufficient carbohydrate intake, the body burns protein for fuel. If carbohydrate intake is adequate, protein can be used to build and repair tissue.

INTESTINAL BACTERIA

Dietary fiber remains in the gastrointestinal tract longer than other nutrients. Undigestible fibers, such as lignin, cellulose, and hemicellulose, may be fermented by microflora in the large intestine. Fermentation produces gas and volatile fatty acids, which the cells lining the colon use for energy. This encourages the growth of bacteria that synthesize certain vitamins (some of the B-complex vitamins and vitamin K).

GASTROINTESTINAL MOTILITY

Dietary and certain functional fibers, particularly those that are poorly fermented, improve fecal bulk and laxation and ameliorate constipation in addition to other functions listed in Table 3-2. Dietary fiber and functional fibers *accelerate* the transit rate (the time it takes for waste products to move through the intestine) in individuals with a slow transit time (constipation). **Viscous fiber** *decreases* the transit rate in individuals with a rapid transit time (diarrhea). The ability of fiber to bind water in the intestine and increase bulk from nondigestible substances decreases the length of time waste products are in the alimentary tract. An *increased transit time* causes tissue exposure to cancer-causing nitrogenous waste products for longer periods. An added benefit of fiber is its stool-softening ability, which helps prevent constipation. These fibers in the colon increase stool bulk, exercising the digestive tract muscles by increasing the radius of the colon and preventing the muscle from being chronically contracted. As muscle tone is maintained and colonic pressure is diminished, the gut is able to resist bulging out into pouches known as *diverticula* (Fig. 3-5).

Viscous fibers, which also are referred to as *soluble fiber,* include pectins, gums, psyllium, mucilages, and algal polysaccharides. They influence the physiology of the upper gastrointestinal tract. Soluble fibers are physiologically important for their gel-forming ability, which results in increased viscosity of chyme and delays gastric emptying. Viscous fibers bind bile acids and decrease serum cholesterol levels. Viscous fibers also tend to improve glucose tolerance. Psyllium, added to many cereals and used as a laxative, is effective in reducing blood cholesterol levels.

Because fiber-rich foods are not calorie-dense and are retained longer in the stomach, they may cause one to feel full on a fewer number of kilocalories. Whether fiber plays a significant role in weight management has yet to be

Table 3-3	Caloric Values of Polyols	
Polyol	**kcal/g**
Sorbitol	2.6
Xylitol	2.4
Maltitol	2.1
Isomalt	2
Lactitol	2
Mannitol	1.6
Erythritol	0.2

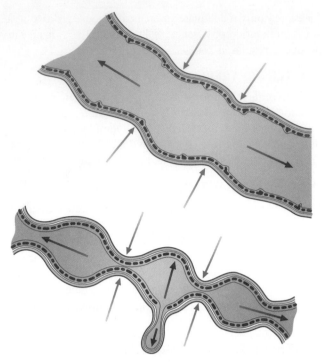

FIGURE 3-5 Mechanism by which low-fiber, low-bulk diets might generate diverticula. Where colon contents are bulk *(top)*, muscular contractions exert pressure longitudinally. If lumen is smaller *(bottom)*, contractions can produce occlusion and exert pressure against colon wall, which may produce a diverticular "blow-out." (From Peckenpaugh NJ: Nutrition Essentials and Diet Therapy, 10th ed. Philadelphia: Saunders, 2007.)

determined. Guidelines for assisting patients in increasing dietary fiber are given in Table 3-4.

OTHER NUTRIENTS

Carbohydrates are normally accompanied by other nutrients. Starchy foods are especially important for their contribution of protein, minerals, and B vitamins. Whole-grain products are superior because they contain fiber plus other nutrients (see Table 1-3); enriched products should always be used in preference to products that are processed but not enriched.

Dental Hygiene Considerations

- Use of carbohydrate requires an adequate supply of B vitamins and two minerals, phosphorus and magnesium. Usually, adequate amounts of these nutrients accompany the increased carbohydrate intake. However, this may not be true if refined sugars and breads are the predominant choices.
- Ketosis can occur in patients with uncontrolled diabetes or in individuals who have inadequate carbohydrate intake, such as individuals who are ill or are following a high-protein, very-low-carbohydrate regimen because they are burning fat rather than carbohydrate. Among other concerns, ketosis creates a disturbance in the acid-base balance of an individual. Patients with acetone or fruity-smelling breath should be questioned about their recent dietary intake.
- Increasing whole grains in the diet without increasing total energy intake may reduce risk of periodontal disease.[8]

Nutritional Directions

- Carbohydrates do not cause obesity. Excessive caloric intake and inadequate energy output are the primary causes of obesity.
- Fiber tends to regulate the transit rate of foods in the gastrointestinal tract. The best source of dietary fiber to relieve constipation is bran, but it must be initiated slowly to avoid severe gas and bloating.
- Enthusiastic patients who eat excessive amounts of bran (50 to 60 g) gain no benefit from the surplus and expose themselves unnecessarily to hazards, such as decreased mineral and vitamin absorption.
- Some vegetables and fruits (e.g., bananas, white potatoes, and apples) are high in pectins, which bind water. They are frequently used to control diarrhea, but also can help relieve constipation by softening the stool.
- Even when an individual is trying to reduce caloric intake, consuming carbohydrates is important, especially vegetables, fruits, and whole-grain breads and cereals, to provide vital nutrients.
- Carbohydrates supply 4 kcal/g and are a less concentrated source of energy than fats (9 kcal/g).

REQUIREMENTS

The recommended dietary allowance (RDA) for carbohydrate is based on providing energy for the body, particularly brain cells. The brain is the only organ requiring glucose. The RDA for digestible carbohydrate is 130 g per day for adults and children. Generally, men typically consume 200 to 330 g per day and women consume 180 to 230 g per day to meet energy requirements without exceeding acceptable levels of fat and protein. No research studies indicate that a specific amount of sugar or starch is required.

The acceptable macronutrient distribution range (AMDR) for carbohydrate is limited to no less than 45% to prevent excess fat intake and no more than 65% to ensure required nutrients from protein and fats that also provide essential micronutrients.[9] The American diet currently furnishes about 50% of the kilocalories from carbohydrates.[10]

For an individual consuming 2000 kcal per day, the maximum amount of added sugars, or 10% of total caloric intake, would be 11 tsp of added sugars (200 kcal). Based on loss-adjusted food availability data in 2005, Americans consumed on average 30 tsp of added sugars and sweeteners daily, or about 24% of the total daily caloric intake for a 2000-kcal diet. This is almost triple the amount recommended.[11] This level of added sweeteners exceeds recommendations in the *Dietary Guidelines for Americans 2005,* which address adequate amounts of vitamins and minerals without consuming excess energy (Box 3-1).

The adequate intake (AI) for total fiber intake is 14 g per 1000 kcal per day, or 38 g for men and 25 g for women

Table 3-4 Guidelines for Developing a High-Fiber Diet

Principles	Guidelines
Before recommending any changes, evaluate the patient's fiber and fluid intake. For patients ≤50 years old, the optimal level of dietary fiber is 38 g for men and 25 g for women; for patients ≥51 years old, 30 g for men and 21 g for women	Fiber normalizes bowel movements to one to two a day by either speeding or slowing the transit rate of food through the gastrointestinal tract. Food preservation methods, such as cooking and freezing, only slightly decrease fiber content; however, grinding or pureeing foods and chewing may have pronounced effects on fiber action
Rather than fiber supplements, foods that contain soluble and insoluble fibers are the best way to increase fiber	Include two to four servings daily of fruits, especially those with skins (figs, pears, apricots, nectarines, raisins, blueberries) and edible seeds (blackberries, raspberries, strawberries). Include three to five servings of vegetables daily, especially sweet potatoes, carrots, mushrooms, raw onions, pumpkin, spinach, turnip greens, kale, Brussels sprouts, parsnips, English peas, beets, okra, and broccoli. Vegetables (mushrooms, peppers, onions, tomatoes) can be added to meatloaf, spaghetti, chili, omelets, or scrambled eggs. Serve raw vegetables with low-fat dip as appetizers or snacks. (Take advantage of ready-to-use vegetables.) Add leafy greens, tomatoes, and sprouts to sandwiches. Include raw vegetables (zucchini, carrots, celery sticks) in brown-bag lunches. Choose fresh fruits and vegetables or plain popcorn instead of fried chips and cookies. Dietary fiber comes principally from whole-grain products; brown color is no guarantee of whole-grain content. Look for breads and cereals that list "whole wheat" or "whole grain" first in the ingredients list. Choose cereals with at least 2 g of fiber (5 g is ideal), but no more than 2 g of fat per serving. Experiment with brown rice, barley, whole-wheat pasta, and bulgur. Supplements made with concentrated or purified dietary fiber lack the nutritional balance provided by a varied diet that contains fruits, vegetables, whole-grain products, and legumes. Large amounts of purified fiber such as lignin and bran may result in important minerals, especially calcium, iron, and zinc, being bound by the fiber and excreted
Fiber absorbs water in the intestines, so adequate fluids are important to keep the intestinal contents moving	Ensure intake of 10-12 cups of water a day to avoid problems such as fecal impactions
Increase high-fiber foods gradually. Begin with 5- to 10-g increments to avoid adverse side effects. At least 6-8 weeks should be allowed for adaptation to prevent flatulence, abdominal cramping, and diarrhea/constipation	Substitute whole-wheat flour for ¼ or ½ of the white flour in baked goods. Add bran, bran flakes, wheat germ, chopped nuts, seeds, or oatmeal to mixed meat dishes, casseroles, salads, cooked cereal, cookies, breads, muffins, and pancake batter. Use whole-grain crackers and unbuttered popcorn. Incorporate beans into soups, casseroles, nachos, or a salad. Use bran flakes for a crispy coating on meats or fish
Increase intake of oat bran, beans, barley, and psyllium to help reduce cholesterol levels	Oat bran, rice bran, and corn bran are effective in reducing serum cholesterol. Use dried beans and peas as the main dish (in place of meat) at least once a week. Soluble dietary fiber is more effective in reducing blood cholesterol levels when the diet is also low in fat

Box 3-1 *Dietary Guidelines for Americans 2005* **Recommendations Related to Carbohydrate Consumption**

Adequate Nutrients within Calorie Needs
- Consume a variety of nutrient-dense foods and beverages within and among the basic food groups, while choosing foods that limit the intake of saturated and *trans* fats, cholesterol, added sugars, salt, and alcohol.

Food Groups to Encourage
- Consume a sufficient amount of fruits and vegetables while staying within energy needs. Two cups of fruit and 2½ cups of vegetables per day are recommended for a reference 2000 kcal intake, with higher or lower amounts depending on the kcalorie level.
- Choose a variety of fruits and vegetables each day. In particular, select from all five vegetable subgroups (dark-green, orange, legumes, starchy vegetables, and other vegetables) several times a week.
- Consume three or more ounce-equivalents of whole-grain products per day, with the rest of the recommended grains coming from enriched or whole-grain products. In general, at least half the grains should come from whole grains.

Carbohydrates
- Choose fiber-rich fruits, vegetables, and whole grains often.
- Choose and prepare foods and beverages with little added sugars or caloric sweeteners, such as amounts suggested by the U.S. Department of Agriculture (USDA) Food Guide and the DASH (Dietary Approaches to Stop Hypertension) Eating Plan (see Chapter 11).
- Reduce the incidence of dental caries by practicing good oral hygiene and consuming sugar- and starch-containing foods and beverages less frequently.

From the Dietary Guidelines for Americans 2005, U.S. Department of Health and Human Services and U.S. Department of Agriculture, 2005. Available at www.healthierus.gov/dietaryguidelines/

daily. This amount is based on the amount needed to prevent coronary heart disease. Average intake of dietary fiber is only 15 g/day in the United States.[12]

SOURCES

Carbohydrates are furnished by the following food groups: milk, grain, fruits, and vegetables. The only animal foods supplying significant quantities of carbohydrate are milk and milk products, which furnish the disaccharide lactose. In cheese making, the lactose is removed as a by-product. Consequently, most cheeses contain only trace amounts of lactose.

Other sugars are furnished by table sugar, syrups, jellies, jams, and honey. Sugars are incorporated into many popular foods (e.g., candy, beverages, cakes and desserts, chewing gum, and ice cream). Only about 25% of the sugar Americans consume is added to foods in the home and by institutions and restaurants; the remainder is added to foods during processing and in canning and freezing. During processing, sugar is added to breakfast cereals; condiments and salad dressings; soft drinks; cookies, crackers, and candies; flavored extracts and syrups; flour and bread products; and milk and milk products. A significant amount of added sweetener intake is from regular soft drinks.

Approximately 18% of the caloric intake is from naturally occuring sugars in fruits and vegetables. (This amount does not include sugar in milk.) Sugars, mainly glucose and fructose, are furnished in fruits and vegetables in varying amounts depending on their maturity (ripe bananas contain more simple sugars than green bananas) and their water content (spinach contains less carbohydrate than potatoes).

Three of the *Dietary Guidelines for Americans 2005* address sugar intake; each encourages limiting intake (see Box 3-1). Because there is no physiological requirement for added sugars, MyPyramid does not include a separate panel for sugars; added sugars are included in the discretionary kilocalories because they contain only kilocalories. Eating sugar in *moderation* implies appropriate balance among foods or nutrients is the overriding consideration in food selection.

Complex carbohydrates or starches are furnished by grain products (wheat, corn, rice, oats, rye, barley, buckwheat, and millet). Some vegetables, especially root and seed varieties (potatoes, sweet potatoes, beets, peas, and winter squashes), also contain considerable amounts of starch. Legumes, or dried beans and peas, are excellent sources of complex carbohydrates.

Dietary fiber, especially hemicellulose and cellulose, is furnished by whole-grain breads and cereals. Cellulose is found principally in the stems, roots, leaves, and seed coverings of plants; unpeeled fruits and leafy vegetables are good sources. Legumes are also a good source of dietary fiber (see Table 3-2). The pectin contributed by fruits and vegetables

Table 3-5	Dietary Fiber Content of Sample Menu

Sample Menu	Dietary Fiber Content (g)
Breakfast	
Oat-bran bagel (1)	2.1
Whipped cream cheese (2 Tbsp)	0
Seedless raisins (¼ cup)	1
1% low-fat milk (8 oz)	0
Coffee (12 oz)	0
Morning Snack	
Fresh orange (1)	4.4
Lunch	
Sandwich	
Tuna salad (¼ cup)	0
Tomato slices (2)	0.5
Thinly sliced cucumber (¼ cup)	0.2
Sliced green bell peppers (¼ cup)	0.4
Whole wheat bread (2 slices)	3.8
Baby carrots (8)	2.3
Fresh apple (1)	4.4
Water (12 oz)	0
Afternoon Snack	
Diet carbonated beverage (12 oz)	0
Dry roasted peanuts (¼ cup)	3.3
Dinner	
Lean roast beef (2 oz)	0
Brown rice (¾ cup)	2.7
Brown gravy (¼ cup)	0.2
Steamed broccoli spears (1 cup)	5.1
Melted reduced fat and sodium cheddar cheese (¼ cup)	0
Mixed green salad (1½ cup)	1.5
Low-calorie salad dressing (2 Tbsp)	0.1
Whole-wheat roll (1)	2.1
Soft margarine (1 Tbsp)	0
Fresh cantaloupe (1 cup)	1.4
Iced tea, unsweetened (12 oz)	0
Evening Snack	
1% low-fat milk (8 oz)	0
Cinnamon graham crackers (4)	1.6
Total	*35.7*

Nutrient data from U.S. Department of Agriculture, Agriculture Research Service. USDA National Nutrient Database for Standard Reference, Release 20. Accessed August 29, 2008.

is an important source of viscous fiber. Small amounts of resistant starches occur naturally in under-ripe bananas, navy beans, lentils, barley, and whole-grain breads. A popular American snack food, popcorn (preferably without butter and salt), is also a whole-grain food.[13] Table 3-5 lists the fiber content of foods in a sample menu.

Dental Hygiene Considerations

- Assess the total sugar intake and the frequency, form, and time of day for carbohydrate intake. (See Chapter 17 for further discussion.)
- Encourage patients to increase fiber intake. Fiber helps reduce constipation and diverticulosis, and may help reduce the risk of some colon cancers (see Table 3-4 for ideas to enhance fiber intake).
- Explain to the patient that a diet with adequate amounts of carbohydrate helps to maintain glycogen reserves; a diet high in fat and low in carbohydrate results in poor glycogen reserves. Another point to emphasize with the patient is the critical need for glycogen stores in the heart for continuous functioning of heart muscles.

Nutritional Directions

- Encourage patients to consume more whole-grain products and less refined sugar.
- A tablespoon of honey has more kilocalories than a tablespoon of sugar and only trace amounts of other nutrients. (Honey is not appropriate for children younger than 1 year old because of the risk of botulism.) Because of its retentive nature, honey is also more cariogenic than refined sugar.
- Food labels indicate the total amount of carbohydrate (starch, sugar, and fiber) in a serving. Because fiber is not absorbed, it does not contribute any kilocalories. A product with 25 g of carbohydrate may have only 80 kcal if at least 5 g of the carbohydrate is from fiber.
- Sugar may be identified as any of the following on food labels: sucrose, fructose, corn sweetener, cane sugar, honey, molasses, high-fructose corn syrup, raw sugar, and maple syrup. Patients trying to reduce added sugars should avoid foods if the first ingredient is any of the aforementioned.

HYPER-STATES AND HYPO-STATES

The role of sugar in nutritional health and behavior continues to be misrepresented by the press and many professionals. Many stories have been published in the media linking sugar to practically every modern-day illness, including malnutrition, hypoglycemia, diabetes mellitus, blood lipid abnormalities, cardiovascular disease, hyperactivity, criminal behavior, obesity, malabsorption syndrome, allergies, gallstones, and cancer. The public's perception of sugar consumption continues to be at odds with scientific facts.

Normal physiological conditions and disease states affect carbohydrate metabolism, which is reflected in serum glucose levels. For adults with diabetes, a blood glucose level that is greater than 130 mg/dL before meals or greater than 180 mg/dL 2 hours after meals is considered to be **hyperglycemia**.[14] A blood glucose level less than 70 mg/dL is known as **hypoglycemia**. Other factors concerning too much or too little carbohydrate are discussed subsequently.

CARBOHYDRATE EXCESS

The preponderance of evidence based on the scientific literature indicates sugar consumption at typical American levels does not directly contribute to any chronic health or behavioral problems, unless excessive sugar consumption results in energy imbalance and weight gain.[15,16] Excessive consumption of added sugars (greater than 25% of total energy) can result in an inadequate intake of micronutrients from foods alone and lack of variety of food intake needed to ensure dietary adequacy. The dietary reference intakes (DRIs) compiled by the Institute of Medicine (IOM) suggest a maximum intake of 25% or less of energy from added sugars.

In 2003, the World Health Organization (WHO) released a comprehensive report on nutrition. This report recommended people limit their added sugar intake to 10% of their total kilocalories (e.g., 12 tsp of added sugars for 2200 kcal).[17] WHO contends added sugars may be helping to fuel the worldwide obesity epidemic. The WHO decision was based on economic, social, and political issues, not on scientific evidence, to prevent and control chronic health problems. The WHO-recommended level of 10% of total kilocalories is contradictory to the 2002 recommendations of the DRIs (less than 25% of total kilocalories). The average intake of added sugars is significantly higher than the WHO-recommended level. Americans need to cut back on their added sugar intake, but the average amount currently consumed is not above the level the IOM deems would result in an inadequate diet or an amount that would contribute to chronic diseases.

Sugars contain no other nutrients (vitamins or minerals) and, when consumed as soft drinks and hard candies, provide nothing other than pleasure and energy. With increasing frequency, soft drinks are substituted for milk. Since 1977, soda has been the most popular beverage in the United States, with consumption of an average of 21 oz a day.[18] The effect of increased soda intake on milk consumption is shown in Figure 3-6. Children older than 5 years old consume more regular soft drinks than 100% fruit juice; adolescents consume more soft drinks than 100% fruit juice, milk, or fruit drinks and –ades (e.g., limeade, lemonade).[19] Consumers are drinking enormous amounts of kcalories in liquid form. Americans are now consuming almost 50 more kcalories daily of sweetened beverages compared to two decades ago.[20]

Sugar increases palatability and may improve choices of certain foods otherwise disliked. Combining sugar with other nutritious foods, as in milk used for pudding, may increase the variety of foods consumed and enjoyed.

CARBOHYDRATE DEFICIENCY

Frequently, complex carbohydrates are eliminated in an effort to lose weight. This elimination can result in an insufficient intake of B vitamins, iron, and fiber. Vitamins and

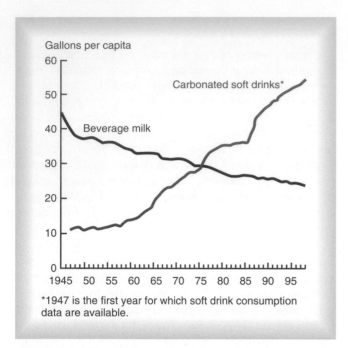

Gallons per capita

*1947 is the first year for which soft drink consumption data are available.

FIGURE 3-6 Milk consumption compared with soft drink consumption. 1947 is the first year for which soft drink consumption data are available. (From USDA's Economic Research Service. In Putnam JJ: Major trends in U.S. food supply, 1909-99. Food Rev 2000; 23[1]:8-15. Available at http://www.ers.usda.gov/publications/foodreview/jan2000/frjan2000b.pdf.)

Table 3-6	Destructive Effects of Soda versus Juices	
Type of Beverage	**Sugar (tsp)***	**pH†**
Soda (12 oz)		
Mountain Dew	11	3.16
Diet Mountain Dew	0	3.29
Surge	10.1	2.42
Coke	9.7	2.47
Diet Coke	0	3.19
Pepsi	9.8	2.51
Diet Pepsi	0	3.06
Sprite	9.4	3.24
Diet Sprite	0	3.35
Fruit Juices (12 oz)		
Orange juice	2.5	3.3-4.1
Tomato juice	<1	4.1
Lemon juice	0	2.3

*Information from National Soft Drink Association.
†Neutral pH = 7.

minerals are necessary for the body to use sugar, but these nutrients do not need to be present in the same foods. Only when sugar consumption interferes with or replaces a well-balanced intake does the diet become inadequate. When that occurs, sugar warrants the designation of "empty calorie," which indicates it is inadequate in vitamins, minerals, and trace elements. Fortification of foods has a positive effect on **nutrient density** of the diet. Nutrient density is the amount of nutrients of a food relative to the number of kilocalories it provides.

DENTAL CARIES

For many years, sucrose, the most frequently consumed form of sugar, has been considered the "arch-villain" in dental caries formation. Sucrose and other carbohydrates have unusual biochemical properties that promote bacterial growth. The presence of sucrose and other carbohydrates in the mouth increases the volume and rate of plaque biofilm formation. Even low amounts of sucrose in the mouth promote production of polysaccharides (glucans) by **Streptococcus mutans**, the bacteria that facilitate adherence of plaque biofilm to a tooth. These glucans help provide a matrix supporting communities of microorganisms collectively referred to as **plaque biofilm**. Sucrose can lower the pH of plaque biofilm, hastening the dissolution of hydroxyapatite crystals of the enamel. Glucose available from sucrose or any other carbohydrate food can be used for energy by oral bacteria in plaque biofilm.

Many health professionals and consumers falsely believe that removing sucrose from the diet would largely eliminate

dental caries. The American Dental Association (ADA) recognizes carbohydrates provide energy required for optimal nutrition. However, the ADA has recommended fermentable carbohydrates consumed frequently or repeatedly (chewable tablets, cough drops, breath mints) be replaced with products containing noncariogenic sweeteners, preferably xylitol.[21]

Despite differences in the carbohydrate content of carbonated beverages, fruit drinks, juices (about 10% carbohydrates), sport drinks (about 46% to 48% carbohydrates), energy drinks (about 9% to 10% carbohydrates), flavored coffees and teas, and powdered drinks, all of these beverages seem to have similar cariogenic potential.[22] Although federal regulations prohibit sale of soft drinks to students during lunch in most high schools, vending machines are accessible to students throughout the day. Adolescent boys consume an average of 1.5 cans of soda daily, and teenage girls consume 1 can a day. Regular sodas and energy drinks contain fermentable carbohydrates and are highly acidic (Table 3-6). Tooth erosion occurs when the enamel gradually dissolves and the outer layer is removed with frequent exposure to acidic liquids. Research suggests enamel erosion with various beverages occurs in the following order: energy drinks, sports drinks, regular soda, and diet soda.[23]

Other monosaccharides and disaccharides, such as glucose, fructose, maltose, and lactose, are also readily metabolized by oral microorganisms, with resultant demineralization of tooth enamel. These sugars diffuse rapidly into plaque biofilm to become available for bacteria. In laboratory tests, fructose and glucose rapidly lower plaque biofilm pH similar to sucrose; they are considered as cariogenic as sucrose. Substituting glucose or fructose for sucrose would not be significantly effective in reducing caries rates. Lactose is less cariogenic than other sugars. The kind of sugar is not significant; the concentration or quantity of sugar in a foodstuff is not critical to its cariogenic potential.

Most studies of large populations have correlated caries rates with total sugar consumption. Conversely, no clear-cut relationship has been shown between total carbohydrate consumption of individuals and caries. Starches can cause acid production in the plaque biofilm when consumed as part of a mixed diet containing fermentable carbohydrates. Some foods, such as potato chips or crackers, containing a high-carbohydrate, low-sugar content can be active participants in the caries process when salivary amylase hydrolyzes the complex carbohydrate to simple sugars. The starch molecule is large and cannot penetrate into plaque biofilm. Cooked and refined cereal grains are readily hydrolyzed by salivary amylases to produce maltose, which can lower the pH and demineralize enamel. Some foods high in sugar are removed quicker and do not lower the pH of plaque biofilm as much as starchy foods with less sugar. Starches, such as breads and pasta, are considered less cariogenic than sugars, but may tend to prolong the caries attack after it has been initiated, especially when sugar is added, as in sweet breads and cookies.

The total amount of dietary fermentable carbohydrate seems to be of less importance than the form in which it is eaten and the frequency of consumption. This may be related to variables influencing the length of time carbohydrate is in contact with the teeth and its potential for promoting growth of caries-forming, acid-producing bacteria. (See Chapter 17 for further discussion.)

Because of the belief that sucrose restriction would curtail dental caries, some popular snack products contain sweeteners that are less cariogenic than sucrose. Sugar alcohols may decrease the risk of dental caries through any of the following mechanisms: (1) inhibiting the growth of *S. mutans,* (2) not promoting the synthesis of plaque biofilm, or (3) not lowering plaque biofilm pH. The ADA has approved the use of the ADA seal on sugarless gums by a gum manufacturer, based on several studies. One study using sugarless gum showed 8% fewer cavities over a 3-year period, and another study showed a 39% decrease in caries over a 2-year period.[24]

Sorbitol causes only a slight pH decrease in plaque biofilm. Bacteria in plaque biofilm are able to ferment sorbitol and mannitol, but only at a very slow rate over several weeks. After a period of adaptation, however, acid production increases.

Xylitol is anticariogenic because oral bacteria lack the enzymes to ferment it; plaque biofilm pH does not decrease. An **anticariogenic** substance reduces the risk of caries by preventing bacteria from recognizing a cariogenic food. Xylitol stimulates secretion of saliva, which contains a larger number of bicarbonate ions to neutralize acid. Xylitol may inhibit growth of *S. mutans.*[5] Certain mixtures of sorbitol and xylitol may be more protective against dental caries than sorbitol alone.

Lactitol cannot be metabolized by bacteria in plaque biofilm and may provide a protective effect for teeth. However, it is only about one-third as sweet as sucrose. Saccharin inhibits tooth decay in rats. Aspartame does not support the growth of *S. mutans,* acid production, or plaque biofilm formation.

Dental Hygiene Considerations

- Approximately 90% of commonly consumed snack foods contain fermentable carbohydrates (sugars or cooked starch or both).
- Snacks contribute significantly to the nutritional intake of young children and teenagers, who need larger amounts of energy for growth.
- Patients unable to tolerate adequate amounts at meals require snacks to promote healing and avoid loss of lean tissue.
- Although sucrose is a major factor in caries risk, provide factual information that does not overblame or overclaim sugar's role in caries formation.
- Some foods, such as milk and aged cheese, actually protect the teeth by increasing the pH of the mouth and inhibiting acid production. If snacks are needed when oral hygiene cannot be performed, suggest snacks consisting of low-fat milk products or aged cheese.
- Total elimination of sweets permanently is unrealistic. The best advice is to (1) use sugar in moderation, (2) limit the frequency of sugar exposure, and (3) brush the teeth after consuming sugar-containing products. If brushing cannot be performed, chew xylitol-containing gum.
- Encourage nutrient-dense beverages (100% fruit juice, milk) and water as a part of a varied diet.
- Excessive intake (more than 20 g per day) of sorbitol-containing sugar-free gum and sweets may lead to unintended weight loss as a result of chronic diarrhea.[25] One stick of sugar-free gum contains about 1.25 g sorbitol.

Nutritional Directions

- Counsel patients that they can maintain healthy teeth and still include sweet-tasting foods without increasing the risk of caries.
- The most important cause of dental caries is the frequency of intake of fermentable carbohydrates, which supply substrate to the caries-producing oral bacteria.
- The potential for caries exists every time a carbohydrate is eaten because most foods promote acid formation if no procedures are taken to remove food debris or plaque biofilm, to buffer the acid produced, or to interfere with acid production.
- The amount of carbohydrate in a food is unrelated to its caries-forming potential; all carbohydrate foods are potentially cariogenic. Proteins and fats are **cariostatic**, or cannot be metabolized by microorganisms in plaque biofilm, and are caries-inhibiting.
- Natural sugars, primarily fructose and glucose, in unprocessed foods, such as bananas and raisins, are potentially as cariogenic as sucrose.
- Vegetables such as lettuce, celery, and broccoli contain carbohydrate (5 g per serving), but do not cause acid production or demineralization of enamel in humans.
- Sugar alcohols are less likely to promote caries; xylitol seems to prevent caries formation.
- Highly acidic foods may prevent bacterial fermentation, but cause enamel erosion.
- Replacing potentially cariogenic snacks with foods such as fresh fruits and vegetables; low-fat cottage cheese, cheese, and yogurt; peanuts; or low-fat popcorn can decrease caries and promote other health-conscious nutritional habits.

- To prevent dental caries, (1) always brush after eating, and (2) eat fermentable carbohydrates as part of a meal rather than as snacks.
- Using a straw with beverages such as carbonated drinks may lessen contact with the teeth and may lessen the risk of caries.[26]
- Consumption of sodas should be limited to 8 oz or less daily with a meal. If brushing teeth after drinking the soda is not possible, rinse the mouth with water or chew gum containing xylitol.
- High-carbohydrate foods, especially complex unrefined carbohydrates, are high in fiber and other nutrients.

OBESITY

A common misperception is that sugar is uniquely fattening. Because the taste of sugar is so pleasant, some rationalize that sugar becomes irresistible to the point of overconsumption or addiction. However, most individuals have a limit as to how sweet they like their foods and how much they can consume in a given period.

No evidence exists that carbohydrates or sugars are a cause of obesity. A higher intake of whole grains (about three servings daily) was associated with healthier body weights and fat stores.[27] Excessive caloric intake leads to obesity, whether from carbohydrates, proteins, fats, or alcohol. Although excessive energy intake from sugar may lead to obesity, epidemiological studies and several individual studies have shown that obese patients actually consume less sugar than thin patients.[15] Many sweet foods contain large amounts of fat. Too much carbohydrate is likely to be consumed when fat is limited and overall food intake is not restricted to some degree.

Dental Hygiene Considerations

Scientific studies do not support the claim that sugars interfere with bioavailability of vitamins, minerals, or trace nutrients, or the notion that dietary imbalances are preferentially caused by increased sugar consumption.[15] Do not assume that because a patient is obese, increased sugar intake is the culprit.

Nutritional Directions

- A well-balanced diet that contains adequate nutrients with appropriate amounts of fruits and vegetables and milk and dairy products is advisable.
- Several organs depend on glucose to function. A change to a minimal-carbohydrate, high-protein, high-fat diet may result in an inadequate intake of numerous nutrients.

SUGAR SUBSTITUTES

The practice of flavoring foods without additional kilocalories is one of many approaches to the problems of excess energy intake and a sedentary lifestyle. The use of sugar substitutes also has beneficial ramifications for dental hygiene. The desire to decrease sugar consumption is being met through widespread and increasing use of numerous sugar substitutes. Consumption of low-calorie sweeteners is increasing faster than that of caloric sweeteners.

These products are used principally for their sweetening power, but they also make some foods more palatable. The large variety of sweeteners is desirable because each has certain advantages and limitations. Because each sweetener has different properties, the availability of various products helps satisfy various flavor and texture requirements in foods and beverages. Sweeteners may be combined because of their **synergistic** effect—that is, when combined, sweeteners yield a sweeter taste than that provided by each sweetener alone.

Although taste buds may be fooled by their sweetness, non-nutritive sweeteners do not produce a prolonged feeling of satiety and could prompt overeating. An emerging body of scientific evidence suggests artificial sweeteners offer little help to dieters and may help promote weight gain.[28] Concerns have been expressed that nonnutritive sweeteners may promote energy intake and contribute to obesity. Most of the possible mechanisms by which this occurs are not supported by available evidence. Resolution of this important issue will require long-term randomized controlled trials.[29]

Use of these non-nutritive sweeteners may or may not decrease the total kilocaloric intake, depending on other food choices. Making compensatory food choices, such as drinking a diet carbonated beverage to permit a piece of cheesecake, is ineffective in weight control, whereas replacing a high-calorie food with a low-calorie food, watching other food intake, and engaging in some form of exercise may be beneficial.

Many patients question the safety of these products. All products on the market have been extensively researched and are safe for most people if consumed in moderation except for aspartame. Aspartame should be avoided by patients who have **phenylketonuria**, a genetic disorder characterized by an inability to metabolize the amino acid phenylalanine. Table 3-7 summarizes information regarding sugar substitutes.

Dental Hygiene Considerations

- Sugar substitutes can reduce the energy content and decrease cariogenicity of a product. Used in moderation, sugar substitutes are beneficial for many people, especially patients with diabetes.
- Because aspartame contains phenylalanine, aspartame-containing products are labeled to warn patients with phenylketonuria to avoid their use.
- Use of sugar substitutes is especially advocated for between-meal snacks to decrease frequency of exposure of the teeth to sugar. For individuals who do not need to decrease energy intake, sugar alcohols may be recommended.
- Sugar substitutes are nonfermentable and do not promote caries formation; antimicrobial activity has not been observed. Saccharin and aspartame exhibit microbial inhibition and caries suppression.

Nutritional Directions

- Non-nutritive sweeteners may not have cariogenic potential. However, bulking ingredients that allow them to pour and measure more like sugar and other constituents of a product may have cariogenic potential because of the presence of fermentable carbohydrates.
- Non-nutritive sweeteners do nothing to appease the appetite, but they do provide the pleasure of sweetness. They may enable patients to choose a wide variety of foods while managing their caloric or cariogenic intake.
- When deciding whether a young child should be given foods sweetened with a non-nutritive sweetener, consider the child's body weight, and limit the sweetener to below recommended levels (500 mg/day for saccharin, 50 mg/kg body weight for aspartame, and 15 mg/kg body weight for Acesulfame-K).
- One packet of Sweet 'n Low (Cumberland Packing Corp) contains 40 mg of saccharin; one packet of Sweet One (Stadt Corp), 50 mg of acesulfame; and one packet of Equal (Nutrasweet Co), 35 mg of aspartame. (Because there are no known side effects for sucralose, no maximum limits have been established for children). Remember, children need energy for growth and development.
- Combinations of sweeteners can produce a sweet taste more similar to that of sugar than can a single high-intensity sweetener.
- During pregnancy, saccharin is not recommended because it is known to cross the placenta. Refer a pregnant patient to her obstetrician for counseling about use of any non-nutritive sweeteners.

HEALTH APPLICATION 3   High-Fructose Corn Syrup

In recent years, the lay press has drawn a lot of attention to several studies regarding high-fructose corn syrup (HFCS) and its association with the current obesity epidemic, diabetes mellitus, and other maladies. HFCS has been labeled "the devil's candy," "the crack of sweeteners," and "a sinister invention." Consumers are specifically concerned about HFCS; many of their changes in food choices are driven by an effort to lose weight.

HFCS was so named because it is made from corn; however, it is different from regular corn syrup, which is composed of glucose and glucose polymers. Some of the glucose molecules in corn are changed into fructose, making HFCS sweeter. The enzymatic processes involved in the production of HFCS are used to produce other foods and ingredients that are considered natural. The U.S. Food and Drug Administration (FDA) has stated that HFCS may be labeled as a natural ingredient.

HFCS has a ratio of fructose to glucose identical to sucrose and honey; in other words, it contains nearly equal amounts of fructose and glucose. It is comparable to sugar and honey in its sweetness and the way it is processed in the body. It was designed to be equal to sucrose in sweetness so that they could be used interchangeably in foods and beverages. HFCS has been used principally in carbonated beverages and fruit preparations because of its stability in acidic products. After fructose and glucose (from sucrose, HFCS, or honey) are absorbed from the intestinal tract, each enters into its own metabolic pathway, just as the fructose and glucose molecules from sucrose. After

fructose and glucose reach the bloodstream, the human body cannot distinguish these sweeteners from one another. Many studies have shown that HFCS does not prompt the production of hormones that help regulate appetite and fat storage, and scientific evidence does not indicate that HFCS alters metabolism uniquely to promote deposition of body fat.[30-35] Fructose can produce elevated levels of triglycerides, which have been linked to an increased risk of heart disease.

The Center for Food, Nutrition and Agriculture Policy organized an expert panel to discuss the relationship between the consumption of HFCS or "soft drinks" and weight gain. After studying the published scientific literature, the expert panel concluded that HFCS does not seem to contribute to overweight and obesity any differently than do other energy sources.[36]

HFCS currently accounts for about 10% of sweeteners used around the world. Many other countries are seeing increasing rates of obesity and diabetes even though little or no HFCS is present in their food supply.[37] As a result of the availability of HFCS, sucrose use has declined from 80% of total caloric sweetener in 1970 to 40% in 1997.[38] Body mass index (BMI) values continued to increase between 1997-2004, whereas per capita consumption of HFCS remained stable (see Fig. 3-2).[2] Overconsumption of either sweetener, or any caloric-containing food or beverage, along with fats and decreased physical activity contribute to weight gain.

Table 3-7	Non-nutritive Sweeteners					
	Acesulfame K	**Aspartame**	**Neotame**	**Saccharin**	**Sucralose**	**Stevia (Rebaudioside A)**
Description	Noncaloric crystalline sweetener; 200 times sweeter than sucrose	Non-nutritive noncaloric sweetener made from two amino acids, phenylalanine and aspartic acid; 200 times sweeter than sucrose	Noncaloric sweetener; derivative of two amino acids, aspartic acid and phenylalanine; 7000-13,000 times sweeter than sucrose	Noncaloric sweetener; 300 times sweeter than sucrose	Noncaloric sweetener made from sucrose; 600 times sweeter than sucrose	Noncaloric sweetener derived from a South American plant; more than 300 times sweeter than sucrose
Assets	Clean, quickly perceptible sweet taste; no aftertaste; excellent shelf life; synergistic effect with other low-calorie sweeteners; stable under high temperatures; does not promote tooth decay	Clean, quickly perceptible sweet taste; no aftertaste; intensifies and extends flavors; does not promote tooth decay	Clean, sugar-like taste; unique flavor enhancement properties	Stable shelf life; synergistic effect with other low-calorie sweeteners	Clean, quickly perceptible sweet taste that tastes like sugar; no aftertaste; retains sweetness over a wide range of temperature and storage conditions and in solutions over time; can replace sugar in equal amounts; does not promote tooth decay, cancer, genetic changes, birth defects	Extremely sweet; slower onset and longer duration than sucrose; works synergistically with other sweeteners; readily soluble in water
Limitations	Blended with other low-calorie sweeteners, provides improved taste	Loses sweetness with lengthy heating or baking; not recommended for clients with phenylketonuria	None identified	Slight aftertaste	None identified	Exhibits a menthol-like or liquorice aftertaste

Safety	Tested in approximately 90 studies; JECFA† established an ADI‡ of 15 mg/kg of body weight	Most thoroughly studied ingredient in the food supply; more than 3 decades in more than 500 studies indicate aspartame is safe.§ ADI of 50 mg/kg of body weight/day	More than 100 scientific studies show its safety	Over a century of safe human use; research indicates that saccharin is unlikely to cause cancer in humans, based on more than 30 human studies that found no association between saccharin and bladder cancer	More than 100 studies over a 20-year period show the safety of sucralose	Little to no stevia is absorbed; used for decades in Japan, Korea, Taiwan, Thailand, Malaysia, Paraguay, Brazil, and Uruguay to flavor beverages, desserts, and sauces
Status	Approved by FDA in July 1988 and reaffirmed its safety by broadening its approval	Approved for use by regulatory bodies of more than 100 countries	Approved by FDA in 2002; approved for use in Australia and New Zealand	Warning label removed in 1977; government, scientists, and industry agree that saccharin is safe	Approved for use in the U.S. in 1998, approving it as a "general purpose" sweetener in 1999; approved in more than 40 countries	Approved by FDA in December 2008 for use as a general-purpose sweetener in foods, excluding meat and poultry products‖

Data from Low-Calorie Sweeteners fact sheets: Downloaded from www.caloriecontrol.org. Calorie Control Council, 5775 Peachtree-Dunwoody Road, Ste 500-G, Atlanta, GA 30342. Accessed February 2, 2008.
†JECFA, Joint Expert Committee on Food Additives.
‡ADI, acceptable daily intake.
§Magnuson BA, et al: Aspartame: a safety evaluation based on current use levels, regulations, and toxicological and epidemiological studies. Crit Rev Toxicol 2007 Sep; 37(8):629-727.
‖Center for Food Safety and Applied Nutrition, U.S. FDA. Agency response letter GRAS Notice No GRN 000253. Available at www.cfsan.fda.gov/~rdb/opa-g253.html. Accessed January 16, 2009.)

CASE APPLICATION FOR THE DENTAL HYGIENIST

A healthy patient needs information on how to eat less refined sugar and more complex carbohydrates. He knows this regimen is encouraged, but does not know all the health reasons. Fiber intake is also important to him, but he is not knowledgeable about the types of food needed or the benefits.

Nutritional Assessment
- Willingness/motivation to learn
- Usual dietary habits; focus especially on carbohydrate
- Basic knowledge of carbohydrate and carbohydrate principles
- Usual food/nutrient intake
- Financial status, employment status, and where most of the food is consumed
- Support system—family, friends, coworkers
- Use of community resources
- Food shopping practices

Nutritional Diagnosis
Health-seeking behavior related to lack of knowledge concerning carbohydrate and carbohydrate principles for optimal nutrition.

Nutritional Goals
The patient will consume a high-fiber food and complex carbohydrate foods daily, and state three principles concerning carbohydrate.

Nutritional Implementation
Intervention: Explain that (1) the main function of carbohydrate is to provide energy for the body; (2) that excessive amounts of carbohydrate by themselves do not cause obesity, but excessive overall caloric intake increases body fat (and consequently weight); and (3) the role of carbohydrate in the dental caries process and enhancing plaque biofilm formation.
Rationale: Knowledge corrects misinformation.
Intervention: (1) Follow suggestions in Table 3-4. (2) Explain the importance of fiber. Recommend 30 to 38 g of fiber daily, and help the patient plan a diet that will provide this amount, incorporating his food preferences. Stress the importance of adequate fluid intake.
Rationale: These suggestions increase fiber in the diet. Fiber increases stool bulk, exercising digestive tract muscles and

preventing them from being chronically contracted. Muscle tone is maintained, colonic pressure is diminished, and the gut is able to resist bulging out into pouches. Additionally, fiber slows starch hydrolysis and delays glucose absorption.
Intervention: Explain sources of complex carbohydrates and fiber sources, and provide the patient with a list of these foods. Emphasize the importance of increasing fiber intake gradually and increasing noncariogenic, noncaloric fluid intake when increasing fiber.
Rationale: The patient's increased knowledge will encourage him to increase consumption of complex carbohydrate and fiber.
Intervention: (1) Recommend substituting non-nutritive sweeteners for sugar, especially at snacktime. (2) Read a label with the patient to determine how to recognize sugars (they usually end in *-ose*). (3) Recommend substituting fresh fruit for juices to increase fiber. (4) Instruct him to limit products that contain complex carbohydrates and sugar, such as cookies and pastries.
Rationale: He wanted to reduce refined sugar intake, and these measures will help meet this personal goal.
Intervention: Refer him to a registered dietitian and county extension agencies.
Rationale: These will provide expert knowledge and community resources for continued compliance.
Intervention: Review labeling: (1) "no sugar added" means sugar was not added, although the product may naturally contain sugar; (2) "sugar-free" means the product contains no added sucrose, but may have other sugars added, such as sorbitol; (3) a high-fiber food has been defined as containing 5 g or more per serving; (4) incorporate foods with 3 g or more of fiber per serving.
Rationale: Knowing the meaning of these terms facilitates making healthy food choices.

Evaluation
The patient consumes a bran muffin, beans, or other high-fiber foods daily and verbalizes that carbohydrates provide energy and fiber, carbohydrate has several roles in maintaining gut functioning, and most sugars end in *-ose*. Other indicators of success include reading a label correctly, modifying intake of refined sugars, and using the community resources.

STUDENT READINESS

1. Differentiate between the three classes of carbohydrates.
2. Identify sources of complex carbohydrates in the diet.
3. What are the main sources of fiber in the American diet? What are the main sources of starch?
4. List three of your favorite foods high in added sugar. What realistic modifications can you make to your diet with respect to these high-sugar foods?
5. Explain the functions of sugars and fiber in the diet in terms a patient can understand.

6. From cereal boxes at the local grocery store, identify some of the products that claim to be high in fiber: (a) evaluate the source of fiber on the ingredient label to determine if those are soluble or insoluble fibers, and (b) rank the cereals according to the amount of dietary fiber they contain. Which would you recommend?
7. Based on ready-to-eat cereals available at the grocery store, list five that name a whole grain as the first ingredient.
8. Discuss why a diet with limited amounts of carbohydrate is neither healthy nor wise.
9. How would you advise a mother who has been told she should never give her infant anything that contains sugar because the infant will develop a sweet tooth?

10. Match the carbohydrates on the left with the appropriate answer in the right column.

Dextrose	Cannot be used by the body
Glycogen	Milk
Fructose	Sweetest sugar
Lactose	Glucose
Cellulose	Storage form of carbohydrate in the body

CASE STUDY

A 22-year-old African-American man presents with four carious lesions acquired since his last dental hygiene recall appointment. While questioning the patient, you learn that he frequently skips meals and relies heavily on snacks to get him through the day.

1. What further information about his dietary intake do you need?
2. Could the patient's snacking habits be related to his increase in dental caries?
3. Which types of foods should be suggested as snack foods and why?
4. What other precautions could the patient practice that might be helpful in preventing further caries problems?

References

1. Wells HF, Buzby JC: Dietary assessment of major trends in U.S. Food consumption, 1970-2005, Economic Information Bulletin No. 33, ERS, USDA, March 2008.
2. Wells HF, Buzby JC: High fructose corn syrup usage may be leveling off. Amber Waves (serial online): www.ers.usda.gov/AmberWaves/February08/Findings/HighFructose.htm. Accessed February 8, 2008.
3. USDA, ERS Briefing rooms, sugar and sweeteners data tables. Available at www.ers.usda.gov/Briefing/Sugar/Data.htm. Accessed August 29, 2008.
4. Phipps K, Bruer B: Caries prevention arsenal. Dimens Dental Hyg 2004; 2(16):16-18.
5. Maguire A, Rugg-Gunn AJ: Xylitol and caries prevention: is it a magic bullet? Br Dent J 2003; 194:429-436.
6. Mäkinen KK, et al: Thirty-nine-month xylitol chewing-gum program in initially 8-year-old school children: a feasibility study focusing on mutans streptococci and lactobacilli. Int Dent J 2008 Feb; 58(1):41-50.
7. Lemes U, et al: Effects of resistant starch type III polymorphs on human colon microbiota and short chain fatty acids in human gut models. J Agric Food Chem 2008 Jul 9; 56(13):5415-5421.
8. Merchant AT, et al: Whole-grain and fiber intakes and periodontitis risk in men. Am J Clin Nutr 2006; 83:1395-1400.
9. Institute of Medicine (IOM), National Academy of Sciences: Dietary Reference Intakes for Energy, Carbohydrates, Fiber, Fat, Protein, and Amino Acids (Macronutrients). Washington, DC: National Academy Press, 2002. Available at http://www.nap.edu./books/0309085373/html/.
10. U.S. Department of Agriculture, Agricultural Research Service: Nutrient intakes from food: mean amounts and percentages of calories from protein, carbohydrate, fat, and alcohol, one day, 2003-2004. Available at www.ars.usda.gov/ba/bhnrc/fsrg. Accessed August 29, 2008.
11. Wells HF, Buzby JC: Dietary assessment of major trends in U.S. food consumption, 1970-2005. Economic Information Bulletin No. 33. Economic Research Service, U.S. Department of Agriculture, March 2008.
12. Slavin JL: Position of the American Dietetic Association: Health implications of dietary fiber. J Am Diet Assoc 2008 Oct; 108(10):1716-1731.
13. Grandjean AC, et al: Popcorn consumption and dietary and physiological parameters of US children and adults: Analysis of the National Health and Nutrition Examination Survey (NHANES) 1999-2002 dietary survey data. J Am Diet Assoc 2008 May; 108(5):853-856.
14. American Diabetes Association: Standards of medical care in diabetes—2009. Diabetes Care 2009 Jan; 32(Suppl 1): S13-S61.
15. International Food Information Council Foundation (IFIC): The science of sugars. Food Insight, May/Jun 2008.
16. ADA Reports: Position of the American Dietetic Association: use of nutritive and nonnutritive sweeteners. J Am Diet Assoc 2004 Feb; 104(2):255-275.
17. Joint FAO/WHO Expert Consultation: Diet, Nutrition, and the Prevention of Chronic Diseases. Geneva, Switzerland: World Health Organization, 2003. Available at ftp://ftp.fao.org/es/esn/nutrition/diet_prevention_disease.pdf.
18. Popkin BM, et al: A new proposed guidance system for beverage consumption in the United States. Am J Clin Nutr 2006 Mar; 83(3):529-542.
19. Rampersaud GS, Bailey LB, Kauwell GP: National survey beverage consumption data for children and adolescents indicate the need to encourage a shift toward more nutritive beverages. J Am Diet Assoc 2003 Jan; 103(1):97-100.
20. Bleich SN et al. Increasing consumption of sugar-sweetened beverages among US adults: 1988-1994 to 1999-2004. Am J Clin Nutr 2009 Jan; 89(1):372-381.
21. Touger-Decker R, Mobley CC; American Dietetic Association: Position of the American Dietetic Association: oral health and nutrition. J Am Diet Assoc 2007 Aug; 107(8):1418-1428.
22. Oliver MM, Drause PR: Powering up with sports and energy drinks. J Pediatr Health Care 2007 Jun; 21(6): 413-416.
23. Owens BM, Kitchens M: The erosive potential of soft drinks on enamel surface substrate: an in vitro scanning electron microscopy investigation. J Contemp Dent Pract 2007 Nov 1; 8(7):11-20.
24. Horovitz B: Dentists smile on sugarless gums' impact. Available at www.usatoday.com/money/industries/food/2007-09-24-gum_N.htm. Accessed September 25, 2007.
25. Bauditz J, et al: Lesson of the week: severe weight loss caused by chewing gum. BMJ 2008 Jan 12; 336:96-97.
26. Bassiouny MA, Yang J: Influence of drinking patterns of carbonated beverages on dental erosion. Gen Dent 2005 May-Jun; 53(3):205-210.
27. Harland JI, Garton LE: Whole-grain intake as a marker of healthy body weight and adiposity. Public Health Nutr 2008 Jun; 11(6):554-563.
28. Hampton T: Sugar substitutes linked to weight gain. JAMA 2008 May 14; 299(18):2137-2138.
29. Mattes RD, Popkin BM. Nonnutritive sweetener consumption in humans: effects on appetite and food intake and their putative mechanisms. Am J Clin Nutr 2009 Jan; 89(1):1-14.
30. Stanhope KL, et al: Twenty-four-hour endocrine and metabolic profiles following consumption of high-fructose corn syrup-, sucrose-fructose-, and glucose-sweetened beverages with meals. Am J Clin Nutr 2008 May; 87(5): 1194-1203.
31. Soenen S, Westerterp-Plantenga MS: No differences in satiety or energy intake after high-fructose corn syrup, sucrose

or milk preloads. Am J Clin Nutr 2007 Dec; 86(6): 1586-1594.

32. Akhavan T, Anderson GH: Effects of glucose-to-fructose ratios in solutions on subjective satiety, food intake, and satiety hormones in young men. Am J Clin Nutr 2007 Nov; 86(5):1254-1263.

33. Monsivais P, Perrigue MM, Drewnowski A: Sugars and satiety: Does the type of sweetener make a difference? Am J Clin Nutr 2007 Jul; 86(1):116-123.

34. Melanson KJ, et al: Effects of high-fructose corn syrup and sucrose consumption on circulating glucose, insulin, leptin, and ghrelin and on appetite in normal-weight women. Nutrition 2007 Feb; 23(2):103-112.

35. Wylie-Rosett J: Hot topic: high fructose corn syrup. American Dietetic Association. Available at http://www.eatright.org/ada/files/Hot.pdf. Accessed August 29, 2008.

36. Forshee RA, et al: A critical examination of the evidence relating high fructose corn syrup and weight gain. Crit Rev Food Sci Nutr 2007; 47(6):561-582.

37. White JS, Foreyt JP: Ten myths about high-fructose corn syrup. Food Technology 2006 Oct; 60(10):96.

38. USDA: U.S. per Capita Food Consumption. Beltsville, MD: U.S. Department of Agriculture, Economic Research Services, 2006.

Chapter 4

Protein: The Cellular Foundation

OUTLINE

AMINO ACIDS

CLASSIFICATION

PHYSIOLOGICAL ROLES

REQUIREMENTS

SOURCES

UNDERCONSUMPTION AND HEALTH-RELATED
PROBLEMS

OVERCONSUMPTION AND HEALTH-RELATED
PROBLEMS

LEARNING OBJECTIVES

*Upon completion of this chapter, the student will be able
to achieve the following objectives:*
- List the possible fates of amino acids.
- Classify foods as sources of high-quality or lower-
  quality proteins.
- Explain how protein foods can be used to complement
  one another.
- Plan menus to include the recommended protein level
  for a meat-containing diet and a vegetarian diet.

- Explain why various physiological states require
  different amounts of protein.
- State the problems associated with protein deficiency
  or excess.
- Assess a patient's protein consumption in terms of
  deficiency or excess.
- Incorporate nutrition principles regarding food intake
  to prevent protein deficiency and protein excess into
  patient counseling.

KEY TERMS

Ad libitum
Amino acids
Bioavailability
Collagen
Complementary foods
Conditionally essential amino acids
Dipeptide
Erythema
Essential amino acids (EAAs)
Flexitarians

High-quality protein
Immune response
Immunocompromised
Immunoglobulins
Interstitial
Kwashiorkor
Lactovegetarian
Low-quality protein
Marasmus
Necrosis

Necrotizing ulcerative gingivitis (NUG)
Nitrogen balance
Nonessential amino acids (NEAAs)
Noma
Ovolactovegetarian
Ovovegetarian
Periodontium
Polypeptide

Protein digestibility corrected amino acid (PDCAA)
  score
Protein-energy malnutrition (PEM)
Radical group
Sarcopenia
Secretory immunoglobulin A (sIgA)
Thermogenesis
Vegan

 Test Your NQ

1. **T/F** A protein deficiency during childhood may lead to increased caries susceptibility related to alterations in tooth development and diminished salivary flow.
2. **T/F** Brown-shelled eggs are more nutritious than white-shelled eggs.
3. **T/F** Gelatin is a good source of high-quality protein.
4. **T/F** Older patients require less protein than younger adults.
5. **T/F** High protein intake strengthens the enamel of the tooth.
6. **T/F** An increase in protein intake without decreasing intake of other energy-containing nutrients may lead to an increase in fat stores rather than muscle.
7. **T/F** Amino acids are the building blocks of proteins.
8. **T/F** Marasmus is a protein-deficiency disorder.
9. **T/F** Lactovegetarians eat eggs and plant foods.
10. **T/F** Positive nitrogen balance occurs during periods of growth.

Until the middle of the 19th century, many scientists thought all life was composed of a single basic chemical: protein. Protein is present in each living cell, making up almost half of the dry weight of a cell. Second to water, protein is the most plentiful substance in the body. The United States is a nation of meat eaters, more so now than ever. Most Americans are unable or unwilling to plan a balanced meal without a meat entree. High-protein diets have been increasingly popular for weight reduction for many years, contributing to increased protein consumption. Although chicken and fish are being chosen more often, beef is still the major source of animal protein (Fig. 4-1).

AMINO ACIDS

Proteins are very large molecular structures containing the elements carbon, hydrogen, oxygen, nitrogen, and sometimes sulfur and phosphorus. **Amino acids** are the basic building blocks for proteins. All the billions of proteins associated with life are made from combinations of 20 different amino acids. Amino acids can be compared to letters of the alphabet used in different sequences and combinations to make billions of words. An amino acid contains a basic, or amino, grouping (—NH$_2$) and an acidic, or carboxyl,

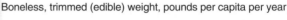
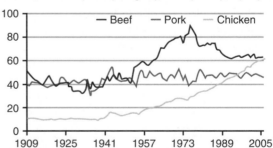

Boneless, trimmed (edible) weight, pounds per capita per year

Note: Food availability data serve as proxies for actual food consumption. Figures are calculated on the basis of raw and edible meat. Excludes edible offals, bones, and viscera for red meat. Includes skin, neck, and giblets for poultry (chicken and turkey). Excludes game consumption for red meat. Excludes use of chicken for commercially prepared pet food.

FIGURE 4-1 The amount of chicken available for consumption has steadily increased in the past 30 years. (Data from the U.S. Department of Agriculture and Economic Research Service. In Buzby J, Farah H: Chicken consumption continues longrun rise. Amber Waves 2006 Apr; [serial online]: www.ers.usda.gov/AmberWaves/April06/Findings/Chicken.htm.)

grouping (—COOH). The general design of an amino acid is as follows:

$$\text{Radical group---}\underset{\underset{\text{H}}{|}}{\overset{\overset{\text{NH}_2\quad(\text{amino group})}{|}}{\text{C}}}\text{---COOH}\quad(\text{acid group})$$

The distinguishing feature of amino acids is the amine group, which is the body's source of nitrogen. The fundamental constituent of the protein molecule, called a **radical group**, is the part of the structure that varies to form 22 different amino acids.

Amino acids combine with each other to make long chains. Two amino acids together form a **dipeptide**, as shown:

$$\text{Radical---}\underset{\underset{\text{H}}{|}}{\overset{\overset{\text{NH}_2}{|}}{\text{C}}}\overset{\overset{\text{O}}{\|}}{}\text{---NH---}\overset{\overset{\text{H}}{|}}{}\overset{\overset{\text{O}}{\|}}{\text{C}}\text{---C---OH}$$

Peptide linkage

Several amino acids bound together form a **polypeptide**. Food and body proteins contain polypeptides. The number of amino acids in proteins varies greatly (from 100 to 300), but each protein has a specific number.

CLASSIFICATION

A very important classification of amino acids is whether they are essential or nonessential. **Essential amino acids (EAAs)** are required in the diet. **Nonessential amino acids (NEAAs)** are essential for the body, but because they can be made from EAAs, they are not required in the diet. The nine EAAs are listed in Box 4-1. If any one of the EAAs is unavailable when the cell needs it for protein synthesis, the protein cannot be produced. The body is able to make adequate amounts of NEAAs if a sufficient amount of protein is available to furnish the nitrogen needed and enough kilocalories are present to spare the catabolism (breakdown) of amino acids. Other amino acids, called **conditionally essential amino acids**, are essential in certain nutritional or disease states or in certain stages of development; these are arginine, cysteine, tyrosine, glutamine, glycine, and proline.

The amount of EAAs furnished by a food determines its ability to support growth, maintenance, and repair. A food with all the EAAs present is identified as a complete protein food. When the nine EAAs are provided from a food in amounts adequate to maintain nitrogen balance (Box 4-2) and permit growth, the food is referenced as providing **high-quality protein**. **Nitrogen balance** refers to the balance of reactions in which protein substances are broken down or destroyed and rebuilt. Healthy individuals excrete (in feces, in urine, and from skin) the same amount of protein as is consumed from their food. A patient with a burn or illness excretes more nitrogen than is ingested. In periods of growth, as in a child or pregnant woman, the body is in a positive

---

Box 4-1 | Classification of Amino Acids

Essential Amino Acids (9)
Histidine
Isoleucine
Leucine
Lysine
Methionine
Phenylalanine
Threonine
Tryptophan
Valine

Nonessential Amino Acids (11)
Alanine
Arginine*
Aspartic acid
Asparagine
Cysteine (cystine)*
Glutamic acid
Glutamine*
Glycine*
Proline*
Serine
Tyrosine*

*Sometimes essential in certain coditions.

Box 4-2 | Nitrogen Balance*

N balance: body protein constant

$$\text{N intake} = \text{N excretion}$$

Positive N balance: increase in body protein

$$\text{N intake} > \text{N excretion}$$

Negative N balance: decrease in body protein

$$\text{N intake} < \text{N excretion}$$

Positive N Balance	Negative N Balance
Growth	Inadequate intake or protein (fasting, gastrointestinal tract diseases)
Pregnancy/lactation	Inadequate energy intake
Recovery from illnesses, surgery, or trauma	Illnesses, such as fevers, trauma, infections, or wasting diseases
Medications	Routine intake of glucocorticoids
Athletic training	Injury or immobilization
	Deficiency of EAAs
	Accelerated protein loss (albuminuria, protein-losing gastroenteropathy)
	Burns
	Increased secretion of thyroxine and glucocorticoids

*Because nitrogen is a unique component of protein metabolism, measurements of nitrogen and nitrogenous constituents in the blood and urine assess protein equilibrium in the body. Although "nitrogen balance" means that the output is equal to input, the amount of excreted nitrogen atoms is usually not the same as that ingested. For nitrogen equilibrium, not only must the diet contain the required amounts of protein, but also energy intake must be adequate to prevent protein being used for energy.

nitrogen balance (more protein is retained than is lost daily).

Complete protein foods have all the EAAs present in balanced amounts in terms of human physiological requirements. If the quantity of one or more of the EAAs in a food is insufficient for optimal protein synthesis, the food is a source of lower quality protein. **Low-quality proteins**, if fed as the only protein source, support life, but not normal growth. These include proteins found in legumes, nuts, and grains. The amino acid in short supply relative to need is referred to as the "limiting amino acid." High-quality proteins are well balanced in their EAA content.

The World Health Organization (WHO) and the U.S. Food and Drug Administration (FDA) have established a new method of evaluating protein quality.[1] **Protein digestibility corrected amino acid (PDCAA) score** is the official method of evaluating protein quality for humans. It is based on amino acid requirements of young children and corrects for digestibility. After the digestibility adjustments, proteins containing amino acids equal to or greater than requirements receive a PDCAA score of 1. Table 4-1 lists PDCAA scores for common protein in foods. Proteins not containing EAAs in adequate amounts to support life have a low PDCAA score. Vegetable and some grain proteins are less well digested than animal protein, partly because the protein is encased in cell walls that make it less available to digestive enzymes. Vegetables and grains contain all the EAAs, but because one or more EAAs are present in a very low ratio, the protein they furnish has a low PDCAA score.

Dental Hygiene Considerations

Inquire about the patient's use of amino acid supplements because toxicity and amino acid imbalance syndromes may occur when an excess of one amino acid is ingested. For example, when large doses of tryptophan are taken, toxic metabolites build up, causing an unusual autoimmune disorder.

Table 4-1	Protein Digestibility Corrected Amino Acid Score
Casein (milk protein)	1.00
Whey	1.00
Egg white	1.00
Soy bean isolate	0.99
Beef protein	0.92
Kidney beans	0.68
Garbanzo beans	0.66
Rolled oats	0.57
Lentils	0.52
Peanuts	0.52
Whole wheat	0.40

From UCLA Center for Human Nutrition. Fundamentals of Human Nutrition. Available www.cellinteractive.com/ucla/physician_ed/fund-nut.html.

Nutritional Directions

- The PDCAA score indicates how well the body can digest and use a particular protein. The higher the number, the higher the protein quality because it contains all the EAAs in adequate amounts that are easily digested and absorbed.
- Foods from animal and fish sources (except for gelatin) are high-quality proteins, but are not essential to an adequate diet.

PHYSIOLOGICAL ROLES

Proteins perform many important physiological roles. However, protein is not the only important nutrient because others are essential for the body to fully use available protein. Proteins are the principal source of nitrogen for the body and are fundamental components of all body cells. Proteins are necessary for many physiological functions, which can be classified into the following seven categories:

1. *Generation of new body tissues.* Because protein is a constituent of all cells, it is necessary for growth. During periods of increased growth (infancy, childhood, adolescence, and pregnancy) and in periods of wound healing or recovery (illness, surgery, burns, or fever), the need for protein to build new tissues is increased. In some individuals, moderately high protein consumption may stimulate muscle protein growth, favoring retention of lean muscle mass, while improving metabolism.[2]
2. *Repair of body tissues.* Body proteins are continuously being broken down, necessitating their replacement. Assessment of recent and usual protein intake is important.
3. *Production of essential compounds.* Amino acids and proteins are constituents of regulatory enzymes, hormones, and other body secretions. The structural compound **collagen** is a protein substance of connective tissue that helps support body structures, such as skin, bones, teeth, and tendons. A low protein intake may affect all of these functions.
4. *Regulation of fluid balance.* Protein dissolved in water forms a colloidal solution; in other words, it attracts water. Blood albumin (a protein) draws water from **interstitial** (space between tissue cells) fluid or cells to maintain blood volume. During protein deficiency, a decreased amount of protein in the blood causes a loss of osmotic balance, resulting in an accumulation of interstitial fluid (edema).
5. *Resistance to disease.* Antibodies, or **immunoglobulins**, the body's main protection from disease, are proteins. Low protein levels may negatively affect an individual's **immune response**, resulting in an inability to fight bacteria and other harmful organisms.
6. *Transport mechanisms.* Proteins enable insoluble fats to be transported through the blood.

Table 4-2	Recommended Dietary Allowances for Protein		
Life Stage/ Gender	Age (years)	Protein (g/kg)	Protein (g/d)
Infants	0-6 mo	1.52	9.1*
	7-12 mo	1.2	11
Children	1-3	1.05	13
	4-8	0.95	19
Males	9-13	0.95	34
	14-18	0.85	52
	19->70	0.80	56
Females	9-13	0.95	34
	14-18	0.85	46
	19->70	0.80	46
Pregnant	All ages	1.1	71 (+25 g/day)
Lactating	All ages	1.3	71 (+25 g/day)

Data from Institute of Medicine (IOM) of the National Academies: Dietary Reference Intakes for Energy, Carbohydrates, Fiber, Fat, Protein, and Amino Acids. Washington, DC: National Academy Press, 2002.

*Adequate intake (AI), based on 0.8 g protein/kg body weight for reference body weight. For healthy breastfed infants, the AI is the mean intake.

Table 4-3	Protein Recommendations for Adults*		
	g/d	g/kg	% kcal
Dietary Guidelines for Americans	90 @ 2000 kcal	—	18
IOM	56 g/day (males) 46 g/day (females)	RDA 0.8; EAR† 0.66	AMDR 10-35
DASH Diet	105 @ 2000 kcal	—	21

*Adults 19-70 years old.
†Estimated average requirement.

7. *Energy.* When the nitrogen grouping is removed, the remaining carbon skeleton can be used for energy, furnishing 4 kcal/g. Although this is not one of its main functions, protein is used in this manner when (a) caloric intake from carbohydrate and fat is inadequate, (b) protein intake exceeds requirements, and (c) EAAs are unavailable for synthesis of proteins.

REQUIREMENTS

Protein requirements for health are based on body size and rate of growth. (The body needs more protein during growth periods or for maintenance and repair of a larger body mass.) To a certain extent, the better the quality of protein (higher PDCAA score), the less quantity is required. Protein requirements are based on the assumption that EAAs and kilocalories are provided in adequate amounts.

The recommended dietary allowances (RDAs) for protein vary proportionately for different ages and stages of life to adjust for growth rates. The Institute of Medicine (IOM) has determined the daily minimum requirement of protein for adults is about 0.6 g/kg. Using 0.6 g/kg, a patient weighing 150 lb (68.2 kg) would require 41 g of protein. Because RDAs provide a margin of safety, the IOM has established 0.8 g/kg daily as the RDA. With this standard, a patient weighing 150 lb (68.2 kg) requires 56 g protein. The RDAs for protein for various stages of life are listed in Table 4-2.

Based on the *National Health and Nutrition Examination Survey* (NHANES), 2003-2004 data, protein intake averaged approximately 91 g in adults 19 to 30 years old, and decreased to about 66 g/day in elderly adults. This repre-

sents approximately 15% of total kilocalories, within the recommended amount of acceptable macronutrient distribution range (AMDR) of 10% to 35%. (See summary of protein recommendations in Table 4-3.) Males consume more protein than females. Approximately 7% to 8% of adolescent girls and 7.2% to 8.6% of elderly women consume protein levels below their estimated average requirement. Very few individuals consume protein amounts close to the highest AMDR of 35% for their age/sex group.[3]

Recent research indicates many adults may benefit from eating more than the minimum requirement, and investigators have requested that the IOM revisit protein recommendations. The conclusions of the Protein Summit in 2007 were presented in the May 2008 Supplemental issue of the *American Journal of Clinical Nutrition*.[4] Findings presented indicate higher protein diets are linked with a lower risk for chronic diseases, such as type 2 diabetes, coronary heart disease (CHD), and osteoporosis, and sarcopenia. **Sarcopenia** is the loss of muscle mass and strength with aging, a condition many believe is normal for elderly individuals.

The conclusion of the investigators at the Protein Summit was that overweight or obese and older Americans may benefit by consuming 35% of their kilocalories from protein. It was also recommended that the revised 2010 *Dietary Guidelines for Americans* address protein as a required nutrient.

When any condition of health or disease causes a significant protein loss, an increased protein intake (greater than the RDAs) prevents excessive loss of tissue and plasma proteins. Although these states increase protein requirements, RDAs have not been established for these conditions. Providing additional amounts for supplementation with high-quality proteins can help prevent protein malnutrition and shorten recovery periods. While updating the macronutrients in 2002, the IOM reviewed scientific evidence for protein requirements for healthy adults undertaking resistance or endurance exercise. They found no compelling evidence for additional protein requirements, especially because Americans commonly ingest significantly more protein than is recommended.

Ordinarily, dietary protein is restricted only in some physiological disease states affecting the liver and kidney because these organs are heavily involved in protein use and excretion of protein waste products. If the liver and kidney are diseased, excessive amounts of protein cannot be properly handled without further organ damage.

SOURCES

Foods with a high protein content are readily available in the United States. Table 4-4 lists the average protein content of some foods. Meat and milk food groups furnish most of the protein. Soy is a good source of protein and has other health benefits. An increased intake of cereal products boosts protein intake. The protein content of items from the sample menu displayed in Figure 1-2 is shown in Figure 4-2.

Depending on sex, size, and activity level, MyPyramid recommends 5 to 7 oz of cooked lean meat, poultry, or fish daily for adults. About 3 Tbsp of chopped/ground meat, or the size of a small matchbox, equals 1 oz of meat; a small chicken drumstick or thigh is equivalent to 2 oz of meat; and a deck of cards or the size of your palm is approximately 3 oz. One-half cup, or the amount that can fit in a cupped hand, of beans or 1 Tbsp of peanut butter (size of a ping-pong ball) can be substituted for 1 oz of meat.

In most cases, digestibility and nutritional value are favorably affected by cooking procedures. Proper cooking

Table 4-4 Protein Content of Selected Foods

Food	Quantity	Protein (g)
Chicken, light meat, cooked	2 oz	20
Chicken, dark meat, cooked	2 oz	18
Pork chop, lean, cooked	2 oz	16
Beef, cooked, lean cuts	2 oz	15
Pinto beans, cooked	1 cup	15
Cottage cheese	½ cup	14
Cheddar cheese	2 oz	14
Cod fish, cooked	2 oz	13
Egg, hard cooked	2	13
Thick milkshake	11 oz	12
American processed cheese	2 oz	10
Milk, whole, reduced fat, or low fat	1 cup	10
Peanut butter	2 Tbsp	8
Nonfat dried skim milk powder	⅓ cup	8
Macaroni, cooked	1 cup	7
Oatmeal, cooked	1 cup	6
Rice, white, cooked	1 cup	4
Rice, brown, cooked	1 cup	5
Ice cream, 10% fat	1 cup	5
Corn muffin, small	1	4
Enriched white bread	1 slice	2
Vegetables	½ cup	1-2
Fruits	½ cup	0.1-1

Data from USDA, Agricultural Research Service, USDA National Nutrient Database for Standard Reference, Release 20, 2008. Available at www.nal.gov/fnic/foodcomp/. Accessed February 26, 2008.

Dental Hygiene Considerations

- Most Americans consume almost twice as much protein as recommended in the RDAs.
- When assessment indicates a normal consumption of 1.5 g/kg or more above the RDA for protein, this is considered a high-protein diet. Further increases may not be beneficial and may contribute to increased fat stores and dehydration.
- An inadequate protein intake could affect any or all of the physiological functions of protein in the body. If dietary intake seems inadequate, evaluate the patient's status in the areas described in the section on Physiological Roles.
- Assessment of protein intake of patients with periodontal issues is especially important. Protein deficiencies may compromise the physiological systemic response to inflammation and infection, and periodontal problems may increase the protein requirement to promote healing in patients with inadequate or marginal protein intake.
- One rule of thumb is protein should provide 10% to 35% of caloric intake. If protein intake seems inappropriate, determine caloric or protein intake or both. The adequacy of intake can be established by using one of two methods. As an example, based on consumption of 2200 kcal/day, the *amount of protein based on total energy intake* is calculated as follows:

  $$2200\,kcal \times 0.35\,(\text{maximum recommended \% of total kilocalories from protein}) = 770\,kcal \text{ from protein or less}$$

  $$770\,kcal \div 4\,(kcal/g\,protein) = 193\,g \text{ or less of protein recommended}$$

  The intake of 193 g of protein is the highest level recommended. Because 35% is the upper limit, protein consumption above this level may jeopardize adequate intakes of nutrients provided from other food sources.

  For the second method for calculating, if protein intake is 55 g, and caloric intake is 2200 kcal, the *percentage of protein based on the actual protein intake* can be determined as follows:

  $$55\,(g\,protein) \times 4\,(kcal/g\,protein) = 220\,kcal \text{ from protein}$$

  $$220\,(\text{kilocalories from protein}) \div 2200\,(\text{total kilocalorie intake}) \times 100\,(\%) = 10\% \text{ of total kilocalories from protein}$$

  Because 10% is the lower limit, this patient's protein may be inadequate, and professional counseling may be warranted. Refer the patient to a registered dietitian.
- Do not overemphasize animal sources of protein to patients on restricted incomes (elderly, homeless, and impoverished individuals). Too much emphasis on high-protein foods may result in inadequate amounts of other nutrients in the diet, especially when the food budget is low. Complementary sources of protein (described in Health Application 4), which are less expensive, can provide adequate protein.
- Healthy patients are in nitrogen balance appropriate for their stage of life if their diet contains adequate kilocalories with the recommended number of servings from all MyPyramid food groups. Evaluate food intake by gathering data from the patient and comparing them with the recommended servings from MyPyramid for the stage of growth, and DRIs for kilocalories and protein needed.

Sample menu	Protein content (g)	Ovolactovegetarian menu*	Protein content (g)
Breakfast		*Breakfast*	
Oat bran bagel (1)	6.1	Oat bran bagel (1)	6.1
Whipped cream cheese (2 Tbsp)	0.7	Whipped cream cheese (2 Tbsp)	0.7
Seedless raisins (1/4 c)	0.8	Seedless raisins (1/4 c)	0.8
1% Low-fat milk (8 oz)	9.9	1% Low-fat milk (8 oz)	9.9
Coffee (12 oz)	0	Coffee (12 oz)	0
Morning snack		*Morning snack*	
Fresh orange (1)	1.6	Fresh orange (1)	1.6
Lunch			
Sandwich with:		Sandwich with:	
Tuna salad (1/4 c)		Low-fat monterey jack cheese (1 oz)	7.6
Tomato slices (2)	8.1	Cherry tomatoes (5)	0.4
Thinly sliced cucumber	0.4	Thinly sliced cucumber	0.2
Sliced green bell peppers (1/4 c)	0.2	Sliced green bell peppers (1/4 c)	0.2
Whole wheat bread (2 slices)	0.2	Whole wheat bread (2 slices)	6.0
Baby carrots (8)	6.0	Baby carrots (8)	0.5
Fresh apple (1)	0.5	Fresh apple (1)	0.5
Water (12 oz)	0.5	Water (12 oz)	0
	0		
Afternoon snack		*Afternoon snack*	
Diet carbonated beverage (12 oz)	0	Diet carbonated beverage (12 oz)	0
Dry roasted peanuts (1/4 c)	6.0	Dry roasted peanuts (1/4 c)	6.0
Dinner			
Lean roast beef (2 oz)	21.4	Vegetarian stew (1 c)	42.0
Brown rice (3/4 c)	3.0	Brown rice (¾ c)	3.0
Brown gravy (1/4 c)	2.2	Steamed broccoli spears (1 c)	3.2
Steamed broccoli spears (1 c)	3.2	Salad with garbanzo beans (1/4 c)	3.5
Melted reduced fat and sodium	6.0	Low calorie salad dressing (2 Tbsp)	0.1
cheddar cheese (1/4 c)		Whole wheat roll (1)	2.2
Mixed green salad (1 1/2 c)		Soft margarine (1 Tbsp)	0
Low calorie salad dressing (2 Tbsp)	0.5	Fresh cantaloupe (1 c)	0
Whole wheat roll (1)	0.1	Iced tea, unsweetened (12 oz)	0
Soft margarine (1 Tbsp)	2.2		
Fresh cantaloupe (1 c)	0		
Iced tea, unsweetened (12 oz)	0		
	0		
Evening snack		*Evening snack*	
1% Low-fat milk (8 oz)	9.9	1% Low-fat milk (8 oz)	9.9
Cinnamon graham crackers (4)	3.1	Cinnamon graham crackers (4)	3.1
Totals	92.6		107.5

*Only items changed are listed; all others are the same.

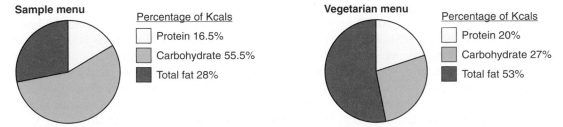

Sample menu

Percentage of Kcals
- Protein 16.5%
- Carbohydrate 55.5%
- Total fat 28%

Kilocalories 1989; carbohydrate, 283 g; protein, 92 g; fat, 64 g

Vegetarian menu

Percentage of Kcals
- Protein 20%
- Carbohydrate 27%
- Total fat 53%

Kilocalories 2125; carbohydrate, 281 g; protein, 107 g; fat, 65 g

FIGURE 4-2 Protein content of sample menu and modifications for ovolactovegetarian diet. (Nutrient data from U.S. Department of Agriculture, Agriculture Research Service. U.S. Department of Agriculture, National Nutrient Database for Standard Reference, Release 20, 2008. Available at www.nal.gov/fnic/foodcomp/ Accessed August 29, 2008.)

sometimes facilitates digestion and use. Cooking makes egg albumin more readily digestible, and cooking soybeans increases amino acid bioavailability. **Bioavailability** indicates the amount of nutrient available to the body after absorption. Processing affects proteins in cereal by binding lysine (an amino acid), making it unusable by the body.

UNDERCONSUMPTION AND HEALTH-RELATED PROBLEMS

Although protein supplies in the United States are plentiful, and drastic protein deficiency is uncommon, several groups of individuals are susceptible to insufficient intakes: (1) elderly individuals, (2) individuals with low income, (3) strict vegetarians, (4) individuals with a lack of education or who are unwilling to shop wisely, and (5) patients who are chronically ill or hospitalized (e.g., patients with AIDS, anorexia nervosa, or cancer). Fewer than 10% of U.S. adults older than 70 years of age get less than the recommended 0.8 g/kg body weight per day.[3] Consumption of protein by older Americans may be related to cost, inability to prepare nutritious meals, depression, difficulty chewing, or concerns about the fat and cholesterol content of meats. Inadequate amounts of dietary protein contribute to sarcopenia.[5]

Certain physiological conditions and impaired digestion or absorption cause excessive protein losses and may precipitate **protein-energy malnutrition (PEM)**. Although PEM is uncommon in the United States, given the above-mentioned conditions, malnutrition is frequently unrecognized. PEM is usually accompanied by other nutritional deficiencies. Separating the effects of different nutrient deficiencies by observing clinical symptoms is often difficult. PEM affects the whole body, including every component of the orofacial complex.

The occurrence of PEM during critical developmental stages, including the prenatal and postnatal periods, may affect developing tissues and can lead to irreversible changes affecting oral tissues. During tooth development, mild-to-moderate protein deficiency results in smaller molars, significantly delayed eruption, and retardation during development of the mandible. Smaller salivary glands result in diminished salivary flow; this saliva is different in its protein composition and amylase and aminopeptidase activity, compromising the immune function of the saliva.

Poor nutrition results in delayed eruption and delayed exfoliation of deciduous teeth. In addition to the increased rate of caries in malnourished children, the peak caries experience is delayed by approximately 2 years. The increased caries rate may simply be related to the length of time a tooth is in the oral cavity; if the delay in exfoliation is greater than the delay in eruption, the tooth is in the mouth a longer time, and it is exposed to caries-producing bacteria longer. Children with malnutrition (e.g., in developing countries and in many urban and rural areas in developed countries) have different dietary habits overall and oral environments that are not conducive to dental caries. However, the teeth in these populations are highly susceptible to dental caries.[6] Increased caries susceptibility may be related to alterations in structure of tooth crowns and diminished salivary flow, or changes in saliva composition may be related to malnutrition issues.

Epithelium, connective tissue, and bone also may be poorly developed. An increase in acid solubility associated with chemical alterations of the exposed enamel surface may contribute to increased caries susceptibility.

The **periodontium** includes the hard and soft tissues surrounding and supporting the teeth: gingival, alveolar mucosa, cementum, periodontal ligament, and alveolar bone. An insufficient intake of protein results in negative nitrogen balance depleting nitrogen reserves, reducing blood protein levels, and decreasing resistance of the periodontium to infections. In addition, the ability of the periodontium to withstand the stress of injury or surgery is reduced, and recovery periods are longer. In malnourished children, **secretory immunoglobulin A (sIgA)** levels are depressed. sIgA is the predominant immunoglobulin, or antibody, in oral, nasal, intestinal, and other mucosal secretions, and provides the first line of defense in the oral cavity. Low sIgA levels in malnourished children probably play a role in their increased susceptibility to mucosal infections.

PEM may be a major reason for the increased incidence of **noma** and **necrotizing ulcerative gingivitis (NUG)**, conditions that are clearly associated with depressed immune responses caused by nutritional deficiencies, stress, and infection (see Figure 18-6 in Chapter 18). Noma is a severe gangrenous process usually manifesting as a small ulcer on

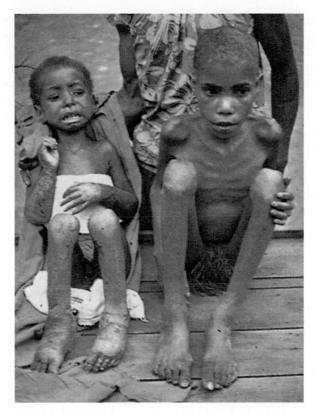

FIGURE 4-3 Kwashiorkor and marasmus in brothers. The younger brother, on the left, has kwashiorkor with generalized edema, skin changes, pale reddish yellow hair, and an unhappy expression. The older child, on the right, has marasmus, with generalized wasting, spindly arms and legs, and an apathetic expression. (From Peters W, Pasvol G [eds]: Tropical Medicine and Parasitology, 5th ed. London: Mosby, 2002.)

Dental Hygiene Considerations

- When assessing for marasmus or kwashiorkor, remember the main difference between the two conditions is the presence of some subcutaneous fat tissue in individuals with kwashiorkor and edema, especially in the abdomen, feet, and legs. Fat stores and edema are absent in marasmus. Assess the patient's financial status because poverty is a major cause of PEM and has been identified in rural and urban inner city areas.
- To assess for inadequate protein intake, look for or identify frequent or extended periods of fasting, medications that cause anorexia, abnormal food intake, nausea and vomiting, and problems with hair (dull, dry, brittle, breaks easily), skin (flaky and dry), or fingernails (dry and cracked, spoon-shaped).
- Treatment of malnutrition requires referral to a healthcare provider or a registered dietitian.
- Malnourished patients take longer to heal and regain strength and are at risk for frequent infections. Adequate infection control procedures are particularly important for these patients.
- The protein requirement of older individuals is the same as that of young adults; however, older individuals are frequently not motivated to eat because of low income level, transportation problems, depression and loneliness, edentulous status, and gustatory (taste and smell) changes. Decreased protein intake is common as a result of ill-fitting dentures or edentulousness. Closely assess protein intake of older patients.
- In the United States, noma-like lesions may occur in patients with cancer whose immune systems have been severely impaired by chemotherapy.

the gingiva that becomes necrotic and spreads to produce extensive destruction of the lips, cheek, and tissues covering the jaw. NUG is characterized by **erythema** (marginated redness of the mucous membranes caused by inflammation) and **necrosis** (degeneration and death of the cells) of the interdental papillae. This painful gingivitis is generally accompanied by a metallic taste and foul oral odor. Cratered papillae often remain after treatment of the disease.

A scenario in which NUG occasionally occurs is in college students who are under a great deal of psychological stress and have poor eating habits. It also can be observed in individuals who live in developed countries and are severely debilitated or **immunocompromised** (having an immune response that has been weakened by a disease or pharmacological agent), or in children 2 to 6 years old who live in developing countries, are malnourished, and have recently experienced a stressful event, such as a viral disease.

NUG is possibly precipitated by emotionally stressful situations that affect eating patterns, leading to acute deficiencies, and lowering the immune response to bacteria normally found in most oral cavities. Decreased host resistance to infection may permit gingival lesions to spread rapidly

into adjacent tissues, producing extensive necrosis and destruction of orofacial tissues, whereas in a healthy individual, the lesion is limited to the gingiva alone. Wound healing is also delayed (see Chapter 18 for further discussion).

In other areas of the world, where quantities of high-quality protein and kilocalories are insufficient, PEM is commonly seen. **Kwashiorkor** develops when young children receive adequate kilocalories, but not enough high-quality protein (Fig. 4-3). It usually appears after the child has been weaned from breast milk. **Marasmus** occurs in infants when protein and kilocalories are deficient in the diet.

Kwashiorkor and marasmus are very serious health problems that have received much attention by the United Nations and the WHO. Incaparina, a food powder made from corn, cottonseed, and sorghum with mineral and vitamin supplements; skim milk powder; and the addition of lysine to cereal products have been used to improve nutritional status in developing countries. However, most of these efforts to improve the status of nutrition worldwide have not been well accepted for various reasons, and the protein-energy problems in the world still exist.

OVERCONSUMPTION AND HEALTH-RELATED PROBLEMS

An upper limit for safe levels of protein intake has not been determined. Most patients believe no upper limits for protein exist. Americans frequently eat 150% to 200% of the RDA for protein. Excessive protein intake can contribute to obesity because any energy-providing nutrient consumed in excess of physiological needs is converted to fat and stored.

One concern regarding high protein intake is its effect on calcium balance. The adequate intakes (AIs) established for calcium in the United States are approximately double the recommendations for most other nations. For many years, general consensus in the medical community was that high protein intake had a negative impact on calcium and bone metabolism. Numerous studies contradict this theory, however, and research generally indicates meat intake may have a favorable impact on bone health if calcium intake is adequate, at least in older men and women.[7,8]

When protein intake is excessive, fluid imbalances may occur in all age groups, but especially in infants. Metabolism of 100 kcal of protein requires 350 g of water compared with 50 g of water for a similar amount of carbohydrates or fats. Water requirements are increased as well as the end products of protein metabolism in the bloodstream.

It is controversial whether the popular high-protein diets are excessive in protein content. Regardless, this trend has stimulated scientific research that has expanded the scientific knowledge base in this realm. Higher protein diets are beneficial for weight control by enhancing loss of body fat with less muscle loss and improved control of blood glucose levels. Dietary protein may aid in weight loss by increasing satiation; increasing muscle mass, which burns more kilocalories and increases **thermogenesis** (production of body heat); and decreasing energy efficiency.[6-16] Protein intake generally increases satiety to a greater extent than carbohydrate or fat and may facilitate a reduction in **ad libitum** (as desired) energy consumption.[2] Obtaining adequate protein, or within the upper range of recommended amounts, is an important dietary concern, especially for weight loss or management or for physical activity.

Clinicians are concerned about the long-term effects of a high-protein diet, especially when the principal source of protein is red meat and regular dairy products because of their large cholesterol and saturated fat content. A study involving 29,000 postmenopausal women found subjects who reported the highest protein intakes from red meat and dairy products had approximately a 40% higher risk of dying of heart disease than subjects with the lowest intake of these foods.[17] Although high protein intake is not associated with kidney function decline in individuals with healthy kidneys, protein intake three times the RDA can lead to kidney problems in patients with mild kidney impairment.[18,19] The American Diabetes Association recommends limiting protein intake to less than 20% of total kilocalories (100 g protein for a 2000-kcal diet).[20]

HEALTH APPLICATION   4   Vegetarianism

Despite the fact that protein is not limited in the U.S. food supply, some people choose plant sources of protein for health reasons or because of their philosophical, ecological, or religious convictions. The large numbers of vegetarian cookbooks and meatless "veggie" burgers and sausage-style products would lead one to believe vegetarianism is a growing consumer movement. The Vegetarian Resource Group indicates only 2% to 3% of the population are true vegetarians; in 2006, 6.7% of adults said they never eat meat.[21]

Technically, the major types of vegetarian diets differ in the types of foods included. In a **lactovegetarian** diet, dairy products are consumed in addition to plant foods (*lacto-* comes from the Latin word for milk, *lactis*). Meat, poultry, fish, and eggs are excluded. Milk and cheese products, which complement plant foods and enhance the amino acid content, are included. The **ovolactovegetarian** diet is supplemented with milk, cheese, and eggs (*ovo-* comes from the Latin word for egg, *ovum*). Only meat, poultry, and fish are excluded. If adequate quantities of eggs, milk, and milk products are consumed, all nutrients are likely to be provided in sufficient quantities. Strict supervision is not warranted. The **ovovegetarian** diet consists of foods from plants with the addition of eggs. Meat, poultry, fish, and dairy products are excluded. The **vegan** (or strict vegetarian) diet is the strictest type and contains only food from plants, including vegetables, fruits, and grains. No foods of animal origin are allowed (e.g., meat, milk, cheese, eggs, butter). Some "self-described" vegetarians are not true vegetarians because they occasionally eat fish and poultry. These people are known as "semi-vegetarians" or **flexitarians**.[22]

Some groups, especially Seventh-Day Adventists, supplement protein intake with many textured vegetable protein (TVP) products. These meat substitutes are produced from vegetable proteins, usually soybeans. The protein in TVP products is of good quality, but these products may have a high sodium content.

EAAs can be provided by plants, but larger amounts of these plant products must be consumed to match the protein obtained from animal sources. EAAs present in low levels in grains are abundant in other plants, such as legumes. Beans are low in methionine and tryptophan, and corn is low in lysine and threonine. When eaten together, as in pinto beans and cornbread, they are said to be **complementary foods**, and less volume is required.

Protein from a single source is seldom consumed alone. Foods are usually combined without awareness they are complementary to each other (e.g., beans are usually combined with rice, bread, or crackers [wheat], or tortillas or cornbread [corn]). When a combination of plant proteins is eaten throughout the day, the amino acids provided by each complement each other—that is, the deficiencies of one are offset by the adequacies of another. Additionally, small amounts of high-quality proteins can be combined with plant foods, as in macaroni and cheese or cereal and milk, to provide adequate amounts of EAAs. If caloric requirements are met, protein requirements are met when a variety of protein-containing foods are eaten throughout the day. The foods providing complementary amino acids do not have to be consumed at the same time.

With some basic nutrition knowledge, vegetarian foods can be selected that are healthy and nutritionally balanced. The major difference is the protein source. The Vegetarian Food Guide Pyramid and Vegetarian Food Guide Rainbow (Fig. 4-4) are designed specifically to address the nutrient inadequacies and reduced mineral bioavailability of vegetarian diets. Vegetarian diets generally result in lower dietary intake of saturated fat and cholesterol, and high levels of carbohydrate, fiber, magnesium, boron, folate, and vitamins C and E.[23] Key nutrients that may fall short of the DRI in the vegetarian diet include zinc, calcium, riboflavin, vitamins D and B_{12}, and n-3 fatty acids.[24,25] Laboratory tests show reduced blood levels of vitamins B_{12} and D and the minerals calcium, zinc, and iron in vegetarians.[26] Commonly available fortified foods (i.e., fortified breakfast cereals and nondairy soymilks) are emphasized to ensure good sources of vitamins B_{12} and D and calcium.

Box 4-3 summarizes information that can be used in planning healthy and nutritionally balanced vegetarian diets that meet calcium and vitamins B_{12} and D requirements of adults. Table 4-5 indicates changes in number of servings from the vegetarian food groups shown in Figure 4-4 to meet nutrient needs for various life stages. By using a variety of principally unrefined foods, and enough kilocalories to promote good health, protein quality and quantity and other nutrients can be adequate for most individuals.

Because of the difficulty of consuming adequate volumes of food to meet kilocaloric requirements, the vegan diet is not recommended for infants, children, or pregnant/lactating women. Breastfed infants of two vegan mothers in the United States developed brain abnormalities as a result of vitamin B_{12} deficiency.[27]

Much can be said of the healthy aspects of vegetarian diets. Vegetarian diets can meet the DRIs as long as the variety and amounts of foods are adequate. The fact that vegetarian diets and lifestyles seems to be conducive to good health is exemplified by vegetarians exhibiting better weight control, improved gastrointestinal function, fewer breast and colon cancers, better glucose control, a lower incidence of gallstones, lower blood pressure, and a decreased rate of coronary heart disease; they also live longer.[28,29] These advantages are not attributed solely to avoidance of meat products, but benefits from additional plant food selections. For instance, beans, legumes, and whole-grain products help with blood glucose control; plant foods are associated with a lower risk of cardiovascular disease. When working with a vegetarian patient, keep lines of communication open by respecting their decision, unless eating habits are potentially harmful. Patients who have an interest in pursuing a vegetarian diet should be encouraged to do so; all patients should be encouraged to have more meatless meals and to consume more plant foods.

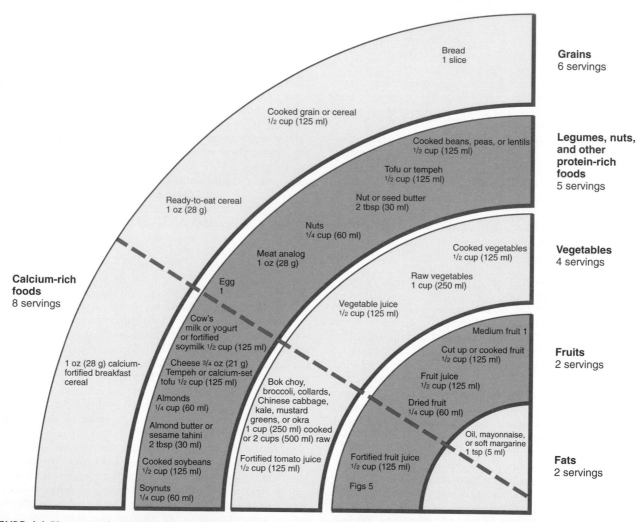

FIGURE 4-4 Vegetarian food guide rainbow. Notice the slice of the rainbow calling attention to the foods in each group that are good sources of calcium. (Redrawn from Messina V, Melina V, Mangels AR: A new food guide for North American vegetarians. J Am Diet Assoc 2003 Jun; 103[6]:771-775.)

Box 4-3	**Eight Tips for Meal Planning**

1. Choose a variety of foods.
2. The number of servings in each group is for minimum daily intakes. Choose more foods from any of the groups to meet energy needs.
3. A serving from the calcium-rich food group provides approximately 10% of adult daily requirements. Choose eight servings per day. These also count toward servings from the other food groups in the guide. For example, ½ cup (125 mL) of calcium-fortified fruit juice counts as a calcium-rich food and counts toward servings from the fruit group.
4. Include two servings every day of foods that supply n-3 fats (see Chapter 5). Foods rich in n-3 fat are found in the legumes/nuts group and in the fats group. A serving is 1 tsp of flaxseed oil, 3 tsp of canola or soybean oil, 1 Tbsp of ground flaxseed, or ¼ cup walnuts. For the best balance of fats in your diet, olive and canola oils should be chosen for cooking.
5. Nuts and seeds may be used in place of servings from the other choices in the fats group.
6. Be sure to get adequate vitamin D from daily sun exposure or through fortified foods or supplements. Cow's milk and some brands of soymilk and breakfast cereals are fortified with vitamin D.
7. Include at least three good food sources of vitamin B_{12} in your diet every day. These include 1 Tbsp of *Red Star* Vegetarian Support Formula nutritional yeast, 1 cup fortified soymilk, ½ cup cow's milk, ¾ cup yogurt, 1 large egg, 1 oz of fortified breakfast cereal, or 1½ oz of fortified meat substitute. If these foods are not consumed regularly (at least three servings per day), take a daily vitamin B_{12} supplement of 5 to 10 µg or a weekly vitamin B_{12} supplement of 200 µg.
8. If you include sweets or alcohol in your diet, consume these foods in moderation. Get most of your daily kilocalories from foods in the vegetarian food guide.

Adapted from Messina V, Melina V, Manges AR: A new food guide for North American vegetarians. J Am Diet Assoc 2003 Jun; 103(6):771-775.

Table 4-5	Modifications to the Vegetarian Food Rainbow (Fig. 4-4) for Children, Adolescents, and Pregnant and Lactating Women

	Food Group*		
Life Cycle	Vitamin B₁₂–rich Foods (servings)	Beans/Nuts/Seeds/Egg (servings)	Calcium-rich Foods (servings)
Child (4-8 years)	2	5	6
Adolescent (9-13 years)	2	6	10
Adolescent (14-18 years)	3	6	10
Pregnancy	4	7	8
Lactation	4	8	8

From Messina V, Melina V, Mangels AR: A new food guide for North American vegetarians. J Am Diet Assoc 2003 Jun; 103(6):771-775.
*The number of servings in each group is the minimum amount needed. The minimum number of servings from other groups is not different from the vegetarian food guide (see Fig. 4-4). Additional foods can be chosen from any of the groups in the vegetarian food guide to meet energy needs.

CASE APPLICATION FOR THE DENTAL HYGIENIST

A single mother of two children comes to the clinic complaining about sensitivity to hot and cold foods and bleeding gums. She has recently lost her job, and child support payments are irregular. She is very concerned about the limited amount of protein foods she is able to purchase with her food stamps. Based on her diet diary, her caloric intake is 1800 kcal, and protein is about 50 g. Food intake is principally pastas, tortillas, chips, sweet pastries, and sodas.

Nutritional Assessment
- Willingness to learn
- Knowledge base of protein, carbohydrate, and fat principles for optimal nutrition
- Cultural beliefs
- Recent percentage of kilocalories from protein (11%)
- Types of protein intake and total nutrient intake
- Overall nutrient intake
- Carbonated beverage intake

Nutritional Diagnosis
Altered health maintenance and limited nutrition knowledge related to insufficient funds to purchase foods to provide adequate nutrients.

Nutritional Goals
The patient will verbalize three principles concerning protein as well as the benefits from other nutrients. The patient will consume foods providing complementary protein and incorporate some fruits and dairy products into her menus.

Nutritional Implementation
Intervention: Teach (1) the seven functions or roles of protein, (2) the difference between EAAs and NEAAs, (3) the difference between high-quality and lower quality protein, and (4) how to incorporate complementary protein into menus.
Rationale: Knowledge corrects inaccurate information.

CASE APPLICATION FOR THE DENTAL HYGIENIST—cont'd

Intervention: Discuss cheaper sources of protein.
Rationale: Good sources of protein do not have to be high-priced meats.
Intervention: Encourage the use of milk and milk products.
Rationale: Dairy products are an excellent source of protein and provide other nutrients important to maintain health.
Intervention: Encourage incorporating fruits and vegetables into the menus.
Rationale: Protein is not the only nutrient needed to maintain good oral health. In addition, consumption of more fruits and vegetables models healthy eating to her children.
Intervention: Refer her to a social worker.
Rationale: The social worker will be knowledgeable about local and federal programs she is eligible for and can direct her to local food banks and other resources.

Evaluation

The patient should understand protein is important, but it is possible to purchase cheaper sources of protein providing all the essential amino acids. To determine this, have the patient repeat three of the principles she remembers from your teaching. The patient should also state plans to use complementary proteins to provide adequate amounts of amino acids, which will provide other nutrients necessary for health, and purchase some dairy products, fruits, and vegetables each week.

STUDENT READINESS

1. Define amino acid, essential amino acid, nitrogen balance, high-quality protein, and complementary proteins for a patient.
2. Name the functions of proteins.
3. Using your desirable body weight, how many grams of protein should you consume?
4. Given a patient weighing 180 lb who has a caloric intake of 2500 kcal, if the diet averages 15% protein, how many kilocalories are provided by protein? How many grams of protein is this? How does this compare with the RDA for this patient?
5. What would you tell a strict vegetarian parent about feeding her infant?
6. What are the oral effects of too much protein in the diet? What are the oral effects of too little protein in the diet?
7. Explain the relationship between kilocalories and protein.
8. What are two methods of obtaining the EAAs from vegetarian foods? List two food combinations for each type of vegetarian diet that would provide adequate amounts of EAAs.
9. If a patient eats more protein than his or her body needs, what happens to the excess protein?
10. Using Table 4-4, what suggestions would you offer to help a patient reduce the amount of money spent on food without compromising protein intake? Would this significantly affect intake of other nutrients?

References

1. Schaafsma G: The protein digestibility-corrected amino acid score. J Nutr 2000 Jul; 130(6):1876S-1877S.
2. Paddon-Jones D, et al: Protein, weight management, and satiety. Am J Clin Nutr 2008 May; 87(5):1558S-1561S.
3. Fulgoni VL: Current protein intake in America: Analysis of the National Health and Nutrition Examination Survey, 2003-2004. Am J Clin Nutr 2008 May; 87(5):1554S-1557S.
4. Protein Summit 2007: Exploring the impact of high-quality protein and optimal health. Am J Clin Nutr 2008; 87(Suppl):1551S-1583S.
5. Houston DK, et al: Dietary protein intake is associated with lean mass change in older, community-dwelling adults: the Health, Aging, and Body Composition (Health ABC) Study. Am J Clin Nutr 2008 Jan; 87(1):150-155.
6. DePaola DP, et al: Nutrition and dental medicine. In Shils ME, et al (eds): Modern Nutrition in Health and Disease, 10th ed. Philadelphia: Lea & Febiger, 2005, pp 1152-1178.
7. Bonjour JP: Dietary protein: an essential nutrient for bone health. J Am Coll Nutr 2005 Dec; 24(6 Suppl):526S-536S.
8. Dawson-Hughes B, et al: Effect of dietary protein supplements on calcium excretion in healthy older men and women. J Clin Endocrinol Metab 2004; 89(3):1169-1173.
9. Clifton PM, Keogh JB, Noakes M: Long-term effects of a high-protein weight-loss diet. Am J Clin Nutr 2008 Jan; 87(1):23-29.
10. Johnstone AM, et al: Effects of a high-protein ketogenic diet on hunger, appetite, and weight loss in obese men feeding ad libitum. Am J Clin Nutr 2008 Jan; 87(1):44-55.
11. Veldhorst M, et al: Protein-induced satiety: effects and mechanisms of different proteins. Physiol Behav 2008 May 23; 94(2):300-307.
12. Krieger JW, et al: Effects of variation in protein and carbohydrate intake on body mass and composition during energy restriction: a meta-regression. Am J Clin Nutr 2006 Feb; 83(2):260-274.
13. Appel LJ, et al: Effects of protein, monounsaturated fat, and carbohydrate intake on blood pressure and serum lipids: results of the OmniHeart randomized trial. JAMA 2005 Nov 16; 294(19):2455-2464.
14. Layman DK, et al: Dietary protein and exercise have additive effects on body composition during weight loss in adult women. J Nutr 2005 Aug; 135(8):1903-1910.
15. Noakes M, et al: Effect of an energy-restricted, high-protein, low-fat diet relative to a conventional high-carbohydrate, low-fat diet on weight loss, body composition, nutritional status, and markers of cardiovascular health in obese women. Am J Clin Nutr 2005 Jun; 81(6):1298-1306.
16. Westerterp-Plantenga MS, Lejeune MP: Protein intake and body-weight regulation. Appetite 2005 Oct; 45(2):187-190.
17. Kelemen LE, et al: Associations of dietary protein with disease and mortality in a prospective study of postmenopausal women. Am J Epidemiol 2005 Feb 1; 161(3):232-249.

18. Lentine K, Wrone EM: New insights into protein intake and progression of renal disease. Curr Opin Nephrol Hypertens 2004 May; 13(3):333-336.

19. Knight EL, et al: The impact of protein intake on renal function decline in women with normal renal function or mild renal insufficiency. Ann Intern Med 2003 Mar 18; 138(6):I51.

20. American Diabetes Association: Nutrition recommendations and intervention for diabetes. Diabetes Care 2009 Jan; 32:(Suppl 1):S98.

21. Stahler C: How many adults are vegetarian? Vegetarian Journal 2006, Issue 4(serial online): www.vrg.org/journal/vj2006issue 4/vj2006issue4poll.htm. Accessed March 8, 2008.

22. Aronson D: Vegetarian nutrition: what every dietitian should know. Today's Dietitian 2005; 7(3):32.

23. American Dietetic Association: Position of the American Dietetic Association and Dietitians of Canada: vegetarian diets. J Am Diet Assoc 2003 Jun; 103(6):748-761.

24. Larrson CL, Johansson GK: Dietary intake and nutritional status of young vegans and omnivores in Sweden. Am J Clin Nutr 2003 Jul; 76(1):100-106.

25. Messina V, Melina V, Mangels AR: A new food guide for North American vegetarians. J Am Diet Assoc 2003 Jun; 103(6):771-775.

26. Venti CA, Johnston SC: Modified food guide pyramid for lactovegetarians and vegans. J Nutr 2002; 132(5):1050-1054.

27. Muhammad R, et al: Neurologic impairment in children associated with maternal dietary deficiency of cobalamin, Georgia, 2001. MMWR Morb Mortal Wkly Rep 2003; 52:61-64.

28. Barnard ND, et al: The medical costs attributable to meat consumption. Prev Med 1995; 24:646-655.

29. Dwyer JT: Health aspects of vegetarian diets. Am J Clin Nutr 1988; 48:712-738.

Chapter 5

Lipids: The Condensed Energy

OUTLINE

CLASSIFICATION

CHEMICAL STRUCTURE
Saturated Fatty Acids
Monounsaturated Fatty Acids
Trans Fatty Acids
Polyunsaturated Fatty Acids

CHARACTERISTICS OF FATTY ACIDS

COMPOUND LIPIDS
Phospholipids
Lipoproteins

CHOLESTEROL

PHYSIOLOGICAL ROLES
Energy
Satiety Value
Palatability

Complementary Relationships
Fat Storage

DIETARY FATS AND DENTAL HEALTH

DIETARY REQUIREMENTS

SOURCES
Food Choices

OVERCONSUMPTION AND HEALTH-RELATED PROBLEMS
Obesity
Blood Lipid Levels
Cancer

UNDERCONSUMPTION AND HEALTH-RELATED PROBLEMS

FAT REPLACERS

LEARNING OBJECTIVES

Upon completion of this chapter, the student will be able to achieve the following objectives:
- Identify the basic structural units of dietary lipids.
- Describe how fatty acids affect the properties of fat.
- Name the essential fatty acids and some of their functions.
- List the functions of fats in the body, and explain how these affect oral health.
- List dietary sources for saturated, monounsaturated, polyunsaturated, omega-3 and *trans* fatty acids, and cholesterol.

- State the number of kilocalories provided per gram of fat.
- Plan appropriate interventions when dietary modification of fat intake has been recommended to a patient.
- Identify nutritional directions for patients concerning fats.

KEY TERMS

Adipose tissue
α-linolenic acid
Atherosclerosis
Calorie-dense foods
Cholesterol
Compound lipids
Conjugated linoleic acid (CLA)
Docosahexaenoic acid (DHA)
Eicosapentaenoic acid (EPA)
Essential fatty acid (EFA)
Fatty acids (short-chain, medium-chain, long-chain)
Hydrogenation
Hyperlipidemia
Interesterification
Interesterified fats
Linoleic acid

Lipids
Lipoproteins
Melting point
Monounsaturated fatty acids (MUFAs)
Oils
Omega-3 fatty acids
Omega-6 fatty acids
Phospholipids
Plant sterols
Polyunsaturated fatty acid (PUFA)
Protein-sparing
Saturated fatty acids (SFAs)
Structural lipids
Trans fatty acid
Triglycerides
Unsaturated

 Test Your NQ

1. **T/F** No food containing more than 35% of its kilocalories from fat can be considered healthy.
2. **T/F** Fats containing vitamin E deteriorate and become rancid rapidly.
3. **T/F** A product containing more unsaturated fatty acids than saturated fatty acids is a healthier food choice than one containing a higher proportion of saturated fatty acids.
4. **T/F** Dietary fat intake should be less than 20% of total kilocalories.

5. **T/F** Bananas and avocados contain cholesterol.
6. **T/F** Oils are less fattening than solid fats.
7. **T/F** Fat intake has been linked more frequently to cancer than any other dietary factor.
8. **T/F** Nuts and cheeses are nutritious foods that should be recommended to all patients for snacks because they reduce caries rate.
9. **T/F** Fats contain 9 kcal/g.
10. **T/F** Omega-3 fatty acids are polyunsaturated fatty acids.

Unsweetened coconut, mayonnaise, sour cream, blue cheese salad dressing, almonds, pecans, olives, avocados, and sausages—what do all these foods have in common? More than 50% of the kilocalories in each of these food items comes from fat, a vital nutrient in our diet.

As shown in Figure 5-1, added fats and oils provide more kilocalories in the average American's diet than any other food group. Examination of food supply trends in the United States indicates an increase in added fat intake with a greater portion of the fat coming from vegetable fats, whereas saturated fat and cholesterol intake has decreased. Consumer concerns about healthy food choices explain these changes. Food manufacturers, producers, and grocers have responded by (1) trimming fat from meats, (2) providing leaner cuts of beef and pork, (3) replacing tropical oils in processed foods, and (4) manufacturing foods containing less fat. In addition, consumers have increased their consumption of fish and poultry and substituted lower fat milk for whole milk. The fat content of very lean beef and pork cuts currently compares favorably with a skinless chicken breast.

CLASSIFICATION

Fats in the diet should actually be called **lipids**. Lipids contain the same three elements as carbohydrates: carbon, hydrogen, and oxygen. Lipids contain less oxygen in proportion to hydrogen and carbon than carbohydrates. Because of their structure, they provide more energy per gram than either carbohydrates or proteins.

The two classes of water-insoluble substances are (1) simple lipids or **triglycerides**, which occur in foods and in the body, and (2) **structural lipids**, which are produced by the body for specific functions. The structural component of lipids is **fatty acids**. Triglycerides with at least one of the fatty acids replaced with carbohydrate, phosphate, or nitrogenous compounds are called **compound lipids**. Dietary lipids usable by the body include triglycerides, fatty acids, phospholipids, and cholesterol. Lipoproteins are found solely in the body.

CHEMICAL STRUCTURE

Triglycerides are composed of fatty acids and glycerol, as shown:

Monoglycerides = glycerol + one fatty acid

Diglycerides = glycerol + two fatty acids

Triglycerides = glycerol + three fatty acids

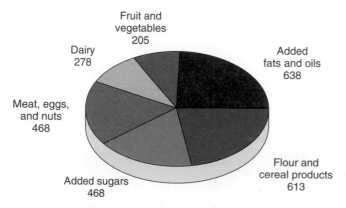

Note: Food availability data serve as proxies for actual food consumption. Added fats and oils and added sugars are added to foods during processing or preparation. They do not include naturally occurring fats and sugars in food (e.g., fats in meat or sugars in fruits).

FIGURE 5-1 Added fats and oils provide more calories per day for the average American than any other food group in 2006. (Data from the U.S. Department of Agriculture and Economic Research Service. Available at http://www.ers.usda.gov/Briefing/DietQuality/fatsandoils.jpg.)

A fatty acid is a chain of carbon atoms attached to hydrogen atoms with an acid grouping on one end. Glycerol is the alcohol portion of a triglyceride to which the fatty acids attach. Triglycerides are the most common fat present in animal or protein foods (Fig. 5-2). Monoglycerides and diglycerides are found in the small intestine and result from the breakdown of triglycerides during digestion. Free fatty acids, monoglycerides, and glycerol can cross cell membranes.

All three fatty acids attached to the triglyceride can be different; they can be long, medium, or short, and saturated or unsaturated. Medium-chain and short-chain fatty acids are readily digested and absorbed, but most fats in foods (especially vegetable fats) contain predominantly long-chain fatty acids. **Short-chain fatty acids** contain less than six carbon atoms, **medium-chain fatty acids** contain 6 to 10 carbon atoms, and **long-chain fatty acids** contain 12 or more carbon atoms.

SATURATED FATTY ACIDS

Fatty acids are classified according to their degree of saturation. Saturation of a fatty acid depends on the number of hydrogen atoms attached to the carbon. **Saturated fatty acids (SFAs)** contain only single bonds, with each carbon atom having two hydrogen atoms attached to it (Fig. 5-3). Palmitic and stearic acids are the two most prevalent SFAs. They are structural components of tooth enamel and dentin.

MONOUNSATURATED FATTY ACIDS

When adjacent carbon atoms are joined by a double bond because two hydrogen atoms are lacking, there is a gap between the hydrogen atoms in the chain; the fatty acid is **unsaturated**. **Monounsaturated fatty acids (MUFAs)** contain only one double bond (see Fig. 5-3). The most abun-

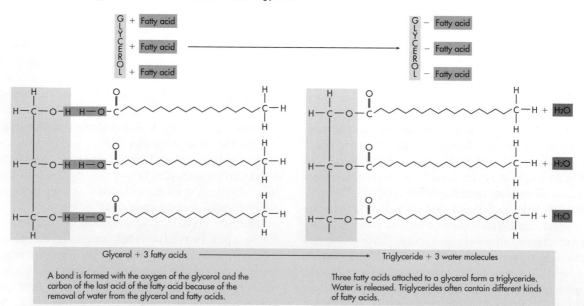

FIGURE 5-2 Formation and structure of a triglyceride. (Adapted from Grodner M, Long S, DeYoung S: Foundations and Clinical Applications of Nutrition: A Nursing Approach, 4th ed. St Louis: Mosby, 2007.)

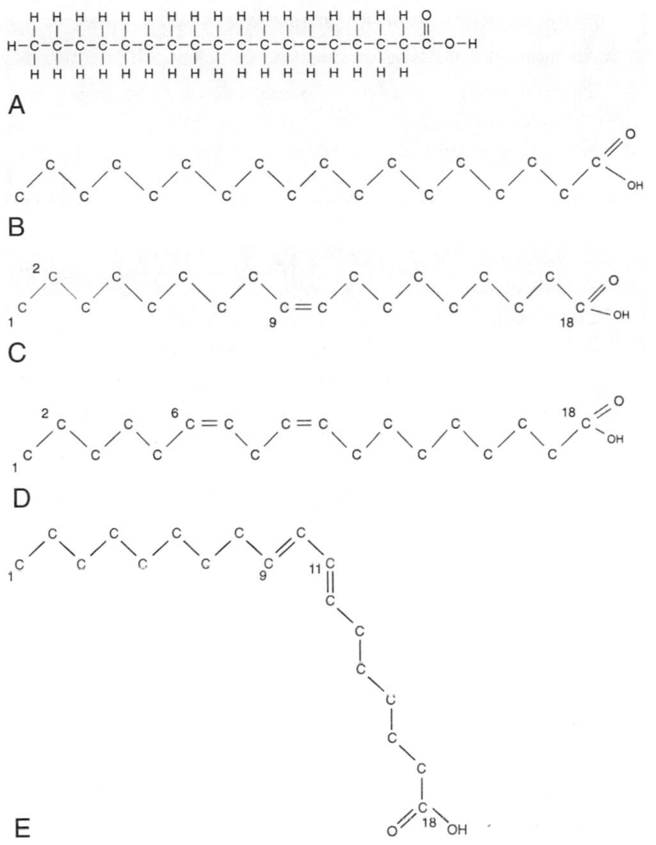

A

B

C

D

E

FIGURE 5-3 Structure of a fatty acid. Saturated fatty acid: stearic acid, an 18-carbon fatty acid (18:0). These numbers indicate the number of carbon atoms and how many double bonds are present. Stearic acid, a saturated fatty acid containing 18 carbon atoms and no double bonds, is labeled 18:0. **A,** Detailed structure. **B,** Simplified structure. Each of the C's at the corners of the zigzag lines represents a carbon atom with two atoms of hydrogen attached. The structure can rotate around single bonds and is constantly twisting and bending. **C,** Structure of oleic acid, a monounsaturated fatty acid. A flat space with an extra line indicates a double bond. **D,** Structure of linoleic acid, a polyunsaturated fatty acid. **E,** Structure of conjugated linoleic acid.

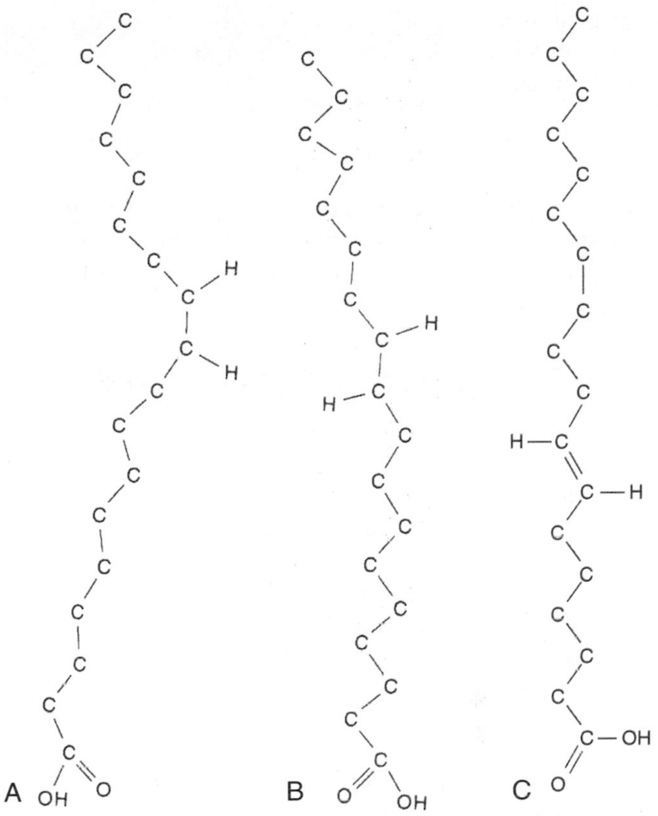

FIGURE 5-4 Note structural differences of *trans* and *cis* fatty acids. **A,** *Cis* configuration. **B,** *Trans* configuration. **C,** Naturally occurring *trans* fatty acid.

dant MUFA is oleic acid. Oleic acid is also a structural component of the tooth.

TRANS FATTY ACIDS

Hydrogenation is a commercial process in which vegetable oil is converted to a solid margarine or shortening by adding hydrogen to the oil. This process results in naturally unsaturated vegetable oils being changed to an SFA by changing unsaturated bonds to saturated bonds. Hydrogenation can be controlled, so "tub" or "soft" margarine is "partially hydrogenated," or not completely saturated. The hydrogenation process not only increases the proportion of SFAs, but also the shape of the fatty acid. When the hydrogen atoms are rotated so that they are on opposite sides of the bond, in the "*trans*" position (Fig. 5-4), the fatty acid is called a ***trans* fatty acid**. Partial hydrogenation results in large numbers of fatty acids having this altered shape. Foods with *trans* fatty acids have a longer shelf life, and flavors are stable. The

most common *trans* fatty acid is elaidic acid, found in partially hydrogenated vegetable oils, such as tub margarines and cooking oils. A naturally occurring *trans* fatty acid with double bonds on adjacent carbons is present in small amounts in milk and meat of ruminants (cows, sheep, and deer).

POLYUNSATURATED FATTY ACIDS

When numerous carbons in a fatty acid are connected by double bonds, the fatty acid is polyunsaturated. A **polyunsaturated fatty acid (PUFA)** has two or more double bonds (see Fig. 5-3). Linoleic, arachidonic, and a conjugated linoleic acid are PUFAs. These PUFAs are **omega-6 fatty acids**. They have their first double bond on the sixth carbon from the omega (terminal) end; they are also referred to as n-6 PUFAs.

PUFAs naturally occur in what is called the "*cis*" configuration (i.e., the carbon chain bends so that hydrogens stick out on the same side of the molecule). These *trans* PUFAs, called **conjugated linoleic acid (CLA),** have naturally occurring double bonds on adjacent carbons. CLAs are a derivative of linoleic acid and have different physiological functions than commercially produced *trans* fatty acids.

Omega-3 fatty acids, or α-linolenic acids, make up another class of PUFAs. As shown in Figure 5-5, these fatty acids are unique in that the first double bond is located three carbon atoms from the omega end of the molecule; hence

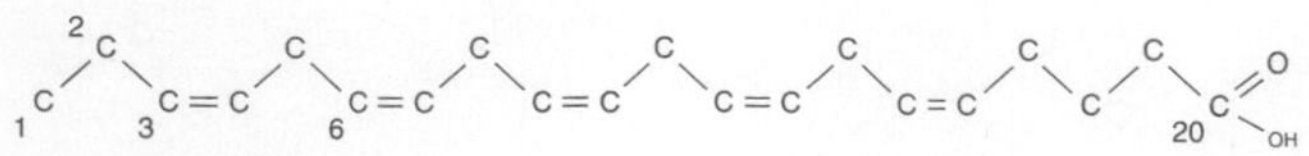

FIGURE 5-5 Structure of eicosapentaenoic acid (EPA), an omega-3 fatty acid.

they are called *omega-3's* or *n-3's*.* Omega-3 fatty acids include **α-linolenic acid,** which has 18 carbon atoms and two double bonds, **eicosapentaenoic acid (EPA),** which has 20 carbon atoms and five double bonds.

CHARACTERISTICS OF FATTY ACIDS

The carbon chain length and degree of saturation determine various properties of fats, including their flavor and hardness or **melting point** (the temperature at which a product becomes a liquid). Most SFAs are solid at room temperature; because most animal fats are predominately saturated fats, they are solid at room temperature. Short-chain fatty acids (12 carbon atoms or less), MUFAs, and PUFAs that are liquid at room temperature are called **oils.** Milk fat contains a large amount of short-chain SFAs.

Fats with a high proportion of unsaturated fatty acids may deteriorate or become rancid, resulting in unpleasant flavors and odors. Fats become rancid when subject to high temperatures and exposure to light, which cause oxidation and decomposition of fats. The decomposition results in peroxides that may be toxic in large amounts. Vitamin E, a fat-soluble vitamin, is an antioxidant and, to some degree, protects the oil to which it is added; however, in doing so, vitamin E is inactivated so that it cannot be used by the body. Other antioxidants, such as butylated hydroxyanisole (BHA) and butylated hydroxytoluene (BHT), are added to commercially processed fats and oils to prevent their spoilage.

COMPOUND LIPIDS

PHOSPHOLIPIDS

Phospholipids contain phosphorus and a nitrogenous base in addition to fatty acids and glycerol. Fats from plant and animal foods contain phospholipids, but they are not required in the diet because the body produces adequate amounts of phospholipids. These substances cannot be absorbed intact; they are broken down into their chemical components before absorption. As a structural component of cell membranes, tooth enamel, and dentin, they are the second most prevalent form of fat in the body. As such, these substances are not used for energy, even in a state of severe starvation. Although the mechanism is not fully understood, phospholipids are

---

*Fatty acids are identified by numbers to indicate the position of any double bonds. The double bond can be designated in two ways: (1) if the structure is numbered from the carboxyl group (C-OH), the symbol "Δ" is used, or (2) if carbon atoms are numbered from the omega end, this is indicated by "n-" or "ω" (omega is the final letter in the Greek alphabet).

🦷 Dental Hygiene Considerations

- Lipids are an integral part of many foods and are important physiologically.
- The primary form of fat in the body is triglyceride, not cholesterol.

Nutritional Directions

- Frying foods at low temperatures causes the food to absorb excessive amounts of fats, whereas frying at very high temperatures results in decomposition of some fats, which can be irritating to the intestine and cause gastrointestinal discomfort after meals containing fried foods.
- The relatively small amounts of *trans* fatty acids that occur naturally in meat and milk products do not seem to be harmful.
- BHA and BHT are added to processed foods to retard or prevent spoilage.

involved in the initiation of calcification and mineralization in teeth and bones, and are present in higher amounts in the enamel matrix of teeth than in dentin.

Phospholipids are important in fat absorption and transport of fats in the blood. Phospholipids can mix with either fat-soluble or water-soluble ingredients and transport these products across membrane barriers.

Phospholipids include lecithin, cephalin, and sphingomyelins. Lecithin, the most widely distributed phospholipid, is present in all cells. Lecithin supplements have been marketed as reducing the risk of atherosclerosis. However, the value of lecithin in this role is questionable because lecithin is digested before it is absorbed. Cephalin is present in thromboplastin, which is necessary for blood clotting. Sphingomyelins are important constituents of brain tissue and of the myelin sheath around nerve fibers. Phospholipids, especially lecithin, are used as additives in commercial products to prevent fat and water components from separating.

LIPOPROTEINS

Lipoproteins are produced by the body to transport insoluble fats in the blood. Lipoproteins are compound lipids composed of triglycerides, phospholipids, and cholesterol combined with protein. The liver and intestinal mucosa produce lipoproteins. Four different types of lipoproteins are present in the blood: high-density lipoproteins (HDLs), low-density lipoproteins (LDLs), very-low-density lipoproteins (VLDLs), and chylomicrons.

The ratio of lipid to protein in lipoproteins varies widely; these variations affect their density. Density increases as lipids decrease and the protein increases. Lipoproteins can be classified according to their density and composition, as shown in Figure 5-6. Phospholipids in lipoproteins are present in approximately the same proportions in all individuals.

HDLs, which are protective against the development of heart disease, contain larger amounts of protein and less

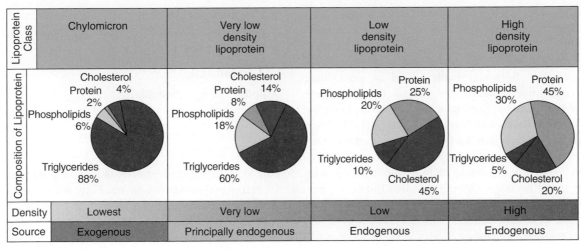

Lipoprotein Class	Chylomicron	Very low density lipoprotein	Low density lipoprotein	High density lipoprotein
Composition of Lipoprotein	Cholesterol 4% Protein 2% Phospholipids 6% Triglycerides 88%	Cholesterol 14% Protein 8% Phospholipids 18% Triglycerides 60%	Protein 25% Phospholipids 20% Triglycerides 10% Cholesterol 45%	Protein 45% Phospholipids 30% Triglycerides 5% Cholesterol 20%
Density	Lowest	Very low	Low	High
Source	Exogenous	Principally endogenous	Endogenous	Endogenous

FIGURE 5-6 Characteristics of lipoproteins.

FIGURE 5-7 Complex ring structure of cholesterol.

lipid. LDL cholesterol typically constitutes 60% to 70% of the total blood cholesterol. It is considered the main agent in elevated serum cholesterol levels, or the "bad" cholesterol. Serum HDL, LDL, and VLDL are important predictors of heart disease, which is discussed in Health Application 5.

CHOLESTEROL

Cholesterol is a fatlike, waxy substance classified as a sterol (lipid) with a complex ring structure (Fig. 5-7). Because the body can produce all the cholesterol it needs, cholesterol intake is not essential. Cholesterol has important functions as a constituent of brain, nervous tissue, and bile salts; a precursor of vitamin D and steroid hormones; and a structural component of cell membranes and teeth. Lipoproteins transport cholesterol in the blood.

PHYSIOLOGICAL ROLES

ENERGY

Dietary fats are a concentrated source of energy, furnishing 9 kcal/g. Foods high in fats are generally referred to as calorie-dense, which has its merits in some cases. **Calorie-dense foods** are usually high in fats (or fat and sugar) and low in vitamins and minerals and other nutrients. A charac-

teristic of calorie-dense foods is that less volume of food is needed to furnish energy requirements. As an energy source, fats are also referred to as **protein-sparing** because they allow protein to be used for the important functions of building and repairing tissues.

SATIETY VALUE

Dietary fats are important for their satiety value. Fats contribute to a feeling of fullness for a longer time than carbohydrates or protein because digestion of high-fat meals is slower than other energy-containing nutrients. This fact has given rise to such descriptions as "sticks to the ribs" in reference to rich meals. The higher the fat content of a meal, the longer the food remains in the stomach. Nevertheless, about 95% of the ingested fats is absorbed. Soft fats that are liquids at body temperature (e.g., margarine) are digested more quickly than hard fats (e.g., meat fats).

PALATABILITY

Fats contribute to palatability and flavor of foods. Their use in cooking improves texture. A receptor has been identified on the tongue that detects dietary fat, which may affect food preferences.[1] Preference for high-fat foods develops at an early age and persists through adulthood.

COMPLEMENTARY RELATIONSHIPS

Fat-soluble vitamins and linoleic acid are generally found in foods containing fat. The absorption of fat-soluble vitamins is facilitated by the presence of fats in the gastrointestinal tract.

Linoleic acid, an omega-6 fatty acid with 18 carbon atoms and two double bonds (see Fig. 5-3), cannot be synthesized by the body and must be supplied from dietary sources. If linoleic acid is not furnished in the diet, signs of deficiency, including growth retardation, skin lesions, and reproductive failure, result. For this reason, linoleic acid is an **essential fatty acid (EFA)**.

Arachidonic (18-carbon chain with four double bonds) and linolenic (18-carbon chain with three double bonds) acids are also considered EFAs, but healthy individuals can produce them from sufficient quantities of linoleic acid. Linolenic acid can be converted rapidly into omega-3 fatty acids in the body. The conversion of linolenic acid to EPA (see Fig. 5-4) and linoleic acid to arachidonic acid is competitive because the process uses the same enzyme. When intake of linoleic acid is substantially higher than intake of linolenic acid, less EPA is available. Linolenic acid may be a protective factor against coronary heart disease.

Omega-3 fatty acids are used to produce compounds regulating blood pressure, clotting, immune responses, gastrointestinal secretions, and cardiovascular functions; they also prevent heart arrhythmias and decrease triglyceride levels. The presence of omega-3 fatty acids in the diet has been linked to reduction or amelioration of several chronic diseases, including **atherosclerosis** (a complex disease of the arteries in which the interior lining of arteries becomes roughened and clogged with fatty deposits that hinder blood flow) and atherosclerotic plaque, rheumatoid arthritis, psoriasis, inflammatory and immune disorders, and serious eye problems such as macular degeneration (Table 5-1).

Naturally occurring *trans* PUFAs, also called CLAs, in foods have unique biological effects. Scientific studies in animals have shown CLAs to decrease fat deposits; decrease risk of different types of cancer and cardiovascular disease;

and improve bone health, insulin resistance, and immune response. Human research on CLA is promising, but limited at this time.[2,3]

FAT STORAGE

Adipose tissue, or body fat, has several roles: (1) it provides a concentrated energy source, (2) it protects internal organs, and (3) it maintains body temperature.

Energy

Excess dietary carbohydrates and protein are converted to fat and stored in adipose tissue. Fatty acids can be used as an energy source by all cells except red blood cells and central nervous system cells. People have been known to survive total starvation for 30 to 40 days with only water to drink.

Protection of Organs

Fatty tissue surrounds vital organs and provides a cushion, protecting them from traumatic injury and shock.

Insulation

The subcutaneous layer of fat functions as an insulator that preserves body heat and maintains body temperature. Excessive layers of fat can also deter heat loss during hot weather.

Table 5-1	Common Food Sources and Physiological Actions of Fatty Acids	
Fatty Acid Classification	**Common Food Sources**	**Physiological Action**
Saturated fatty acids (SFA)	Coconut oil, butter fat, most fats and oils, cocoa butter, fully hydrogenated vegetable oils	Raises (except stearic acid) total, LDL and HDL cholesterol
Monounsaturated fatty acids (MUFA)		
Cis configuration	Some fish oils, beef fat, most fats and oils, nuts, seeds, avocados	Decreases total and LDL cholesterol when substituted for saturated fatty acids and decreases total cholesterol compared with dietary carbohydrate
Trans configuration	Partially hydrogenated vegetable oils	Raises total and LDL cholesterol similar to saturated fatty acids, decreases HDL more than saturated fatty acids, and raises total-to-HDL ratio more than saturated fatty acids
Trans configuration	Dairy fat, meat from ruminating animals (beef, lamb)	May have beneficial health effects; more research needed
Polyunsaturated fatty acids (PUFA)		
n-6 fatty acids		
Linoleic acid	Liquid vegetable oils, nuts, seeds	Decreases total and LDL cholesterol
Arachidonic acid	Meat, poultry, fish, eggs	Precursor for important biologically active substances
Conjugated linoleic acid	Butterfat, meat	Anticancer properties, decreases body fat in growing animals
n-3 fatty acids		
α-linolenic acid	Flaxseed, canola oil, soybean oil, walnuts	Decreases cardiovascular risk
Eicosapentaenoic acid (EPA)	Fish oil, algae	Decreases risk of sudden death from cardiovascular conditions and has beneficial effects on nervous system development and health
Docosahexaenoic acid (DHA)		

Adapted from Kris-Etherton P, Innis S: Position of the American Dietetic Association and Dietitians of Canada: dietary fatty acids. J Am Diet Assoc 2007 Sep; 107(9):1599-1611.

DIETARY FATS AND DENTAL HEALTH

Dietary fats are essential for oral health because they are incorporated into the tooth structure. There is some evidence from epidemiological and laboratory studies that fats may have a cariostatic effect.[4] Eskimos, whose diet may contain 80% fat from animal and seafood sources, have a very low incidence of dental caries. Another factor that may affect caries rate in Eskimos is a low carbohydrate intake. Dietary fats probably have local rather than systemic influence because fats added to foods protect the teeth more than foods naturally high in fat. Precisely how fats reduce the caries rate is unknown; however, several hypotheses have been explored, as follows:

1. Some fatty acids, specifically oleic acid, are growth factors for lactic acid bacteria, whereas streptococcal organisms are inhibited by lauric acid (Lauricidin).
2. Long-chain fatty acids may reduce dissolution of hydroxyapatite by acids.
3. Oral food retention is reduced by increasing fat intake.

Dental Hygiene Considerations

- Although fat intake may have a positive effect on dental health, the medical history of the patient needs to be considered when providing nutritional counseling.
- Lipids provide a source of energy, 9 kcal/g, whereas carbohydrates and proteins provide 4 kcal/g.
- Fish consumption may have a favorable effect on blood platelets and other blood clotting mechanisms, reducing the risk of clot formation.
- Interview the patient to evaluate total fat intake. Everyone needs adequate amounts of fat to allow protein to perform its functions of building and repairing. If total energy intake is inadequate, healing is slower. Also, inadequate fat intake could lead to secondary deficiencies of fat-soluble vitamins.
- Foods such as nuts and certain cheeses (cheddar, Monterey Jack, Swiss) may protect teeth against acid attack, especially when consumed after fermentable carbohydrates. Even though they are generally considered nutritious foods, they have a relatively high fat content.
- Because omega-3 fatty acids may be beneficial to health, determine the patient's frequency of fish consumption. An increase in fish consumption is recommended for most patients, but some fish, especially mackerel and tuna, should be consumed in moderation because of their mercury content.
- Do not advocate indiscriminate use of omega-3 fatty acid supplements. Fish oils may have a negative effect on blood glucose levels in patients with diabetes mellitus. If the patient is consuming omega-3 fatty acid supplements, inquire about the quantity. Intakes of more than 3 g should be under a healthcare provider's supervision.
- If the patient is taking anticoagulants or aspirin, evaluate use of omega-3 fatty acids. These patients may be prone to bleeding problems or poor wound healing.
- Structural differences among the various trans fatty acids result in different health effects.

Nutritional Directions

- Although the digestion of fried foods takes longer, the process is as complete as that of other foods in most individuals if food is fried at the proper temperature.
- Fats act as a lubricant in the intestines, decreasing constipation.
- Foods containing trans fats include stick margarine, vegetable shortening, peanut butter, commercially baked goods (cookies, crackers, biscuits, cake, and breads), potato chips, salad dressing, and fast foods (French fries, doughnuts, and other fried foods). The use of products containing hydrogenated or partially hydrogenated (or trans) fats should be limited because trans fats behave like saturated fat in the body.
- Encourage patients to consult their healthcare provider or a registered dietitian before taking an omega-3 fatty acid supplement.
- Counsel patients to read labels of omega-3 fatty acid supplements. Supplements made from liver should be avoided because high levels of pesticides or heavy metals may be present.
- The potential relationship between periodontal disease and heart disease emphasizes important health reasons for good dental hygiene.
- Partially hydrogenated oils are trans fats, but fully hydrogenated fats do not contain trans fats.
- Avoid choosing a product with less trans fats but more saturated fat because both have undesirable effects on blood lipids.

4. Fats may lubricate the tooth surface and prevent penetration of acid to the enamel (i.e., the "greased" tooth is impervious to acid, protecting caries-susceptible areas).
5. Fats may produce a film on the food particles and prevent partial digestion of food particles in the mouth.
6. Dietary fat delays gastric emptying, enhancing fluoride absorption and increasing tissue fluoride concentration.

Bacterial inflammation and the systemic immune response are believed to play a central role in the initiation and propagation of atherosclerosis.[5-7] When bacteria are allowed to grow rampantly in the mouth, inflammation may occur throughout the body, including in plaque forming on the lining of the arteries. This inflammation may serve as a base for development of arterial atherosclerotic plaques. Research is ongoing to determine how these conditions are related, but some researchers believe gingivitis is a risk factor for coronary artery disease.

DIETARY REQUIREMENTS

A certain amount of fat is needed to provide adequate amounts of fat-soluble vitamins and EFAs. The acceptable macronutrient distribution range (AMDR) for fat is estimated to be 20% to 35% of energy intake for adults (Table 5-2). The lower limit for fat intake was established to minimize the increase in blood triglyceride levels and decreases in HDL cholesterol levels that occur with higher intakes of

Table 5-2   Fat Recommendations for Adults*

Classification of Fat	Dietary Guidelines	IOM† Reference Dietary Allowance (RDA)/Adequate Intake‡ (AI)	IOM† Acceptable Macronutrient Distribution Range (AMDR)	American Heart Association§	American Diabetes Association¶	Canadian Diabetes Association**
Total fat	20-35% kcal	—	20-35% kcal	25-35%	—	≤ 30%
Saturated fatty acids (SA)	<10% kcal	Minimize	Minimize	<7% kcal	<7% kcal	≤ 10%
Trans fatty acids (TFA)	<1%	Minimize¶	Minimize¶	<1% kcal	Minimize¶	Limit
Omega-6 fatty acids (n-6 PUFA)		14 g/day for males; 11 g/day for females	5-10% kcal			
α-linolenic acid		1.6 g/day for males; 1.1 g/day for females	0.6-1.2% kcal			
Omega-3 fatty acids (DHA and EPA)	2 servings fish/wk††			2 servings oily fish/wk (8 oz/wk)		Fish rich in omega-3 fatty acids at least weekly
Plant sterols				~2 g/day		

*Adults 19-70 years old.

†Institute of Medicine: Dietary Reference Intakes for Energy, Carbohydrate, Fiber, Fat, Fatty Acids, Cholesterol, Protein, and Amino Acids. Washington, DC: The National Academies Press, 2002.

‡AI—observed median intake

§Lichtenstein AH, et al: American Heart Association Nutrition Committee, Diet and lifestyle recommendations revision 2006: a scientific statement from the American Heart Association Nutrition Committee. Circulation 2006 Jul 4; 114(1):82-96.

¶American Diabetes Association: Standards of Medical Care in Diabetes—2009: A position statement of the American Diabetes Association. Diabetes Care 2009 Jan; 32:S13-S41.

¶Minimize while consuming a nutritionally adequate diet.

**Wolever T et al. Guidelines for the nutritional management of diabetes mellitus in the new millennium: A position statement by the Canadian Diabetes Association. Can J Diab Care 2008: 23(3):56-69. Available: www.diabetes.ca/cpg2008/cpg-2008.pdf. Accessed January 17, 2009.

††Two servings fish/wk = 450-500 mg DHA and EPA.

Box 5-1   Calculating Total Daily Fat Recommendations for Specific Caloric Levels*

To Calculate Dietary Fat

1. Determine caloric level of the diet (RDA tables can be used) (e.g., patient needs 2000 kcal).
2. Multiply the kilocalories by 0.35 to determine the number of kilocalories of fat the diet can contain (e.g., 2000 kcal × 0.35 [% of total kilocalories]) = 700 kcal from fat.
3. Divide the answer by 9 to determine the grams of fat allowed daily (e.g., 700 kcal from fat ÷ 9 kcal/g of fat = 77.7 g of fat).

Kilocalorie Level	Grams of Fat per Day
1200	<46
1500	<58
1800	<70
2000	<78
2200	<86
2400	<93

*Total fat intake limited to less than 35% of the total daily kilocalories.

carbohydrates. The upper limit of 35% kcal from fat was based on information indicating higher fat intake is associated with a greater intake of energy and SFA, which may be detrimental to health. A method for calculating the recommended amount of dietary fat is shown in Box 5-1.

Between 1971-2000, the percentage of kilocalories from total fat decreased to about 33%. This decrease was because of an increase in total kilocalories consumed; actually, the total fat consumed increased.[8] The World Health Organization (WHO) recommends a range of 15% to 30% of total kilocalories from fats.[9]

The dietary reference intake (DRI) also recommends SFA and *trans* fatty acid be as low as possible while consuming a diet providing an adequate intake of all essential nutrients. The percentage of saturated fat in a 2000-kcal diet is currently about 11%.[8]

The adequate intake (AI) established for linoleic acid is 17 g per day for men and 12 g per day for women 19 to 50 years old, and 14 g per day for men and 11 g per day for women older than 51 years. When dietary intake is high, linoleic acid is stored in the tissues.

Table 5-3	Fatty Acid and Cholesterol Content of Selected Foods					
Food	Portion	Total Fat (g)	SFA (Saturated Fatty Acids) (g)	MUFA (Monounsaturated Fatty Acids) (g)	PUFA (Polyunsaturated Fatty Acids [Total]) (g)	Omega-3 Fatty Acids (20:5, 22:5, and 22:6) (g)	Cholesterol (mg)
Milk and Milk Products							
Cheddar cheese	1 oz	9.4	6	2.7	0.27	0	30
Monterey Jack cheese	1 oz	8.6	5.4	2.5	0.26	0	25
2% cottage cheese	½ cup	2.2	1.4	0.6	0.07	0	9
Cream cheese	1 oz	10	6.2	2.8	0.40	0	31
1% milk	1 cup	2.4	1.6	0.7	0.09	0	12
2% milk	1 cup	4.9	3.1	1.4	0.18	0	20
Whole milk	1 cup	7.9	4.6	2	0.48	0	24
Ice cream, 10% fat	1 cup	14.5	9	4	0.60	0	58
Meats, Fish, and Eggs							
Lean beef tenderloin	3 oz	9.45	3.7	3.9	0.35	0	71
Beef liver	3 oz	4.7	1.5	0.6	0.58	0	351
Chicken breast (without skin)	3 oz	3.2	0.9	1.1	0.69	0.36	76
Chicken breast (with skin)	3 oz	7	2	2.7	1.5	0.045	76
Skinless chicken thigh	3 oz	9.8	2.7	3.7	2.2	0.08	86
Lean pork chop, center loin	3 oz	7.5	2.5	3.1	0.82	0	59
Lean veal loin	3 oz	6.3	2.2	2.2	0.51	0.09	95
Canned salmon	3 oz	4.4	0.8	0.8	1.21	1.044	74
Sockeye salmon	3 oz	9.3	1.6	4.5	2.05	1.16	74
Shrimp	3 oz	0.9	0.3	0.2	0.37	0.284	166
Whole egg, large	1	5.3	1.6	2	0.71	0.022	212
Egg white	1	0.1	0	0	0	0	0
Fats and Oils							
Butter	1 Tbsp	11.5	7.3	3	0.43	0	31
Half-and-half cream	¼ cup	7	4.3	2	0.26	0	22
Vegetable oil margarine, stick	1 Tbsp	8.6	1.6	4.2	2.4	0	0
Corn oil margarine, soft	1 Tbsp	8.4	1.6	2.7	3.7	0	0
Corn and canola oil	1 Tbsp	13.6	1.8	3.8	7.4	0	0
Shortening, hydrogenated soybean and cottonseed oil	1 Tbsp	12.8	3.2	5.7	3.3	0	0
Mayonnaise-type salad dressing	1 Tbsp	11.7	1.6	2.7	6.8	0	0

Data from USDA, Agricultural Research Service, USDA National Nutrient Database for Standard Reference, Release 20, 2008. Available at www.nal.usda.gov/fnic/foodcomp/search/. Accessed February 26, 2008.

SOURCES

Selected foods containing SFAs, MUFAs, and PUFAs, including omega-3 fatty acids, are itemized in Table 5-3. Of the food groups, animal products contribute the largest proportion of fat, although their share has been declining. The most important sources of saturated fats are the meat and milk groups; cocoa butter and coconut and palm oils also are high in saturated fat. SFAs are found in animal fats, butter fat, coconut oil, cocoa butter, coffee creamers and fully hydrogenated vegetable oils (see Table 5-1). Animal products and canola and olive oils supply approximately 50% of MUFAs. Oleic acid, the most prevalent MUFA, is present in most fats, oils, nuts, seeds, and avocados.

PUFAs from the n-6 series are derived from land plants, especially foods from the grain group, and additional fats and oils. Linoleic acid is the most prevalent PUFA in the food supply. Safflower, soybean, and corn oils provide the most linoleic acid; food sources are nuts and seeds. Approximately 80% of all vegetable oil consumed in the United States is soybean oil.[10] CLAs are natural components of beef, lamb, and dairy products. Linolenic acid is present in flaxseed, canola, and soybean oils; soybeans; walnuts; flaxseed; and wheat germ. The long-chain n-3 fatty acids (EPA and **doxosahexaenoic acid [DHA]**) are provided from seafood, including fatty fish such as mackerel, Atlantic salmon, and albacore tuna (presented in order of highest to lowest), and fish oils. These foods are also low in saturated

---

Box 5-2   Wise Choices of Dietary Fats

Purchasing and Planning

- Read nutrition labels on foods to determine the amount of fat and saturated fat in a serving. Low fat is less than 3 g fat per serving.
- Choose fats and oils with 2 g or less saturated fat per tablespoon, such as liquid and tub margarines and canola and olive oil. Liquid vegetable oil should be listed as the first ingredient. Avoid saturated fats such as butter, lard, and palm and coconut oils.
- Avoid foods containing hydrogenated or partially hydrogenated fats because they contain *trans* fatty acids. Such foods include shortening, chips, doughnuts, cookies, snack crackers, cakes, fried foods, and some processed and convenience foods.
- Foods containing partially hydrogenated fats may have some redeeming factors if they contain canola or soybean oil that contain trace amounts of partially hydrogenated oil.
- Watch for reformulated products with lower *trans* fats.
- Substitute plain low-fat yogurt for mayonnaise or sour cream or purchase light sour cream (compare fat content on labels).
- Choose two or three servings of lean meat, skinless poultry, or fish, with a daily total of about 6 oz.
- Choose a vegetarian entree (dry beans and peas) at least once a week.
- Include fish (not fried) at least twice a week.
- Include all types of meat; producers breed animals to produce leaner beef and pork.
- Choose beef graded "select" because it contains fewer kilocalories as a result of less fat marbling. The fat content of the meat also depends on the type of cut; leaner cuts include flank steak, sirloin or tenderloin, loin pork chops, and 85% or greater lean ground beef.
- Use low-fat ground turkey or extra-lean ground beef in casseroles, spaghetti, and chili.
- Moderate the use of egg yolks (maximum of four egg yolks weekly) and organ meats (liver, brains, and kidney).
- Choose tuna packed in water, not in oil (compare fat content on labels).

- Choose cheeses with 6 g or less of fat per ounce (90% of the kilocalories in cream cheese are from fat).

Food Preparation

- Use fats and oils sparingly in cooking (roast, bake, grill, or broil when possible). Baste meats with broth or stock.
- Use nonstick cookware and an aerosol cooking spray.
- Use the paste method for making gravy or sauces: add flour or cornstarch to cold liquids slowly and blend well.
- Season with herbs, lemon juice, or stock rather than lard, bacon, ham, margarine, or fatty sauces.
- Remove skin from poultry and visible fat from beef and pork products.
- Skim fat from homemade soups or stews by chilling and removing the fat layer that rises to the top.
- Include healthful fats, such as olive, canola, soybean, and flaxseed oils; nuts; avocados; and olives.
- Use jam, jelly, or marmalade instead of butter or margarine.
- Rely on mustard and salad greens to add moisture to sandwiches rather than fat-laden spreads.
- Marinate leaner cuts of meat in lemon juice, flavored vinegars, or fruit juices.
- Sauté with olive oil instead of butter. Substitute olive oil for vegetable oil in salad dressings and marinades. Use canola oil for baking.
- Sprinkle slivered nuts or flaxseed or sunflower seeds on salads instead of bacon bits.
- Choose a handful of nuts rather than chips or crackers.
- Place meat or poultry on a rack to allow the fat to drain.
- Steam, simmer or boil, broil, bake, or microwave foods rather than fry.
- Use smaller servings of oil-based or low-fat salad dressings.
- Use whole-grain flours to enhance flavors of baked goods made with less fat.
- Choose nonhydrogenated peanut butter or other nut-butter spreads on celery, banana, or rice or popcorn cakes.
- Add avocado slices rather than cheese to a salad or sandwich.

---

fat. The American Heart Association (AHA) Guidelines recommend consumption of fish at least two times a week.[11]

Approximately 52% of the soybean oil used in the United States was partially hydrogenated in 2003-2004.[10] *Trans* fats are present in shortening; stick margarine; deep-fried fast foods such as French fries and commercially baked pastries and desserts such as doughnuts, cookies, and crackers. Box 5-2 details how to limit the total amount of fat in the diet, focusing on reducing foods high in saturated and *trans* fats and choosing more foods containing unsaturated fats.

Only animal products contain cholesterol (see Table 5-3); it is not found in egg whites or plant foods (i.e., vegetable oils). It is highest in egg yolks, liver, and other organ meats.

FOOD CHOICES

The percentage of fat by weight is widely used on food labels and advertising. Although this information is correct,

it is misleading to the American public. The recommendation that fat intake should be limited to 35% refers to the percentage of fat based on the total kilocalories of the product. As shown in Table 5-4, the percentage of fat in whole milk is 49% of the total kilocalories, not 3.25% as the label indicates.

The Nutrition Facts Label on foods (see Fig. 1-6) indicates the grams and % Daily Value for fat, saturated fat, and *trans* fats in a serving of the food. All *trans* fats, including those from ruminant animals, are included on the Nutrition Facts Label; only CLAs are excluded. In 2003, before *trans* fats were added to the nutrition label, average consumption was 5.8 g, or 2.6% of kilocalories.[12] Because a specific amount of *trans* fats has not been recommended, consumers find it difficult to interpret whether the product contains a high level or not. Even a motivated consumer may misinterpret a label indicating 4 g of *trans* fats as being acceptable. A claim such as "zero" *trans* fat is more helpful than the

	Kilocalories (1 cup)	Total Fat (g)	Percentage of Fat by Weight	Percentage of Fat by Kilocalories
Table 5-4 Analysis of Fat Content of Milk				
Type of Milk				
Whole milk (3.25%)	146	7.9	3.3	49
Low-fat milk (2%)	122	4.8	2	35
Low-fat milk (1%)	102	2.4	1	21
Skim milk	83	0.20	<1	2

Data from USDA, Agricultural Research Service, USDA National Nutrient Database for Standard Reference, Release 20, 2008. Available at www.nal.usda.gov/fnic/foodcomp/search/. Accessed February 26, 2008.

information on the Nutrition Facts Panel. The AHA recommends less than 2 g of *trans* fat daily, but zero *trans* fat intake is best. The Nutrition Facts Label may indicate the product has no *trans* fats, but the ingredient label indicates "partially hydrogenated" oil. This is because the U.S. Food and Drug Administration (FDA) allows manufacturers to label a food as "zero" *trans* fats if the product contains less than 0.5 g per serving. Canadian regulations set the labeling threshold at 0.2 g per serving.

For most people, a decrease in red meat consumption is probably desirable, but the decision to eliminate it completely from the diet is not advisable. In recent years, through improvements in breeding and feeding livestock,

Dental Hygiene Considerations

- Use Box 5-1 when assessing fat recommendations.
- Patients frequently consume more fat than they realize because of the "invisible" fats in dairy and meat products. Interview patients to assess their intake of these foods.
- Foods having a higher fat content are more calorie-dense. For example, ¼ cup of peanuts and seven whole carrots have the same number of kilocalories (210 kcal). Carrots have only a trace of fat; peanuts contain 18 g of fat per ¼ cup. Knowledge of fat content of foods is necessary to assess for fat intake.
- Have patients read a nutrition label to determine whether the product is a good buy as well as a healthy choice with regard to fat.
- Encourage intake of fruits and vegetables, whole-grain foods, and low-fat dairy products, and discourage intake of fatty meats, fried foods, and processed foods that are low in fiber and high in saturated and *trans* fats.

Nutritional Directions

- Butter contains more saturated fats than most margarines; it also contains cholesterol, whereas most margarines do not. However, it does not contain *trans* fatty acids similar to many margarines.
- An easy way to determine whether a food is low in fat is to hold up one finger for every 50 kcal in the food (based on the food label); if the total number of fingers you are holding is more than the total fat grams on the label, the item is low fat; if the total number of fingers you are holding is less than the total fat grams on the label, the item is high fat.[13]
- Purchase processed foods that contain more PUFAs and MUFAs than SFAs. If the food label contains only the total fat, saturated fat, and *trans* fat content, subtract the total

number of grams of saturated fat and *trans* fat from the total fat. For example, if the product contains 8 g of fat with 2 g of saturated fat and 1 g of *trans* fat, the 5 g of MUFAs and PUFAs is more than the 3 g from saturated and *trans* fats. This product is acceptable, but if there is another similar product that contains less than 3 g of saturated and *trans* fats, that product would be a wiser choice.

- Tropical oils, including palm, palm kernel, and coconut oils, are saturated fats, and their consumption should be limited. In transitioning away from *trans* fats, it is important to avoid reverting to using alternatives, such as palm or coconut oils, that are MUFAs and increase the risk of coronary heart disease (CHD).
- High-fat foods should not replace more nutritious foods, such as fruits, vegetables, or whole-grain foods.
- A few fruits and vegetables contain a small amount of fat. Bananas contain a trace of fat (0.55 g or 0.5% fat by weight and 6% of the kilocalories); avocados contain 31 g of fat (15% by weight and 86% of the kilocalories). Both are good sources of several vitamins and minerals.
- Increasing intake of good dietary sources of omega-3 fatty acids is recommended over taking supplements.
- Teach patients to read labels and to understand the percentage of fat should be determined based on the total kilocalories, not the weight, of the food. To determine fat content, use either of the following formulas:
  1. Grams of fat × 9 – kilocalories provided by fat, *or*
  2. Kilocalories of fat ÷ total kilocalories of the product × 100 = % fat content of the product.
- Based on the above formula, if the food contains less than 35% fat, it is generally a wise choice.
- Fats and oils that are 100% fat are necessary to provide adequate PUFAs and fat-soluble vitamins; food items are averaged together to determine if an item exceeding 35% fat would cause the day's or week's intake to exceed the overall 35% desired fat level.
- Children younger than age 2 years are growing rapidly; fat restriction is potentially unsafe for this age group because of uncertainties about the amounts of energy, cholesterol, and EFAs required for growth. After 2 years of age, the *Dietary Guidelines for Americans 2005* are applicable.
- If vegetable oil is the first ingredient on the label, the *trans* fatty acid content will be lower than if the first ingredient listed is partially hydrogenated oil.

these products are lower in fat, saturated fat, kilocalories, and cholesterol. Other important nutrients are present in beef, pork, and lamb; moderate use of these products is encouraged for everyone. Loin (sirloin, tenderloin, or center loin) and round cuts (top, bottom, eye, or tip) and lean or extra lean ground beef contain the least amount of fat. More important than the fat content of a product is its saturated and *trans* fatty acid content.

OVERCONSUMPTION AND HEALTH-RELATED PROBLEMS

Some conditions related to fat intake are observed in dental hygiene practice. The following conditions suggest alteration of the amount or type, or both, of fat in the diet: obesity, diabetes mellitus, **hyperlipidemia** (elevated concentrations of any or all of the blood lipids, especially triglycerides and LDL cholesterol), fatty infiltration of the liver, and certain types of cancer.

OBESITY

Excessive fat stores are a common disorder in the United States (as discussed in Health Application 1). Although the cause is usually overconsumption of all energy nutrients, kilocalories from fat are so concentrated that relatively small quantities may rapidly increase caloric intake.

BLOOD LIPID LEVELS

Elevated blood lipids are related to diet. Hyperlipidemia is associated with heart disease. Although many factors can affect blood lipid levels, the strongest dietary determinant of the blood cholesterol level is the saturated fat content of the diet. Based on results of metabolic and epidemiological studies, *trans* fatty acids act like SFAs by increasing the risk of heart disease considerably (2.5- to 10-fold),[14] and have a negative influence on blood glucose.[15] Because of the unfavorable publicity about the harmful effects of *trans* fatty acids and food labels disclosing how much is in the product, commercial food producers have developed product alternatives to partially hydrogenated fats. Preserving the structural characteristics and palatability of these food products is not easy.

Many of the *trans* fatty acid alternatives, especially those made from tropical fats containing SFA, may not have a desirable effect on blood lipids. In some cases, the hydrogenation process has been modified to reduce the amount of *trans* fatty acid to less than 10% of the oil content.[16]

A process called **interesterification** produces customized fats with properties suitable for foodservice applications. Highly saturated hard fats are blended with oils to produce fats with intermediate characteristics. Some zero *trans* fat margarines may have a higher amount of SFA compared with conventional margarines with *trans* fatty acid.[17] In short studies comparing the effects of *trans* fatty acid and **interesterified fats**, these new fats negatively affect blood lipids, but not as severely as *trans* fats.[18,19] Needless to say, more research is needed to determine the potential consequences of the products being used to replace *trans* fatty acids.

In contrast, stearic acid, found in beef and cocoa butter, has no detrimental effect on serum cholesterol.[20] Total fat content also affects serum lipid levels, but to a lesser extent. Reduction of the total dietary fat content may help reduce saturated fat content of the diet. Factors and dietary modifications influencing serum lipid levels are discussed in more detail in Health Application 5.

CANCER

Annually, 33% of the more than 500,000 deaths that occur in the United States because of cancer can be attributed to diet and physical activity. Research continues to examine whether the association between high-fat diets and various cancers is due to the total amount of fat, the particular type of fat, the kilocalories contributed by fat, or some other factor associated with high-fat foods. Diets high in fat also are high in energy and contribute to obesity, which has been associated with increased risk of cancer of the breast and ovaries, and possibly other sites.[21] Evidence linking dietary fat and particular fatty acids with risk of cancer has elicited considerable interest and debate because of the diversity of findings. Different mechanisms may be involved in tumor development

🦷 Dental Hygiene Considerations

- To distinguish obesity from edema, when the skin of an obese subject is palpated, it has a flabby consistency, in contrast to the mushy or spongy consistency found in edematous skin.
- Ask adult patients if they know their blood lipid levels. A high serum HDL level is desirable to prevent heart disease, whereas elevated levels of cholesterol, triglycerides, LDL, and VLDL increase the risk of heart disease.
- Ask adult patients about a family history of cardiovascular disease and other risks associated with heart disease.
- Stay current on research differentiating the health effects of commercially produced and naturally occurring *trans* fatty acids.
- Teach patients to read the Nutrition Facts Label for saturated and *trans* fats to avoid substituting one unhealthy fat for another.

Nutritional Directions

- Advise patients 10% of the total caloric intake should come from linoleic acid. Serum cholesterol can be reduced by a diet low in total fat and higher in MUFAs and PUFAs (see Table 5-1).
- Reduce dietary cholesterol intake to less than 300 mg daily by limiting meats, whole milk and cheese, and eggs.
- "Low cholesterol" on a food label can be misleading. A cholesterol-free product, such as stick margarine, can still be high in saturated and *trans* fatty acids, which elevates blood cholesterol.
- Dietary saturated and *trans* fatty acids have a greater effect on serum cholesterol than dietary cholesterol.
- The consumption of soluble fibers may decrease serum cholesterol.
- Wise food choices to prevent heart disease are unsaturated fats found in liquid vegetable oils, nuts, and seeds, and omega-3 unsaturated fats found in fatty fish such as salmon, sardines, and shellfish.
- Saturated and *trans* fats can increase total cholesterol and LDL cholesterol; both types should be limited.
- Interesterified fat may be listed on food labels as fully hydrogenated oil.

at different sites and stages of the cancer. Despite many uncertainties about a relationship between dietary fat and cancer risk, the consensus of opinion is to limit total fat intake by increasing fish and lean meat consumption, while concurrently decreasing high-fat meats and foods.

UNDERCONSUMPTION AND HEALTH-RELATED PROBLEMS

Overconsumption of fat is a primary concern in health care, whereas underconsumption of fats is virtually nonexistent in the United States without medical or dietary intervention. However, clinical symptoms of fat deficiency may occur, especially in patients with malabsorption syndromes such as cystic fibrosis or patients in later stages of AIDS. EFA defi-

Dental Hygiene Considerations

- If a patient has a poor reserve of subcutaneous fat, monitor temperature closely. These patients are unable to regulate temperature as effectively as patients who have subcutaneous fat reserves.
- A patient with inadequate fat intake is thin, has dry skin and dull hair, and is sensitive to cold temperatures. If these signs and symptoms are noted, suggest examination by a health-care provider.

Nutritional Direction

Although much is heard about the problems of fat consumption, fats have important physiological functions, and a certain amount must be provided in the diet.

ciency results in poor growth, dermatitis, reduced resistance to infection, and poor reproductive capacity.

When overall food intake, including fats, is poor, patients lose weight, and the subcutaneous fat stores needed to maintain body temperature are depleted. Patients with anorexia nervosa are especially of concern.

FAT REPLACERS

As a result of health concerns regarding dietary fats, numerous foods are being manufactured containing less fat. Because of the possible connection between excessive fat intake and chronic diseases, fat replacers may be helpful in reducing fat and energy consumption. Most of the formulations to replace fat are carbohydrate- and protein-based, but lipid-based materials are available. Each of these fat replacers possesses diverse sensory, functional, and physiological properties that affect their incorporation into various types of products (Table 5-5). Low-calorie salad dressing, low-fat

Table 5-5 Fat Replacers

Generic Name (Trade Name)	kcal/g	Appropriate Uses
Carbohydrate-based		
Cellulose	0	Dairy-type products, sauces, frozen desserts, salad dressings
Dextrins	4	Salad dressings, puddings, spreads, dairy-type products, frozen desserts
Fiber	0	Baked goods, meats, spreads, extruded products
Gums	0	Salad dressings, desserts, processed meats
Inulin	1-1.2	Yogurt, cheese, frozen desserts, baked goods, icings, fillings, whipped cream, dairy products, fiber supplements, processed meats
Maltodextrins	4	Baked goods, dairy products, salad dressings, spreads, sauces, frostings, fillings, processed meats, frozen desserts
Nu-Trim	Unknown	Baked goods, milk, cheese, ice cream
Oatrim	1-4	Baked goods, fillings and frostings, frozen desserts, dairy beverages, cheese, salad dressings, processed meats, confections
Polydextrose	1	Baked goods, chewing gums, confections, salad dressings, frozen dairy desserts, gelatins, puddings
Polyols	1.6-3	Bulking agent
Starch and modified food starch	1-4	Processed meats, salad dressings, baked goods, fillings and frostings, sauces, condiments, frozen desserts, dairy products
Z-Trim	0	Baked goods, burgers, hot dogs, cheese, ice cream, yogurt
Protein-based		
Microparticulated protein (Simplesse)	1-2	Dairy products (ice cream, butter, sour cream, cheese, yogurt), salad dressings, margarine- and mayonnaise-type products, baked goods, coffee creamers, soups, sauces
Modified whey protein concentrate		Milk/dairy products (cheese, yogurt, sour cream, ice cream), baked goods, frostings, salad dressings, mayonnaise-type products
Fat-based		
Emulsifiers	9	Cake mixes, cookies, icings, vegetable dairy products
Salatrim	5	Confections, baked goods, dairy products
Esterified propoxylated glycerol (EPG)*		Formulated products, baking and frying
Olestra (Olean)	0	Salty snacks, crackers, fried products
Sorbestrin*	1.5	Fried foods, salad dressings, mayonnaise, baked goods

Data from Fat Replacers: Food ingredients for health eating: Glossary of fat replacers. © 2007 Calorie Control Council. Available at www.caloriecontrol.org/frgloss.html. Accessed February 2, 2008.
*May require FDA approval.

yogurt, and imitation margarine are made by using modified starches and gums to reduce the oil or fat in the product.

Countless other fat replacers are expected to be available in the future. By substituting fat replacers for fats, total fat intake can be reduced, and some weight loss may be achieved. However, an overall weight loss program is still needed to effect weight loss. By consuming large portions of lower fat products, an individual can potentially negate the caloric and fat savings of the replacement foods. Fat substitutes seem to pose little risk to health, but data are sparse regarding possible benefits under conditions of normal consumer use.

Dental Hygiene Considerations

- Assess use of fat replacers.
- Evaluate overall dietary habits because a patient may think using fat replacers will make a desirable change in health without considering other aspects of the diet.
- If a patient exhibits symptoms such as gastrointestinal distress after consuming a product containing a fat substitute, recommend avoidance of that fat substitute.

Nutritional Directions

- Patients allergic to eggs or cow's milk could be at risk for an allergic reaction to Simplesse because it is made from egg white and milk protein.
- Intake of fat replacers needs to be balanced with variety and moderation in food choices to achieve an overall healthy, nutritious diet.

HEALTH APPLICATION 5 Hyperlipidemia

Despite years of research and copious studies, cardiovascular disease (CVD) is still a major concern in the United States. Cardiovascular disorders include hypertension, CHD, stroke, congenital cardiovascular defects, and congestive heart failure. The Centers for Disease Control and Prevention (CDC) reported in January 2008 that CHD and stroke-related deaths were significantly lower than in 1999.[22] The AHA's 2010 strategic goal for reducing deaths from CVD has already been achieved, and the goal for reducing deaths related to stroke has almost been met.[23] However, almost 325,000 people die each year either out of the hospital or in hospital emergency departments because of CVD.[22] Heart disease and stroke remain the number one and three causes of death in the United States.

Hyperlipidemia, or increased plasma cholesterol and LDL levels, seems to be a major risk factor in CHD. The *Third Report of the Expert Panel (NCEP) on Detection, Evaluation, and Treatment of High Blood Cholesterol in Adults* (ATP III)[24] and the AHA[11] routinely re-evaluate guidelines and update recommendations for healthcare professionals to help prevent CVD. Continual scientific research provides more information allowing refinement of recommendations on detection and management of established risk factors, including evidence against the safety and efficacy of interventions previously thought promising. Most cardiovascular disease is preventable by helping people adopt healthy diet and lifestyles.

The AHA and NCEP encourage a fasting lipoprotein profile (total cholesterol, LDL and HDL cholesterol, and triglycerides) for all adults older than 20 years old every 5 years along with assessment for risk factors. LDL cholesterol levels less than 100 mg/dL throughout life are associated with a very low risk for CHD; LDL cholesterol greater than 100 mg/dL is the primary target of therapy. Reducing LDL cholesterol produces favorable outcomes for coronary lesions and reduces the likelihood of acute coronary syndromes. Table 5-6 shows levels that are considered desirable.

In 2006, the AHA updated recommendations for cardiovascular risk reduction, incorporating new scientific data that are more readily understood (Box 5-3). Maintaining a healthy diet and lifestyle offers the greatest potential of all known approaches for reducing the risk for CVD in the general public. For all individuals without CHD or CHD risk equivalents whose LDL cholesterol is less than 100 mg/dL, adoption of healthy life habits, including avoidance or cessation of cigarette smoking, a healthy diet, weight control, and increased physical activity, is recommended as well as routine medical checkups for blood pressure and cholesterol. These general recommendations also can be applied to patients with or at risk of CHD. Patients at high risk may need more intense therapy.

Based on risk category and LDL goals shown in Table 5-7, therapeutic lifestyle changes, which include dietary changes, weight management, and increased physical activity, are initiated. With implementation of the therapeutic lifestyle changes, it is estimated that LDL cholesterol can decrease 20% to 30%. Other dietary recommendations shown in Boxes 5-4 and 5-5 also have a positive effect on prevention of heart disease. Natural food sources generally are recommended for most of the nutrients rather than supplements.[25]

Many other dietary factors have been proposed to help reduce risk of CVD. Some of these are generally unproven or have uncertain effects on CVD. Although antioxidants seem to prevent CVD, antioxidant vitamin supplements or other supplements such as selenium are not recommended to prevent CVD. Rather, foods containing antioxidants from a variety of fruits and vegetables, whole grains, and vegetable oils are recommended. Phytochemicals found in fruits and vegetables may be important in reducing the risk of atherosclerosis. Until more is known about the mode of action of these compounds, the most prudent practice to ensure optimum consumption of bioactive compounds is by increasing intake of fruits and vegetables.

Plant sterols are bioactive compounds, found in all vegetable foods, which inhibit cholesterol absorption. Consumption of soy protein–rich foods, a source of plant sterols, may indirectly reduce CVD risk if they replace animal and dairy products that contain saturated fat and cholesterol. Small quantities of sterols are present in a

HEALTH APPLICATION 5 Hyperlipidemia

variety of foods, including fruits, vegetables, nuts, seeds, cereals, and legumes. Plant sterols are absorbed at the same sites in the small intestine as cholesterol, and interfere with cholesterol absorption, resulting in a 15% reduction of LDL cholesterol.[26] An intake of approximately 2 g is needed to produce maximum effects. To sustain LDL cholesterol reductions from sterols, daily intake is necessary, as with medications. Scientists have incorporated a plant sterol into fat products and other foods to provide this beneficial product in a readily available source so that dietary intake of sterols can be increased. In the United States, sterols are added to margarine spread, orange juice, and other products (Table 5-8). A low-fat diet increases the effectiveness of these products.

The AHA recommends patients without CHD eat a variety of fish, preferably oily fish, at least twice a week. Individuals who already have CHD are advised to consume at least 1 g of EPA and DHA daily, preferably from oily fish, but the healthcare provider may recommend supplements.

Average cholesterol intake in the United States is 341 mg daily.[27] The body synthesizes approximately two to four times more cholesterol than it obtains from exogenous sources. Of all the dietary changes recommended, cholesterol intake probably has the least effect on plasma cholesterol concentrations in most individuals because of less endogenous cholesterol production in response to cholesterol absorption. The AHA recommendations do not limit the number of eggs as long as total dietary cholesterol is limited to about 200 mg per day. One large egg contains 212 mg of cholesterol.

Most studies have found that reductions in total dietary fat reduce serum cholesterol. Because fat consumption generally coincides with decreased saturated fat intake, changes in blood lipids may be related more to type of fat consumed rather than to total fat. However, a low-cholesterol, low-fat diet rarely reduces cholesterol more than 15%, and medications may be needed to reduce blood lipids further. A diet limiting fat to 35% of kilocalories with 10% from PUFAs and 10% from SFAs and *trans* fatty acids reduces total and LDL cholesterol concentrations in most patients with hyperlipidemia. By replacing some SFAs with MUFAs and some PUFAs, and decreasing total fat, LDL is lowered without decreasing HDL concentrations. These changes result in a more palatable diet that is better received by Americans.

Table 5-6	Optimal Blood Lipid Levels
Lipid	**Optimal Level (mg/dL)**
LDL	<100
HDL	>40-60
Triglyceride	200

Data from National Cholesterol Education Program (NCEP): Third Report of the National Cholesterol Education Program (NCEP) on Detection, Evaluation, and Treatment of High Blood Cholesterol in Adults (Adult Treatment Panel III), Final Report. Publication No. 02-5125. Bethesda, MD: National Institutes of Health, National Heart, Lung, and Blood Institute, 2002.

Box 5-3	American Heart Association 2006 Diet and Lifestyle Goals for Cardiovascular Disease Risk Reduction

- Consume an overall healthy diet.
- Aim for a healthy body weight.
- Aim for recommended levels of LDL cholesterol, HDL cholesterol, and triglycerides.
- Aim for a normal blood pressure.
- Aim for a normal blood glucose level.
- Be physically active.
- Avoid use of and exposure to tobacco products.

From Lichtenstein AH, et al: AHA Scientific Statement: Diet and Lifestyle Recommendations Revision 2006. A scientific statement from the American Heart Association Nutrition Committee. Circulation 2006 Jul 4; 114(1):82-96.

Table 5-7	Thresholds for Lifestyle and Drug Interventions*		
Risk Category	**LDL Goal (mg/dL)**	**LDL (mg/dL) Threshold for Initiating Lifestyle Changes**	**LDL (mg/dL) Threshold to Consider Drug Therapy**
High (confirmed CHD or CHD risk equivalent)	<100	≥100	≥130 (optional if 120-129)
Intermediate (≥2 major risk factors)	<130	≥130	≥160
Low (0 or major risk factors)†	<160	≥160	≥190

Data from National Cholesterol Education Program (NCEP): Third Report of the National Cholesterol Education Program (NCEP) on Detection, Evaluation, and Treatment of High Blood Cholesterol in Adults (Adult Treatment Panel III), Final Report. Publication No. 02-5125. Bethesda, MD: National Institutes of Health, National Heart, Lung, and Blood Institute, 2002.
*Clinical or laboratory assessment is needed to rule out whether elevated LDL is related to diabetes, hypothyroidism, obstructive liver disease, renal failure, or certain drugs before initiating therapy.
†Almost all people with 0-1 risk factor have a 10-year risk of 10%; 10-year risk assessment in people with 0-1 risk factor is unnecessary.

Box 5-4 | **American Heart Association 2006 Diet and Lifestyle Recommendations for Cardiovascular Disease Risk Reduction**

- Balance kilocalorie intake and physical activity to achieve or maintain a healthy body weight.
- Consume a diet rich in vegetables and fruits.
- Choose whole-grain, high-fiber foods.
- Consume fish, especially oily fish, at least twice a week.
- Limit intake of saturated fat to less than 75% of energy, *trans* fat to less than 1% of energy, and cholesterol to less than 300 mg per day by
  - Choosing lean meats and vegetable alternatives;

- Selecting fat-free (skim), 1% fat, and low-fat dairy products; and
  - Minimizing intake of partially hydrogenated fats.
- Minimize intake of beverages and foods with added sugars.
- Choose and prepare foods with little or no salt.
- If you consume alcohol, do so in moderation.
- When you eat food that is prepared outside of the home, follow the AHA Diet and Lifestyle Recommendations (Box 5-5).

From Lichtenstein AH, et al: AHA Scientific Statement: Diet and Lifestyle Recommendations Revision 2006. A scientific statement from the American Heart Association Nutrition Committee. Circulation 2006 Jul 4; 114(1):82-96.

Box 5-5 | **Practical Tips to Implement American Heart Association 2006 Diet and Lifestyle Recommendations**

Lifestyle

- Know your caloric needs to achieve and maintain a healthy weight.
- Know the kilocalorie content of the foods and beverages you consume.
- Track your weight, physical activity, and kilocalorie intake.
- Prepare and eat smaller portions.
- Track and, when possible, decrease screen time (e.g., watching television, surfing the Web, playing computer games).
- Incorporate physical movement into habitual activities.
- Do not smoke or use tobacco products.
- If you consume alcohol, do so in moderation (equivalent of no more than 1 drink in women or 2 drinks in men per day).

Food Choices and Preparation

- Use the nutrition facts panel and ingredients list when choosing foods to buy.
- Eat fresh, frozen, and canned vegetables and fruits and added salt and sugars.
- Replace high-kilocalorie foods with fruits and vegetables.
- Increase fiber intake by eating beans (legumes), whole-grain products, fruits, and vegetables.
- Use liquid vegetable oils in place of solid fat.
- Limit beverages and foods high in added sugars. Common forms of added sugars are sucrose, glucose, fructose,

maltose, dextrose, corn syrups, concentrated fruit juice, and honey.
- Choose food made with whole grains. Common forms of whole grains are whole wheat, oats, oatmeal, rye, barley, corn, popcorn, brown rice, wild rice, buckwheat, triticale, bulgur (cracked wheat), millet, quinoa, and sorghum
- Cut back on pastries and high-kilocalorie bakery products (e.g., muffin, doughnuts).
- Select milk and dairy products that are either fat free or low fat.
- Reduce salt intake by
  - Comparing the sodium content of similar products (e.g., different brands of tomato sauce) and choosing products with less salt;
  - Choosing versions of processed foods, including cereals and baked goods, that are reduced in salt; and
  - Limiting condiments containing a lot of salt (e.g., soy sauce, ketchup).
- Use lean cuts of meat, and remove skin from poultry before eating.
- Limit processed meats that are high in saturated fat and sodium.
- Grill, bake, or broil fish, meat, and poultry.
- Incorporate vegetable-based meat substitutes into favorite recipes.
- Encourage the consumption of whole vegetables and fruits in place of juices.

From Lichtenstein AH, et al: AHA Scientific Statement: Diet and Lifestyle Recommendations Revision 2006. A scientific statement from the American Heart Association Nutrition Committee. Circulation 2006 Jul 4; 114(1):82-96.

Table 5-8	Sterol/Stanol Content of Selected Food Products		
Product	Serving Size	Amount of Sterols or Stanols per Serving	Kilocalories per Serving
Benecol Spread*	1 Tbsp	0.85 g plant stanol esters	70
Benecol Light Spread*	1 Tbsp	0.85 g plant stanol esters	50
Benecol Smart Chews*	1 chew	0.85 g plant stanol esters	20
Promise Buttery Spread†	1 Tbsp	1.7 g plant sterol esters	80
Promise Light†	1 Tbsp	1.7 g plant sterol esters	45
Smart Balance Omega PLUS Butter Spread‡	1 Tbsp	0.45 g plant sterols	80
Minute Maid Heart Wise Orange Juice§	8 oz	1 g plant sterols	110
Nature Valley Heart Healthy Granola Bar¶	1 bar	0.4 g plant sterols	160

From Horn LV, et al: The evidence for dietary prevention and treatment of cardiovascular disease. J Am Diet Assoc 2008 Feb; 108(2):287-331.
*McNeil Nutritionals, Fort Washington, PA.
†UnileverUSA, Inc, Englewood Cliffs, NJ. Take Control Spread is now known as Promise Active Buttery spread. Take Control Light is now known as Promise Active Light Spread.
‡Smart Balance, Inc, Paramus, NJ.
§The Coca-Cola Company, Atlanta, GA.
¶General Mills, Inc, Minneapolis, MN.

CASE APPLICATION FOR THE DENTAL HYGIENIST

A 50-year-old patient complains to his dental hygienist he has recently been having chest pain. He says a recent testing at his grocery store indicated his blood cholesterol level was elevated. A healthcare provider told him several years ago his cholesterol was slightly elevated, and he probably should lower his cholesterol intake. No formal diet education was ordered, and no follow-up work has been done. His blood pressure is 145/90 mm Hg.

He continues to eat anything he wants. He realizes some foods are high in fat and should be avoided, but he is unable to identify these foods. When questioned about fat requirements and different types of fat, he says that he does not understand all of those big medical terms. He also indicates his parents ate what they wanted without all these problems and concerns.

Nutritional Assessment
- Readiness/willingness to learn
- Knowledge level concerning fat principles and how these relate to his diagnosis
- Total amount of fat intake
- Typical foods eaten
- Type of dietary habits: who purchases and prepares the food, where he lives, where most meals are eaten
- Blood pressure
- Serum lipids, if known
- Family medical history (parents still living, cause of death)

Nutritional Diagnosis
Altered health maintenance related to lack of knowledge of fat principles; diet and how it relates to the condition.

Nutritional Goals
The patient will adhere to a low-fat, low-cholesterol diet; list foods high and low in fat; and state how disease may improve or deteriorate with diet.

Nutritional Implementation
Intervention: Emphasize the importance of having a thorough examination annually by a healthcare provider and a confir-

mation of laboratory work with a complete fasting lipid profile.
Rationale: Dietary changes and lifestyle changes are probably indicated; however, the best individuals to diagnose and prescribe treatment are a healthcare provider and registered dietitian.
Intervention: Explain how diet and lifestyle affect his condition: (1) saturated fat increases rate of fatty deposits in the arteries, (2) high cholesterol intake also adversely affects this process, (3) roles of fat (see pp. 88–90 for more details), (4) smoking increases risk of heart disease, and (5) maintaining a body mass index (BMI) within normal range decreases risk.
Rationale: Knowledge increases compliance.
Intervention: Explain the difference between PUFAs and SFAs: (1) use actual food labels; (2) provide a list of foods high and low in these two types of fat; (3) keep fat intake to less than 35% of total kilocalories—less than 10% of kilocaloric intake from SFAs and *trans* fatty acids, up to 20% from MUFAs, and up to 10% from PUFAs.
Rationale: If the patient knows the difference between the two types of fat, he can make informed choices to help reduce the likelihood of heart disease.
Intervention: Explain the difference between the types of lipids and cholesterol: (1) provide a list of foods high and low in cholesterol; (2) limit daily cholesterol intake to 200 mg or less; (3) explain that "cholesterol-free" does not mean "fat-free."
Rationale: Reducing serum cholesterol levels may help slow effects of heart disease.
Intervention: Inquire at each recall appointment if the patient has had a blood lipid profile check recently (HDL, greater than 35 mg/dL for men; LDL, less than 100 mg/dL). Use these as motivators to stay on a healthy diet.
Rationale: These values can provide concrete evidence for motivation and compliance.
Intervention: Monitor blood pressure values at each recall appointment. Inform the patient that hypertension is another

CASE APPLICATION FOR THE DENTAL HYGIENIST—cont'd

risk factor for heart disease. Refer to the healthcare provider for elevated values.

Rationale: If the patient is aware of his blood pressure and the harmful effects of blood pressure elevation, he will make attempts to lower it.

Intervention: Teach the patient how to read nutrition labels (use an actual food label for teaching); use a margarine brand that lists the first ingredient as liquid oil. Explain the different claims on labels, such as "fat-free," "low-fat," and "reduced-fat." (See Box 1-3.)

Rationale: Labels can be confusing. Accurate information can promote healthy food choices, and reduce the incidence of heart disease.

Intervention: Suggest the patient decrease the amount of dietary fat and saturated fats: advise him to (1) eat smaller servings of meat; (2) trim visible fat from meats; (3) consume more poultry and fish; (4) avoid fried foods; and (5) use less salad

dressing, change the type of fat (use olive oil), or reduce the amount of fat in the salad dressing (fat-free or low-fat).

Rationale: These are all ways to decrease intake of fat, decreasing progression of atherosclerosis. The use of more fish increases intake of omega-3 fatty acids.

Evaluation

If the patient lists foods higher and lower in fat and makes better choices to consume a low-fat, low-cholesterol diet, dental hygiene care was effective. In addition, dental hygiene care was successful if the patient can identify the healthiest low-fat, low-cholesterol choices from three food labels; state how fat and cholesterol can lead to further deterioration of his disease; and verbalize that fat speeds up the progression of fatty deposits. Other factors to evaluate include whether (1) blood lipid levels improve, (2) blood pressure is within normal values, and (3) patient has begun a smoking cessation program.

STUDENT READINESS

1. Define the terms "lipid," "hydrogenation," "triglyceride," and "*trans* fatty acid."

2. A patient wants to know foods to consume to (1) increase PUFAs, (2) increase MUFAs, and (3) decrease saturated fats. Name three sources of each.

3. In observing physical properties of fats, how could you make an intelligent guess about the polyunsaturated and saturated fat content of a food?

4. What unsaturated fatty acid is essential in the diet? What are the functions of unsaturated fatty acids in the body?

5. Compare the labels of three brands of stick margarine, three brands of tub margarine, two brands of diet margarine, and two brands of spray margarines. How do they differ in their polyunsaturated-to-saturated fat ratio? List the first ingredient of each.

6. List the functions of fat in the diet.

7. Evaluate one day of your intake for types of foods consumed and amounts of cholesterol, *trans* fatty acid, and saturated fat. If that day represented your average cholesterol and saturated fat intake over an extended period, determine whether the cholesterol or saturated fat content of intake should be reduced. List some simple, realistic suggestions for decreasing their intake.

8. Describe the role of cholesterol in the body.

9. Calculate the caloric value of the following items:
   2 slices bacon (8 g of fat, 4 g of protein)
   1 Tbsp margarine (12 g of fat)
   1 Tbsp whipped margarine (8 g of fat)
   1 Tbsp mayonnaise (6 g of fat)
   1 Tbsp lard (13 g of fat)

10. A patient asks if it is possible to lose or gain 1 lb of body fat every day. What would you say?

11. Calculate the grams of fat a patient could consume on (1) a 1500-kcal diet and (2) a 2000-kcal diet to meet the Dietary Guidelines.

12. List five points you think a patient should know about fats in general.

References

1. Laugerette F, et al: CD36 involvement in orasensory detection of dietary lipids, spontaneous fat preference, and digestive secretions. J Clin Invest 2005; 115:2695.

2. Bhattacharya A, et al: Biological effects of conjugated linoleic acids in health and disease. J Nutr Biochem 2006 Dec; 17(12):789-810.

3. Badinga L, Greene ES: Physiological properties of conjugated linoleic acid and implications for human health. Nutr Clin Pract 2006 Aug; 21(4):367-373.

4. Bowen WH: Food components and caries. Adv Dent Res 1994 Jul; 8(2):215-220.

5. Gotsman I, et al: Periodontal destruction is associated with coronary artery disease and periodontal infection with acute coronary syndrome. J Periodontol 2007 May; 78(5):849-858.

6. Janket SJ, et al: Asymptotic dental score and prevalent coronary heart disease. Circulation 2004 Mar 9; 109(9):1095-1100.

7. Meurman JH, et al: Dental infection and serum inflammatory markers in patients with and without severe heart disease. Oral Surg Oral Med Oral Pathol Oral Radiol Endod 2003 Dec; 96(6):695-700.

8. Wright JD, et al: Trends in intake of energy and macronutrients—United States, 1971-2000. MMWR Morb Mortal Wkly Rep 2004 Feb 6; 53(04):80-82. Available at www.cdc.gov/MMWR/preview/mmwrhtml/mm5304a3.htm. Accessed March 22, 2008.

9. Joint FAO/WHO Expert Consultation: Diet, Nutrition, and the Prevention of Chronic Diseases. Geneva, Switzerland: World Health Organization, 2003. Available at ftp://ftp.fao.org/docrep/fao/005/ac911e/ac911eoo.pdf. Accessed on March 22, 2008.

10. Graf PA, Lemke S, DiRienzo M: Reducing the trans-fatty acid content in foods. Nutr Today 2008 Mar/Apr; 43(2):46-51.

11. Lichtenstein AH, et al: AHA Scientific Statement: Diet and Lifestyle Recommendations Revision 2006. A scientific statement from the American Heart Association Nutrition Committee. Circulation 2006 Jul 4; 114(1):82-96.

12. FDA: Revealing trans-fats. FDA Consumer. 2003 Sept-Oct (serial online): www.fda.gov/FDAC/features/2003/503_fats.html. Accessed March 15, 2008.

13. Renkilo M: Nutritional approaches to type 2 diabetes control. Presented at Old Questions, New Hope: Type 2 Diabetes Prevention and Control. Thirty-First Annual Texas Human Nutrition Conference; College Station, Texas, February 6, 2004.

14. Carson JS, Burke FM, Hark LA: Cardiovascular Nutrition: Disease Management and Prevention. Chicago, IL: American Dietetic Association, 2004.

15. Sundram K, Karupaiah T, Hayes K: Stearic acid rich interesterified fat and trans-rich fat raise the LDL/HDL ratio and plasma glucose relative to palm, olein in humans. Nutr Metab (Lond) 2007; 4:10.

16. Tarrago-Trani MT, et al: New and existing oils and fats used in products with reduced trans-fatty acid content. J Am Diet Assoc 2006 Jun; 106(6):867-880.

17. Satchithanandam S, et al: Trans, saturated, and unsaturated fat in foods in the United States prior to mandatory trans-fat labeling. Lipids 2004; 39:11-18.

18. Sundram K, Karupaiah T, Hayes K: Stearic acid-rich interesterified fat and trans-rich fat raise the LDL/HDL ratio and plasma glucose relative to palm olein in humans. Nutr Metab (Lond) 2007; 4:3.

19. Noakes M, Clifton PM: Oil blends containing partially hydrogenated or interesterified fats: differential effects on plasma lipids. Am J Clin Nutr 1998 Aug; 68(2):242-247.

20. Mensink RP, et al: Effects of dietary fatty acids and carbohydrates on the ratio of serum total to HDL cholesterol and on serum lipids and apolipoproteins: A meta-analysis of 60 controlled trials. Am J Clin Nutr 2003 May; 77(5):1146-1155.

21. Prentice RL, et al: Low-fat dietary pattern and cancer incidence in the Women's Health Initiative Dietary Modification Randomized Controlled Trial. J Natl Cancer Inst 2008 Feb 20; 100(4):284-285.

22. American Heart Association, American Stroke Association: Know the facts, get the stats, 2007 (website). Available at www.americanheartassoc.org. Accessed March 28, 2008.

23. AHA: Heart and stroke death rates steadily decline; risks still too high. AHA News (online). Available at www.americanheart.org/print_presenter.jhtml?identifier=3052335. Accessed March 28, 2008.

24. National Cholesterol Education Program: Third Report of the National Cholesterol Education Program (NCEP) Expert Panel on Detection, Evaluation, and Treatment of High Blood Cholesterol in Adults. NIH Publication No. 02-5215. Bethesda, MD: National Institutes of Health, 2002. Available at http://www.nhlbi.nih.gov/guidelines/chol/index.html.

25. Kris-Etherton PM, Hill AM: N-3 fatty acids: Food or supplements? J Am Diet Assoc 2008 Jul; 108(7):1125-1130.

26. Grundy SM: Stanol esters as a component of maximal dietary therapy in the National Cholesterol Education Program Adult Treatment Panel III report. Am J Cardiol 2005; 96:47D-50D.

27. Briefel RR, Johnson CL: Secular trends in dietary intake in the United States. Ann Rev Nutr 2004; 24:401-431.

Chapter 6

Use of the Energy Nutrients: Metabolism and Balance

OUTLINE

METABOLISM

ROLE OF THE LIVER

ROLE OF THE KIDNEYS

CARBOHYDRATE METABOLISM

PROTEIN METABOLISM
Anabolism
Catabolism

LIPID METABOLISM

ALCOHOL METABOLISM

METABOLIC INTERRELATIONSHIPS

METABOLIC ENERGY
Measurement of Potential Energy
Energy Production

BASAL METABOLIC RATE
Factors Affecting the Basal Metabolic Rate

TOTAL ENERGY REQUIREMENTS
Thermic Effect of Food
Voluntary Work and Play
Estimated Energy Requirements

ENERGY BALANCE
Physiological Factors
Psychological Factors
Energy Expenditure

INADEQUATE ENERGY INTAKE

LEARNING OBJECTIVES

Upon completion of this chapter, the student will be able to achieve the following objectives:

- Calculate energy needs according to the patient's weight and activities.
- Explain physiological sources of energy.
- Identify factors affecting the basal metabolic rate.
- Assess factors affecting energy balance.
- Describe the effects of inadequate energy intake.
- Explain the principles for regulating energy balance to a patient.

KEY TERMS

Adenosine triphosphate (ATP)
Anabolism
Appetite
Basal energy expenditure (BEE)
Basal metabolic rate (BMR)
Calorimeter
Catabolism
Coenzyme
Cofactor
Gluconeogenesis
Glycemic effect
Glycogenesis

KEY TERMS—cont'd

High-energy phosphate compounds	**Kilocalorie (kcal)**
Hormones	**Lipolysis**
Hunger	**Metabolism**
Indirect calorimetry	**Oxidation**
Insulin	**Pedometer**
Ketoacidosis	**Postabsorptive state**
Ketonuria	**Renal failure**
Ketosis	**Thermic effect**

Test Your NQ

1. **T/F** Insulin is a hormone that decreases blood glucose levels.
2. **T/F** Even during sleep, the body requires energy.
3. **T/F** BMR stands for blood malnutrition reaction.
4. **T/F** A malnourished patient would have a low BMR.
5. **T/F** The hypothalamus controls hunger and satiety.
6. **T/F** Hunger is the same as appetite.
7. **T/F** Fats are a good source of quick energy.
8. **T/F** The kidneys play an important role in maintaining nutrient balance within the body.
9. **T/F** Ketoacidosis can occur as a result of strict carbohydrate restriction.
10. **T/F** Vitamins are a source of energy.

After foods are chewed and digested, the macronutrients (carbohydrate, protein, fat, and alcohol) supplying physiological energy for the body are converted to glucose, fatty acids, and amino acids. These basic nutrient units are delivered to cells where, at the direction of specific enzymes, they can be used.

Recall from earlier chapters that no single nutrient can be isolated from the others because nutrients are concurrently distributed in foods and share many points of interaction in digestion, absorption, and metabolism. **Metabolism** encompasses the continuous processes whereby living organisms and cells convert nutrients into energy, body structure, and waste.

METABOLISM

In metabolic activity, the two major chemical reactions are catabolism and anabolism. **Catabolism** is splitting complex substances into simpler substances; **anabolism** is using absorbed nutrients to build or synthesize more complex compounds. Anabolism and catabolism are continuous reactions in the body. Cells in the epithelial lining of the oral and gastrointestinal mucosa are replaced approximately every 3 to 7 days. Despite this rapid turnover, the rate of catabolism is usually equal to that of anabolism in a healthy adult. During certain stages of life, such as growth periods or pregnancy, more anabolism is occurring than catabolism. Conversely, when illness or stress occurs, excessive catabolism is evident.

Other phases of metabolism include delivery of nutrients to the cells where they are needed, and delivery of wastes to sites where they can be excreted. After absorption of the macronutrients, glucose, fatty acids, and amino acids can be used via a common pathway within the mitochondria of cells

to yield energy (Fig. 6-1). The catabolic end products of carbohydrates, proteins, and fats are carbon dioxide, water, and energy. Nitrogen is an additional end product of protein.

The Krebs cycle (also called citric acid cycle or tricarboxylic acid cycle [TCA]) converts glucose, fatty acids, and amino acids to a usable form of energy, requiring many enzymes. For activation of some of the enzymes, vitamins or minerals or both must be available. An enzyme needing vitamins for activation is called a **coenzyme**. Thiamin, riboflavin, and niacin are B vitamins essential as coenzymes in the Krebs cycle. An enzyme may also require a cofactor. A **cofactor** functions in the same way as coenzymes, but the molecule required is a mineral or electrolyte.

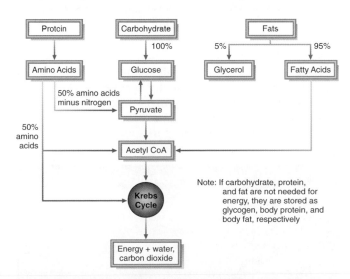

FIGURE 6-1 Metabolic pathways. (From Peckenpaugh NJ: Nutrition Essentials and Diet Therapy, 10th ed. Philadelphia: Saunders, 2007.)

Anabolic processes require energy. Examples of anabolism are the building of new muscle tissue or bone and the secretion of cellular products such as hormones. **Hormones** are "messengers" produced by a group of cells that stimulate or retard the functions of other cells. Hormones principally control different metabolic functions that affect growth and secretions. Anabolism involves the use of glucose, amino acids, fatty acids, and glycerol to build various substances that make up the body itself and the other substances necessary for the body to function. All nutrients are intertwined in this process. For instance, nonessential amino acids are ordinarily used to build proteins, but glucose can be the basis for anabolism of amino acids and fatty acids.

ROLE OF THE LIVER

The liver plays a major regulatory role by controlling the kinds and quantities of nutrients in the bloodstream. All monosaccharides are converted to glucose in the liver to provide an energy supply for the cells. The polysaccharide glycogen also can be broken down to glucose and released into the circulating blood as needed. Other end products of digestion may be oxidized to provide energy; converted to glucose, protein, fat, or other substances; or released to circulate at prescribed levels in the blood for use by cells throughout the body.

ROLE OF THE KIDNEYS

Kidneys perform the important metabolic task of removing waste products from the blood, and along with the liver, control the levels of many nutrients in the blood. Metabolic end products from cells, unnecessary substances absorbed from the gastrointestinal tract, potentially harmful compounds that have been detoxified by the liver, and drugs all are removed from the blood by the kidneys.

The kidneys accomplish this task by a process of filtration and reabsorption. Glucose, amino acids, vitamins, water, and various minerals are reabsorbed or excreted by the kidneys, depending on the body's need. Excess nitrogen from protein catabolism also is excreted by the kidneys. Kidneys help maintain nutrient balance within the body. Other routes of excretion of waste products are through the bowel; the skin, which excretes water and electrolytes; and the lungs, which remove carbon dioxide and water.

Dental Hygiene Considerations

- The goal of nutrition in a dental setting is to promote anabolism for growth or healing.
- Uncontrolled blood glucose levels may cause numerous complications, such as poor wound healing and increased risk of infection for patients with diabetes.
- The kidneys' ability to reabsorb nutrients may be altered by certain medications, especially diuretics, or a kidney disorder. Function also depends on fluid balance.

Nutritional Directions

- The liver is a vital organ for metabolism of food and drugs.
- The kidneys help the body dispose of waste products and drugs. Adequate fluid intake (9 to 11 cups per day) facilitates this process.
- If the kidneys are not working properly, drugs and nutrients may be retained or lost. Both are undesirable.

CARBOHYDRATE METABOLISM

Monosaccharides are transported through the portal vein to the liver for **glycogenesis**, a process in which sugars, including fructose, galactose, sorbitol, and xylitol, are stored as glycogen. Glucose is the circulating sugar in the blood; it is the major energy supply for cells. The level of circulating glucose is closely monitored by the liver and is constantly maintained at a level between 70 and 100 mg/dL in normal individuals. **Insulin** is a hormone that lowers blood glucose levels. Blood glucose levels peak at 140 mg/dL 30 to 60 minutes after a meal and return to normal within 3 hours in individuals with normal secretion and use of insulin. This consistent blood glucose level is significant, indicating the necessity of a certain amount of glucose in the blood for normal functioning of body tissues (Fig. 6-2). Hyperglycemia, elevated blood glucose, and hypoglycemia, decreased blood glucose, are very serious conditions that could be fatal; the precipitating cause for either should be identified. Many patients with diabetes who take insulin or an antidiabetic medication that causes hypoglycemia, or both, may exhibit symptoms related to hypoglycemia or be asymptomatic if they have not eaten within a 4- to 5-hour time span. These patients need to be treated with a carbohydrate source before continuing treatment (see Health Application 6).

In the past, it was assumed all sugars produced a higher blood glucose response than starches. However, the blood glucose response to different foods and different combinations of food cannot be accurately predicted from the amount of simple sugars or complex carbohydrates ingested. White bread, potatoes, and white rice have a glycemic effect similar to sucrose. **Glycemic effect** is the rate at which glucose increases in the bloodstream after a particular food is eaten.

A complex hormonal system maintains a constant blood glucose level. Insulin is the primary hormone that lowers blood glucose levels. When hyperglycemia occurs, insulin is secreted to decrease blood glucose levels. Conversely, hypoglycemia elicits the secretion of several hormones (thyroid hormone, epinephrine, glucagon, and growth hormone) to increase blood glucose levels. Blood glucose levels can be elevated by converting amino acids from protein, and glycerol from fats to glucose. The process of synthesizing glucose from noncarbohydrate sources is known as **gluconeogenesis**.

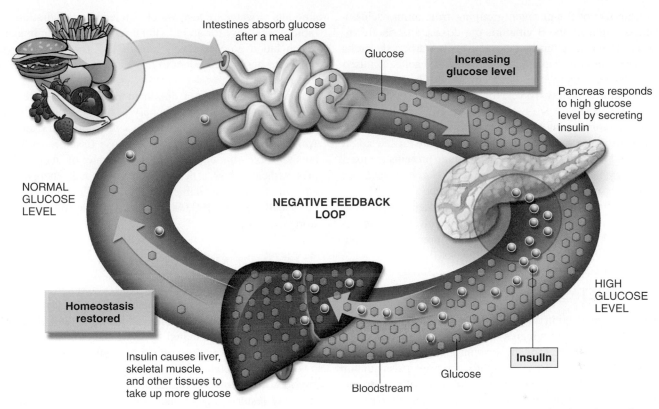

Intestines absorb glucose after a meal

Glucose

Increasing glucose level

Pancreas responds to high glucose level by secreting insulin

NORMAL GLUCOSE LEVEL

NEGATIVE FEEDBACK LOOP

HIGH GLUCOSE LEVEL

Homeostasis restored

Insulin

Insulin causes liver, skeletal muscle, and other tissues to take up more glucose

Glucose

Bloodstream

FIGURE 6-2 Role of insulin. Insulin operates in a negative feedback loop that prevents blood glucose concentration from increasing too far above the normal, or set-point, level. Insulin promotes uptake of glucose by all cells of the body, enabling them to catabolize it, store it, or both. The liver and skeletal muscles are especially well adapted for storage of glucose as glycogen. Excess glucose is removed from the bloodstream. If the glucose level falls below the set-point level, hormones such as glucagon promote the release of glucose from storage into the bloodstream. (From Thibodeau GA, Patton KT: Anatomy and Physiology, 6th ed. St Louis: Mosby, 2007.)

Dietary carbohydrates ensure optimal glycogen stores and are digested faster than other energy nutrients. The body can catabolize glycogen to glucose. The amount of energy available from glycogen stores is generally less than a day's energy expenditure, or about 1200 to 1800 kcal. Brain cells, red blood cells, and cells of the renal medulla require glucose as their energy source.

PROTEIN METABOLISM

Amino acids are transported through the portal vein into the liver. The liver is an "aminostat," monitoring the intake and breakdown of most of the amino acids. Individual amino acids are released by the liver to enter the general circulation at specific levels, so each amino acid is available as needed to synthesize each individual protein. Amino acids transported in the blood are rapidly removed for use by cells. If individual amino acids increase above a specific level in the blood, they are removed and oxidized for energy.

Protein metabolism is in a constant dynamic state, with catabolism and anabolism occurring continuously to replace worn-out proteins in cells. Even during anabolic periods such as growth, muscle catabolism is elevated as each cell remodels itself. Anabolic and catabolic processes are controlled by the liver and by hormones. Insulin, thyroxine, and growth hormone stimulate protein synthesis.

ANABOLISM

A small reservoir of amino acids, which is called the "amino acid metabolic pool," is available for anabolism and to maintain the dynamic state of equilibrium. This metabolic pool, containing about 70 g of amino acids, is less than most Americans consume in a day and could hardly be classified as a large storage of protein. Increasing muscle size is considered an increase in body mass, not protein storage. High-protein diets are neither safe nor effective as a means to increase muscle mass in athletes without physical activity or exercise to promote muscle development. To maintain a satisfactory protein status, a daily supply of essential amino acids obtained from the diet is necessary.

Anabolism depends on the presence of all essential amino acids simultaneously. It is not a stepwise process in which a protein can be started and completed when the needed amino acid appears.

Protein synthesis is also affected by caloric intake. If caloric intake is inadequate, tissue proteins are used for energy, resulting in increased nitrogen excretion. This process requires the B vitamin, pyridoxine.

CATABOLISM

Amino acids are catabolized principally in the liver, but metabolism also occurs to some extent in kidney and muscle.

The removal of the nitrogen grouping from amino acids, a process requiring the B vitamins pyridoxine and riboflavin, yields carbon skeletons and ammonia. The carbon skeletons can be (1) used to make nonessential amino acids, (2) used to produce energy via the Krebs cycle, or (3) converted to fats and stored as fatty tissue. Not all ingested protein is used to build muscle.

When amino acids are not needed for protein anabolism, and energy is not needed, they are converted to fat and stored in the body. If caloric intake is inadequate, proteins are used for energy rather than to build or repair lean body mass or produce essential protein-based compounds.

Urea is the major waste product of protein catabolism. Ammonia is a toxic substance the liver converts to urea to be excreted by the kidneys. The levels of urea and ammonia vary directly with dietary protein levels.

LIPID METABOLISM

Hormones involved in carbohydrate metabolism also control fat metabolism. Insulin increases fat synthesis, whereas thyroxine, epinephrine, growth hormone, and glucocorticoids increase fat mobilization. The liver is the principal regulator of fat metabolism and lipoprotein synthesis. Fatty acids can be hydrolyzed or modified by shortening, lengthening, or adding double bonds before their release from the liver into the circulation. The liver produces cholesterol, removes it from the blood, and uses it to make bile acid.

Metabolism of chylomicrons in the liver results in triglycerides being transported to the tissues for energy or other uses or carried to adipose tissue to be stored. Serum triglycerides are the result of not only absorption from foods, but also the conversion of carbohydrates and proteins into fats. Triglycerides can be synthesized in the intestinal mucosa, adipose tissue, and liver. Fats are synthesized in the process of lipogenesis and broken down during **lipolysis**. These continual processes are in equilibrium when energy needs are balanced.

The process of hydrolyzing triglycerides into two-carbon entities to enter the Krebs cycle for energy production is known as **oxidation**. During oxidation, 1 lb of fat results in the release of 3500 kcal for energy—more than most individuals use in a 24-hour period. When excessive amounts of fats are oxidized for energy, the liver is overwhelmed, and acidic metabolic products, or ketones, are formed. Ketones are not oxidized in the liver, but are carried to the skeletal and cardiac muscles, where, under normal circumstances, they are rapidly metabolized.

If the glucose supply is reduced, the capacity of the tissues to use ketone bodies may be exceeded. Accumulation of ketone bodies in the blood is known as **ketosis** or **ketoacidosis**. Ketoacidosis can be a dangerous condition for several reasons. Bases must neutralize these strong acids to maintain acid-base balance in the blood. Ketones are excreted in the urine, a condition known as **ketonuria**, along with sodium. If adequate amounts of base are not available, acidosis may result. In addition to the loss of sodium ions, large

amounts of water are lost, which can lead to dehydration (or rapid weight loss for an individual reducing caloric intake). When blood glucose levels remain low for several days, brain and nerve cells adapt to use ketones for some of their fuel requirements.

Carbohydrates play a dominant role in heavy exercise when the muscle's oxygen supply is limited, but triglycerides provide about half the energy with continued exercise. Although fats can be stored as adipose tissue in virtually inexhaustible amounts, their slower rate of metabolism makes them a less efficient source of quick energy. The amount of energy available is highly variable in individuals, but usually at least 160,000 kcal is available from body fat stores.

ALCOHOL METABOLISM

Although alcohol is considered a drug or toxin, the kilocalories it provides can be used by the body for energy, providing approximately 7 kcal per gram. Caloric content of alcoholic beverages can be calculated by using the equations in Box 6-1. Alcoholic beverages contain negligible nutrients.

Alcohol is metabolized primarily by the liver. Alcohol provides an alternative fuel that is oxidized instead of fat; this may result in accumulation of lipids in the liver. Not much is known about safe amounts of alcohol consumption without risk of liver damage.

A well-balanced diet accompanied by habitual consumption of alcoholic beverages in excess of energy needs can be a risk factor for weight gain. However, excessive amounts of alcohol in a person who is an alcoholic tend to result in poor appetite for food and may lead to weight loss and malnutrition. In addition to causing liver damage, alcohol can interfere with the transport, activation, catabolism, and storage of almost every nutrient. Alcohol has a marked effect on blood pressure and risk of hypertension.[1]

The *Dietary Guidelines for Americans 2005* advise moderation in alcohol consumption: one drink a day for women and no more than two drinks a day for men. (An alcoholic beverage is defined as 12 oz of regular beer, 5 oz of wine, or $1\frac{1}{2}$ oz of 80-proof distilled spirits.) For middle-aged and

---

Box 6-1	**Calculation of Energy Value of Alcoholic Beverages**

The equation for determining energy (caloric) value of liquors is as follows:

$$\text{Ounces of beverage} \times \text{proof} \times 0.8\,\text{kcal/proof/1 oz}$$

Example: $1.5\,\text{oz} \times 86\ \text{proof} \times 0.8\,\text{kcal/proof/1 oz} = 103.2\,\text{kcal}$

The equation for determining energy (caloric) value of beer and wines is as follows:

$$\text{Ounces of beverage} \times \% \text{ of alcohol} \times 1.6$$

Example: $12\,\text{oz} \times 5\% \times 1.6 = 96\,\text{kcal}$

From Gastineau CF: Nutrition note: alcohol and calories. Mayo Clin Proc 1976 Feb; 51(2):88.

older adults, one to two drinks daily results in the lowest mortality rate.[2] This is perhaps due to the protective effects of moderate alcohol consumption on coronary heart disease. Alcohol consumption seems to provide little, if any, health benefit for younger individuals. Alcoholic beverages should be avoided by women who may become pregnant or are pregnant or breastfeeding.

METABOLIC INTERRELATIONSHIPS

The body is an overwhelmingly complex system. Whether excessive food intake is in the form of protein, carbohydrate, alcohol, or fat, most excess energy intake is stored as adipose tissue (Fig. 6-3). (Glycogen is another storage form of energy; however, the amount of glycogen stored in the body is limited.)

Protein from the metabolic pool of amino acids and in lean muscle mass is generally not considered a good source of energy, but it can be used for energy if caloric intake is below caloric expenditure. Fat is a good source of energy, but carbohydrate is the preferred fuel. However, the body cannot metabolize excessive quantities of fat without some side effects—ketoacidosis, hyperlipidemia, and accumulation of fat in the liver.

Carbohydrates can be used in forming nonessential amino acids. Proteins contribute to synthesis of some lipids (e.g., lipoproteins). Although lipids do not contribute significantly to the synthesis of amino acids, the glycerol from triglycerides can be used for synthesis of carbohydrates. Fatty acids and some amino acids can be converted to glucose.

Catabolism of all classes of foodstuffs involves oxidation through the Krebs cycle to produce energy. The quantity of kilocalories in the diet from carbohydrate or lipids influences protein metabolism. In some situations, one nutrient can be substituted for another because of their interrelationship. For example, a decrease in carbohydrate intake increases lipolysis; protein excess can be used for energy. Because the body can easily adapt to shifts in either carbohydrate or fat as the main source of energy, and in view of substantial body fat stores, large variations in macronutrient

intake (energy sources) and energy expenditure are well tolerated.

In addition to energy-providing nutrients, vitamins and minerals are essential for the digestion, absorption, and metabolism of carbohydrate, protein, and fat. Although vitamins and minerals are not required in large quantities, as are the macronutrients, their presence is just as important. When

Dental Hygiene Considerations

- Glycogen stores are depleted with a carbohydrate-poor diet even when high levels of fat and protein are eaten. A patient who ingests a carbohydrate-poor diet has decreased energy reserves and is prone to prolonged healing periods and fatigue.
- Blood glucose concentrations are increased only slightly when fructose, sorbitol, or xylitol is given because these sugars are absorbed more slowly; less insulin is required for their metabolism. Caution with portion size is still a consideration for individuals with diabetes.
- Patients with compromised liver or renal function may postpone progression of their condition by avoiding excessive amounts of protein.
- Ketoacidosis does not result from the rapid breakdown of adipose tissue alone; severe curtailment of carbohydrate intake must occur simultaneously. Ensure patients are consuming an adequate amount of carbohydrate.
- Ketoacidosis frequently occurs in patients with uncontrolled diabetes mellitus (see Health Application 6) or who are not eating (as a result of illness or weight reduction) because they are burning fat rather than carbohydrate. Question patients with fruity-smelling breath about recent food and fluid intake, weight loss, and conditions such as diabetes mellitus.
- High ketone levels may be associated with starvation or high-protein, low-carbohydrate, low-calorie diets. These result in decreased appetite and occasionally nausea, which can worsen the condition.
- Symptoms of hypoglycemia include weakness or light-headedness, confusion, pale color, sweating, and rapid, shallow breathing, or the patient may have no symptoms, yet have low blood glucose levels.

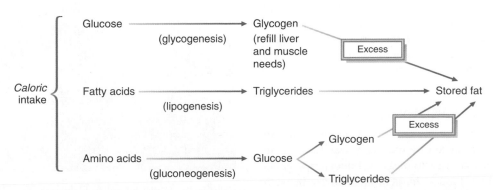

FIGURE 6-3 Metabolic pathways of excess energy. (From Nix S: Williams' Basic Nutrition and Diet Therapy, 12th ed. St Louis: Mosby, 2005.)

a deficiency occurs, reactions do not proceed normally. For example, although protein may be consumed alone (as in liquid protein supplements), many other nutrients, including vitamins and minerals, must be present for the protein to be used by cells. Each nutrient has its specific function; all the nutrients must be present simultaneously for optimal benefits.

A detailed discussion of metabolic interrelationships is beyond the scope of this text. These interrelationships are important, and for optimal use of nutrients, food sources of all the nutrients should be incorporated into every diet. The easiest way to obtain optimal nutrition is to include a variety of foods from all the food groups.

METABOLIC ENERGY

Without energy from chemical reactions, people could not bat an eye, wiggle a toe, or think a thought. Energy is required for all physiological functions. Energy from food is converted into forms the body can use: electrical for the brain and nerves, mechanical for muscles, thermal for body heat, and chemical for synthesis of new compounds.

The potential energy value of foods and energy exchanges within the body are expressed in terms of the kilocalorie. A **kilocalorie (kcal)** is the amount of heat required to increase the temperature of 1 kg of water 1° C. A kilocalorie is 1000 times larger than the small calorie. Although *kilocalorie* is the proper term, it is commonly used interchangeably with calorie or Calorie (abbreviated *Cal*).

Carbohydrate, fat, protein, and even alcohol provide energy for humans. (Vitamins and minerals are not energy sources, but are necessary for energy-producing reactions.) Physiological energy values commonly used are 4 kcal/g carbohydrate, 9 kcal/g fat, 4 kcal/g protein, and 7 kcal/g alcohol.

MEASUREMENT OF POTENTIAL ENERGY

The amount of energy, or kilocalories, available in a food may be precisely calculated by placing a weighed amount of food inside a device used to measure kilocalories, called a **calorimeter**. As a food is burned, an increase in water temperature indicates the heat given off or potential (free) energy of that food.

ENERGY PRODUCTION

The metabolism of basic nutrients results in production of cellular energy, which is stored as **adenosine triphosphate (ATP)**. ATP is an instant source of cellular energy for mechanical work, transport of nutrients and waste products, and synthesis of chemical compounds generated from the Krebs cycle. ATP units, also called **high-energy phosphate compounds**, are the currency or "money" the body uses for energy. Because ATP can be metabolized without oxygen, the reaction is classified as anaerobic. The body must always have a supply of ATP, and several systems within the body ensure a constant supply.

Increasing kilocaloric intake from carbohydrates and fats would not produce optimal energy without adequate protein intake. Energy use is remarkably sensitive to the quantity and the quality of dietary protein.

BASAL METABOLIC RATE

Even during sleep, the body requires energy for the obvious minimum tasks of respiration and circulation, and many intricate activities within each cell. **Basal metabolic rate (BMR)** indicates the energy required for involuntary physiological functions to maintain life, including respiration, circulation, and maintenance of muscle tone and body temperature. A patient's BMR is lowest while lying down, awake, rested, and relaxed in a comfortable environment, not having eaten for 12 to 15 hours. The BMR can be measured in a clinical setting using **indirect calorimetry,** which indirectly measures the rate of oxygen used while the person is resting (Fig. 6-4). Because digestion and absorption require energy, the BMR is the amount of energy required when the body is in a **postabsorptive state** (digestive and absorptive processes are minimal).

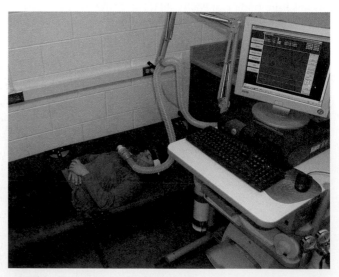

FIGURE 6-4 Measuring basal metabolic rate. (From Nix S: Williams' Basic Nutrition and Diet Therapy, 12th ed. St Louis: Mosby, 2005.)

FACTORS AFFECTING THE BASAL METABOLIC RATE

Various factors can increase or decrease the BMR, which determines energy needs.

Sleep

Metabolic rate is lowest after a few hours of sleep because muscles are more relaxed. About 10% less energy is needed for the BMR during this relaxed state.

Age

From birth through age 2, growth results in the highest BMR, which then decreases until the puberty growth spurt, and is followed by a gradual decline for the rest of the life cycle (Fig. 6-5).

Pregnancy and Lactation

During the last trimester of pregnancy, the BMR increases about 15% to 30%. The amount of energy necessary to produce milk for lactation can increase the BMR 40%.

Surface Area

The more body surface area, the greater the BMR. Because of greater surface area, a tall, thin person requires more energy than a short, heavy one of similar weight.

State of Health

Illnesses and diseases may increase or decrease the BMR. Patients recovering from a wasting illness require extra energy to build new tissue. Additionally, the activity level may be influenced by such conditions as lack of sleep, exhaustion, tenseness, fatigue, or depression.

Body Composition and Gender

In adulthood, lean body mass is the best single predictor of the BMR. Because cells in muscles and glands are more active than cells in bone and fat, body composition influences the BMR. The amount of lean body tissue versus fat tissue in adults is a distinguishing factor; normally, women have more fat tissue and use fewer kilocalories. Differences in the BMR may be primarily related to typical variations in body composition, rather than directly related to gender.

Muscle tone is an important factor in metabolism; the state of tension or relaxation also has an effect. An athlete who has better muscle tone than a sedentary individual of similar size and shape requires more kilocalories.

Endocrine Glands: Chemical Messengers

Thyroxine, the iodine-containing hormone from the thyroid gland, has a greater influence on the rate of metabolic processes than secretions from any other gland. However, obesity as a result of thyroid problems is rare.

Adrenal glands affect metabolism to a lesser degree. Stimulations by fright, excitement, or even joy can cause a temporary increase in the BMR by releasing catecholamines, particularly epinephrine. The pituitary gland accounts for about a 15% to 20% increase in the BMR during growth of children and adolescents.

Temperature

The BMR can be affected by body temperature or climate. The BMR is slightly higher in cooler climates to maintain normal body temperature. The BMR increases when fever is present.

Fasting and Starvation

Patients who are undernourished or fasting for long periods have a lower than normal BMR. This is a result of decreased muscle mass and an adaptive body process to conserve energy. Numerous studies indicate the body responds to dieting the way it does to famine, by decreasing the BMR.

TOTAL ENERGY REQUIREMENTS

Basal energy expenditure (BEE) includes kilocalories necessary to maintain BMR, plus additional kilocalories needed for thermic effect, voluntary activities, and any increased needs from catabolic (disease states, fever) or anabolic (growth, pregnancy) processes for a 24-hour period. The **thermic effect** of food refers to increased energy expenditure resulting from the consumption of food or the number of kilocalories needed to digest the food.

BMR can be estimated using several methods based on a patient's age, gender, and body size. For most patients, the BMR accounts for 65% to 70% of the body's total energy requirement. Determining a patient's precise BMR is still

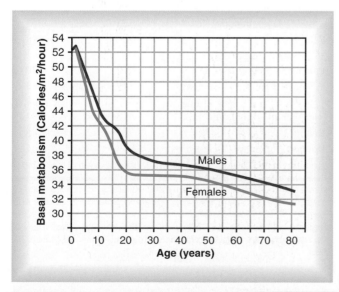

FIGURE 6-5 Normal basal metabolic rates at different ages for each sex. (From Guyton AC, Hall JE: Textbook of Medical Physiology, 11th ed. Philadelphia: Saunders, 2006.)

inexact, but many general guidelines have been formulated. One quick guideline for adults is as follows:

$$10-11\times \text{ideal weight (lb)} = \text{kilocalories needed for BMR daily}$$

THERMIC EFFECT OF FOOD

Food digestion requires energy. The thermic effect of a mixed diet is estimated to be about 10% of the energy required for BMR. Many times this factor is omitted in calculations determining total energy expenditure (TEE).

VOLUNTARY WORK AND PLAY

The most variable factor affecting total energy needs is muscle activity, which is influenced by the physical activity level (Table 6-1). Mental activity uses almost no extra energy (about 3 to 4 kcal per hour). Activity level normally accounts for 20% to 30% of the daily energy requirement. A quick easy estimation of caloric requirements can be determined using the following calculations:

$$3\times \text{ideal weight (lb)} = \text{kilocalories for inactive, bedfast, or obese individuals}$$

$$5\times \text{ideal weight (lb)} = \text{kilocalories for sedentary individuals or individuals older than 55 years}$$

$$10\times \text{ideal weight (lb)} = \text{kilocalories for thin or very active individuals}$$

The *Dietary Guidelines for Americans 2005* and MyPyramid guidelines address the need for regular physical activity. The Institute of Medicine (IOM) initially recommended a minimum of 30 minutes a day of moderate exercise most days of the week, but in the fall of 2008, the Physical Activities Guidelines from USHSS indicated the $2^{1}/_{2}$ hours per week should be moderate intensity for substantial health benefits.[3] The exercise or activity should be one the individual enjoys to enhance the likelihood the activity will be maintained.

ESTIMATED ENERGY REQUIREMENTS

The estimated energy requirements (EERs) established by the IOM indicate the daily kilocalorie intake needed to maintain energy balance in healthy individuals of a specific age, gender, weight, height, and level of physical activity (see p. i). These levels are recommended to sustain body weights in the desired range for good health (body mass index [BMI] 18.5 to 25 kg/m^2), while maintaining a lifestyle including adequate levels of physical activity. A recommended dietary allowance (RDA) was not established because energy intakes greater than the EER could result in weight gain. Weight gain resulting in a BMI greater than 25 kg/m^2 is associated with an increased risk of early mortality. Numerous studies substantiate a morbidity risk of type 2 diabetes, hypertension, coronary heart disease (CHD), stroke, gallbladder disease, osteoarthritis, and some types of

Table 6-1 Energy Expenditure during Various Activities

Activity (1 hour)	130 lb	155 lb	190 lb
Aerobics, general	354	422	518
Aerobics, low impact	295	352	431
Bicycling, 14-15.9 mph, vigorous effort	590	704	863
Bicycling, stationary, general	295	352	431
Bicycling, stationary, vigorous effort	620	739	906
Billiards	148	176	216
Bowling	177	211	259
Calisthenics, home, light/moderate effort	266	317	388
Carpentry, general	207	246	302
Cleaning, house, general	207	246	302
Construction, outside, remodeling	325	387	474
Cooking or food preparation	148	176	216
Dancing, aerobic, ballet or modern, twist	354	422	518
Dancing, ballroom, fast	325	387	474
Dancing, ballroom, slow	177	211	259
Electrical work, plumbing	207	246	302
Fishing, general	236	281	345
Football or baseball, playing catch	148	176	216
Football, competitive	531	633	776
Football, touch, flag, general	471	563	690
Frisbee playing, general	177	211	259
Golf, carrying clubs	325	387	474
Handball, general	708	844	1035
Health club exercise, general	325	387	474
Hiking, cross country	354	422	518
Horseback riding, general	236	281	345
Jogging, general	413	493	604
Judo, karate, kick boxing, tae kwon do	590	704	863
Marching, rapidly, military	387	457	561
Mowing lawn, general	325	387	474
Painting, papering, plastering, scraping	266	317	388
Polo	472	563	690
Pushing or pulling stroller with child	148	176	216
Racquetball, casual, general	413	493	604
Raking lawn	236	281	345
Rowing, stationary, light effort	413	493	604
Rowing, stationary, vigorous effort	561	669	819

Adapted from NutriStrategy Software. Kilocalories are calculated based on research data from *Medicine and Science in Sports and Exercise*, The Official Journal of the American College of Sports Medicine. Copyright © 2004 by NutriStrategy. Available at http://www.nutristrategy.com/activitylist4.htm. Accessed March 29, 2008.

cancer for BMIs greater than 25 kg/m². The IOM suggests that at the end of adolescence, BMI should be around 22 kg/m² to allow for a moderate weight gain in midlife without exceeding the 25 kg/m² threshold.[4]

Dental Hygiene Considerations

- Encourage intake of adequate amounts of protein and energy to spare protein for growth or healing, as needed. If energy is insufficient, healing is prolonged.
- Low-carbohydrate diets are not as effective in supporting high activity levels as a high intake of complex carbohydrates. For athletic patients, advise increased intake of complex carbohydrates.
- For healthy men, the BMR usually ranges from about 1580 to 1870 kcal daily, whereas approximately 1150 to 1440 kcal is needed for women. If energy intake is inadequate, physical status may deteriorate. A referral to a healthcare provider or registered dietitian is needed to improve nutrient intake.
- Increased thyroxine activity (hyperthyroidism) may double the BMR and can cause vitamin deficiencies because the quantity of many of the enzymes is increased (vitamins are essential parts of some of these coenzymes).
- A naturally higher BMR is a reason why children and pregnant women do not feel as cold as adults under the same weather conditions. Do not overdress children based on an adult's perception.
- Unless physical activity is above average, the BMR represents the largest proportion of a patient's energy requirement. Determination of the BMR can be used to evaluate adequacy of caloric intake.

Nutritional Directions

- The BMR may be elevated or depressed. A high BMR requires more kilocalories; fewer kilocalories are needed for a low BMR.
- Because the BMR decreases about 2% every 10 years after age 25, many patients gain weight because previous eating habits are maintained without increasing activity.

ENERGY BALANCE

The proper energy balance for stable weight is maintained when the caloric intake equals the amount of energy needed for body processes and physical activities (Fig. 6-6). Energy balance is maintained when the kilocalorie intake equals the amount of energy needed for body processes and physical activities. This statement sounds simple, but very few Americans are able to maintain energy balance at an appropriate body weight. Many factors enter into this unbalanced equation; because it is a complex system, there are no easy answers. An alarming and increasing number of Americans are overweight; energy consumption increased by more than 168 kcal per day for men and approximately 335 kcal for women between 1971-2000.[5] The estimated 1877 kcal per day for women and 2618 kcal per day for men are signifi-

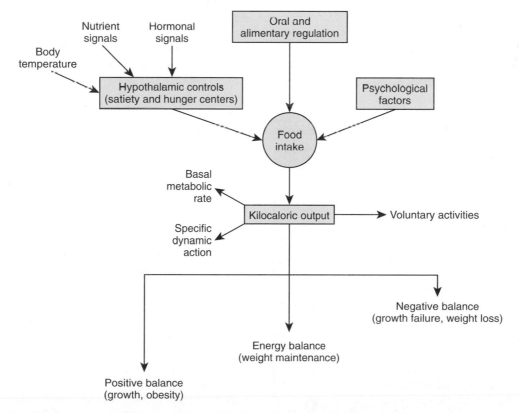

FIGURE 6-6 Factors affecting energy balance. (From Davis JR, Sherer K: Applied Nutrition and Diet Therapy for Nurses, 2nd ed. Philadelphia: Saunders, 1994.)

cantly above the government recommendation of 1600 kcal per day for women and 2200 kcal per day for men. Dental hygienists need to have an awareness of the complexities of maintaining energy balance to be more understanding of patients who have problems managing their weight.

Many healthy patients are able to control energy intake to balance energy output with little effort; their **appetite**, or the desire to eat, controls food intake to balance energy expenditure. **Hunger**, or the physiological drive to eat, is regulated by a complex network of factors (see Fig. 6-6). Appetite is frequently used in the same sense as hunger, but it usually implies desire for specific types of food and is related to the pleasurable sensation of eating.

Hunger and appetite greatly affect weight balance. When more kilocalories are consumed than the body needs, the excess is stored as fat, resulting in weight gain. One pound of body fat is equivalent to 3500 kcal. Overweight patients have a very difficult time losing extra pounds and maintaining their energy balance to keep off unwanted pounds. Weight control can be approached by either decreasing the number of kilocalories consumed or increasing physical activities. A combination of both is most effective (Box 6-2).

Intake has generally been regarded as the key to weight regulation. Most patients' weight tends to remain stable for long periods with only a 1- to 5-lb gain or loss of adipose tissue over a year. Even small daily deviations from balance could result in gradual significant fluctuations in fat stores. For instance, an additional 100 kcal daily would result in a 10-lb weight gain over a year's time and a 100-lb gain over 10 years.

PHYSIOLOGICAL FACTORS

The hypothalamus, located in the middle of the brain, is especially important in controlling hunger. A satiety center and a hunger or feeding center are present within the hypothalamus.

Stimulation of the hunger center causes insatiable hunger; damage to this area results in no desire for food. Stimulation of the satiety center results in complete satiety. If the satiety center of the hypothalamus is destroyed, the appetite becomes voracious, resulting in obesity. The feeding center stimulates the drive to eat, whereas the satiety center inhibits the feeding center.

Metabolic factors control the feeding center. The knowledge that hypoglycemia causes hunger has led to the glucostatic theory of hunger and feeding regulation. An increase in blood glucose activates the satiety center and deactivates neurons in the hunger center. A high-protein, very-low-carbohydrate diet reduces hunger, reducing food intake significantly more than high-protein diets containing larger amounts of carbohydrate.[6]

Usually the body discerns food characteristics such as sweetness and viscosity to gauge intake. The body may use this information to determine how much food is needed to meet its caloric requirements. Many have hypothesized that the use of noncaloric sweeteners may confuse the body's ability to discern that the taste and feel of food in the mouth is providing caloric intake. It is possible by substituting noncaloric sweetened foods and beverages for natural sweeteners, the body learns it can no longer use the taste sense to gauge kilocalories, resulting in increased caloric intake.[7,8] More research is needed to determine the effect low-calorie products have on the appetite. When food comes into contact with the stomach mucosa and small intestine muscles, gut peptides are secreted affecting satiety.

Several mechanisms affect the amount eaten at a particular meal. Distention of the stomach results in inhibitory signals that suppress the feeding center, reducing the desire to eat. The release of cholecystokinin in response to fat in the duodenum has a strong direct effect on the feeding center, causing the person to cease eating. Food in the stomach and duodenum causes the secretion of glucagon and insulin, both of which suppress the feeding center.

Additionally, the hypothalamus is responsive to body temperature. Cold temperatures lead to increased food intake, resulting in a higher metabolic rate and more fat stores for insulation.

The relationship between exercise and food intake is unclear. Exercise has been reported to increase, decrease, or have no effect on appetite. These findings cannot be explained, but may be related to timing or duration of the exercise, individual metabolic differences, or some unknown reason. Generally, acute exercise decreases food intake after the activity, but regular exercise promotes increased energy intake.

Nutrient and hormonal signals affect the brain and liver to stimulate satiety and feeding centers in the brain (Table 6-2). Numerous studies have shown physiological control of energy intake is unreliable. Energy balance must be adjusted through some other mechanism.

Box 6-2	**Equation for Weight Loss**

The TEE for a sedentary individual 67 inches tall, weight 191 lb (BMI = 30) is 2235 kcal.

For 1 lb weight loss per week, decrease caloric intake by 500 kcal per day:

$$2235 - 500 = 1735 \text{ kcal per day}$$

The result of a 500-kcal deficit in 1 week:

$$500 \times 7 = 3500 \text{ kcal}$$

A kilocalorie reduction combined with exercise to lose 2 lb per week can be accomplished by increasing caloric expenditure by 500 kcal per day.

Cycling at a rate of 15 mph or running at a rate of 10 minutes per mile for 45 minutes = 525 kcal:

$$525 \times 7 = 3675 \text{ kcal}$$

This would result in a weight loss of 2 lb per week or 8 lb per month.

Table 6-2	Stimuli Affecting Food Intake	
	Food Intake	
Signal	**Increased**	**Decreased**
Food odors	Pleasant	Repulsive
Taste	Desirable	Offensive
Climate (temperature)	Cold	Hot
Gastrointestinal	Hunger pains	Distention Cholecystokinin Glucagon
Glucose level	Low	High
Lipoprotein	High	Low
Nutrient stores	Decreased	Increased

From Davis JR, Sherer K: Applied Nutrition and Diet Therapy for Nurses, 2nd ed. Philadelphia: Saunders, 1994.

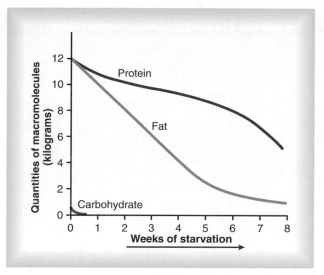

FIGURE 6-7 Effects of starvation on the body. Three major macromolecules serve as primary energy sources: carbohydrates, fats, and proteins. During starvation, the carbohydrate stores (glycogen) are rapidly depleted. However, stored lipids can mobilize and provide much of a person's energy needs for several weeks. Eventually, lipid stores run low, and the body starts using proteins as a major source of energy—causing the breakdown of muscle and other protein-rich tissues. Muscle damage during starvation usually leads to death. (From Guyton AC, Hall JE: Textbook of Medical Physiology, 11th ed. Philadelphia: Saunders, 2006.)

PSYCHOLOGICAL FACTORS

Appetite is affected by the fact that eating is rewarding or pleasurable and makes us feel good. The eating behavior of obese individuals is thought to be influenced more by external cues, including time, taste, smell, and sight of food, than it is in individuals of normal weight. Greater weight usually means the individual is responding to feelings and emotions rather than actual hunger. Boredom and stress are frequently factors affecting eating habits of obese individuals.

ENERGY EXPENDITURE

Contrary to popular opinion, obese women have a similar or higher metabolic rate than thinner women. The effect of this is less weight gain for a given increase in caloric intake. Genetics may also play a role in the BMR. Some families have low metabolic rates, but not all individuals with a low BMR are obese.

Exercise tolerance of obese individuals is less than normal, but any activity uses more kilocalories because of the amount of additional mass that has to be moved. Not all inactive patients are obese, so activity level does not seem to be a principal determinant in the development of obesity. Because of differences in body composition (percentage of muscle and fat), the BMR affects energy expenditure for various activities. Weight loss resulting from a specific energy deficit is invariably smaller than expected. Conversely, overconsumption fails to produce weight gains anticipated. Adjustments in energy expenditure seem to be adaptive.

Because food is abundant in the United States, and many Americans enjoy eating, physical activity of most individuals needs to increase to balance energy intake. Walking is a physical activity that has been emphasized because it is inexpensive and convenient, and most individuals are physically able to walk, even if they initially need to walk at a slow rate. Numerous studies have shown use of a **pedometer** (a small meter worn at the waist that monitors the number of steps a person takes) results in significant improvements in the number of steps per week.[9-11] Usually the goal is 10,000 steps a day, but individuals are encouraged to start at a comfortable pace and distance, and gradually increase intensity and distance.

INADEQUATE ENERGY INTAKE

A deficiency in energy intake may result in a depressed rate of growth in children and weight loss in adults. Intentional weight loss may be helpful or harmful, depending on the methods used for losing weight. Decreased fat stores are normally the goal, but loss of muscle may be an undesirable side effect (Fig. 6-7).

Inadequate energy intake may result in malnutrition and become a serious problem in the face of a physiologically stressful situation. Inadequate intake may be intentional, as in the case of anorexia nervosa, a psychological disorder in which one's undernourishment is not perceived. Inadequate intake causes a vicious downward spiral in which metabolic imbalances decrease hunger and may become life-threatening without proper treatment.

Dental Hygiene Considerations

- Observe emotional factors. Depression and stress as well as other emotional factors result in overeating and decreased activity in some patients. Referral to a healthcare provider may be indicated.
- A positive energy balance is desirable during periods of growth; a proportionately larger amount of energy is needed by pregnant and lactating women and children.
- When nutrient stores decrease, the feeding center of the hypothalamus becomes active, and the patient becomes hungry; when nutrient stores are abundant, the patient feels satiated and loses the desire to eat. If the hypothalamus is injured in any way (as in a head injury or stroke), hunger and satiety may be altered.
- If kilocalories are underestimated, the body must use stored energy (fat and protein), making the patient at risk for malnutrition. If excessive kilocalories are given, the body converts excess kilocalories to fat.
- A patient with a BMI between 18.5 kg/m^2 and 25 kg/m^2 has approximately 13 to 44 lb of body fat, which could provide 50,000 to 200,000 kcal.

Nutritional Directions

- Exercise may enhance the BMR by increasing the amount of lean body mass, which uses more energy.
- To gain 1 lb of fat, a patient must consume 3500 kcal more than are used.
- To lose 1 lb of weight, energy intake must be 3500 kcal less than the number of kilocalories used.
- A decrease from prior activity level or additional caloric intake may result in weight gain.
- Large variations from energy balance are well tolerated, but may be reflected in gains or losses of fat.
- Although quitting smoking is linked to an increased risk of weight gain, encourage patients who smoke to enroll in a smoking cessation program along with a weight loss program. Remind the patient that the benefits of not smoking outweigh the potential risk factor of weight gain associated with quitting smoking.

HEALTH APPLICATION 6   Diabetes Mellitus

Diabetes mellitus is a heterogeneous group of metabolic abnormalities in which carbohydrates, proteins, fats, and insulin are ineffectively metabolized, leading to disturbances in fluid and electrolyte balances (Fig. 6-8). It is a chronic, lifelong disease. Diabetes mellitus is specifically related to hormonal pancreatic secretions, but involves the entire endocrine system.

Diabetes mellitus is presently one of the most common diseases, with rates increasing at an alarming pace, especially in children and adolescents. African Americans, Hispanic Americans and Native Americans have the highest incidence of diabetes mellitus of all population groups. In addition to metabolic complications secondary to diabetes mellitus, life expectancy is about 70% to 80% that of the general population. The Centers for Disease Control and Prevention (CDC) estimates more than 18.2 million individuals in the United States, or 6.3% of the population, have diabetes mellitus; 57 million have prediabetes, and an additional 5.2 million have diabetes but are not aware of it.[12] Type 2 diabetes mellitus can be prevented or delayed by changes in lifestyles of high-risk individuals.[6,7] Exercise improves the body's sensitivity to insulin and helps the body metabolize glucose better, preventing development of diabetes in individuals who are at high risk.

The two most prevalent types of diabetes mellitus are characterized by different metabolic defects and can appear to be very different conditions (Table 6-3). Type 1 diabetes mellitus, which affects 5% to 10% of individuals with the disease, is distinguished by little or no endogenous insulin production. This condition most commonly manifests in young people but can occur at any age. (Type 1 diabetes mellitus was formerly known as *juvenile* or *insulin-dependent diabetes*; the name was changed because adults also develop type 1 diabetes.) Onset is sudden with all the clinical symptoms associated with this condition. Patients are prone to ketosis and must receive exogenous insulin for life.

Approximately 90% to 95% of Americans with diabetes have type 2 diabetes mellitus, which results from insulin resistance, usually with a relative insulin deficiency. Family history, age, history of gestational diabetes, obesity (BMI greater than 27 kg/m^2), and sedentary lifestyle are risk factors associated with diabetes. For obese patients, increased fat stores cause some degree of insulin resistance. In many cases, insulin is secreted in adequate or higher-than-normal amounts, but glucose uptake by body cells (except for the brain) is decreased.

Abnormalities in insulin levels precipitate clinical manifestations. Insulin deficiency or defects in insulin action or both result in hyperglycemia, the main manifestation of type 2 diabetes mellitus. Symptoms of hyperglycemia include thirst, frequent urination, hunger, blurry vision, fatigue, frequent infections, and dry, itchy skin; or the patient can be asymptomatic.

Treatment should be implemented as soon as possible after diagnosis to prevent complications of metabolic alterations secondary to diabetes mellitus. Elevated blood glucose levels can damage almost every major organ of the body. Early, tight control of diabetes can postpone and minimize many of these severe complications. Chronic complications develop slowly over long periods as body tissues are adversely exposed to hyperglycemia and hypoglycemia. Hyperglycemia in type 2 diabetes mellitus causes macrovascular and microvascular disease (involving large and small vessels) and can damage almost every major organ of the body. Patients with uncontrolled diabetes experience slow wound healing, frequent abscesses, periodontal disease, a predisposition to bacterial infections, a compromised immune system, skin irritations, pruritus

Normal

Carbohydrates

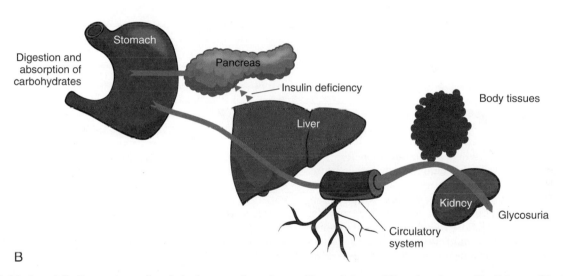

A

Diabetes Mellitus (type 1)

Carbohydrates

B

FIGURE 6-8 **A** and **B,** Comparison of carbohydrate use in patients without diabetes (**A**) and patients with diabetes (**B**). (Adapted from What Is Diabetes? Indianapolis: Eli Lilly & Co, 1973.)

HEALTH APPLICATION   **6**   Diabetes Mellitus—cont'd

(itching), numbness and tingling of the extremities, and visual disturbances. The American Diabetes Association defines uncontrolled blood glucose levels as three consecutive readings at 200 mg/dL or greater.[13] Because of the increased risks of hyperglycemia on the oral cavity, the patient may need to be rescheduled when his or her blood glucose levels are in a safer range (70 to 200 mg/dL).

Obtaining a blood glucose level using a glucometer (meter used to self-monitor capillary blood glucose levels) provides a day-to-day, minute-to-minute reading. It is a "snapshot" of the blood glucose level at the time it is taken. This is valuable information to obtain before a dental procedure because blood glucose levels can vary throughout the day. It is measured in milligrams per deciliter or millimoles per liter.

Another valuable reading is the glycosylated hemoglobin (A_{1C}) assay, a widely accepted and reliable measure of a blood glucose level over the past 3 months. It provides a guide for long-term planning and possible adjustments to diabetes treatment. However, hemoglobin A_{1C} does not show the ups and downs in a given day, just an average level over 3 months. It is used to evaluate metabolic control and to determine whether the target range is maintained.[14]

Hyperlipidemia and hypertension are common risks for individuals with diabetes, and are often treated more

Table 6-3   Comparison of Type 1 and Type 2 Diabetes Mellitus

	Type 1	Type 2
Prevalence	About 5-10% of cases	90-95% of cases (1 in 5 adults >65 years old)
Age at onset	Most frequently during childhood or puberty, but may occur at later ages	Frequently >40, but occurring more frequently in overweight children and adolescents
Precipitating cause	Genetic, autoimmune destruction of the pancreatic cells that produce insulin	Obesity and inactivity
Type of onset	Sudden, but may develop slowly in adults	Usually gradual; may go undetected for years
Family history of diabetes	Frequently positive	Usually positive
Nutritional status at time of onset	Normal weight with recent weight loss, but occasionally obese	Usually overweight (BMI >25) with increased percentage of body fat predominantly in the abdominal region
Symptoms	Polydipsia, polyphagia, ketoacidosis, weight loss	Glycosuria without ketonuria; absent or mild polyuria and polydipsia
Blood glucose stability	Fluctuates widely in response to changes in insulin, diet, exercise, infection, and stress	Fluctuations less marked
Control of diabetes	Difficult	Easy, especially if diet is followed
Ketosis	Frequent	Seldom
Plasma insulin	Negligible or absent	May be low (not absent) or high, with insulin resistance
Vascular complications and degenerative changes	Occur after diabetes present for about 5 years	Increased risk of macrovascular and microvascular complications
Medical nutrition therapy	Required	May eliminate need for hypoglycemic agents or insulin or both
Medication	Insulin required for all	Usually can be controlled with hypoglycemic agents; insulin may be necessary for some

HEALTH APPLICATION 6   Diabetes Mellitus—cont'd

aggressively than in individuals without diabetes. For example, a patient with diabetes who has a blood pressure of 130/80 mm Hg or greater begins treatment for hypertension, whereas someone without diabetes receives the same treatment when blood pressure readings are 140/90 mm Hg or greater.[13] Changes in capillary membranes result in renal complications (leading to **renal failure,** or inability of the kidneys to maintain their normal function of excreting toxic waste materials), obstruction of circulation in the extremities (leading to gangrene), and progressive blood vessel damage in the retina of the eye (leading to blindness). Neuropathy, or deterioration of nervous tissue, also is frequently seen in diabetes mellitus. Abnormalities of the gastrointestinal tract causing nausea, early satiety, and frequent vomiting interfere with food intake and absorption.

Hypoglycemia, or low blood glucose levels (less than 70 mg/dL) can occur when a patient is taking insulin or an antidiabetic medication whose side effect is hypoglycemia. Signs and symptoms include a fast heartbeat, hunger, shakiness, blurry vision, sweating, fatigue, dizziness, and irritability. However, the patient may have no symptoms, so it is valuable to obtain blood glucose readings before treatment to prevent a medical emergency. A patient whose blood glucose level is less than 70 mg/dL should be treated with 10 to 15 g of a carbohydrate source, such as 3 glucose tablets, 1 tube of glucose gel, 8 hard candies (disk), 4 oz of regular soda, or 4 oz of fruit juice. Wait 15 minutes and retest. If the blood glucose level is still less than 70 mg/dL

or symptoms remain, repeat. When the blood glucose level is greater than 70 mg/dL, continue with treatment, and offer a meal or snack within 30 minutes. If the patient is experiencing severe hypoglycemia (e.g., uncooperative, unable to take fluids, or unconscious), administer glucagon to bring the blood glucose value into an appropriate range. Call the community emergency medical services (EMS) for assistance.

Consensus supports medical nutrition therapy as the cornerstone for preventing hyperglycemia and hypoglycemia and decreasing chronic complications. No single dietary plan can be appropriate for all individuals with different personalities and lifestyles. The objective of the meal plan is to empower patients to maintain good control of their diabetes or to promote near-normal blood glucose, lipid, and blood pressure levels. Additionally, food choices should promote overall health by providing optimal nutrition and allowing physical activity; achieving or maintaining an ideal body weight; and preventing or delaying development or progression of periodontal disease, and cardiovascular, renal, retinal, neurological, and other complications associated with diabetes, insofar as these are related to metabolic control. The meal plan should be flexible to allow personal and cultural preferences and lifestyles, while respecting the individual's wishes and willingness to make changes.

Beginning in 2002, the American Diabetes Association's nutritional recommendations were assigned a grade (A, B, C, or E) based on the weight of the scientific evidence that

| HEALTH APPLICATION | 6 | Diabetes Mellitus—cont'd |

supports it. An *A* rating means supportive evidence is based on multiple, well-conducted studies; *B* is an intermediate rating signifying some supporting evidence is available; *C* means supporting evidence is limited; *E* means the recommendation is based on expert consensus. These are reviewed annually, and grades are re-evaluated based on new research. Table 6-4 lists some of the more than 51 nutrition recommendations.

The American Diabetes Association, the American Dietetic Association, and the U.S. Public Health Service compiled the exchange system to allow flexibility of the meal plan in addition to achieving a reasonable constancy of carbohydrate, protein, fat, and energy intake. These exchange lists divide foods into six groups; within each group, all food items are approximately equal in carbohydrate, protein, and fat content. Serving sizes vary so that foods in each list are calorically equivalent. Foods within any group can be traded, or exchanged, with other foods in the same group. Use of the exchange system is not essential, but it is a good tool for teaching macronutrient content of foods, is easy for patients to follow, and can be adapted easily to meet the individual's needs.

Because of increased awareness of nutrient metabolism in diabetes, the "diabetes meal plan" has been liberalized in favor of modifying the patient's usual eating habits to be more consistent with the *Dietary Guidelines for Americans* and MyPyramid. When kilocalorie content is controlled, all foods containing carbohydrate, protein, fat, and alcohol are limited because these sources of energy are potential sources of glucose.

Carbohydrate counting focuses on total carbohydrate consumption. Because carbohydrate is the major factor in blood glucose fluctuations, the given amount of carbohydrate affects insulin requirements more than the protein and fat content. Carbohydrate counting provides greater precision in estimating carbohydrate intake than the diabetic food exchange lists.

For individuals with a healthy weight and normal lipid profile, the American Diabetes Association recommends the same guidelines as advocated by the National Cholesterol Education Program (NCEP), discussed in Chapter 5. Because of undesirable lipid levels for many patients with diabetes, a moderate increase in monounsaturated fat with a moderate intake of carbohydrate is recommended.

| Table 6-4 | American Diabetes Association Nutritional Recommendations |

A-C, E Rating*	Recommendation
Diabetes Prevention	
A	Among individuals at high risk for developing type 2 diabetes, structured programs that emphasize lifestyle changes including moderate weight loss (7% body weight) and regular physical activity (150 min/wk), with dietary strategies including reduced calories and reduced intake of dietary fat can reduce risk for developing diabetes and are recommended
B	Individuals at high risk for type 2 diabetes should be encouraged to achieve the U.S. Department of Agriculture (USDA) recommendation for dietary fiber (14 g fiber/1000 kcal) and foods containing whole grains (one-half of grain intake)
Carbohydrates	
A	Monitoring carbohydrate, whether by carbohydrate counting, exchanges, or experienced-based estimation, remains a key strategy in achieving glycemia control
A	Sucrose-containing foods can be substituted for other carbohydrates in meal plan or, if added to meal plan, covered with insulin or other glucose-lowering medications. Care should be taken to avoid excess energy intake
A	Sugar alcohols and non-nutritive sweeteners are safe when consumed within daily intake levels established by U.S. Food and Drug Administration (FDA)
B	A dietary pattern that includes carbohydrate from fruits, vegetables, whole grains, legumes, and low-fat milk is encouraged for good health
B	The use of glycemic index and load may provide modest additional benefit over that observed when total carbohydrate is considered alone
B	As for the general population, patients with diabetes are encouraged to consume a variety of fiber-containing foods. Evidence is lacking to recommend a higher fiber intake for patients with diabetes than for the population as a whole
Protein	
A	For patients with type 2 diabetes, ingested protein can increase insulin response without increasing plasma glucose concentrations. Protein should not be used to treat acute hypoglycemia or prevent nighttime hypoglycemia
E	For patients with diabetes and normal renal function, there is insufficient evidence to suggest that usual protein intake (15-20% of energy) should be modified

Table 6-4   American Diabetes Association Nutritional Recommendations—cont'd

A-C, E Rating*	Recommendation
E	High-protein diets are not recommended as a method for weight loss at this time. Long-term effects of protein intake >20% of calories on diabetes management and its complications are unknown. Although such diets may produce short-term weight loss and improved glycemia, it has not been established that these benefits are maintained long-term, and long-term effects on kidney function for patients with diabetes are unknown
Fats	
A	Limit saturated fat to <7% of total calories
B	Two or more servings of fish per week (with the exception of commercially fried fish filets) provide n-3 polyunsaturated fatty acids and are recommended
B	Intake of *trans* fat should be minimized
E	In patients with diabetes, limit dietary cholesterol to <200 mg per day
Energy Balance, Overweight, and Obesity	
A	In overweight and obese insulin-resistant patients, modest weight loss has been shown to improve insulin resistance. Weight loss is recommended for all such individuals who have or are at risk for diabetes
A	For weight loss, either low-carbohydrate or low-fat, calorie-restricted diets may be effective in the short-term (up to 1 year)
B	Physical activity and behavior modification are important components of weight loss programs and are most helpful in maintenance of weight loss
B	Bariatric surgery may be considered for some patients with type 2 diabetes and BMI ≥35 kg/m^2 and can result in marked improvements in glycemia. Long-term benefits and risks of bariatric surgery in patients with prediabetes or diabetes continue to be studied
Micronutrients	
A	There is no clear evidence of benefit from vitamin or mineral supplementation in patients with diabetes (compared with the general population) who do not have underlying deficiencies
A	Routine supplementation with antioxidants, such as vitamins E and C and carotene, is not advised because of lack of evidence of efficacy, and concern related to long-term safety
E	Benefit from chromium supplementation in individuals with diabetes or obesity has not been shown; chromium supplementation cannot be recommended
Alcohol	
B	In individuals with diabetes, moderate alcohol consumption (when ingested alone) has no acute effect on glucose and insulin concentrations, but carbohydrate co-ingested with alcohol (as in a mixed drink) may increase blood glucose
E	If adults with diabetes choose to use alcohol, daily intake should be limited to a moderate amount (≤1 drink per day for women and ≤2 drinks per day for men)
E	To reduce risk of nocturnal hypoglycemia in individuals using insulin or insulin secretogogues, alcohol should be consumed with food

Data from American Diabetes Association: Nutrition recommendations and interventions for diabetes. Diabetes Care 2008 Jan; 31(Suppl 1):S61-S78; and American Diabetes Association: Summary of revisions for the 2009 clinical practice recommendation. Diabetes Care 2009 Jan; 32 (suppl 1): S3-S5.

*ABC rating—evidence based on research criteria: *A,* strong supporting evidence; *B,* some supporting evidence; *C,* limited supporting evidence; *E,* based on expert consensus.

CASE APPLICATION FOR THE DENTAL HYGIENIST

On a routine recall appointment, Ronnie, who is 10 years old, reports that he was diagnosed with type 2 diabetes about a year ago. He appears to be about 100 lb overweight. After talking with him, you learn that he does not want to be labeled as "different" from his friends, so he eats when and what they do. Typically, they eat cheeseburgers, pizza, French fries, shakes, and regular sodas throughout the day. He says he does not have time to eat breakfast. He does not floss his teeth, has numerous caries, and has bleeding on probing.

Nutritional Assessment
- Observe height, weight, BMI, and age
- Knowledge of diabetes guidelines

- Motivation level
- Food/nutrient intake
- Eating habits
- Support from family and friends
- Activity level

Nutritional Diagnosis
Altered nutrition: Body requirements less than kilocalorie intake in relation to energy expenditure.

Nutritional Goals
The patient will have gradual weight loss until a BMI for age is below the 85th percentile.

CASE APPLICATION FOR THE DENTAL HYGIENIST—cont'd

Nutritional Implementation

Intervention: Provide Ronnie and his parents with the name of a registered dietitian who can provide necessary nutritional counseling.

Rationale: Well-balanced food choices that naturally contain a large amount of vitamins and minerals rather than high-calorie foods are needed to maintain his health and promote growth. A dietitian's knowledge of nutrition and expertise in counseling is recommended to provide adequate nutrients safely and effectively without affecting his linear growth.

Intervention: Explain that some of his food choices are not good for his overall physical or oral health.

Rationale: Consuming too many carbohydrates at meals and snacks affects his blood glucose level and increases the risk of caries.

Intervention: Explain carbohydrates, proteins, and fats all provide kilocalories, but fats are the most concentrated source of energy.

Rationale: To maintain his weight while still growing, wise food choices are advisable. Foods high in fat and sugar will not help him in his attempts to look handsome and may worsen his diabetes status.

Intervention: Stress the importance of consuming complex carbohydrate and fiber, and reducing intake of fat and kilocalories.

Rationale: Complex carbohydrate and fiber intake is effective in helping maintain a lower caloric intake without excessive hunger. Fat reduction enhances weight maintenance because a lower fat intake may help reduce energy intake and decrease risk of developing heart disease.

Intervention: Discuss the benefits of eating at routine times.

Rationale: This is important for control of his diabetes and may allow him time to brush his teeth after eating and reduce his risk of caries.

Intervention: Discuss the importance of a plan incorporating diet, exercise, and behavior modification.

Rationale: This combination of therapies has proven more effective for long-term weight control.

Intervention: Explain that good oral hygiene is very important for patients with diabetes because of an exaggerated response to plaque bacteria.

Rationale: Knowledge may help increase compliance.

Intervention: Suggest becoming involved in some sports, or increasing his activity level by walking to friends' homes, or participating in some recreational activity such as skating.

Rationale: Weight and diabetes control is improved when energy expenditure is increased along with decreased caloric intake. Additionally, physical activity helps increase muscle mass and improves strength.

Evaluation

The patient consulted with the dietitian and did not gain any weight before the next recall visit. Additionally, no new caries developed.

STUDENT READINESS

1. Define the terms "energy," "thermogenic effect," "basal metabolism," and "basal energy expenditure."
2. Calculate your total caloric needs for 1 day (BMR plus estimated voluntary energy expenditures plus thermogenic effect).
3. Assuming height and weight are the same, is the BMR higher or lower in:
   Men or women?
   An athlete or a sedentary person?
   A 40-year-old or a 20-year-old?
   A woman who is not pregnant or a woman who is pregnant?
4. How many kilocalories of protein, fat, and carbohydrate are in 1 cup of homogenized milk that contains 8.5 g of protein, 8.5 g of fat, and 12 g of carbohydrate?
5. A boxer achieved a dramatic weight loss of about 18 kg (39.6 lb) in about 60 days. A strict diet, heavy exercise, thyroid supplements, and a diuretic drug produced his large weight loss. His defeat in a boxing match shocked some of his fans. What happened to his physical condition? Explain.

CASE STUDY

Jay G. is a 16-year-old high school athlete on the football and baseball teams. He recently developed three dental caries. His classmates have encouraged him to eat a high-protein, low-carbohydrate diet. His mother is concerned about this and talks to her best friend, who is a dental hygienist.

1. What points do you think the dental hygienist should mention to this mother?
2. For increased energy expenditure, what should be the primary source of nutrients?
3. Would decreasing the carbohydrate content of the diet have a positive effect on the rate of dental caries?
4. What is the effect of a high protein intake?
5. On a high-protein, low-carbohydrate diet (approximately 120 g of protein, 80 g of carbohydrate, 2800 kcal), where would most of his energy requirements come from? Is this good or bad?
6. Which vitamins are important in the production of energy?
7. Is the diet varied? Does the diet provide recommended amounts of fruits, vegetables, grains, and other nutrients?

References

1. Chen L, et al: Alcohol intake and blood pressure: a systemic review implementing a mendelian randomization approach. PLoS Med 2008 Mar 4; 5(3):e52.
2. King DE, Mainous AG 3rd, Geesey ME: Adopting moderate alcohol consumption in middle age: subsequent cardiovascular events. Am J Med 2008 Mar; 121(3):201-206.
3. USHHS. 2008 Physical Activity Guidelines for Americans. Available online: www.health.gov/paguidelines. Accessed January 10, 2008.
4. Institute of Medicine (IOM), National Academy of Sciences: Dietary Reference Intakes for Energy, Carbohydrates, Fiber, Fat, Protein and Amino Acids (Macronutrients). Washington, DC: National Academy Press, 2002. Available at: http://www.nap.edu/books/0309085373/html
5. Wright JD, et al: Trends in intake of energy and macronutrients—United States, 1971-2000. MMWR Weekly (serial online): www.cdc.gov/MMWR/preview/mmwrhtml/mm5304a3.htm. Accessed March 22, 2008.
6. Johnstone AM, et al: Effects of a high-protein ketogenic diet on hunger, appetite, and weight loss in obese men feeding ad libitum. Am J Clin Nutr 2008 Jan; 87(1):44-55.
7. Swithers SE, Davidson TL: A role for sweet taste: calorie predictive relations in energy regulation by rats. Behav Neurosci 2008 Feb; 122(1):161-173.
8. Davidson TL, Swithers SE: Food viscosity influences caloric intake compensation and body weight in rats. Obes Res 2005 Mar; 13(3):537-544.
9. Rowland K, Schumann SA: Have pedometer, will travel. J Family Pract 2008 Feb; 57(2):90-93.
10. Faghri PD, et al: E-technology and pedometer walking program to increase physical activity at work. J Prim Prev 2008 Jan; 29(1):73-91.
11. Crotera KA, et al: Effect of a pedometer-based intervention on daily step counts of community-dwelling older adults. Res Q Exerc Sport 2007 Dec; 78(5):401-406.
12. Centers for Disease Control and Prevention: National Diabetes Fact Sheet: General Information and National Estimates on Diabetes in the United States, 2007. Atlanta, GA: U.S. Department of Health and Human Services, Centers for Disease Control and Prevention, 2008.
13. American Diabetes Association: Standards of medical care in diabetes—2009. Diabetes Care 2009; 32(suppl 1):S13-S61.
14. Nathan DM, et al: Translating the A_{1C} assay into estimated average glucose values. Diabetes Care 2008 Aug; 31(8):1473-1478.

Chapter 7

Vitamins Required for Calcified Structures

LEARNING OBJECTIVES

Upon completion of this chapter, the student will be able to achieve the following objectives:
- List the fat-soluble vitamins.
- Compare the characteristics of water-soluble vitamins with those of fat-soluble vitamins.
- Identify functions, deficiencies, surpluses, and toxicities and oral symptoms for vitamins A, D, E, K, and C.

- Select food sources for vitamins A, D, E, K, and C.
- Identify dental hygiene considerations for vitamins A, D, E, K, and C.
- Discuss nutritional directions for patients regarding vitamins A, D, E, K, and C.

KEY TERMS

Alopecia
Ameloblasts

Anticoagulant
Antioxidants

Calcitonin
Collagen
Diplopia
Enamel hypoplasia
Epiphyses
Fibroblasts
Follicular hyperkeratosis
Hematopoiesis
Hormone
Hypercarotenemia
Hypervitaminosis A
Leukoplakia
Lysosomes
Meta-analysis
Night blindness
Odontoblasts

Osteoblasts
Osteocalcin
Osteoclasts
Osteomalacia
Petechiae
Prostaglandins
Prothrombin
Retinoic acid
Rhodopsin
Scorbutic
Tocopherols
Tocotrienols
Vitamins
Xeroderma
Xerophthalmia

Test Your NQ

1. **T/F** Fat-soluble vitamins are stored in the body.
2. **T/F** Vitamins do not provide energy.
3. **T/F** Vitamin E is found in vegetable oils and green leafy vegetables.
4. **T/F** Fat-soluble vitamins include A, D, E, and K.
5. **T/F** Animal foods are the principal dietary source of beta carotene.
6. **T/F** Xerophthalmia occurs with a deficiency of vitamin A.
7. **T/F** The liver and kidney help convert vitamin D to its active form.
8. **T/F** An excess of vitamin D causes rickets.
9. **T/F** Vitamin K is essential for regulation of blood calcium and phosphorus levels.
10. **T/F** Vitamin C is needed for wound healing.

OVERVIEW OF VITAMINS

Nutrients never work single-handedly, but in partnership with each other. **Vitamins** are catalysts for all metabolic reactions using proteins, fats, and carbohydrates for energy, growth, and cell maintenance. Because only small amounts of these chemical substances obtained from food facilitate millions of processes, they may be regarded as "miracle workers."

Eating fats, carbohydrates, and proteins without enough vitamins means the energy from these nutrients cannot be used. The opposite is also true. Vitamins do not provide energy, and they cannot be used without an adequate supply of fats, carbohydrates, proteins, and minerals. Most vitamins come in several forms; each form may perform a different task. Vitamins are easily destroyed by the heat, oxidation and chemical processes used in their extraction. In this text, water-soluble vitamins, fat-soluble vitamins, and minerals are presented based on their function in calcified structures (teeth and periodontium) or their role in oral soft tissues (oral mucous membranes and salivary glands) to familiarize you with nutrients that might be involved when oral changes are observed. Most dental hygiene students are well aware of the role of several minerals in calcified structures in the oral cavity, but the vitamins presented in this chapter are also important for healthy teeth and the periodontium (Box 7-1).

Most nutrients have various functions; some are involved in both calcified and soft oral tissues. Oral physiological roles for these nutrients are presented in appropriate chapters, but information such as requirements and food sources is found only when the vitamin is first discussed. Fat-soluble and water-soluble vitamins differ in many ways, but a basic understanding of their fundamental similarities can facilitate learning.

REQUIREMENTS

Although vitamins are vital to life, they are required in minute amounts. Vitamins are similar to hormones because of their potent effects, but they must come from an outside source because they either cannot be produced by the body or cannot be produced in adequate amounts to meet body needs. Each vitamin is essential, although the amount needed may vary from 2.4 µg per day for vitamin B_{12} to 425 to 550 mg per day for choline.

Although the dietary reference intakes (DRIs) list the amounts of vitamins for different ages and sexes, many factors (e.g., smoking; use of alcohol, caffeine, or drugs; and stress) modify an individual's requirements. Periods of rapid growth, pregnancy or lactation, fever, and recovery from

Box 7-1	**Vitamins Required for Calcified Structures**

Fat-Soluble Vitamins
Vitamin A
Vitamin D
Vitamin E
Vitamin K

Water-Soluble Vitamins
Vitamin C

Box 7-2	**Groups at Potential Risk of Nutritional Deficiencies**

- Older adults
- Impoverished, low income
- Vegans
- Chronic disease states
- Alcoholics
- Inadequate intake
- Smokers
- Excessive caffeine use
- Polypharmacy
- Physiological stress
- Periods of rapid growth
  - Pregnancy
  - Lactation
  - Infants, children, adolescents
- Medical conditions causing
  - Inadequate absorption
  - Inadequate use
  - Excessive excretion
  - Destruction
- Physical stress
  - Surgery
  - Accidents
  - Disease
  - Burns
  - Fever

accidents, disease, surgery, and burns all are considered stressful. Requirements for most vitamins, especially water-soluble vitamins, are increased during periods of stress because of elevated metabolic activity (Box 7-2).

DEFICIENCIES

If adequate amounts of the nutrient are unavailable to sustain biochemical functions, a nutritional deficiency occurs. A nutritional deficiency as a result of decreased intake is called a *primary deficiency*. A vitamin deficiency caused by inadequate absorption or use, increased requirements, excretion, or destruction is called a *secondary deficiency*. Nutrients are codependent; a deficiency of one may cause deficiency symptoms of another because it relies on a metabolic product unavailable owing to the initial vitamin deficit.

Although specific vitamin deficiency syndromes are rare in the United States, several groups are at risk (see Box 7-2).

Vitamin levels in the blood are often unmeasurable, so a nutritional deficiency may be identified on the basis of clinical signs and symptoms and their response to vitamin supplementation. However, one of the peculiarities of vitamins is that the symptoms of a deficiency frequently resemble the symptoms caused by an overdose, making definitive diagnosis difficult.

CHARACTERISTICS OF FAT-SOLUBLE VITAMINS

Although the four fat-soluble vitamins (A, D, E, and K) differ in function, use, and sources, they have several similar characteristics: (1) they are soluble in fat or fat solvents; (2) they are fairly stable to heat, as in cooking; (3) they are organic substances (contain carbon); (4) they do not contain nitrogen; (5) they are absorbed in the intestine along with fats and lipids in foods; and (6) they require bile for absorption.

Fat-soluble vitamins are different from water-soluble vitamins mainly because larger amounts can be stored in the body. Vitamins A and D are stored for long periods, so minor shortages may not be identified until drastic depletion has occurred. For example, vitamin A can be stored in the liver to meet basic needs for at least 1 year. Observable signs and symptoms of a dietary deficiency are often not identified until they are in an advanced state. Dietary deficiencies occur when foods consumed do not provide necessary amounts of a nutrient.

Because several forms of each of the fat-soluble vitamins can be used by the body, vitamins A, D, and E were previously measured by their biological activity based on the growth of animals. International units (IU) reflect this biological activity in animal studies and do not always represent absorption rates in humans. Because of this, the retinol activity equivalents (RAE) standard was created for vitamin A. The recommended dietary allowances (RDAs) for vitamins A and E were determined based on the biological effectiveness of each form because the different forms of these vitamins have varying activity levels. After measurement of all active forms of the vitamins, the measurements are converted to micrograms or milligrams and totaled to indicate the amount of the vitamin in that food. RAE reflect vitamin A activity of foods. Although previous food tables listed international units, more accurate weight measurements in micrograms or milligrams are now used.

CHARACTERISTICS OF WATER-SOLUBLE VITAMINS

B-complex vitamins and vitamin C are water-soluble and are organic substances. In contrast to vitamin C and fat-soluble vitamins, B-complex vitamins contain nitrogen. Water-soluble vitamins have vital roles as coenzymes, which are necessary for almost every cellular reaction in the body. Vitamin C is discussed in this chapter with the fat-soluble vitamins because of its vital role as a structural component of the tooth; it is also important in oral soft tissues. B-complex vitamins are discussed in Chapter 10.

Most water-soluble vitamins are readily absorbed in the jejunum. High concentrations of these vitamins result in decreased absorption efficiency. The body stores very small amounts of each of these vitamins; few water-soluble vitamins produce toxic symptoms. Because of their limited storage, daily intake is important.

Dental Hygiene Considerations

- Assessment is crucial to determine requirements for vitamins. Assess for the following: smoking, alcohol use, excessive caffeine use, medications, physiological stress, or surgery. If any of the aforementioned is present, vitamin requirements in the diet may be increased.
- Dietary and physical assessments are more diagnostic for vitamin deficiencies than laboratory values.
- Evaluate nutrient intake of groups at high risk for developing nutritional deficiencies; older adults, impoverished/low-income patients, and patients with chronic diseases should be questioned. If indicated, refer the patient to a registered dietitian.

Nutritional Directions

- No vitamin contains kilocalories, but some vitamins, especially the B-complex vitamins, are essential to the production of energy.
- The use of mineral oil as a laxative can interfere with the absorption of fat-soluble vitamins.

VITAMIN A (RETINOL, CAROTENE)

Retinol is the dietary source of vitamin A from animal sources, and beta carotene is the principal carotenoid present in plant pigments. Retinoic acid is the most biologically active form of vitamin A.

PHYSIOLOGICAL ROLES

Vitamin A has many hormone-like roles in the body. It is also required for normal bone growth and development, and for facilitating the transcription of DNA into RNA.

Vision

Retinol is converted to retinal in the eye. Retinal combines with opsin, a protein in the eye, to form the visual pigment, **rhodopsin**. **Night blindness** may result from inadequate vitamin A to permit rhodopsin production. This condition takes years to develop in adults, but occurs much sooner in children because they have fewer body stores.

Growth

Vitamin A is necessary for growth of soft tissues and bones. In skeletal tissue, vitamin A is necessary for resorption of old bone and synthesis of new bone. **Retinoic acid,** produced by the body from retinal, is the form of vitamin A involved in the development of teeth, especially in the formation of **ameloblasts** (in enamel) and **odontoblasts** (in dentin) along with growth of bone. Vitamin A deficiency during pre-eruptive stages of tooth development leads to enamel hypoplasia and defective dentin formation. Vitamin A also is involved with normal teeth spacing and promotes osteoblast function of the alveolar bone. The main functions relating to health and integrity of the body openings and their linings are discussed in Chapter 10.

Cancer

Vitamin A and carotene have consistently been associated with cancer prevention because of their importance to the development and integrity of cells. The antioxidant role of vitamin A is discussed in Health Application 7. **Antioxidants** prevent cell membrane damage by free radicals that are produced by cells and tissues using free oxygen. Unchecked by an antioxidant, free radicals can damage the structure and impair the function of cell membranes. Research is inconclusive in regard to the use of beta carotene to prevent cancer. Early studies suggest vitamin A, retinoids, and beta carotene may resolve oral leukoplakia, but relapse is common. **Leukoplakia** (see Figs. 16-10 and 16-11) is a white plaque that forms on oral mucous membranes. Despite the potential to resolve leukoplakia, evidence does not indicate that any of these nutrients prevent malignant transformation.[1] Currently, it is uncertain whether beta carotene or some other components in fruits and vegetables leads to the resolution of leukoplakia. Supplementation is not advised other than increasing consumption of fruits and vegetables because some studies show an increased risk of lung cancer among smokers using beta carotene supplements.[2]

REQUIREMENTS

As shown in Table 7-1, the RDA for vitamin A is 900 μg RAE for men and 700 μg RAE for women (1 RAE = 1 μg = 12 μg beta carotene = 3.3 IU). The tolerable upper intake level (UL) is 3000 μg RAE per day. The need for vitamin A is increased during periods of rapid growth, when gastrointestinal problems affect its absorption or conversion (e.g., cystic fibrosis, celiac disease, Crohn's disease, chronic diarrhea), and in hepatic diseases that limit vitamin A storage or conversion of beta carotene to its active form. Although no UL has been established for beta carotene, the Institute of Medicine (IOM) does not advise supplements for healthy people.[3]

Average intake in the United States meets the RDA, and because vitamin A can be stored in the liver, most adults have sufficient quantities to maintain health. Inadequate intake occurs in lower socioeconomic groups as a consequence of inadequate vegetable and fruit intake.

SOURCES

Vitamin A, as preformed retinol, is found in milk, cheese, butter, eggs, meat, cod liver oil, liver, and fortified foods (e.g., breakfast cereals, bread, crackers). Sometimes retinol

Table 7-1	Institute of Medicine Recommendations for Vitamin A					
	EAR (µg/d)†		RDA (µg/d)‡			
Life Stage	*Male*	*Female*	*Male*	*Female*	AI (mg/d)§	UL (µg/d)¶¶
0-6 mo					400	600
7-12 mo					500	600
1-3 yr	210	210	300	300		600
4-8 yr	275	275	400	400		900
9-13 yr	445	420	600	600		1700
14-18 yr	630	485	900	700		2800
>18 yr	625	500	900	700		3000
Pregnancy						
14-18 yr		530		750		2800
19-50 yr		550		770		3000
Lactation						
14-18 yr		885		1200		2800
19-50 yr		900		1300		3000

Data from Institute of Medicine (IOM), Food and Nutrition Board: Dietary Reference Intakes for Vitamin C, Vitamin K, Arsenic, Boron, Chromium, Copper, Iodine, Iron, Manganese, Molybdenum, Nickel, Silicon, Vanadium, and Zinc. Washington, DC: National Academy Press, 2000.

†EAR (estimated average requirement)—the intake that meets the estimated nutrient needs of half of the individuals in a group.

‡RDA (recommended dietary allowance)—the intake that meets the nutrient needs of almost all (97-98%) individuals in a group.

§AI (adequate intake)—the observed average or experimentally set intake by a defined population or subgroup that seems to sustain a defined nutritional status, such as growth rate, normal circulating nutrient values, or other functional indicators of health. An AI is used if insufficient scientific evidence is available to derive an EAR. For healthy human milk–fed infants, the AI is the mean intake. *The AI is not equivalent to an RDA.*

¶UL (tolerable upper intake level)—the highest level of daily nutrient intake that is likely to pose no risk of adverse health effects to almost all individuals in the general population. As intake increases above the UL, the risk of adverse effects increases. Unless specified otherwise, the UL represents total nutrient intake from food, water, and supplements.

¶Preformed vitamin A.

is added to skim milk and margarine. Beta carotene or pro-vitamin A is also present in yellow, orange, and green leafy vegetables (e.g., spinach, turnip greens, broccoli) (Table 7-2). Although not as well absorbed as from animal sources and fortified foods, beta carotene is still a valuable source of this vitamin. Beta carotene is deep red in pure form and derives its name from carrots, from which it was first isolated. Chlorophyll disguises the carotenoids in green vegetables. Most yellow, orange, and dark green fruits and vegetables are high in carotene or vitamin A content. The deeper the color, the more vitamin A activity in a fruit or vegetable.

ABSORPTION AND EXCRETION

Absorption is optimal when body stores are depleted, and when adequate amounts of other interrelated nutrients are present. The presence of vitamin E and the hormone thyroxine also enhances use of vitamin A.

The liver stores approximately 90% of vitamin A. Adequate serum proteins are necessary to mobilize vitamin A from the liver. Vitamin A is not readily excreted by the body, but a small amount is lost in the urine.

HYPER-STATES AND HYPO-STATES

Extreme levels of vitamin A (high or low) can cause serious problems, even resulting in death (Fig. 7-1).

Toxicity

When present in high concentrations, unbound vitamin A causes damage to cell membranes, especially in red blood cells (RBCs) and **lysosomes** (small bodies occurring in many types of cells). Large amounts of vitamin A supplements can exceed the storage capacity of the liver. If this occurs, free vitamin A enters the bloodstream and exerts toxic effects on cell membranes. High levels of vitamin A in the body are referred to as **hypervitaminosis A**.

Maternal consumption of vitamin A supplements before conception and during the first trimester of pregnancy has been associated with fetal birth defects (see Fig. 7-1). Toxicity is evident in infants by bulging of the fontanelle as a result of increased cerebrospinal fluid pressure. Other clinical symptoms include headache; vomiting; **diplopia** (double vision); **alopecia** (hair loss); dryness of the mucous membranes; reddened gingiva (Fig. 7-2); thinning of the epithelium; cracking and bleeding lips; and increased activity of **osteoclasts** (cells associated with bone resorption), which leads to decalcification, desquamation of oral mucosa, bone growth retardation, softening of the skull, and liver abnormalities (Fig. 7-3). Toxicity symptoms usually appear only when excessive intakes occur over a sustained period.

A review of 20 clinical studies suggested excess vitamin A (primarily in the form of retinol) may have a negative impact on bone health. Amounts only twice the RDA have

Table 7-2 Food Sources of Vitamin A

Food	Portion	Vitamin A (μg RAE)
Beef liver	3 oz	8498
Chicken liver	3 oz	3583
Sweet potato, baked	1	1096
Margarine	1 Tbsp	819
Special K	1 cup	743
Collard greens, cooked	1 cup	595
Butternut squash, baked	½ cup	572
Raw carrots, shredded	½ cup	509
Spinach, cooked	½ cup	472
Cantaloupe	1 cup	299
Turnip greens, cooked	½ cup	274
Winter squash, baked	½ cup	268
Mustard greens, cooked	½ cup	221
Dandelion greens, cooked	½ cup	180
Skim milk (fortified)	1 cup	150
Spinach, raw	1 cup	141
Romaine lettuce	1 cup	136
Broccoli, cooked	1 cup	120
Apricots, dried	10 halves	119
Butter	1 Tbsp	97
Whole egg	1	84
Whole milk (unfortified)	1 c	68
Apricot, raw	1	34

Data from U.S. Department of Agriculture, Agricultural Research Service, USDA Nutrient Data Laboratory, USDA National Nutrient Database for Standard Reference, Release 20, 2008. Available at http://www.nal.usda.gov/fnic/foodcomp/search/. Accessed February 25, 2008.

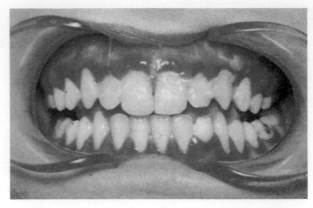

FIGURE 7-2 Hypervitaminosis A. Bright red marginal discoloration of the gingiva shown here is characteristic. (Courtesy of Dr. M.D. Muenter. From McLaren DS: A Colour Atlas and Text of Diet-related Disorders, 2nd ed. London: Mosby–Year Book Europe Limited, 1992.)

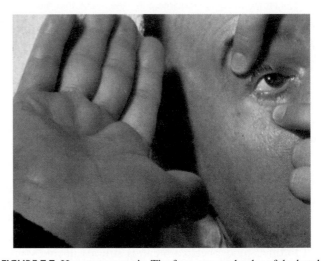

FIGURE 7-3 Hypercarotenosis. The face, eye, and palm of the hand. The sclerae remain clear, distinguishing the condition from jaundice. (Courtesy of Dr. I.A. Abrahamson, Sr. From McLaren DS: A Colour Atlas and Text of Diet-related Disorders, 2nd ed. London: Mosby–Year Book Europe Limited, 1992.)

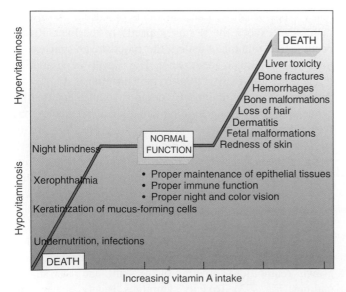

FIGURE 7-1 Vitamin A intake. This chart shows how changing the amount of vitamin A in the diet can lead to hypovitaminosis A or hypervitaminosis A. In extreme, either condition can lead to death. (From Thibodeau GA, Patton KT: Anatomy and Physiology, 6th ed. St. Louis: Mosby, 2007.)

been implicated in reducing bone mineral density (BMD) and increasing the risk for fracture.[4] How this change in BMD may affect alveolar bone is unknown.

Toxicity from excessive intake of vitamin A food sources is possible, but most cases are a result of oversupplementation. Beta carotene is much less toxic than vitamin A. The body converts only the amount of carotenoids it needs into vitamin A. Although beta carotenes are not toxic, overconsumption may result in **hypercarotenemia**, yellow pigmentation of the skin occurring first on the palms of the hands and soles of the feet, which is caused by carotene storage in fatty tissue (see Fig. 7-3). This condition subsides when ingestion of beta carotene is diminished.

Deficiency

Inadequate dietary intake is the primary reason for vitamin A deficiency, found most commonly in children younger than 5 years of age. It also may result from chronic fat malabsorption. Vitamin A deficiency is rarely seen in the United States, but it is a major nutritional problem in developing countries. Mild vitamin A deficiency may contribute to a depressed immune response.

Inadequate vitamin A intake results in degeneration of epithelial cells in the eye and cessation of tear secretion. Lids are swollen and sticky with pus, and eyes are sensitive to light in **xerophthalmia**, sometimes resulting in permanent blindness. The first symptom of xerophthalmia is night blindness, followed by the occurrence of xerotic spots on the conjunctiva, called Bitot's spots. These ulcers of the eye may spread and result in blindness if left untreated (Fig. 7-4).

Degeneration of epithelial cells results in an inability to produce mucus (Fig. 7-5A). This occurs not only in epithelial cells, but also in the intestines and lungs. **Xeroderma** can progress until the whole body is covered with dry, flaky, scaly skin similar to dandruff. It is followed by **follicular hyperkeratosis**, in which the skin is thickened, dry, and wrinkled (Fig. 7-5B). Keratinization may also affect the oral mucosa and the respiratory and gastrointestinal tracts. In these areas, degeneration of epithelial cells results in increased risk of infection and delayed or impaired wound healing.

Severe vitamin A deficiency may result in enamel hypoplasia and defective dentin formation in developing teeth. **Enamel hypoplasia** involves defects in the enamel matrix and incomplete calcification of the enamel and dentin. Odontoblasts lose their ability to arrange themselves in normal parallel linear formation, resulting in degeneration and atrophy of ameloblasts. The normal deposition of dentin is altered.

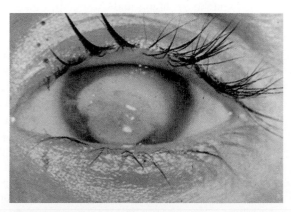

FIGURE 7-4 Xerophthalmia. (From McLaren DS: A Colour Atlas and Text of Diet-related Disorders, 2nd ed. London: Mosby–Year Book Europe Limited, 1992.)

🦷 Dental Hygiene Considerations

- Vitamin A or beta carotene supplements are not recommended for most healthy adults.
- Assess for signs of vitamin A deficiencies (loss of night vision, keratomalacia, corneal ulceration, or Bitot's spots), especially in young and older patients. When in doubt, refer to a healthcare provider or dietitian.
- In contrast to vitamin A, beta carotene is not toxic, but large amounts can cause a temporary change in skin color. Hypercarotenemia may be distinguished from jaundice because the sclera retains its normal white color.
- Jaundice or any disorder affecting fat absorption also affects fat-soluble vitamin absorption, making these patients prone to vitamin A deficiency.
- Drugs such as orlistat (Alli) used for weight loss and food components such as olestra negatively affect fat and fat-soluble vitamin absorption, especially the absorption of vitamin A and beta carotene. Patients taking orlistat should follow a low-fat diet and take a multivitamin 2 hours before or after taking the drug.
- An alcoholic or alcoholic-cirrhotic patient may be deficient in vitamin A because of the effects of ethanol and impaired liver function.
- Vitamin A toxicity can be masked, especially when protein-energy malnutrition is present.
- Excessive intake of vitamin E or vitamin C may decrease absorption of vitamin A. Do not encourage use of vitamin E and vitamin C supplements or vitamin E–rich or vitamin C–rich foods if the patient is at risk of vitamin A deficiency.

✏️ Nutritional Directions

- Vitamin A from animal or fortified foods is used better by the body than beta carotene.
- Vegans need to consume a minimum of five servings of dark green, yellow, and orange fruits and vegetables daily to receive the recommended amount of vitamin A.
- Fortified foods and vitamin supplements should be used judiciously; severe, life-threatening liver damage or increased risk of hip fractures can result from chronic use in excess of the RDA.
- Discourage patients from taking more than the RDA in over-the-counter vitamin preparations unless specifically advised to do so by a healthcare provider or registered dietitian.
- Recommend storing vitamins in a cool, dark place to prevent deterioration.
- Women of childbearing age need to limit intake of preformed vitamin A (retinol, retinyl, and retinoyl acetate) found in liver and fortified foods (breakfast cereals and dietary supplements) to about 100% of the daily value (DV) because of the increased risk of neural defects during the first trimester of pregnancy.

VITAMIN D (CALCIFEROL)

Although vitamin D has been called a vitamin, it is more appropriately classified as a **hormone** (a compound that is secreted by one type of cell that acts to control the function of another type of cell). Skin cells are able to make vitamin

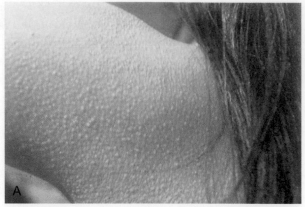

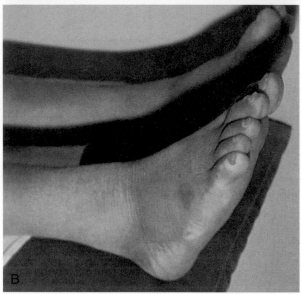

FIGURE 7-5 **A,** Follicular hyperkeratosis caused by vitamin A deficiency. **B,** Hyperkeratosis. The skin over parts of the body is thickened, dry, and wrinkled, associated with vitamin A deficiency. (From McLaren DS: A Colour Atlas and Text of Diet-related Disorders, 2nd ed. London: Mosby–Year Book Europe Limited, 1992.)

D when the precursor 7-dehydrocholesterol, present in the skin, is exposed to ultraviolet (UV) light or sunshine. Vitamin D from food, ergocalciferol (vitamin D_2) or cholecalciferol (vitamin D_3), is biologically inert. Further processing occurs in the liver with conversion of vitamin D_2 or vitamin D_3 into 25-hydroxycholecalciferol (calcidiol) and a final change to the active form of 1,25-dihydroxycholecalciferol (calciferol) primarily by the kidney (Fig. 7-6).

Until more recently, vitamin D was viewed primarily as a protective agent against bone disease, such as rickets. Research has shown, however, that vitamin D receptors are present in approximately 36 different types of cells, and the hormone is involved in the maintenance of more than 200 human genes.[5-7] Reports from many nations have highlighted a variety of vitamin D insufficiency and deficiency diseases. More research is needed to learn about the impact of vitamin D on different stages of the life cycle and in racial and ethnic groups.[8]

PHYSIOLOGICAL ROLES

Vitamin D is intricately related to calcium and phosphorus, each being required for optimal use of the other. Vitamin D helps the body absorb and regulate calcium. The primary role of vitamin D is mineralization of bones and teeth, and regulation of blood calcium and phosphorus levels. It functions with the parathyroid and thyroid (**calcitonin**) hormones to regulate intestinal absorption of calcium and phosphorus, enhance renal calcium and phosphorus reabsorption, and regulate skeletal calcium and phosphorus reserves.

Vitamin D may also be involved in the functioning of cells involved in **hematopoiesis** (the formation of RBCs), the skin, cardiovascular function, and immune responses. Its regulatory role helps keep serum calcium in the appropriate range to maintain cardiac and neuromuscular function. Calciferol (1,25-dihydroxycholecalciferol) interacts with **osteoblasts** (cells that help produce collagen, and build and reform new bone) to increase the withdrawal of **osteocalcin** (calcium-binding noncollagen protein in bone) and other bone-building compounds, or interacts with parathyroid hormone to mobilize calcium stores from the skeleton when calcium is needed.

REQUIREMENTS

The vitamin D requirement is difficult to determine. When sufficient sunlight is available, people do not require an exogenous source of vitamin D. Because many Americans have limited exposure to sunlight, however, and because many factors can interfere with UV light–dependent synthesis of vitamin D in the skin, vitamin D is considered an essential dietary nutrient.

The IOM determined that an adequate intake of vitamin D for all adults younger than 51 years old is 5 µg; the recommended amount increases with age (Table 7-3). ULs for various life stages also were established for vitamin D. One microgram is equivalent to 40 IU. Medical researchers and the American Medical Association have been raising strong doubts about the adequacy of the current DRI for vitamin D.[9] The American Academy of Pediatrics has recommended that vitamin D intake by infants and children be doubled, or 400 IU daily, to prevent rickets and deficiency, and possible links with diabetes and cancer prevention.

To date, IOM members have not been convinced of assertions for the health-promoting potential of vitamin D. One reason they are hesitant to act is because of potential toxicity from vitamin D. Research should validate the health benefits and the appropriate level of vitamin needed. Because U.S. residents comprise different ethnicities and locations and sensitivities, a "one-size-fits-all" recommendation may not be appropriate.

American and Canadian diets do not provide sufficient vitamin D.[8,12] A study involving healthy children and adolescents indicates low vitamin D blood concentrations are prevalent related to low intake, race, and season.[13] The National Osteoporosis Foundation urges adults older than

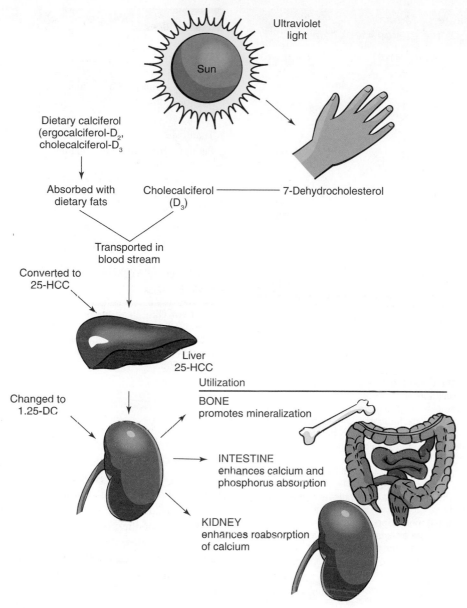

FIGURE 7-6 Vitamin D metabolism. (Adapted from Davis JR, Sherer K: Applied Nutrition and Diet Therapy for Nurses, 2nd ed. Philadelphia: Saunders, 1994.)

age 50 to get at least 800 to 1000 IU in the form of vitamin D_3 supplements to prevent fractures.

SOURCES

Sunlight

The body's ability to produce adequate amounts of vitamin D from sunlight is the reason the sun has been considered as a source of health. UVB rays are the principal cause of sunburn and cellular damage that leads to skin cancer. UVB radiation penetrates uncovered skin and converts a precursor of vitamin D to previtamin D_3, which becomes vitamin D_3. Most people experience an increase in vitamin D levels during the summer months, which decrease during the winter because of less sun exposure. During summer months, 10

minutes a day without sunblock on hands and face can replete the body's supply.

Many people in the northern hemisphere (above a line approximately between the northern border of California and Boston), especially older adults and darker-skinned individuals, may lack sufficient exposure to UVB, especially mid-October through mid-March. Complete cloud cover reduces UV energy needed for vitamin D conversion by 50%; shade or severe pollution reduces UV energy by 60%. UV radiation does not penetrate glass. Sunscreens with a sun protection factor (SPF) of 8 or more seem to block UVB rays.[14] Sunscreen is much more effective in blocking the formation of vitamin D_3 than its labeled SPF for preventing sunburn.[15] Dermatologists continue to advise sunscreen and

Table 7-3	Institute of Medicine Recommendations for Vitamin D	
Life Stage†	AI (μg/d)‡§¶	UL (μg/d)¶
0-6 mo	5	25
7-12 mo	5	25
1-3 yr	5	50
4-8 yr	5	50
9-13 yr	5	50
14-18 yr	5	50
19-30 yr	5	50
31-50 yr	5	50
51-70 yr	10	50
>70 yr	15	50
Pregnancy		
≤18-50 yr	5	50
Lactation		
≤18-50 yr	5	50

Data from Institute of Medicine (IOM), Food and Nutrition Board: Dietary Reference Intakes for Calcium, Phosphorus, Magnesium, Vitamin D, and Fluoride. Washington, DC: National Academy Press, 1997.
†All groups except pregnancy and lactation are males and females.
‡AI (adequate intake)—the observed average or experimentally set intake by a defined population or subgroup that seems to sustain a defined nutritional status, such as growth rate, normal circulating nutrient values, or other functional indicators of health. An AI is used if insufficient scientific evidence is available to derive an EAR. For healthy human milk–fed infants, the AI is the mean intake. *The AI is not equivalent to an RDA.*
§As cholecalciferol. 1 μg cholecalciferol = 40 IU vitamin D.
¶In the absence of adequate exposure to sunlight.
¶UL (tolerable upper intake level)—the highest level of daily nutrient intake that is likely to pose no risk of adverse health effects to almost all individuals in the general population. As intake increases above the UL, the risk of adverse effects increases. Unless specified otherwise, the UL represents total nutrient intake from food, water, and supplements.

Table 7-4	Food Sources of Vitamin D	
Food	Portion	Vitamin D (IU)
Cod liver oil	1 Tbsp	1360
Sardines, canned in oil, drained	3 oz	428
Salmon, cooked	3 oz	308
Mackerel, cooked	3 oz	295
Tuna fish	3 oz	200
Pudding, from mix with vitamin D–fortified milk	1 cup	100
Milk (skim or whole), fortified with vitamin D	1 cup	98
Margarine, fortified	1 Tbsp	60
Ready-to-eat cereal (fortified with 10% of the DV for vitamin D)	¾ cup	40
Egg	1	20
Beef liver, cooked	3 oz	13
Cheese, Swiss	1 oz	12

Data from U.S. Department of Agriculture, Agricultural Research Service, USDA Nutrient Data Laboratory, USDA National Nutrient Database for Standard Reference, Release 20, 2008. Available at http://www.nal.usda.gov/fnic/foodcomp/search/. Accessed February 25, 2008.

clothing protection for anyone in the sun more than 20 minutes. Although sunscreen inhibits vitamin D production, its use and moderation in sun exposure are important to protect against skin cancer. By age 70, the skin generally produces vitamin D at only half the level it did at age 20.

Food

Although adequate quantities of vitamin D may be derived from exposure to sunlight, additional food sources are necessary in most cases. Naturally occurring vitamin D content in foods is limited and variable; food tables do not normally list vitamin D content. The U.S. Department of Agriculture (USDA) Nutrient Data Laboratory has requested analysis of specific foods that are important contributors of vitamin D.[16] On completion, the information will be added to the National Nutrient Database for Standard Reference (available at http://www.nal.usda.gov/fnic/foodcomp/search/).

Natural sources include oily fish such as salmon, mackerel, catfish, sardines, and tuna as well as cod liver oil and fish oils (Table 7-4). A diet composed of the best (unfortified) food sources of vitamin D supplies only slightly more than 2.5 μg daily.

Because of the prevalence of vitamin D deficiencies in the United States, the U.S. Food and Drug Administration (FDA) allows vitamin D fortification of orange juice; this provides a good alternative source for people who do not drink milk. Other foods, such as margarine, infant formulas and cereals, prepared breakfast cereals, chocolate beverage mixes, orange juice, and cocoa, also may be fortified with vitamin D (see Table 7-4).

Foods are not legally required to be fortified, but about 98% of the milk in the United States is fortified to provide 10 μg of cholecalciferol per quart. Milk is fortified because of its popular consumption among children. In addition, the calcium and phosphorus content of milk is beneficial for absorption and use of vitamin D. Vitamin D from fortified regular and low-fat cheeses is well used by the body.[17] Because fortification is optional, it cannot be taken for granted.

Foods fortified with vitamin D are often inadequate to satisfy either a child's or an adult's vitamin D requirement.[18] If federal nutrition guidelines were increased, dairies and food manufacturers could add more vitamin D to their products, making it easier for people to get the vitamin from foods.

Nutrition labels can be used to assess daily intake of vitamin D; this information plus the amount of exposure to sunlight must be considered to ensure adequate amounts of vitamin D. Vitamin D is in multivitamins, prenatal vitamins, calcium–vitamin D combinations, and individual vitamin D supplements. Most multivitamins provide 400 IU per dose. Traditionally, supplement manufacturers have used vitamin D_2 (ergocalciferol), but this form is about one-third to one-fourth less effective than vitamin D_3 at increasing calcidiol levels in the blood.[19]

ABSORPTION

As with other nutrients, optimal absorption occurs when all closely interrelated nutrients (particularly calcium and phosphorus) are present in sufficient quantities. Conversely, diets high in fiber can result in less vitamin D absorption.

HYPER-STATES AND HYPO-STATES

Toxicity

Vitamin D has the potential to become toxic at high levels, but the exact level for toxicity has not been determined. It is generally recognized that the toxicity level is much higher than the UL, but research is lacking to ascertain the association between long-term harm and higher doses of vitamin D.[20] However, uncontrolled use of vitamin D supplements by older patients with osteoporosis resulted in occult vitamin D intoxication with the resultant effect being diminished bone mass.[21]

When synthetic vitamin D supplements are taken by mouth in milligram amounts for 6 weeks, toxicity signs occur. Nausea, vomiting, poor appetite, weight loss, constipation, and weakness are signs of vitamin D toxicity. Vitamin D toxicity can also increase blood levels of calcium, causing mental changes and confusion and heart rhythm abnormalities.[22] Calciferol poisoning can result in enhanced bone resorption, leading to deposition of calcium and phosphate in soft tissues and irreversible kidney and cardiovascular damage.[23] Without detection of symptoms and immediate reduction of the vitamin D source, permanent damage results.

The most common reason for vitamin D toxicity is prolonged intake of excessive supplements or cod liver oil; otherwise, toxicity through diet is unlikely. Toxicity from excessive vitamin D intake may occur when a concentrated calciferol preparation is mistakenly given. An infant given a commercial formula and a vitamin supplement can easily ingest vitamin D well above the RDA.

Deficiency

Vitamin D deficiency is now recognized as a pandemic problem with new research suggesting it protects against a wide variety of diseases.[24] Approximately 50% to 60% of older North Americans are lacking in vitamin D.[25] In adults, vitamin D deficiency has been linked in emerging research studies to conditions as diverse as asthma, cardiovascular disease, hypertension, diabetes mellitus, depression, some infectious disease, autoimmune disorders, and schizophrenia.[18,26,27] In addition, 42% of adolescents have been found to be vitamin D deficient.[28] Many vitamin D

researchers believe that by diligently shielding ourselves from sunlight, many benefits of this vitamin may be missed.[29] Also, the melanin that makes skin dark effectively filters out UVB, so dark-skinned individuals are much more likely than fair-skinned individuals to have low levels of vitamin D.

Vitamin D deficiency affects skeletal structure in children and adults. Signs of deficiency are commonly found in children because of increased requirements, decreased stores, decreased exposure to the sun, or use of sunscreens. In elderly patients, deficiencies are created by consuming inadequate diets with little exposure to the sun, reduced skin thickness, inability of the kidney to convert vitamin D to its active form, or inadequate absorption of vitamin D from the gastrointestinal tract. Plasma vitamin D is significantly lower in older patients than in a younger population; it is consistently higher for older men than women. A healthcare provider may recommend vitamin D and calcium supplements to older patients to prevent osteoporosis. When supplementation is recommended, care must be used to prevent toxic overdoses. Vitamin D deficiency is associated with muscle weakness, causing older individuals to tire easily and experience difficulty climbing stairs and rising from a chair. This muscle weakness frequently results in falls.[30]

Rickets. Laboratory values indicating serum calcium or phosphorus above or below normal values, the failure of bones to grow properly in length, and x-ray films showing abnormal **epiphyses**, or growing points of the bones, indicate deficiencies (Fig. 7-7). Because vitamin D is intricately related to calcium and phosphorus functions, a change in any of these three nutrients affects the others.

The name rickets came from the word *wrikken,* meaning "to bend or twist." Rickets, caused by vitamin D deficiency, usually occurs in children 1 to 3 years old and is characterized by weak bones and skeletal deformities. Rachitic deformities such as bowlegs or knock-knees develop (Fig. 7-8A). The epiphyses of bones do not develop normally in children, so bones are twisted and warped. Other bone changes include a row of beadlike protuberances (rachitic rosary) on each side of the narrow, distorted chest (pigeon breast) at the juncture of the ribs and costal cartilage (Fig. 7-8B). A narrow pelvis, making future childbearing difficult in women, is also observed.

Rickets develops during a time of extremely rapid growth when children have had only a brief period to acquire vitamin D stores. Adequate intake of vitamin D during pregnancy and lactation is important because vitamin D is passed from the mother to the infant before birth and in breast milk. However, adequate vitamin D cannot be met solely by breastfeeding. Rickets is occurring in the United States with increasing frequency because of the increased prevalence of breastfeeding and lack of sun exposure.[31,32]

The alveolar bone is affected similar to other bones in the body when rickets occurs. The trabeculae of the alveolar bone also weaken. Delayed dentition and small molars are observed in vitamin D deficiency.

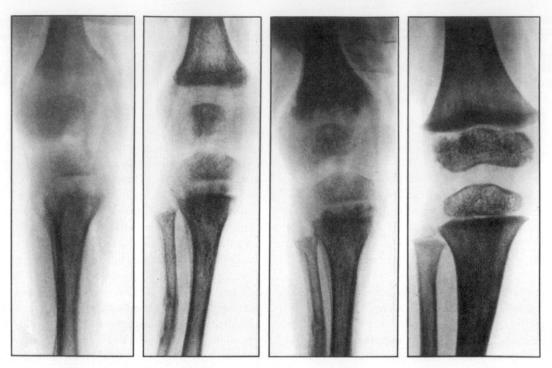

FIGURE 7-7 Active rickets of the knees. The metaphyses of the bones are concave and irregular, and the zone of uncalcified osteoid is enlarged. These x-rays show the progressive changes over 10 months during which healing took place in this case. (Courtesy of Prof. A. Prader. From McLaren DS: A Colour Atlas and Text of Diet-related Disorders, 2nd ed. London: Mosby–Year Book Europe Limited, 1992.)

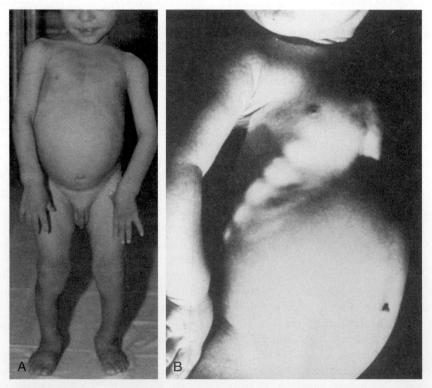

FIGURE 7-8 **A,** Bowlegs in rickets. The typical lateral curvature indicates that the weakened bones have bent after the second year as a result of standing. **B,** Rachitic rosary in a young infant. (**A,** From McLaren DS: A Colour Atlas and Text of Diet-related Disorders, 2nd ed. London: Mosby–Year Book Europe Limited, 1992. **B,** From Kliegman RM, et al: Nelson Textbook of Pediatrics, 18th ed. Philadelphia: Saunders, 2007.)

Enamel Hypoplasia. A few patients with evidence of rickets develop enamel hypoplasia as a result of vitamin D deficiency. Usually these changes are visible only with the aid of a microscope or during clinical assessment. Whether these teeth are more susceptible to dental caries is uncertain. The enamel does not seem to be weakened, but the rougher surface may facilitate adherence of dental plaque and food residue.

Osteomalacia. Vitamin D deficiency in adults is called **osteomalacia**; it is also intricately related to calcium intake. Osteomalacia is characterized by decreased bone mineralization or softening of the bones, which may lead to deformities of the limbs, spine, thorax, and pelvis. The main symptoms are skeletal pain and muscle weakness, resulting in kyphosis or an uneven gait. Oral manifestations include loss of the lamina dura around the roots of the teeth. The condition is more prevalent in women of childbearing age with calcium depletion because of multiple pregnancies or inadequate intake or in women who have little exposure to the sun.

A healthcare provider or dietitian may recommend a vitamin D supplement or a calcium supplement with vitamin D to maximize the absorption of calcium for patients, especially women who are at high risk for osteoporosis because of small frame size. Medication may also be prescribed to prevent further deterioration of BMD.

Osteoporosis. Osteoporosis was previously thought of as a calcium deficiency, but new research has indicated vitamin D levels to be as important as calcium intake. As discussed previously, vitamin D deficiency interferes with mineralization of the skeleton, reducing bone density and increasing the risk of bone fractures. Osteoporosis is a disease characterized by fragile bones and is associated with an increased incidence of bone fractures, especially the hip. Osteoporosis is discussed further in Health Application 8.

Cancer and Cardiovascular Risks. Laboratory, animal, and epidemiologic evidence suggest that vitamin D may be protective against some cancers. Numerous studies indicate that higher vitamin levels in blood are associated with reduced colon and colorectal cancers[33,34] and breast cancer.[35] In animal studies, tumor growth has been reduced by giving vitamin D. The future of vitamin D and cancer is uncertain; evidence from these findings is based on limited data, and more studies are needed to determine the optimal levels and intakes of vitamin D to reduce cancer risk.[36]

New studies indicate vitamin D also is important for heart health. In one study, men with low blood levels of vitamin D were at twice the risk of heart attack as men getting adequate amounts.[37] Another study indicated individuals with lower blood levels of vitamin D had an increased risk of death in general, especially from cardiovascular conditions.[38] More research is needed to determine just how vitamin D affects these conditions and how much vitamin D is needed to promote cardiovascular health.

Dental Hygiene Considerations

- Assess for vitamin D toxicity and deficit, especially in young children, pregnant and lactating women, and older adults.
- Vitamin D supplements should be given only in prescribed dosage because patients vary widely in their susceptibility to vitamin D toxicity. Do not recommend patients buy vitamin D supplements. Refer them to a healthcare provider or dietitian.
- If supplemental doses of vitamin D are used, cloudiness or a red color of the urine may indicate toxicity and should be brought to the healthcare provider's attention.
- Conditions leading to vitamin D deficiency include any abnormalities that (1) interfere with intestinal absorption (e.g., diarrhea, steatorrhea, celiac disease, Crohn's disease, and cystic fibrosis), and (2) abnormalities in calcium balance and bone metabolism caused by disease states such as renal failure. Evaluate the patient's health status for risk of vitamin D deficiency.
- Studies suggest vitamin D intake in excess of current recommendations may be associated with better health outcomes. However, optimal serum concentrations of 25-hydroxycholecalciferol have not been established.[39]
- Patients with no exposure to sunlight should be monitored for adequate vitamin D intake or supplementation or both to maintain adequate vitamin D stores. Evaluate the patient's living environment or hobbies to determine exposure to sunlight.
- Determine the use of sunscreens. Consistent use of sunscreens may contribute to vitamin D deficiency in some patients. Sunscreens with an SPF of 8 or greater block the UV rays from the sun that produce vitamin D.
- Anticonvulsant drugs, such as phenytoin and phenobarbital, inactivate vitamin D, directly affecting skeletal and intestinal metabolism to cause osteomalacia. If a patient is taking these drugs over a long period, vitamin D supplements and some daily exposure to the sun may be beneficial.
- Low skeletal bone mass may also be associated with periodontal bone loss and tooth loss.[40]

Nutritional Directions

- The bright sunlight between 11 a.m. and 2 p.m. offers maximum conversion. For light-skinned individuals, 10 to 20 minutes of daily sun exposure results in adequate conversion.
- Toxicity may result from excess intake of cod liver oil or from taking excessive vitamin D supplements.
- Older individuals, especially individuals living in a long-term care facility, are at high risk for vitamin D deficiency and should receive a daily supplement.
- Read the label on vitamin supplements; select brands that contain vitamin D₃ or cholecalciferol. Ergocalciferol is less effective.

VITAMIN E (TOCOPHEROL)

Eight different compounds are collectively called vitamin E: four **tocopherols** and four **tocotrienols**. Biological activity of each form varies; α-tocopherol is the most active form and is better used by the body.

PHYSIOLOGICAL ROLES

Vitamin E is the most important fat-soluble antioxidant. Vitamin E protects the integrity of normal cell membranes and effectively prevents hemolysis of RBCs. It also protects vitamins A and C, beta carotene, and unsaturated fatty acids from oxidation. Vitamin E supplementation improves the immune response in healthy older patients; this effect may be mediated by increases in **prostaglandins**, which enhance growth of white blood cells. These functions promote resistance of the periodontium to inflammation. In larger amounts, vitamin E is an **anticoagulant**, or blood thinner. The role of vitamin E as an antioxidant is discussed further in Health Application 7.

REQUIREMENTS

The DRIs for vitamin E (adequate intake [AI], RDA, and UL) are based solely on the α-tocopherol form because humans are unable to convert and use other forms. The RDA for vitamin E is 15 mg of α-tocopherol for healthy individuals 14 years old and older except for lactating women (Table 7-5). One milligram of α-tocopherol is the same as 1.5 IU. High intakes of polyunsaturated fatty acids (PUFAs) increase the vitamin E requirement. Most polyunsaturated oils contain vitamin E, but chemical processes may have rendered the antioxidant ineffective. If an individual's systemic stores are low, vitamin E requirement is increased.

The daily UL is 1000 mg of α-tocopherol (1500 IU of natural vitamin E is equivalent to 1000 IU of synthetic vitamin E). The UL was established because of the adverse health effect of bleeding problems. Supplemental amounts in excess of the RDA should not be recommended.[41,42]

Dietary intake of α-tocopherol is inadequate in the typical U.S. diet. Only 8% of men and 2.4% of women in the United States receive the estimated average requirement (EAR) for vitamin E intake from foods alone.[43]

SOURCES

Vitamin E is available from vegetable oils (especially soybean oil) and margarine made from them; whole-grain or fortified cereals; wheat germ; nuts; seeds; green leafy vegetables; and some fruits, such as apples, apricots, and peaches. Meats, fish, and animal fats contain very little vitamin E. Table 7-6 lists the amounts of vitamin E in some foods. Because vitamin E is widely distributed in foods, dietary deficiencies seldom occur if a well-balanced, varied diet is consumed.

Although outdated, food labels list the vitamin E content of the food or supplement in international units because the DV is measured in international units. The DV for vitamin E is 30 IU (or 20 mg of α-tocopherol). Dietary supplements label vitamin E as "dl" α-tocopherol, which means the vitamin E is a synthetic form, in contrast to "d" α-tocopherol, which means it is natural.

ABSORPTION AND EXCRETION

Absorption of vitamin E is inefficient, ranging from 20% to 80% in healthy individuals. Efficiency of absorption depends

| Table 7-5 | Institute of Medicine Recommendations for α-Tocopherol† |

Life Stage	EAR (mg/d)‡	RDA (mg/d)§	AI (mg/d)¶	UL (mg/d)¶
0-6 mo			4	ND**
7-12 mo			6	ND**
1-3 yr	5	6		200
4-8 yr	6	7		300
9-13 yr	9	11		600
14-18 yr	12	15		800
19-70 yr	12	15		1000
>70 yr	12	15		1000
Pregnancy				
≤18 yr	12	15		800
19-50	12	15		1000
Lactation				
≤18 yr	16	19		800
19-50 yr	16	19		1000

Data from Institute of Medicine (IOM), Food and Nutrition Board: Dietary Reference Intakes for Vitamin C, Vitamin E, Selenium, and Carotenoids. Washington, DC: National Academy Press, 2000.
†α-tocopherol includes the only form of α-tocopherol that occurs naturally in foods, and some of the forms that occur in fortified foods and supplements, but not all forms because some that are used in fortified foods and supplements have not been shown to meet human requirements.
‡EAR (estimated average requirement)—the intake that meets the estimated nutrient needs of half of the individuals in a group.
§RDA (recommended dietary allowance)—the intake that meets the nutrient needs of almost all (97-98%) individuals in a group.
¶AI (adequate intake)—the observed average or experimentally set intake by a defined population or subgroup that seems to sustain a defined nutritional status, such as growth rate, normal circulating nutrient values, or other functional indicators of health. An AI is used if insufficient scientific evidence is available to derive an EAR. For healthy human milk–fed infants, the AI is the mean intake. *The AI is not equivalent to an RDA.*
¶Institute of Medicine (IOM), Food and Nutrition Board: Dietary Reference Intakes for Vitamin A, Vitamin K, Arsenic, Boron, Chromium, Copper, Iodine, Iron, Manganese, Molybdenum, Nickel, Silicon, Vanadium, and Zinc. Washington, DC: National Academy Press, 2000.
**Not determinable due to lack of data of adverse effects in this age group and concern about lack of ability to handle excess amounts. Source of intake should be from food and formula in order to prevent high levels of intake.

on the body's ability to absorb fat and seems to decline as the amount of dietary vitamin E increases.

HYPER-STATES AND HYPO-STATES

Scientific studies have suggested this potent antioxidant may reduce the risk for various diseases, including heart disease, some types of cancer, cataracts, age-related macular degeneration, Parkinson's disease, and Alzheimer's disease. However, evidence is not conclusive that vitamin E reduces the risk of heart disease and other chronic diseases. Vitamin E supplements do not seem to reverse any disease, including cancer, and a systematic review suggests that vitamin E supplementation may increase significantly the risk of mortality.[41,44]

Table 7-6	Food Sources of Vitamin E	
Food	**Portion**	**Vitamin E (mg)**
Total cereal	1 cup	45
Wheat germ oil	1 Tbsp	20
Sunflower seeds	¼ cup	8.4
Special K cereal	1 cup	4.7
Safflower oil	1 Tbsp	4.6
Tomato sauce, canned	1 cup	3.5
Peanut butter	2 Tbsp	2.9
Corn oil	1 Tbsp	2
Spinach, cooked	½ cup	1.9
Peach, fresh	1	1.3
Tomato juice, canned	1 cup	0.8
Sweet potato, cooked	½ cup	0.7
Bran cereal	½ cup	0.7
Almonds	1 oz	0.4
Pecans	¼ cup	0.4
Lima beans, cooked	½ cup	0.3
Walnuts	¼ cup	0.3
Hazelnuts	1 oz	0.3

Data from U.S. Department of Agriculture, Agricultural Research Service, USDA Nutrient Data Laboratory, USDA National Nutrient Database for Standard Reference, Release 20, 2008. Available at http://www.nal.usda.gov/fnic/foodcomp/search/. Accessed February 25, 2008.

Higher doses of vitamin E may disturb the balance of beneficial, naturally occurring antioxidants. Individuals who benefit from vitamin E supplementation are premature infants; infants, children, or adults who cannot absorb fats and oils because of diseases in the gastrointestinal tract; individuals with sickle cell anemia; smokers; and individuals consuming an extremely low-fat diet. Low vitamin E levels in the blood are associated with subsequent decline in physical function, but normal levels of vitamin E can be maintained by consuming vitamin E–rich foods.[45]

Dental Hygiene Considerations

- Vitamin E may help the immune system function better, so assess intake of vitamin E in immunocompromised patients.
- Vitamin E supplementation is not recommended, but may be of special concern for patients with vitamin K deficiency or with known coagulation defects, or for patients receiving anticoagulation therapy because it can interfere with vitamin K activity, increasing risk for hemorrhaging.
- In contrast to other vitamins, naturally occurring α-tocopherol from foods is twice as potent as the synthetic form, making it a more desirable choice than synthetic supplements.

Nutritional Directions

- When oils are reused in frying, heavy losses of vitamin E occur.
- An increase in fruits and vegetables provides more low-fat sources of vitamin E.
- Because of widespread publicity of scientific studies linking vitamin E to decreased risk of heart disease, diabetes, cancer, Alzheimer's disease, and cognitive decline, many patients may choose to use supplements. Advise patients to limit vitamin E supplements to the RDA, unless they are instructed otherwise by their healthcare provider.
- Adverse effects of excessive amounts of vitamin E are associated with vitamin E supplements only; food sources of vitamin E are not associated with adverse reactions.
- If vitamin E supplements are recommended by a healthcare provider or registered dietitian, they should be consumed with a meal containing fat to assist with absorption.[46]
- Vitamin E supplements cannot surmount other proven effective ways to reduce disease risks—not smoking, getting regular exercise, maintaining a healthy weight, and eating a well-balanced, healthy diet.

VITAMIN K

Three forms of vitamin K, a fat-soluble vitamin, have been identified, all belonging to a group of chemical compounds known as quinones. The naturally occurring vitamins are K_1 (phylloquinone), which occurs in green plants, and K_2 (menaquinone), which is formed by *Escherichia coli* bacteria in the large intestine and is found in animal tissues. The fat-soluble synthetic compound menadione (vitamin K_3) is two to three times as potent as the natural vitamin.

PHYSIOLOGICAL ROLES

Vitamin K–dependent proteins have been identified in bone, kidney, and other tissues. These proteins bind calcium and may be involved in bone crystalline formation. Vitamin K functions as a catalyst for synthesis of blood-clotting factors primarily in maintaining **prothrombin** levels, which is the first stage in forming a clot. A low prothrombin level results in impaired blood coagulation.

REQUIREMENTS

The RDA is 120 μg for men and 90 μg for women. No UL for vitamin K has been established (Table 7-7).

SOURCES

Although limited amounts of vitamin K are stored in the body, a shortage of vitamin K is unlikely because it is derived from food and microflora in the gut. Green leafy vegetables are high in vitamin K, but meats and dairy products also provide significant amounts (Table 7-8).

Bacterial flora in the jejunum and ileum synthesize vitamin K and provide about half of the body's requirement. However, synthesis of vitamin K by intestinal bacteria does not provide adequate amounts of the vitamin; that is, a restriction of dietary vitamin K can alter clotting factors.

Table 7-7   Institute of Medicine Recommendations for Vitamin K

Life Stage	AI† Male (µg/d)	AI† Female (µg/d)
0-6 mo	2	2
7-12 mo	2.5	2.5
1-3 yr	30	30
4-8 yr	55	55
9-13 yr	60	60
14-18 yr	75	75
>18 yr	120	90
Pregnancy		
≤18 yr		75
19-50 yr		90
Lactation		
≤18 yr		75
19-50 yr		90

Data from Institute of Medicine (IOM), Food and Nutrition Board: Dietary Reference Intakes for Vitamin A, Vitamin K, Arsenic, Boron, Chromium, Copper, Iodine, Iron, Manganese, Molybdenum, Nickel, Silicon, Vanadium, and Zinc. Washington, DC: National Academy Press, 2000.
†AI (adequate intake)—the observed average or experimentally set intake by a defined population or subgroup that seems to sustain a defined nutritional status, such as growth rate, normal circulating nutrient values, or other functional indicators of health. An AI is used if insufficient scientific evidence is available to derive an EAR. For healthy human milk–fed infants, the AI is the mean intake. *The AI is not equivalent to an RDA.*

Table 7-8   Food Sources of Vitamin K

Food	Portion	Vitamin K (µg)
Spinach, cooked	½ cup	444
Kale, raw	½ cup	274
Broccoli, cooked	½ cup	110
Brussels sprouts, cooked	½ cup	109
Loose-leaf lettuce	1 cup	48
Cabbage, raw	½ cup	26
Peas	½ cup	19
Milk	1 cup	0.5

Data from U.S. Department of Agriculture, Agricultural Research Service, USDA Nutrient Data Laboratory, USDA National Nutrient Database for Standard Reference, Release 20, 2008. Available at http://www.nal.usda.gov/fnic/foodcomp/search/. Accessed February 25, 2008.

bone mass density in women, increasing the risk of hip fractures. However, high-dose supplementation with high levels of vitamin K did not stop age-related bone loss.[48]

Newborns may develop hemorrhagic disease secondary to vitamin K deficiency because the gut is sterile during the first few days after birth. Newborns are usually given a single dose of vitamin K intramuscularly immediately after birth to prevent hemorrhage.

ABSORPTION AND EXCRETION

Vitamin K absorption decreases with high levels of vitamin E supplementation. Some vitamin K is stored in the liver, and some becomes a component of lipoproteins. Ordinarily, 30% to 40% of the amount absorbed is excreted via bile into the feces as water-soluble metabolites, with approximately 15% excreted in the urine.

HYPER-STATES AND HYPO-STATES

No toxicity symptoms have been documented from oral intake of vitamin K. Synthetic menadione has caused toxic effects, however.

Primary vitamin K deficiency is uncommon, but disease or drug therapy may cause deficiencies. Any condition of the biliary tract affecting the flow of bile prevents vitamin K absorption. Vitamin K deficiency is common in celiac disease and sprue, which affect absorption in the small intestine, and other diarrheal diseases (e.g., ulcerative colitis) as a result of malabsorption. In vitamin K deficiency or in patients taking anticoagulants, blood-clotting time is delayed, increasing risk of bleeding problems.

Impairment of vitamin K function in bones of postmenopausal women may be a factor in the effects of declining estrogen production. Typical vitamin K intake may be inadequate to support bone health in postmenopausal years.[47] Low dietary intake of vitamin K has been linked to reduced

Dental Hygiene Considerations

- Excessive amounts of vitamin A or vitamin E or both have a detrimental effect on vitamin K absorption.
- Mineral oil interferes with the absorption of vitamin K and should not be consumed close to a meal.
- Vitamin K should never be confused with the symbol "K" used to designate potassium or kosher foods. If information is confusing or unclear, double-check with a healthcare provider or registered dietitian.
- Vitamin K may be used prophylactically before any oral surgery to prevent prolonged bleeding in patients who have a condition that inhibits clotting.
- Frequently, blood-thinning agents may be discontinued for several days before any oral surgery to prevent excessive bleeding, or the patient may be hospitalized for a few days.
- Cholestyramine prescribed for hyperlipidemia binds with bile salts. The presence of bile is required for vitamin K absorption. Patients taking cholestyramine are at risk of vitamin K deficiency, so assess for any bleeding problems, such as **petechiae** (pinpoint, flat red spots) or ecchymosis (bruising).
- Antibiotic therapy inhibits vitamin K–producing intestinal microflora and seems to be a factor in the origin of vitamin K deficiency, especially with impaired hepatic or renal function.
- Patients receiving oral anticoagulants (warfarin) to prevent blood clots from forming may develop serious hemorrhaging problems and should keep vitamin K intake consistent, and should not consume vitamin K supplements.

VITAMIN C (ASCORBIC ACID)

PHYSIOLOGICAL ROLES

As a coenzyme, vitamin C has numerous metabolic roles. It is important in the production of **collagen** (structural protein in connective tissue, cartilage, and bone), which plays a vital role in wound healing. During the development of connective tissue, bones, and teeth, vitamin C is important in the formation of **fibroblasts** (collagen-forming cells), osteoblasts, and odontoblasts. Vitamin C strengthens tissues and promotes capillary integrity. Vitamin C facilitates development of RBCs by enhancing iron absorption and use. It also aids the body in use of folate and vitamin B_{12}. It has a coenzymatic function in the metabolism of amino acids and biosynthesis of bile acids, thyroxine, epinephrine, and steroid hormones. Vitamin C can also affect immune responses because of the high concentration in white blood cells.

Vitamin C functions as an antioxidant in numerous physiologic reactions. In its role as an antioxidant, it protects cells and tissues against damage caused by free radicals, toxic chemicals, and pollutants. More details on the role of vitamin C as an antioxidant are found in Health Application 7.

REQUIREMENTS

The RDA is established at 90 mg daily for men and 75 mg daily for women, increasing during pregnancy and lactation (Table 7-9). The requirement for vitamin C is increased under many situations in which it is directly involved (e.g., stress, healing, and infections). It is detrimentally affected by many drugs (e.g., tobacco, alcohol, oral contraceptives, and aspirin), which increase requirements and is usually the first nutrient to be depleted. Smokers may benefit from an additional intake of 35 mg per day because they are more likely to experience biological processes that damage cells and deplete vitamin C. The UL is 2000 mg per day. Intakes exceeding this amount may result in stomach upset and diarrhea.

SOURCES

The RDA can usually be met by choosing one serving daily of foods known as an excellent source of vitamin C (e.g., citrus fruits and juices, cantaloupe, green and red pepper, broccoli, kiwi, strawberries, and mango). Good sources

Table 7-9	Institute of Medicine Recommendations for Vitamin C						
Life Stage	**EAR (mg/d)†**		**RDA (mg/d)‡**		**AI (mg/d)§**		**UL (mg/d)¶**
	Male	*Female*	*Male*	*Female*	*Male*	*Female*	
0-6 mo					40	50	ND¶
7-12 mo					50	50	ND¶
1-3 yr	13	13	15	15			400
4-8 yr	22	22	25	25			650
9-13 yr	39	39	45	45			1200
14-18 yr	63	56	75	65			1800
19-70 yr	75	60	90	75			2000
>70 yr	75	60	90	75			2000
Pregnancy							
≤18 yr		66		80			1800
19-50 yr		70		85			2000
Lactation							
≤18 yr		96		115			1800
19-50 yr		100		120			2000

Data from Institute of Medicine (IOM), Food and Nutrition Board: Dietary Reference Intakes for Vitamin C, Vitamin E, Selenium, and Carotenoids. Washington, DC: National Academy Press, 2000.
†EAR (estimated average requirement)—the intake that meets the estimated nutrient needs of half of the individuals in a group.
‡RDA (recommended dietary allowance)—the intake that meets the nutrient needs of almost all (97-98%) individuals in a group.
§AI (adequate intake)—the observed average or experimentally set intake by a defined population or subgroup that seems to sustain a defined nutritional status, such as growth rate, normal circulating nutrient values, or other functional indicators of health. An AI is used if insufficient scientific evidence is available to derive an EAR. For healthy human milk–fed infants, the AI is the mean intake. *The AI is not equivalent to an RDA.*
¶UL (tolerable upper intake level)—the highest level of daily nutrient intake that is likely to pose no risk of adverse health effects to almost all individuals in the general population. As intake increases above the UL, the risk of adverse effects increases. Unless specified otherwise, UL represents total nutrient intake from food, water, and supplements.
¶Not determinable due to lack of data of adverse effects in this age group and concern about lack of ability to handle excess amounts. Source of intake should be from food and formula in order to prevent high levels of intake.

include peaches, cabbage, potatoes, sweet potatoes, and tomatoes; at least two servings of these sources a day may be required to meet the RDA (Table 7-10).

HYPER-STATES AND HYPO-STATES

Healthcare professionals in the United States generally consider vitamin C deficiency, or scurvy, to be a disease of only historical significance. Most Americans usually exceed the RDAs for vitamin C. However, vitamin C deficiency and depletion occurred among 5% to 17% and 13% to 23%, respectively, of individuals surveyed in the *National Health and Nutrition Examination Survey* (NHANES). Smokers, individuals who did not use supplements, and non-Hispanic black men had elevated risks of vitamin C deficiency.[49]

Scurvy, caused by vitamin C deficiency, can occur in 20 days. It is characterized by spontaneous gingival hemorrhaging, perifollicular petechiae, follicular hyperkeratosis, diarrhea, fatigue, depression, and cessation of bone growth (Fig. 7-9).

Inadequate amounts of vitamin C during tooth development may result in changes similar to scurvy or **scorbutic** changes in the teeth because of changes in the ameloblasts and odontoblasts. Ameloblasts and odontoblasts atrophy, and there is a decrease in their orderly polar arrangement in a vitamin C–deficient environment. Any new dentin deposits

forming at this time are similar to osteodentin; the pulp also atrophies and is hyperemetic. Dentin deposits completely cease in severe vitamin C deficiency, with hypercalcification of predentin. Dentinal tubules also lack their normal parallel arrangement. In scorbutic adults, the dentin reabsorbs and is porotic.

Gingivitis, caused by ascorbic acid deficiency, also affects the periodontium, resulting in tooth mobility. This effect is probably related to weakened collagen secondary to vitamin C deficiency, which results in resorption of the alveolar bone (Fig. 7-10). Supplemental amounts of vitamin C in excess of the UL can cause gastrointestinal distress and interfere with vitamin B_{12} absorption.

Dental Hygiene Considerations

- Older patients, especially individuals who live alone or who avoid acidic foods to control gastroesophageal reflux, patients undergoing peritoneal dialysis or hemodialysis, smokers, and drug abusers are at greatest risk to become scorbutic. Assess for deficiency: periodontal disease, deep red to purple gingiva, hyperplasia, bleeding on probing, reported nosebleeds, melena (vomitus or stools containing blood), and petechiae (especially lower legs and back).
- Evaluate the amount of vitamin C supplements taken. If vitamin C intake is high, vitamin B_{12} deficiency could occur.
- Vitamin C chewable tablets, syrup, or cough drops are associated with enamel erosion and dentin hypersensitivity.
- Steroids, antibiotics, and salicylates can increase excretion of vitamin C.
- Deficient vitamin C intake (5 mg per day) increases the propensity of the gingiva to become inflamed or bleed on probing, but serum levels and gingiva return to normal with an intake of 65 mg per day.[50]
- Evaluate the vitamin C intake because low vitamin C levels may affect the severity of periodontal disease.[51]

Table 7-10	Food Sources of Vitamin C	
Food	**Portion**	**Vitamin C (mg)**
Papaya	1	188
Guava	1	125
Orange juice, fresh	1 cup	124
Pineapple juice, canned	1 cup	109
Red sweet pepper, raw	1	95
Navel orange	1	83
Grapefruit	1	77
Kiwi	1	71
Cantaloupe	1 cup	59
Mango	1	57
Broccoli, cooked	½ cup	51
Strawberries, fresh	½ cup	49
Brussels sprouts, cooked	½ cup	48
Tomato juice	1 cup	45
Cranberry juice	½ cup	42
Tomato paste	½ cup	29
Raw cauliflower	½ cup	23
Sweet potato, baked	1	22
Potato, baked	1	20
Turnip greens	½ cup	16
Cabbage, raw	½ cup	13

Data from U.S. Department of Agriculture, Agricultural Research Service, USDA Nutrient Data Laboratory, USDA National Nutrient Database for Standard Reference, Release 20, 2008. Available at: http://www.nal.usda.gov/fnic/foodcomp/search/. Accessed February 25, 2008.

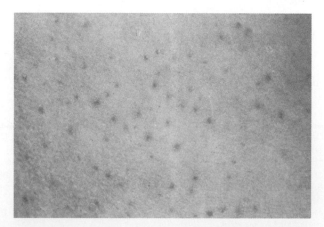

FIGURE 7-9 Perifollicular petechiae. Minimal bleeding into the hair follicles is often one of the earliest clinical manifestations of vitamin C deficiency. (Courtesy of Dr. H.H. Sandstead. From McLaren DS: A Colour Atlas and Text of Diet-related Disorders, 2nd ed. London: Mosby–Year Book Europe Limited, 1992.)

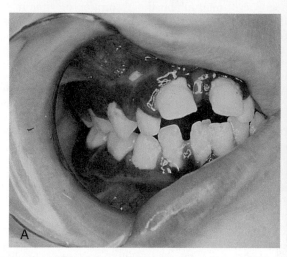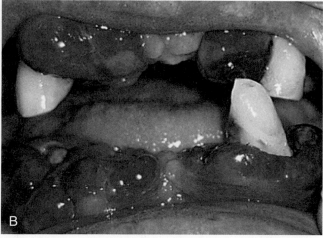

FIGURE 7-10 **A,** Ascorbic acid deficiency. The gums are blue-red and grossly swollen. The earliest changes involve the interdental papillae, which swell and tend to bleed easily. **B,** Effects on the periodontium result in tooth mobility. (From Swartz MH: Textbook of Physical Diagnosis: History and Examination, 5th ed. Philadelphia: Saunders, 2006.)

Nutritional Directions

- Vitamin C requirements are readily available from small amounts of food. One orange contains 98 mg of vitamin C, which is enough vitamin C for healthy nonsmoking adults.
- Patients who smoke need an additional 35 mg of vitamin C daily; a man who smokes should consume 125 mg instead of 90 mg of vitamin C each day.
- Deficiency symptoms may develop within 20 to 40 days after dietary elimination of vitamin C.

- Storage is important to prevent oxidation of vitamin C. Fruit juices should be kept in an airtight container that is appropriate for the amount stored to retain more vitamin C. For example, 2 cups of juice in a pint container with an airtight lid protects the vitamin C content better than 1 pint of juice in a gallon container.
- Ascorbic acid is another name for vitamin C.
- Megadoses of vitamin C (2000 mg or greater per day) can interfere with vitamin B_{12} and copper use.

HEALTH APPLICATION 7 Antioxidants

Free radicals are highly unstable and reactive molecular fragments. They contain one or more unpaired electrons, which try to gain electrons to become more stable. During this process, the free radicals oxidize (damage) body cells. UV radiation from the sun, air pollution, ozone, and smoking are just a few conditions that can generate free radicals in the body. Antioxidants donate electrons to the free radicals to make them stable. This protects the body cells from damage. The antioxidant is oxidized and destroyed. In some situations, an antioxidant can regain or regenerate an electron to allow it to function again.

Although antioxidants have some properties in common, each one has unique properties. A standardized method of measuring antioxidants and the effects of each antioxidant have not been established, so comparing the antioxidants from various foods is virtually impossible.[52] According to one comparative analysis, the best sources of antioxidants are beans (specifically small red, kidney, pinto, and black beans), fruits (particularly blueberries, cranberries, blackberries, prunes, raspberries, strawberries, apples, cherries, and plums), pecans, and potatoes.[53]

Much has been learned about the functions of vitamins C and E, beta carotene, and other phytochemicals (biologically active substances found in plants), and the minerals selenium, zinc, copper, and manganese in their roles as antioxidants. Numerous studies have suggested that

antioxidants may be important in preventing heart disease, cancer, age-related eye disease, and other chronic conditions associated with aging. Ascorbic acid is one of the strongest antioxidants and radical scavengers, serving as a primary defense against free radicals in the blood. However, the connections between vitamin C and these processes have yet to be established. Research has proven vitamin C and other antioxidants in amounts greater than the RDA are desirable. This is especially true if increased levels are achieved by improving food choices.

Increased serum antioxidant concentrations are associated with a reduced risk of periodontitis even in individuals who never smoked.[54] Initially, it was observed that smokers who ate more fruits and vegetables rich in beta carotene had a lower risk of lung cancer. However, two studies using beta carotene supplements were cut short because participants taking beta carotene had a slightly higher risk of lung cancer than participants taking a placebo.[55,56] Research studies have had different outcomes with antioxidants in regard to reduced cardiovascular disease and prevention of other cancers. In 2007, a **meta-analysis** (systematic method that uses statistical analysis to integrate the data from numerous independent studies) published in the *Journal of the American Medical Association* analyzed research studies involving beta carotene, selenium, and vitamins A, C, and E supplementation.[57] This report indicated supplements of beta carotene, vitamin A, and vitamin E significantly increased mortality by 7%, 16%, and 4%, respectively. Vitamin C and selenium had no significant effect on mortality. Additionally, a systematic review of 67 randomized clinical trials found no evidence to support antioxidant supplements to prevent mortality in healthy people or patients with various diseases.[58] Another study in 2005 also found that in patients with vascular disease or diabetes, long-term vitamin E supplementation did not prevent cancer or major cardiovascular events, and possibly had an increased risk of heart failure.[59] In a large, long-term trial of male physicians, neither vitamin E nor vitamin C supplementation reduced the risk of major cardiovascular events.[60]

Apparently the simple image of antioxidants as valiant warriors protecting the body from rampaging free radicals is too simplistic. Currently, the American Heart Association does not recommend antioxidant supplements, awaiting more convincing data.[61] Numerous reports suggest that differences in genes may explain the effect of antioxidants on the risk of disease.[62-64]

Because of the lay-press publicity surrounding the potential health benefits, 30% of Americans are taking some form of antioxidant supplement to prevent chronic diseases.[65] High intake levels of some antioxidants are well tolerated by most individuals, but several known factors must be considered before recommending supplements. Toxic effects occur with vitamin A; organ damage and deaths have been reported. Vitamin E supplements can antagonize vitamin K activity and enhance the effect of anticoagulant drugs. Adverse effects of vitamin C include diarrhea, increased risk of kidney stones, and decreased absorption of vitamin B_{12}. Although vitamin C increases iron absorption, large amounts decrease availability of vitamin B_{12} and copper. Erosion and hypersensitivity of tooth enamel are unique adverse effects of chewable vitamin C tablets. Simultaneous intake of carotenoids with

α-tocopherol may inhibit the absorption of vitamin E by 36%.[62] Possibly unexplored interactions may occur between large amounts of antioxidants and other nutrients. If a patient chooses to take vitamin C supplements, there is no benefit in taking more expensive ones, such as products containing bioflavonoids, over simple ascorbic acid.

Antioxidants may counteract the effects of cell damage produced by metabolic reactions and environmental factors such as pollution, smoking, and toxic chemicals in the diet. However, the health toll of a smoking habit is not corrected by simply eating right or taking vitamins. Recommendations for supplemental amounts of these nutrients should be reserved for claims that have been well substantiated with clinical trials that prove cause and effect and explore related side effects. Patients should also be cautioned about taking megadoses of vitamins and minerals because side effects, nutrient-nutrient interactions, and drug-nutrient interactions can occur. Individuals who are seriously ill with cancer, heart disease, or other conditions should talk with their healthcare provider about everything they put into their bodies, including vitamins, supplements, or herbs.

The *Dietary Guidelines for Americans 2005* emphasize consumption of a varied diet to help prevent several chronic diseases. Dietary patterns high in fruits and vegetables are associated with a lower risk of disease. Advice to patients should be to eat a healthy diet that includes many fruits and vegetables, especially those that are high in vitamin C, vitamin E, and beta carotene. A pill cannot provide what is available from a healthful diet—so the bottom line is to "eat your fruits and veggies." Antioxidant supplements cannot be expected to undo a lifetime of unhealthy living. Adequate intake ideally should be in the form of improving dietary selections rather than supplements because as-yet unidentified components present in food may be beneficial and protective. Beyond diet, decreased exposure to free radicals and increased physical activity are essential.

CASE APPLICATION FOR THE DENTAL HYGIENIST

A healthy patient asks your advice about taking vitamin C supplements to prevent periodontal disease. She is unsure what foods to eat or what to look for if an excess or deficiency develops.

Nutritional Assessment
- Income
- Living arrangements, cooking and storage facilities
- Dietary assessment
- Tobacco and other drug use
- Knowledge level about vitamin C
- Beliefs about water-soluble vitamins
- Knowledge level about periodontal disease
- Physical status, especially any bleeding problems
- Use of over-the-counter or healthcare provider–prescribed supplements or medications
- Emotional state

Nutritional Diagnosis
Health-seeking behavior related to inadequate/insufficient knowledge about vitamin C and periodontal disease.

Nutritional Goals
The patient will consume foods high in vitamin C and state beliefs/information about vitamin C and periodontal disease.

Nutritional Implementation
Intervention: Teach the following about vitamin C: (1) functions, (2) requirements, and (3) sources. Teach the following

about periodontal disease: (1) causes and (2) preventive factors.
Rationale: This provides the patient with a sound knowledge base about vitamin C and periodontal disease.
Intervention: Explain hyper- and hypo-vitamin C states.
Rationale: Large amounts of vitamin C decrease absorption of vitamin B_{12} and cause diarrhea, gastrointestinal distress, and kidney stones. Because vitamin C helps maintain capillary integrity, a vitamin C deficiency results in bleeding problems. Encourage food sources for increasing vitamin C rather than supplements.
Intervention: Provide oral hygiene instruction.
Rationale: The primary cause of periodontal disease is plaque biofilm. Providing education to effectively remove the plaque biofilm is essential. A vitamin deficiency does not cause periodontal disease, but it could exacerbate existing periodontal issues.

Evaluation
The patient should consume citrus fruits, strawberries, cantaloupes, and mangos. Additionally, the patient states that supplements are unnecessary for vitamin C, and large doses may interfere with absorption of other nutrients. She further states that if she does develop any bleeding problems, she will seek help. Lastly, the patient should verbalize information concerning excesses and deficiencies of vitamin C.

STUDENT READINESS

1. How do water-soluble vitamins differ from fat-soluble vitamins? What do these differences mean as you choose foods for your own menu? What do these differences mean as you teach patients about nutrition?

2. Which fat-soluble vitamins are the most toxic? What are the symptoms of toxicity? What treatment is recommended for each?

3. A patient asks why food is fortified with vitamin D. How would you respond?

4. Plan a 1-day menu that meets the RDA for vitamin E.

5. Keep a record of your food intake for 1 day. Use a table of nutrient values of foods (www.nal.usda.gov/fnic/foodcomp) or a nutrient analysis program (www.usda.gov/cnpp) to determine your vitamin A intake. Was your diet adequate? What are some food choices you could make for improvement?

6. Prepare a menu for 1 day that provides adequate amounts of vitamins A and D. Eliminate all sources of milk products and canned fish. What does this do to vitamin D intake? Now remove various types of egg products, green leafy vegetables, and dark yellow vegetables, and see the effect on the vitamin A content of the meal plan.

7. Most fat-soluble vitamins are found in fat sources, but the *Dietary Guidelines for Americans 2005* restrict fat intake to inhibit cardiovascular disease. Discuss the impact of these guidelines on nutritional status if adequate precursor vitamin sources are not consumed.

8. Justify the rationale of vitamin D supplementation of milk products in the United States.

9. What is the role of antioxidants in cancer prevention? What foods are advocated to prevent this condition?

10. Name the deficiency and toxicity conditions associated with vitamins A, D, K, and C.

11. Name five foods other than oranges that are good sources of vitamin C.

12. As a group, discuss the pros and cons of the controversial issue of mandatory food labeling on nutrition supplements.

References

1. Lodi G, et al: Interventions for treating oral leukoplakia. Cochrane Database Syst Rev 2006 Oct 18;(4):CD001829.

2. Goodman GE, et al: The Beta-Carotene and Retinol Efficacy Trial: incidence of lung cancer and cardiovascular disease mortality during 6-year follow-up after stopping β-carotene and retinol supplements. J Natl Cancer Inst 2004;96(23):1729-1731.

3. Institute of Medicine (IOM), Food and Nutrition Board: Dietary Reference Intakes for Vitamin A, Vitamin K, Arsenic, Boron, Chromium, Copper, Iodine, Iron, Molybdenum, Nickel, Silicon, Vanadium, and Zinc. Washington, DC: National Academy Press, 2001.

4. Crandall C: Vitamin A intake and osteoporosis: a clinical review. J Womens Health 2004 Oct; 13(8):939-953.

5. Norman AW: From vitamin D to hormone D: fundamentals of the vitamin D endocrine system essential for good health. Am J Clin Nutr 2008 Aug; 88(2):491S-499S.

6. Cannell JJ, Hollis BW: Use of vitamin D in clinical practice. Altern Med Rev 2008 Mar; 13(1):6-20.

7. Norman AW: From vitamin D to hormone D: fundamentals of the vitamin D endocrine system essential for good health. Am J Clin Nutr 2008 Aug; 88(2):491S-499S.

8. Brannon PM: Overview of the conference "Vitamin D and Health in the 21st Century: an Update." Am J Clin Nutr 2008 Aug; 88(2):483S-490S.

9. Vieth R, et al: The urgent need to recommend an intake of vitamin D that is effective. Am J Clin Nutr 2007 Mar; 85(3):649-650.

10. Wagner C, Greer FR, and the Section on Breastfeeding and Committee on Nutrition. Prevention of rickets and vitamin D deficiency in infants, children, and adolescents. Pediatrics 2008 Nov; 122(5):1142-1152.

11. Svoren BM, Volkenning LK, Wood JR, Laffel LMB: Significant vitamin D deficiency in youth with type 1 diabetes mellitus. J Pediatr 2009 Jan; 154(1):132-134.

12. Wing FL, et al: Risk factors for low serum 25-hydroxy-vitamin D concentrations in otherwise healthy children and adolescents. Am J Clin Nutr 2007 Mar; 86(3):150-158.

13. Beres S: Vitamin D: cancer prevention's sunny future? J Natl Cancer Inst 2008 Mar 5; 100(5):292-293, 297.

14. Wolpowitz D, Gilchrest BA: The vitamin D questions: how much do you need and how should you get it? J Am Acad Dermatol 2006 Feb; 54(2):301-317.

15. Sayre RM, Dowdy JC: Darkness at noon: sunscreens and vitamin D3. Photochem Photobiol 2007 Mar-Apr; 83(2):459-463.

16. Holden JM, Lemar LE: Assessing vitamin D contents in foods and supplements: challenges and needs. Am J Clin Nutr 2008 Apr; 88(Suppl):551S-553S.

17. Wagner D, et al: The bioavailability of vitamin D from fortified cheese and supplements is equivalent in adults. J Nutr 2008 Jul; 138:1365-1371.

18. Holick MF, Chen TC: Vitamin D deficiency: a worldwide problem with health consequences. Am J Clin Nutr 2008 Apr; 87(4):1080S-1086S.

19. Harvard Women's Health Watch: The sunshine D-lemma. (serial online): http://www.health.harvard.edu/press_releases/vitamin-d-has-the-potential-to-ward-off-a-number-of-serious-diseases.htm. Accessed September 5, 2008.

20. Cranney A, et al: Summary of evidence-based review on vitamin D efficacy and safety in relation to bone health. Am J Clin Nutr 2008 Aug; 88(2):512S-519S.

21. Lanske B, Razzaque MS: Vitamin D and aging: old concepts and new insights. J Nutr Biochem 2007 Dec; 18(12):771-777.

22. Office of Dietary Supplements, National Institutes of Health: Dietary supplement fact sheet: Vitamin D. Available at http://ods.od.nih.gov/factsheets/vitamind.asp. Accessed April 15, 2008.

23. Institute of Medicine (IOM), Food and Nutrition Board: Dietary Reference Intakes: Calcium, Phosphorus, Magnesium, Vitamin D, and Fluoride. Washington, DC: National Academy Press, 1997.

24. Holick MF, Chen TC: Vitamin D deficiency: a worldwide problem with health consequences. Am J Clin Nutr 2008 Apr; 87(4):1080S-1086S.

25. Cranney C, et al: Effectiveness and safety of vitamin D. Evidence Report/Technology Assessment No. 158 prepared by the University of Ottawa Evidence-based Practice Center under Contract No. 290-02.0021. AHRQ Publication No 07-E013. Rockville, MD: Agency for Healthcare Research and Quality, 2007.

26. Taylor JA: Defining vitamin D deficiency in infants and toddlers. Arch Pediatr Adolesc Med 2008 Jun; 162(6):583-584.

27. Melamed ML, et al: 25-hydroxyvitamin D levels and the risk of mortality in the general population. Arch Intern Med 2008 Aug 11; 168(15):1629-1637.

28. Brannon PM, et al: Summary of roundtable discussion on vitamin D research needs. Am J Clin Nutr 2008 Aug; 88(2):587S-592S.

29. Gordon CM, et al: Prevalence of vitamin D deficiency among healthy infants and toddlers. Arch Pediatr Adolesc Med 2008 Jun; 162(6):505-512.

30. Janssen H, Samson MM, Verhaar HJJ: Vitamin D deficiency, muscle function and falls in elderly people. Am J Clin Nutr 2002 Apr; 75(4):611-615.

31. Huh SY, Gordon CM: Vitamin D deficiency in children and adolescents: epidemiology, impact and treatment. Rev Endocr Metab Disord. 2008 Jun; 9(2):161-170.

32. Lee WT, Jiang J: The resurgence of the importance of vitamin D in bone health. Asia Pac J Clin Nutr 2008;17(Suppl 1):138-142.

33. Ng K, et al: Circulating 25-hydroxyvitamin D levels and survival in patients with colorectal cancer. J Clin Oncol 2008 Jun 20; 26(18):2984-2991.

34. Pilz S, et al: Low serum levels of 25-hydroxyvitamin D predict fatal cancer patients referred to coronary angiography. Cancer Epidemiol Biomarkers Prev 2008 May; 17(5):1228-1233.

35. Mohr SB, et al: Relationship between low ultraviolet B irradiance and higher breast cancer risk in 107 countries. Breast J 2008 May-Jun; 14(3):255-260.

36. Giovannucci E: The epidemiology of vitamin D and colorectal cancer: recent findings. Curr Opin Gastroenterol 2006 Jan; 22(1):24-29.

37. Giovannucci E, et al: 25-hydroxyvitamin D and risk of myocardial infarction in men. Arch Intern Med 2008 Jun 9; 168(11):1174-1180.

38. Dobnig H, et al: Independent association of low serum 25-hydroxyvitamin D and 1,25-dihydroxyvitamin D levels with all-cause and cardiovascular mortality. Arch Intern Med 2008 Jun 23; 168(12):1340-1349.

39. Bischoff-Ferrari HA, et al: Estimation of optimal serum concentrations of 25-hydroxyvitamin D for multiple health outcomes. Am J Clin Nutr 2006 Jul; 84(1):18-28.

40. Kaye EK: Bone health and oral health. J Am Dental Assoc 2007 May; 138(5):616-619.

41. Bjelakovic G, et al: Antioxidant supplements for prevention of mortality in healthy participants and patients with various diseases. Cochrane Database Syst Rev 2008 Apr 16; (2):21-191.

42. Bjelakovic G, et al: Antioxidant supplements for preventing gastrointestinal cancers. Cochrane Database Syst Rev 2008 Jul 16; (3):CD004183.

43. Maras JE, et al: Intake of α-tocopherol is limited among US adults. J Am Diet Assoc 2004 Apr; 104(4):567-575.

44. Hershman DL, Neugut AI: Anthracycline cardiotoxicity: one size does not fit all! J Natl Cancer Inst 2008 Aug 6; 100(15):1046-1047.

45. Bartoli B: Serum micronutrient concentration and decline in physical function among older persons. JAMA 2008 Jan 23; 299(3):308-315.

46. Leonard SW, et al: Vitamin E bioavailability from fortified breakfast cereal is greater than that from encapsulated supplements. Am J Clin Nutr 2004 Jan; 79(1):86-92.

47. Lukacs J: Differential associations for menopause and age in measures of vitamin K, osteocalcin and bone density: a cross-sectional exploratory study in healthy volunteers. Menopause 2006 Sep/Oct; 13(5):799-808.

48. Cheung AM, et al: Vitamin K supplementation in postmenopausal women with osteopenia (ECKO Trial): a randomized controlled trial. PLoS Med 2008 Oct 14; 5(10):e196.

49. Hampl JS, Taylor CA, Johnston CS: Vitamin C deficiency and depletion in the United States: The Third National Health and Nutrition Examination Survey, 1988 to 1994. Am J Public Health 2004 May; 94(5):870-875.

50. Jacob RA, et al: Experimental vitamin C depletion and supplementation in young men: nutrient interactions and dental health effects. Ann N Y Acad Sci 1987; 498:333-346.

51. Amaliya TMF, et al: Java project on periodontal diseases: the relationship between vitamin C and the severity of periodontitis. J Clin Periodontol 2007 Apr; 34(4):299-304.

52. Huang D, Ou B, Prior RL: The chemistry behind antioxidant capacity assays. J Agric Food Chem 2005 Mar 23; 53(6):1841-1856.

53. Wu X, et al: Lipophilic and hydrophilic antioxidant capacities of common foods in the United States. J Agric Food Chem 2004 Jun 16; 52(12):4026-4037.

54. Chapple IL, Milward MR, Dietrich T: The prevalence of inflammatory periodontitis is negatively associated with serum antioxidant concentrations. J Nutr 2007 Mar; 137(3):657-664.

55. The Alpha-Tocopherol, Beta Carotene Cancer Prevention Study Group: The effect of vitamin E and beta carotene on the incidence of lung cancer and other cancers in male smokers. N Engl J Med 1994 Apr 14; 330(15):1029-1035.

56. Omenn GS, et al: Effects of a combination of beta carotene and vitamin A on lung cancer and cardiovascular disease. N Engl J Med 1996 May 2; 334(18):1150-1155.

57. Bjelakovic G, et al: Mortality in randomized trials of antioxidant supplements for primary and secondary prevention: systematic review and meta-analysis. JAMA 2007 Feb 28; 297(8):842-857.

58. Bjelakovic G, et al: Antioxidant supplements for prevention of mortality in healthy participants and patients with various diseases. Cochrane Database Syst Rev 2008, Apr (2): CD007176.

59. Lonn E, et al: Effects of long-term vitamin E supplementation on cardiovascular events and cancer: a randomized controlled trial. JAMA 2005 Mar 16; 293(11):1338-1347.

60. Sesso HD, et al: Vitamins E and C in the prevention of cardiovascular disease in men. JAMA 2008 Nov 12; 300(18):2123-2133.

61. American Heart Association: Antioxidant vitamins. Available at www.americanheart.org/presenter.jhtml?identifier=4452. Accessed April 25, 2008.

62. Li H, et al: Manganese superoxide dismutase polymorphism, prediagnostic antioxidant status, and risk of clinical significant prostate cancer. Cancer Res 2005 Mar 15; 65(6):2498-2504.

63. Davis DC, Hord NG: Nutritional "omics" technologies for elucidating the role(s) of bioactive food components in colon cancer prevention. J Nutr 2005 Nov; 135(11):2694-2697.

64. Bailey LB: Folate, methyl-related nutrients, alcohol, and the MTHFR 677C?T polymorphism affect cancer risk: intake recommendations. J Nutr 2003 Nov; 133(11 Suppl 1):2748S-2753S.

65. Reboul E, et al: Effect of the main dietary antioxidants (carotenoids, gamma-tocopherol, polyphenols, and vitamin C) on alpha-tocopherol absorption. Eur J Clin Nutr 2007 Oct; 61(10):1167-1173.

Chapter 8

Minerals Essential for Calcified Structures

LEARNING OBJECTIVES

Upon completion of this chapter, the student will be able to complete the following objectives:
- List the minerals found in collagen, bones, and teeth, and describe their main physiological roles and sources.
- Describe causes and symptoms of mineral excesses or deficits.
- Discuss the role of water fluoridation in the prevention of dental caries.

- Describe advantages and disadvantages of mineral supplementation.
- Discuss dental hygiene considerations for patients regarding calcium, phosphorus, magnesium, and fluoride.
- Describe nutritional directions for patients regarding calcium, phosphorus, magnesium, and fluoride.

KEY TERMS

Amenorrhea
Amorphous
Apatite
Bioavailability
Compressional forces

Fluorapatite
Fluorosis
Hydroxyapatite
Hypercalcemia
Hypocalcemia

145

Test Your NQ

1. **T/F** Meats are good sources of phosphorus.
2. **T/F** The only nutrients essential for strong healthy bones are calcium and phosphorus.
3. **T/F** Tooth exfoliation may be an oral sign of osteoporosis.
4. **T/F** Systemic fluoride causes changes in tooth morphology that increase caries resistance.
5. **T/F** To obtain adequate calcium, a teenager needs to drink 2 cups of milk a day.
6. **T/F** Water fluoridation is economically inefficient because very little of the water is actually consumed.
7. **T/F** All women should take calcium supplements to prevent osteoporosis.
8. **T/F** Calcium absorption is increased when a sugar is present.
9. **T/F** Caffeine intake may decrease calcium loss.
10. **T/F** All bottled waters contain fluoride.

BONE MINERALIZATION AND GROWTH

Calcified structures in the body, which include bones and teeth, are composed of a matrix of organic and inorganic substances. Tooth dentin and cementum and bone originate with a protein matrix, or collagen deposition. Collagen is present throughout the periodontium as the primary connective tissue fiber in the gingiva and the major organic constituent of alveolar bone. Collagen is continuously being remodeled (resorption and reformation of bone) throughout growth and development. Defective collagen synthesis affects formation of bones and teeth.

The organic matrix of bone is 90% to 95% collagen fibers, which are secreted by osteoblasts. Formation of collagen requires the presence of a variety of substances, including protein; vitamin C; and the minerals iron, copper, and zinc. When collagen is formed, **apatite**, a calcium phosphate complex, automatically crystallizes adjacent to the collagen fibers.

Bones that have not undergone calcification, **osteoids**, are formed rapidly. Most develop into the finished product, **hydroxyapatite** crystals (inorganic component of bones and teeth).

Immediately after collagen formation, mineralization begins. **Mineralization** is the deposition of inorganic elements (minerals) on an organic matrix (mainly composed of protein in combination with some polysaccharides and lipids). In addition to calcium and phosphorus, numerous other minerals, especially magnesium, sodium, potassium, and carbonate ions, are incorporated into the mineral matrix.

Adequate nutritional components are necessary during the collagen formation and mineral deposition phases to prevent structural imperfections. The crystalline mineral matrix provides great compressional strength similar to marble. The combination of collagen and crystalline mineral matrix forms a material resembling reinforced concrete.

The skeleton is constantly growing, changing, and **remodeling** itself. About 0.4% to 10% of total bone calcium remains in a shapeless or **amorphous** form. This calcium is a reserve source that can be rapidly used when serum calcium levels decrease. Osteoblasts deposit fresh calcium salts where new stresses have developed, and where **osteoclasts** (connected with absorption of bone) are removing calcium deposits. Bone absorption by osteoclasts is controlled by parathyroid hormone (PTH). The rate of osteoblast and osteoclast activity is normally in equilibrium except during periods of growth. In older adults, bone resorption may exceed mineralization, causing osteoporosis.

This dynamic state accommodates the changing demands of the body. Bone strength is adjusted in proportion to the degree of stress on the bone. Continual physical stress stimulates calcification and osteoblastic deposition of bone.

FORMATION OF TEETH

Teeth are composed of three calcified tissues: enamel, dentin, and cementum. Enamel and dentin are principally composed of hydroxyapatite crystals similar to those in bone. Approximately 20% of dentin, cementum, and bone are organic material, principally collagen; only 1% of the enamel is organic material. Dentin lacks the osteoblasts and osteoclasts found in bone; enamel and dentin do not contain blood vessels or nerves. As with bone, the mineral crystallization structure makes teeth extremely resistant to compressional forces; collagen fibers make teeth tough and resistant to tensional forces. Actions in which pressure attempts to diminish a structure's volume are referred to as **compres-**

sional forces; **tensional forces** are actions in which the pressure stretches or strains the structure.

After a tooth erupts, no more enamel is formed, but mineral exchanges occur slowly in response to the oral environment. Changes in mineral composition of enamel occur by exchange of minerals in the saliva, rather than from the pulp cavity. Minerals such as fluoride, sodium, zinc, and strontium can replace calcium ions. Carbonate can be substituted for phosphate; carbonate and fluoride can be substituted for hydroxyl ions. These changes may alter the solubility of apatite. Despite the fact changes can occur in enamel composition, the enamel maintains most of its original mineral components throughout life.

The crystalline structure of enamel is one of the most insoluble and resistant proteins known. This special protein matrix in combination with a crystalline structure of inorganic salts makes enamel harder than dentin, comparable to the hardness of quartz. Enamel is more resistant to acids, enzymes, and other corrosive agents than dentin.

Dentin, the main tissue of the tooth, contains the same constituents as bone, but its structure is more dense. Its principal component is hydroxyapatite crystals embedded in a strong meshwork of collagen fibers. Odontoblasts line the inner surface of the dentin and provide nourishment for the dentin.

Cementum, which covers the dentin in the root area, is another bonelike substance, but because it contains fewer minerals, it is softer than bone. It contains many collagen fibers originating in the alveolar bone. Compressional forces cause the cementum to become thicker and stronger. Cementum exhibits characteristics more typical of bone than enamel and dentin. Minerals are absorbed and deposited at rates similar to that of alveolar bone.

Development of normal, healthy teeth is affected by metabolic factors, such as PTH secretion, and the availability of calcium, phosphate, vitamin D, protein, and many other nutrients. If these factors are deficient, calcification of teeth may be defective and abnormal throughout life.

INTRODUCTION TO MINERALS

Minerals are inorganic elements having many physiological functions. The numerous inorganic elements in the body account for only about 4% of total body weight, or 6 lb for a 150-lb person. Minerals are subdivided into those required in larger amounts (major minerals) and those required in smaller amounts (micronutrients or trace elements) (Box 8-1). Despite the smaller amounts required, trace elements are just as important as major minerals.

CALCIUM

PHYSIOLOGICAL ROLES

At least 99% of the body's calcium is found in the skeleton and teeth. Calcium is indispensable for skeletal function, which requires adequate dietary calcium to achieve full

Box 8-1	**Mineral Elements in the Body**

Major Minerals (greater than 100 mg/d)
Calcium (Ca)*
Phosphorus (P)*
Sodium (Na)
Potassium (K)
Magnesium (Mg)*
Chlorine (Cl)
Sulfur (S)

Trace Elements (less than 100 mg/d)
Iron (Fe)*
Copper (Cu)*
Zinc (Zn)*
Manganese (Mn)*
Iodine (I)*
Molybdenum (Mo)*
Fluorine (F)*
Selenium (Se)*
Chromium (Cr)
Cobalt (Co)

Ultratrace Elements (No Recommended Dietary Allowances [RDAs])
Boron (Bo)*
Arsenic (As)
Nickel (Ni)*
Silicon (Si)
Tin (Sn)
Vanadium (V)*
Cadmium (Cd)
Lead (Pb)
Bromide (Br)
Lithium (Li)
Aluminum (Al)

Data from Institute of Medicine, Food and Nutrition Board: Dietary Reference Intakes for Calcium, Phosphorus, Magnesium, Vitamin D, and Fluoride. Washington, DC: National Academy Press, 1997; Institute of Medicine, Food and Nutrition Board: Dietary Reference Intakes for Vitamin A, Vitamin K, Arsenic, Boron, Chromium, Copper, Iodine, Iron, Manganese, Molybdenum, Nickel, Silicon, Vanadium, and Zinc. Washington, DC: National Academy Press, 2001.
*Tolerable upper intake level (ULs) have been established.

accretion of bone mass prescribed by genetic potential. Calcium (and phosphorus) in the bone functions as a "savings account" for maintaining serum calcium levels. Only 1% of the body's calcium is found in blood, but as such, it controls body functions such as blood clotting, transmission of nerve impulses, muscle contraction and relaxation, membrane permeability, and activation of certain enzymes. Calcium intake has been suggested to be important not only for bone health, but also for reducing the risk of a host of other disorders ranging from hypertension to obesity to colon cancer.

Saliva is supersaturated with calcium; saliva is a source of calcium to mineralize an immature or demineralized enamel surface and reduce susceptibility to caries. Calcium and phosphate in saliva provide a buffering action to inhibit caries formation. This buffer prevents dissolution of minerals in the enamel by plaque biofilm.

REQUIREMENTS

The Institute of Medicine (IOM) established an adequate intake (AI) for calcium rather than an estimated average requirement (EAR) because the scientific data were too weak to set an EAR. The AI was established at 1000 mg per day for adults. During growth periods, primarily from 9 to 18 years of age, the estimated requirement is higher because peak bone mass seems to be related to calcium intake during periods of bone mineralization (Table 8-1). About 85% to 90% of adult bone mass is acquired by age 18 in girls and age 20 in boys.[1] Women may continue to increase bone growth and density through their 20s, but do not achieve the bone mass levels observed in most men. After age 35, and frequently during pregnancy and lactation, bone resorption exceeds formation, resulting in gradual loss of bone mass. Osteoporosis, more prevalent in women than men, is a result of all these factors, combined with the longer life span of

Table 8-1 Adequate Intake for Calcium*

Life Stage Group	AI† (mg/d)	UL‡ (g/d)
Infants (birth–6 mo)	210	ND§
Infants (6-12 mo)	270	ND
Children (1-3 yr)	500	2.5
Children (4-8 yr)	800	2.5
Adolescents (9-18 yr)	1300	2.5
Adults (19-50 yr)	1000	2.5
Adults (>51 yr)	1200	2.5
Pregnancy and lactation	Same as for their age group	2.5

Data from Institute of Medicine (IOM), Food and Nutrition Board: Dietary Reference Intakes for Calcium, Phosphorus, Magnesium, Vitamin D, and Fluoride. Washington, DC: National Academy Press, 1997.

*The observed average or experimentally set intake by a defined population or subgroup that seems to sustain a defined nutritional status, such as growth rate, normal circulating nutrient values, or other functional indicators of health. Adequate intake (AI) is used if insufficient scientific evidence is available to derive an estimated average requirement (EAR). For healthy breastfed infants, AI is the mean intake. All other life stage groups should be covered at the AI value. The AI is not equivalent to a recommended dietary allowance (RDA).

†AI—the experimentally determined estimate of nutrient intake by a defined group of healthy people. AI is used if insufficient scientific evidence is available to derive an EAR. For healthy infants fed human milk, AI is an estimated mean intake. Some seemingly healthy individuals may require higher calcium intake to minimize risk of osteopenia, and some individuals may be at low risk on lower intakes. The AI is believed to cover their needs, but lack of data or uncertainty in the data prevents being able to specify with confidence the percentage of individuals covered by this intake.

‡Tolerable upper intake level (UL)—the highest level of daily nutrient intake that is likely to pose no risk of adverse health effects to almost all individuals in the general population. As intake increases above the UL, the risk of adverse effects increases. Unless specified otherwise, the UL represents total nutrient intake from food, water, and supplements.

§ND—not determinable because of lack of data of adverse effects in this age group and concern with regard to lack of ability to handle excess amounts. Source of intake should be from food only to prevent high levels of intake.

most women. Bone mass loss accelerates after menopause. The IOM has recommended an adequate calcium intake for adults older than 51 years is 1200 mg per day.

In 2004, the U.S. Surgeon General stated "calcium has been singled out as a major public health concern today because it is critically important to bone health, and the average American consumes levels of calcium that are far below the amount recommended."[2] Only one in four Americans achieves the AI for calcium. Women are less likely than men to exceed their AI. The estimated mean calcium intake for women 51 to 70 years old during the 2001-2002 *National Health and Nutrition Examination Survey* (NHANES) was 701 mg per day compared with 874 mg per day for men in the same age category.[3]

Americans consumed only 1.8 cups of milk and milk products per person daily in 2005.[4] Inadequate calcium intake can be attributed to (1) uninformed choices, or not selecting adequate sources of calcium on a daily basis; (2) the mistaken belief that adults do not need milk, or that milk contributes too many kilocalories to the diet; (3) economic hardships, plus a lack of knowledge regarding inexpensive sources of calcium-rich foods; (4) lactose intolerance or allergies to dairy products; (5) access to and consumption of soda; and (6) dislike of calcium-rich foods.

Generally, inadequate calcium intake affects bone mass more than tooth structure. Inadequate calcium and vitamin D intake during tooth formation and maturation may result in hypomineralization of developing teeth. After tooth formation, dietary calcium does not affect caries rate.

Calcium Balance

Despite wide variations in calcium intake, serum calcium is relatively constant because each cell has a vital need for calcium. If the serum calcium level declines, bones are used as calcium reserves. When calcium withdrawal from bones exceeds deposits, calcium imbalance occurs. Decreased bone density caused by insufficient calcium is a slow process.

Calcium-to-Phosphorus Ratio

Serum levels of calcium and phosphorus are inversely related; this relationship is called the serum calcium-to-phosphorus ratio. If the calcium level increases, the phosphorus level decreases, and vice versa. This relationship acts as a protective mechanism to prevent high combined concentrations with subsequent calcification of soft tissue and stone formation.

Sufficient phosphorus intake is necessary to decrease calcium loss. The ideal dietary calcium-to-phosphorus ratio for adults of 1:1 is advisable and needed for mineralization of bone. Excessive intake of phosphorus compared with calcium reduces the serum calcium concentration. Stimulation of PTH results in the possible loss of bone mass. This ratio does not warrant as close attention under normal conditions as in disorders such as renal disease, when dangerously high levels of phosphorus and calcium may cause calcification in soft tissues.

Numerous studies have investigated the relationship of calcium-to-phosphorus ratios and alveolar bone resorption of edentulous patients. Calcium requirements are increased when dietary phosphate is high (typical American diet); a relationship may exist between calcium intake and edentulous ridge resorption.

ABSORPTION AND EXCRETION

Calcium balance, an intake that equals excretion, does not solely depend on adequate calcium intake. Several hormones, including PTH, estrogen, glucocorticoids, and thyroid hormone, help to regulate calcium absorption.[5] Under normal conditions, less than one-third of the calcium consumed is absorbed. Calcium is best absorbed by the body when consumed in smaller amounts and ingested several times throughout the day. In other words, individuals should consume 30% of the daily value (DV) or 300 mg per serving three or four times a day.

Absorption occurs in the upper part of the intestine and is affected by many factors as shown in Figure 8-1. Calcium absorption from various dairy products is similar, whereas calcium present in dark green leafy vegetables is not readily absorbed. During periods of increased need, especially during growth and pregnancy and lactation, calcium absorption may increase to 60% of intake. Calcium absorption decreases with age, probably because of decreased gastric acidity. The rate of absorption is lowest in postmenopausal women because of diminished estrogen levels.

Although several plant foods contain large amounts of calcium, absorption is poor. Oxalates in vegetables and phytates from wheat bran bind with calcium in these foods to reduce absorption, but they do not interfere with calcium absorption from other foods. Excessive dietary fiber (more than 35 g per day) also interferes with calcium absorption.

High-protein intakes typically eaten in the United States have a high phosphorus content. Phosphorus increases the uptake of calcium by bone. The usual intake of protein and phosphorus does not cause calcium loss, whereas a diet low in protein and phosphorus may have adverse effects on calcium balance in older adults. Generally, weight loss causes bone mineral loss. Higher protein diets have been criticized for potential harmful effects on bone because of an elevated urinary calcium. One research study using a reduced-energy, high-protein diet with three dairy servings a day attenuated bone mineral density over a 1-year period. Using a process called radiolabeling, the researchers determined that elevated calcium excretion in the urine was from increased intestinal calcium absorption.[6]

PTH works concurrently with vitamin D to prevent calcium from being excreted and stimulates release of

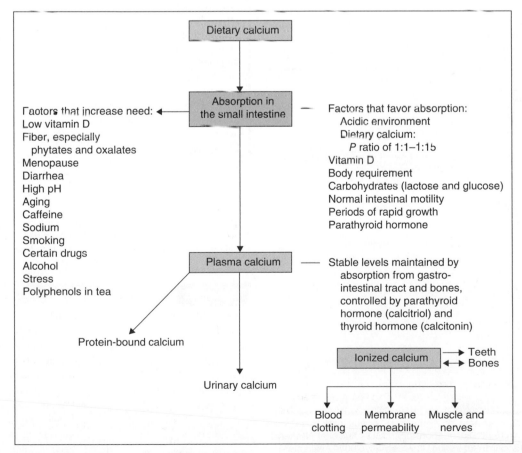

FIGURE 8-1 Calcium absorption and use. (Adapted from Davis JR, Sherer K: Applied Nutrition and Diet Therapy for Nurses, 2nd ed. Philadelphia: Saunders, 1994.)

calcium from the bone when serum levels of calcium are low. Increasing the synthesis of vitamin D by PTH also results in increased absorption of calcium.

SOURCES

Milk and other dairy products supply most of the available calcium (Table 8-2). Not only are they preferred sources of calcium because of their high calcium content, but also their inherent lactose and other nutrient content enhances calcium absorption. Milk also provides other essential nutrients. Calcium from dietary sources positively influences estrogen metabolism, suggesting it has more favorable effects on bone health in postmenopausal women than calcium supplements.[7] Box 8-2 lists portion sizes for various foods that provide approximately 300 mg of calcium.

Since 1999, food manufacturers have been fortifying products such as fruit juices, fruit-flavored drinks, breakfast cereals, and breads with calcium. Numerous calcium-fortified foods introduced to the market have been well received. Food products containing natural or fortified calcium can use terminology on the packaging as shown in Table 8-3.

Consumers in the United States annually spend more than $1 billion on the most popular dietary supplement, calcium.[8] Calcium supplements result in small but significant reductions in bone loss.[9] This strong trend toward the use of calcium supplements is especially evident in the older popu-lation. Benefits may be less than expected, partly because of the limited bioavailability of supplemental calcium. **Bioavailability** refers to the amount of a nutrient available physiologically based on its absorption rate. A calcium supplement contains elemental calcium along with other substances, such as carbonate or gluconate. The amount of elemental calcium varies among supplements. Most calcium supplements are better absorbed when taken with food except for calcium lactate, which is better absorbed when taken on an empty stomach.[10] Calcium-citrate-malate, calcium lactate, calcium citrate, and calcium sulfate have high absorption rates.[5]

HYPER-STATES AND HYPO-STATES

Clinical conditions are associated with excesses and deficiencies of calcium. Hypercalcemia and hypocalcemia (too much or too little calcium) are critical metabolic conditions and can lead to loss of consciousness, fatal respiratory failure, or cardiac arrest. These problems are seldom caused directly by calcium intake; however, bone density can be adversely related to intake.

Box 8-2	Calcium Equivalents

The following foods contain approximately 300 mg of calcium:*†
1 cup milk
1 cup soymilk, calcium fortified
1½ oz cheddar cheese
½ cup ricotta cheese
2 cups cottage cheese
1 cup yogurt
1½ slices processed cheese
1½ cup ice cream
1 cup orange juice, calcium fortified
1½ cup dark green leafy vegetables
4 oz salmon
1½ oz sardines

Data from U.S. Department of Agriculture, Agricultural Research Service, USDA Nutrient Data Laboratory, USDA National Nutrient Database for Standard Reference, Release 20, 2008. Accessed February 28, 2008.
*The RDA for calcium is 1000 mg for individuals 19-50 years old.
†Calcium from vegetable sources is not as easily absorbed by the intestine and is not as effective in fulfilling calcium requirements.

Table 8-2	Calcium and Phosphorus Content of Selected Foods		
Food	**Portion**	**Calcium (mg)**	**Phosphorus (mg)**
Romano cheese	3 oz	905	646
Swiss cheese	3 oz	673	482
Cheddar cheese	3 oz	613	435
American cheese	3 oz	488	641
Yogurt, nonfat plain	1 cup	488	385
Orange juice, calcium fortified	1 cup	351	27
Milk (1%, skim)	1 cup	306	247
Buttermilk	1 cup	284	218
Soy milk, calcium fortified	1 cup	199	151
Salmon, canned	3 oz	181	280
Cottage cheese, low-fat (1%)	1 cup	138	303
Spinach, cooked	½ cup	122	50
Turnip greens	½ cup	99	21
Broccoli, cooked	½ cup	47	51
Shrimp, cooked	3 oz	33	116
Ground beef (83% lean)	3 oz	20	152
Cola	12 oz	7	37

Data from U.S. Department of Agriculture, Agricultural Research Service, USDA Nutrient Data Laboratory, USDA National Nutrient Database for Standard Reference, Release 20, 2008. Available at http://www.nal.usda.gov/fnic/foodcomp/search/. Accessed February 28, 2008.

Table 8-3	Food Labeling for Calcium	
Daily Value (DV) of Calcium in a Food	**FDA-Authorized Labeling Terms**
10% DV of calcium	Calcium enriched / Calcium fortified / More calcium
10-19% DV of calcium	Contains calcium / Provides calcium / Good source of calcium
≥20% DV of calcium	High in calcium / Rich in calcium / Excellent source of calcium

Hypercalcemia

Hypercalcemia, or excessive levels of calcium in the blood, is observed most frequently in infants 5 to 8 months old. It is caused by overdoses of cholecalciferol or excessive amounts of vitamin D preparations. Treatment involves providing a low-calcium diet with no vitamin D. Hyperparathyroidism, certain types of bone disease, vitamin D poisoning, sarcoidosis, cancer, and prolonged excessive intake of milk may cause adult hypercalcemia.

Hypocalcemia

Hypocalcemia, or deficient levels of calcium in the blood, results in **tetany**, a neuromuscular disorder of uncontrollable cramps and tremors involving the muscles of the face, hands, feet, and eventually the heart. Depressed serum calcium levels may be caused by hypoparathyroidism, some bone diseases, certain kidney diseases, and low serum protein levels.

Excessive Calcium Intake

Excessively high calcium intake may cause dizziness, flushing, nausea or vomiting, severe constipation, kidney stone formation, irregular heartbeat, tingling sensations, xerostomia, fatigue, and high blood pressure. It also may inhibit iron and zinc absorption.

Inadequate Calcium Intake

Rickets, discussed in Chapter 7 in connection with vitamin D deficiency, results in porous, soft bones. Rickets is the result of an inadequate amount of calcium deposits in the bone during childhood. Calcium intake may be adequate, but absorption is poor because of inadequate vitamin D.

Osteoporosis is an age-related disorder characterized by decreased bone mass, causing bones to be more susceptible to fracture. It is caused by numerous factors, including decreased estrogen, inadequate calcium or vitamin D intake, and lack of weight-bearing activity. The relationship of calcium intake to bone density indicates a protective effect in women reporting high lifetime calcium intake but not in women who increased intake beginning after menopause. Building bone during the formative years is the best insurance against osteoporosis.

Oral signs of osteoporosis may be loss of calcium in the alveolar bone contributing to tooth exfoliation (Fig. 8-2). The condition usually goes undetected, however, until pain or spontaneous fracture occurs. Osteoporosis is discussed further in Health Application 8. **Periodontal disease**, or the breakdown of healthy periodontal tissue, can be exacerbated by a deficiency of calcium.[11]

PHOSPHORUS

PHYSIOLOGICAL ROLES

Phosphorus is the second most abundant mineral in the body, with about 85% in the skeleton and teeth. Its presence in all body cells is necessary for almost every aspect of metabo-

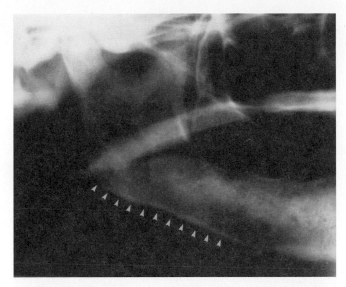

FIGURE 8-2 Radiographic appearance of osteoporosis affecting bone of the maxillofacial complex. This portion of a panoramic radiograph depicts thinning of the gonial and interior cortices of an edentulous mandible (*arrows*). A slight increase in the general size of marrow spaces is also apparent. (Courtesy of Benson BW, DDS, MS, Associate Professor, Department of Diagnostic Sciences, The Texas A&M University System, Baylor College of Dentistry, Dallas, TX.)

Dental Hygiene Considerations

- Lack of physical activity results in immediate bone depletion. In young individuals, recovery of calcium deposits is usually rapid, but older adults may never regain bone density.
- Consumption of calcium in the amounts recommended in the dietary reference intakes (DRIs) is appropriate for fracture healing and should not exceed 2500 mg per day.
- Patients with achlorhydria (the absence of hydrochloric acid in the stomach) may not absorb calcium supplements on an empty stomach and should take them with meals.
- Hyperparathyroidism induces bone disease. Alveolar bone is especially at risk, exhibiting extensive bone resorption.
- Patients who have had gastric bypass surgery for obesity are at risk of decreased bone mineral density as a result of impaired calcium absorption and weight loss.[12]
- Interventions for limiting or preventing further bone loss include encouraging vitamin D–rich and calcium-rich foods and exercise.
- When patients use excessive alcohol or caffeine, or smoke cigarettes, calcium is lost.
- Suggest alternatives for increasing calcium intake for patients with lactose intolerance (see Health Application 2).
- Calcium supplements may inhibit the effects of cellulose sodium phosphate (Calcibind), etidronate (Didronel), phenytoin (Dilantin), and tetracycline. Supplements should be taken 1 to 3 hours before or after taking the drug.
- Poor patient compliance may be expected if several tablets are necessary, the supplement is too expensive, or it causes gastrointestinal problems. More than 500 mg calcium per tablet may cause constipation.

Nutritional Directions

- Adequate daily calcium, phosphorus, and vitamin D intake is important to support bone formation and maintenance.
- Calcium supplement absorption can be enhanced if taken with some form of sugar; lactose, dextrose, and sucrose enhance its absorption.
- Evaluate calcium supplements for their solubility, which affects absorption. For calcium to be absorbed from a supplement, the tablet must first dissolve. To measure how well a calcium tablet would dissolve in the body, drop a tablet in a solution of $4\frac{1}{2}$ oz water and $1\frac{1}{2}$ oz vinegar to produce an environment similar to that of the stomach. Stir occasionally. At least two-thirds of a high-quality tablet dissolves within 30 minutes.
- Compare the amount of elemental calcium provided (actual amount of calcium in the supplement) and cost per tablet. Refer patients who are appropriate candidates for calcium supplementation to a healthcare provider or registered dietitian.
- Decreased calcium intake in women results in lower levels of estrogen production, which can be harmful to the bones. Estrogen helps with calcium absorption and enables the body to use calcium more efficiently.[5]
- Moderate alcohol intake enhances bone density mass as a result of less bone remodeling, but excessive amounts increase the risk of bone loss later in life.
- Weight-bearing exercise has a positive effect on calcium deposition in bone during childhood and adolescence.[13] During adulthood, weight-bearing exercise and resistance training prevent, and in some cases reverse, bone loss.[14,15]
- If a patient's usual calcium intake is low, encourage increased consumption of dairy products. If the patient has an aversion to milk, powdered milk can be added to many items, or other high-calcium foods can be used.
- Do not take calcium supplements within 1 to 2 hours of eating large amounts of fiber, especially foods containing large amounts of phytates and oxalates.
- After menopause, calcium and vitamin D supplements slow bone loss and reduce fractures when coupled with an approved osteoporosis-related therapy, such as estrogen replacement therapy (ERT) or a bisphosphonate or both. If a patient is having an adverse reaction to the osteoporosis medication, encourage the patient to check with the healthcare provider before discontinuing it.
- Antacids and corticosteroids increase urinary excretion of calcium.

lism, including (1) transfer and release of energy stored as ATP; (2) composition of phospholipids, DNA, and RNA; and (3) metabolism of fats, carbohydrates, and proteins.

REQUIREMENTS

The recommended dietary allowance (RDA) of phosphorus for adults older than 18 years of age is 700 mg. The ideal calcium-to-phosphorus ratio is 1:1. Because phosphorus is more readily available than calcium in the United States, intake is generally 1.5 times higher than calcium. Although harmful effects from excessive amounts of phosphorus have not been reported, the IOM established a tolerable

upper intake level (UL) to reflect normal serum levels (Table 8-4).

ABSORPTION AND EXCRETION

Approximately 60% to 70% of dietary phosphorus is absorbed in the jejunum. Its absorption can be inhibited by the same dietary factors affecting calcium absorption: phytate, excessive amounts of fats, iron, aluminum, and calcium. The kidneys excrete excessive amounts of phosphorus to maintain optimal body levels.

SOURCES

Phosphorus is so abundant in foods deficiencies have not been observed. A diet adequate in calcium and protein contains enough phosphorus because all three minerals are present in the same foods (see Table 8-2). In addition to milk products, meats are a good source of phosphorus. Dietary restriction of phosphorus is extremely difficult because of its wide use as a food additive in baked goods, cheese, processed meats, and soft drinks. The daily reference values on nutrition labels is 1000 mg and can be multiplied by the DV to determine the amount of phosphorus in the food.

HYPER-STATES AND HYPO-STATES

Hyperphosphatemia (serum level greater than 2.6 mg/dL) may occur in cases of hypoparathyroidism or renal insufficiency. Excessive amounts of phosphorus bind with calcium, resulting in tetany and convulsions.

Hypophosphatemia may occur with long-term ingestion of aluminum hydroxide antacids, which bind phosphorus, interfering with absorption, or it may occur in certain stress conditions in which the calcium-to-phosphorus balance is disturbed. Intestinal conditions, such as sprue and celiac disease, can result in phosphorus malabsorption deficiencies. The principal clinical symptom of hypophosphatemia is muscle weakness. Even small phosphorus depletions may cause increased calcium excretion, resulting in a negative calcium balance and bone loss.

During tooth development, a phosphorus deficiency can result in incomplete calcification of teeth, failure of dentin formation, and increased susceptibility to caries. The resultant wide dentinal tubules allow bacteria to enter the damaged enamel. This condition responds favorably to treatment with vitamin D and oral phosphate.[16]

Dental Hygiene Considerations

- A phosphorus deficiency is more likely to develop or occur in alcoholics; older adults with inadequate dietary intake; patients with disordered eating, inappropriate weight loss, and long-term diarrhea; and patients taking aluminum-containing antacids or diuretics. Assess the phosphorus status and document any signs or symptoms of a deficiency for these patients. Referrals to the healthcare provider or registered dietitian may be needed.
- Low phosphate intake may lead to an increased rate of caries formation, but additional or supplemental phosphate may not be helpful in preventing dental caries.

Table 8-4	Institute of Medicine Recommendations for Phosphorus			
Life Stage*	**EAR (mg/d)†**	**RDA (mg/d)‡**	**AI (mg/d)§**	**UL (g/d)¶**
Birth–6 mo	—	—	100	ND¶
7-12 mo	—	—	275	ND¶
1-3 yr	380	460	—	3
4-8 yr	405	500	—	3
9-18 yr	1055	1250	—	4
19-70 yr	580	700	—	4
>70 yr	580	700	—	3
Pregnancy				
≤18 yr	1055	1250	—	3.5
19-50 yr	580	700	—	3.5
Lactation				
≤18 yr	1055	1250	—	4
19-50 yr	580	700	—	4

Data from Institute of Medicine (IOM), Food and Nutrition Board: Dietary Reference Intakes for Calcium, Phosphorus, Magnesium, Vitamin D, and Fluoride. Washington, DC: National Academy Press, 1997.
*All groups except Pregnancy and Lactation are males and females.
†EAR (estimated average requirement)—the intake that meets the estimated nutrient needs of 50% of the individuals in a group.
‡RDA (recommended dietary allowance)—the intake that meets the nutrient needs of almost all (97-98%) individuals in a group.
§AI (adequate intake)—for healthy infants fed human milk, AI is the estimated mean intake.
¶UL (tolerable upper intake level)—the UL is the highest level of daily nutrient intake that is likely to pose no risk of adverse health effects to almost all individuals in the general population. As intake increases above the UL, the risk of adverse effects increases. Unless specified otherwise, the UL represents total nutrient intake from food, water, and supplements.
¶ND—not determinable because of lack of data of adverse effects in this age group and concern with regard to lack of ability to handle excess amounts. Source of intake should be from food only to prevent high levels of intake.

Nutritional Directions

Phosphorus is widespread in foods, and a deficiency is unlikely. Educate patients that the goal is to maintain an equal calcium-to-phosphorus ratio. For example, an excessive consumption of soft drinks (more than two to three cans a day) in place of milk can interrupt the calcium-to-phosphorus balance.

MAGNESIUM

PHYSIOLOGICAL ROLES

Bones contain almost two-thirds of the body's magnesium. It is the third most prevalent mineral in teeth, with dentin containing about two times the amount present in enamel. Magnesium has an important function in maintaining calcium homeostasis and preventing skeletal abnormalities. Magnesium is involved in more than 300 enzymatic reactions, including energy metabolism, insulin activity, and glucose use. Some research has suggested that lower intakes of magnesium may lead to insulin resistance or type 2 diabetes mellitus.[17,18] However, the American Diabetes Association does not currently recommend nutrition supplementation of magnesium.[19] Magnesium is vital to the structural integrity of heart muscle and other muscles and nerves. Its role in enzymes is fundamental to energy (ATP) production. It also is crucial to controlling blood pressure.[20]

REQUIREMENTS

The RDA for magnesium ranges from 240 mg per day for children to 420 mg per day for men (Table 8-5). Although it is impossible to get too much magnesium from food alone, excessive amounts can be obtained from supplements. The UL is provided for patients using supplements and other nonfood sources of magnesium.

SOURCES

Whole-grain products, nuts, beans, and green leafy vegetables are some of the best sources of magnesium (Table 8-6). Magnesium (Mg) is part of the chlorophyll molecule (Fig. 8-3); green leafy vegetables are good sources. Bananas are another good source of magnesium. Although whole grains are good sources of magnesium, enrichment of refined grain products does not replace the magnesium lost during processing. Nonfood sources of magnesium include laxatives and antacids.

HYPER-STATES AND HYPO-STATES

Because kidneys regulate plasma magnesium levels, toxicity has been associated with kidney failure. There is no evidence of harmful effects from the overconsumption of magnesium from food sources. A high dose of magnesium acts like a laxative (e.g., milk of magnesia).

In certain diseases or under stressful conditions, deficiencies may occur. Magnesium in bone is not available to replace serum magnesium deficits. A deficiency may result

Table 8-5	Institute of Medicine Recommendations for Magnesium						
	EAR (mg/d)†		RDA (mg/d)‡		AI (mg/d)§		
Life Stage*	Male	Female	Male	Female	Male	Female	UL (g/d)¶
Birth–6 mo	—	—	—	—	30	30	ND¶
7-12 mo	—	—	—	—	75	75	ND¶
1-3 yr	65	65	80	80			65
4-8 yr	110	110	130	130			110
9-13 yr	200	200	240	240			350
14-18 yr	340	300	410	360			350
19-30 yr	330	255	400	310			350
31->70 yr	350	265	420	320			350
Pregnancy							
≤18 yr		335		400			350
19-30 yr		290		350			350
31-50 yr		300		360			350
Lactation							
≤18 yr		300		360			350
19-30 yr		255		310			350
31-50 yr		265		320			350

Data from Institute of Medicine (IOM), Food and Nutrition Board: Dietary Reference Intakes for Calcium, Phosphorus, Magnesium, Vitamin D, and Fluoride. Washington, DC: National Academy Press, 1997.
*All groups except Pregnancy and Lactation are males and females.
†EAR (estimated average requirement)—the intake that meets the estimated nutrient needs of 50% of the individuals in a group.
‡RDA (recommended dietary allowance)—the intake that meets the nutrient needs of almost all (97-98%) individuals in a group.
§AI (adequate intake)—for healthy infants fed human milk, AI is the estimated mean intake.
¶UL (tolerable upper intake level)—the UL is the highest level of daily nutrient intake that is likely to pose no risk of adverse health effects to almost all individuals in the general population. As intake increases above the UL, the risk of adverse effects increases. Unless specified otherwise, the UL represents total nutrient intake from food, water, and supplements.
¶ND—not determinable because of lack of data of adverse effects in this age group and concern with regard to lack of ability to handle excess amounts. Source of intake should be from food only to prevent high levels of intake.

Table 8-6	Magnesium Content of Selected Foods	
Food	Portion	Magnesium (mg)
Sunflower seeds	1 oz	105
Sesame seeds	1 oz	98
Cashew nuts	1 oz	94
Spinach, cooked	½ cup	78
Navy beans	½ cup	48
Lima beans	½ cup	50
Split peas	½ cup	35
Potato, baked	1	48
Yellow corn	½ cup	24
Beets, sliced	½ cup	20
Broccoli, cooked	½ cup	12
Mustard greens	½ cup	10

Data from U.S. Department of Agriculture, Agricultural Research Service, USDA Nutrient Data Laboratory, USDA National Nutrient Database for Standard Reference, Release 20, 2008. Available at http://www.nal.usda.gov/fnic/foodcomp. Accessed February 28, 2008.

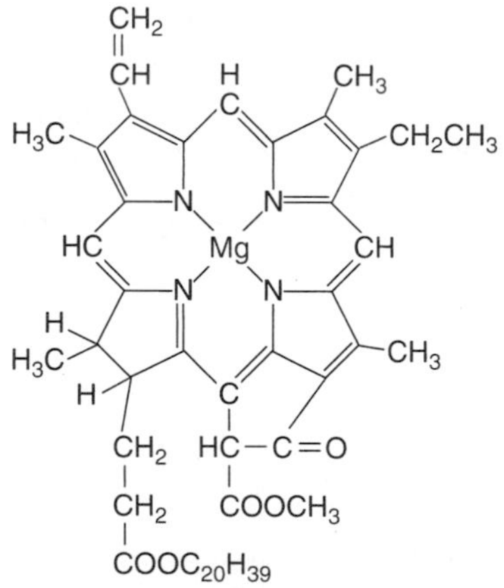

FIGURE 8-3 Structure of chlorophyll. All chlorophyll molecules are essentially alike; they differ only in details of the side chains. Magnesium is basic to all chlorophyll molecules.

from numerous disease states, including gastrointestinal abnormalities with diarrhea, renal disease, general malnutrition, alcoholism, and medications interfering with magnesium conservation. Symptoms of magnesium deficiency are neuromuscular dysfunction, personality changes, muscle spasms, convulsions (especially in infants), tremors, hyperexcitability, anorexia, nausea, apathy, and cardiac arrhythmias.

Dietary deficiencies may affect the teeth and supporting structures. Changes in ameloblasts and odontoblasts result in hypoplasia of the enamel and dentin during development. Alveolar bone formation may be reduced, along with a widening of the periodontal ligament space and gingival hyperplasia.

FLUORIDE

PHYSIOLOGICAL ROLES

In a strict nutritional sense, fluoride is not a nutrient essential for health. Although fluoride is present in low concentrations in soft tissues, it does not have any known metabolic function. However, because of its benefits to dental and bone health, fluoride is considered a desirable element for humans. Saliva contains varying amounts of fluoride; the amount of fluoride ingested has little effect on salivary levels.

Fluoride is advantageous to dental health because of its systemic effects before tooth eruption and topical effects after tooth eruption (Fig. 8-4). The caries-preventing properties of systemic and topical fluoride are cumulative.

Fluoride ions can replace hydroxyl ions in the hydroxyapatite crystal lattice. This fluoridated hydroxyapatite, or **fluorapatite**, is less soluble and makes the tooth more resistant to acid demineralization. Additionally, it enhances remineralization when the tooth is subject to the caries process (Fig. 8-5A). Calcium and phosphate are present in saliva and plaque fluid at higher concentrations than fluoride. When small pits develop in the enamel, fluoride is believed to promote deposition of calcium phosphate to remineralize the enamel surface.

Another, less well recognized effect of systemic fluoride is changes in tooth morphology increasing the tooth's resistance to adherence of plaque biofilm. Numerous investigators have observed that in fluoridated areas, posterior teeth have a distinct gross morphology: surfaces are whiter and more reflective, cusps are rounder, and fissures are more shallow and less penetrable.[21]

Fluoride may be passed from the mother via the placenta and incorporated into developing fetal tooth buds and bones. Fluoride during this stage is probably incorporated in the apatite crystals during formation. Because scientific studies determining optimal levels and benefits are lacking, prenatal fluoride supplementation is not recommended.[22]

Primary teeth benefit from the presence of fluoride during tooth development beginning at 6 months of age.[23] Fluoride

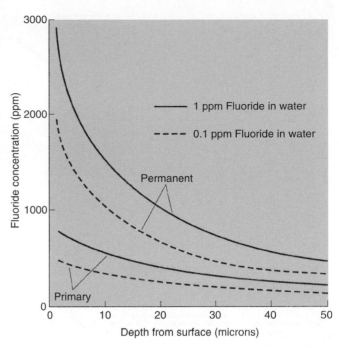

FIGURE 8-4 Concentration gradients of fluoride in outer enamel from permanent and deciduous teeth, from areas with 1 ppm and 0.1 ppm of fluoride in the drinking water. (From Gron P: Inorganic chemical and structural aspects of oral mineralized tissues. In Shaw JH, et al [eds]: Textbook of Oral Biology. Philadelphia: Saunders, 1978, pp 484-507.)

is present in the inner part of the enamel and dentin at lower concentrations; this occurs mainly during the amelogenesis/dentogenesis stage. Enhanced concentration in the surface enamel occurs during the maturation stage of tooth development. Fluoride can be readily incorporated into the apatite crystal from topically available fluoride during the maturation stage, but this reversible process is superficial, rather than distributed throughout the enamel thickness, as shown in Figure 8-5B.

The presence of fluoride in saliva also interferes with the demineralization process. The presence of fluoride generally results in a less cariogenic environment. Topically available fluoride reduces dental caries by inhibiting demineralization, promoting remineralization, and interfering with the formation and function of acidogenic bacteria. Higher concentrations of fluoride inhibit *Streptococcus mutans, Streptococcus sobrinus,* and *Lactobacillus* in plaque biofilm, and accelerate remineralization during early stages of enamel caries development.

The protective effect of fluoride against caries is greatest during the first 6 to 8 years of life, but adults and children continue to benefit from consumption of fluoridated water.[21] Systemic fluoride uptake by calcified tissues is high in infancy through age 16, when mineralization of unerupted permanent teeth occurs. Compared with healthy enamel, demineralized enamel retains more fluoride.

Fluoride stimulates osteoblast proliferation and increases new mineral deposition in cancellous bone, improves the strength of bone, and decreases bone resorption and bone solubility. Concurrent adequate intake of calcium, vitamin

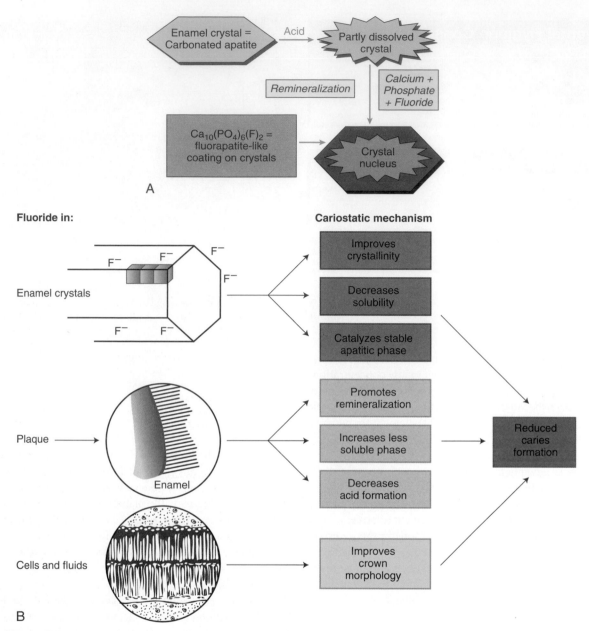

FIGURE 8-5 **A,** Demineralization and remineralization processes that lead to remineralized crystals with surfaces rich in fluoride and low in solubility. **B,** The mechanisms of cariostatic action of fluoride and their interrelationship. (**A,** Modified from Featherstone JDB: Prevention and reversal of dental caries: role of low level fluoride. Community Dent Oral Epidemiol 1999; 27[1]:31-40. **B,** Adapted from Nikiforuk G: Mechanism of cariostatic action of fluorides. In Nikiforuk G [ed]: Understanding Dental Caries Prevention: II. Basel, Switzerland: S. Karger, 1985.)

D, and fluoride is essential. When water fluoride levels are higher than the amount recommended for caries prevention, bone mineral density may increase, but fractures are not reduced and may increase adverse effects.[24]

REQUIREMENTS

Because of its toxicity, AI of fluoride has been established at 3 mg per day for all women and 4 mg per day for men (Table 8-7). Average intake in the United States is 0.9 mg per day in areas with nonfluoridated water and 1.7 mg per day in areas with fluoridation. The UL for healthy individuals age 9 and older is 10 mg per day.

ABSORPTION AND EXCRETION

Most fluoride is absorbed in the stomach, with small amounts also absorbed in the intestine. The rate and degree of absorption depend on the solubility of the source and the amount ingested at a particular time. Absorption of fluoride from sodium fluoride in water is estimated to be 80% to 90%. Incorporation of fluoride into bones and enamel is proportional to total intake and need. Children retain a larger percentage of fluoride in developing bones and teeth, whereas adults retain less in calcified structures. Protein-bound fluoride in foods is not as well absorbed.

| Table 8-7 | Institute of Medicine Recommendations for Fluoride |

Life Stage Group	AI* (mg/d) Male	AI* (mg/d) Female	UL†
Birth–6 mo	0.01	0.01	0.7
7-12 mo	0.5	0.5	0.9
1-3 yr	0.7	0.7	1.3
4-8 yr	1	1	2.2
9-13 yr	2	2	10
14-18 yr	3	3	10
19->70 yr	4	3	10
Pregnancy and Lactation ≤18-50 yr	—	3	10

Data from Institute of Medicine (IOM), Food and Nutrition Board: Dietary Reference Intakes for Calcium, Phosphorus, Magnesium, Vitamin D, and Fluoride. Washington, DC: National Academy Press, 1997.

*AI (adequate intake)—the observed estimate of nutrient intake that reduces the incidence of dental caries maximally in a group of healthy people. For healthy infants fed human milk, AI is the mean intake. The AI is used if insufficient scientific evidence is available to derive an EAR. The AI is believed to cover their needs, but lack of data or uncertainty in the data prevents being able to specify with confidence the percentage of individuals covered by this intake.

†UL (tolerable upper intake level)—the highest level of daily nutrient intake that is likely to pose no risk of adverse health effects to almost all individuals in the general population. As intake increases above the UL, the risk of adverse effects increases. Unless specified otherwise, the UL represents total nutrient intake from food, water, and supplements.

Approximately 60% to 70% of fluoride intake is excreted by the kidneys; about 5% is excreted in the feces. Aluminum (aluminum-containing antacids) and soy (soy-based foods) can bind with fluoride and increase fluoride excretion in the feces. Calcium and fluoride supplements given at the same time inhibit the absorption of both.

SOURCES

Water

The Centers for Disease Control and Prevention (CDC) cites water fluoridation as one of the 10 most important public health measures of the 20th century. Fluoride is available through community water supplies, food, beverages, dentifrices, and other dental products. Fluoridation of community water contributes to fluoride intake and is a practical, cost-effective means of achieving significant decreases in the prevalence of dental caries. Approximately 80% of the fluoride is provided from tap and bottled water and water-based beverages, especially teas. To ensure everyone receives adequate amounts of fluoride, the IOM recommends drinking water contain approximately 1 part per million (ppm) of fluoride (equivalent to 1 mg/L). In warmer climates where water consumption is higher, the optimal level of fluoride may need to be reduced. The range for optimal concentration of fluoride in community water supplies is 0.7 to 1.2 ppm.

In 2006, approximately 69.2% of the U.S. population had access to optimally fluoridated drinking water; the revised goal, as stated by *Healthy People 2010*, targets 75% of the

| Table 8-8 | Fluoride Content of Selected Foods |

Food	Fluoride (µg/100 g)
Black tea, brewed	884
Instant tea	799
White wine	202
Shrimp, canned	201
Crab, canned	178
Carbonated beverage, fruit-flavored	105
Oatmeal, cooked	72
Carrots, canned	49
Corn, canned, cream style	49
Potatoes, mashed	42
Cottage cheese	36
Rice, white, long grain	33
Cheese, American processed	30
Yogurt, plain	27
Tomato sauce	21

Data from U.S. Department of Agriculture, Agricultural Research Service, USDA Nutrient Data Laboratory, USDA National Nutrient Database for Standard Reference, Release 20, 2008. Available at www/nal/usda/gov/fnic/foodcomp. Accessed on February 28, 2008.

population. This *Healthy People 2010* objective has been met by 25 states.[25] Water fluoridation is particularly beneficial for children and adults in economically depressed communities who have less access to oral health care and alternative fluoride resources. Children who do not regularly receive dental care or do not have dental insurance are at high risk of having dental caries. Water fluoridation reduces dental caries in children by 20% or more,[26] and helps prevent root surface caries and tooth loss in adults.

Many households and businesses are using bottled water because of concerns about contamination and quality control of public water supplies. Bottled water is also chosen as a healthy alternative to soft drinks and alcoholic beverages. For water bottled in the United States, the U.S. Food and Drug Administration (FDA) requires fluoride be listed on the label only if the manufacturer adds fluoride during processing. Fluoride amounts in bottled water may or may not be denoted on the label.

In some areas of the United States, the water supply naturally contains much higher levels of fluoride than the recommended amounts. The U.S. Environmental Protection Agency (EPA) allows a maximum level of 4 mg/L. This level could possibly cause adverse health effects. A report submitted to the EPA by the National Academy of Sciences recommends that the maximum allowable fluoride level in water be reduced because of the risk for adverse health effects.[27]

Food

Food is not a major source of fluoride for adults. All foods contain some fluoride, but the amounts provided in vegetables, meats, cereals, and fruits are insignificant (0.2 to 1.5 ppm of fluoride) (Table 8-8). Seafood may contain 5 to

15 ppm of fluoride. Brewed tea provides approximately 1 to 6 ppm of fluoride per cup, depending on the amount of tea, brewing time, and amount of fluoride in the water, but herbal tea has negligible fluoride levels. The process of mechanically deboning poultry results in poultry containing a high concentration of fluoride. Carbonated beverages can be a significant source of fluoride if the water used in the bottling process is fluoridated. It is estimated 77% of soft drinks have fluoride content greater than 0.6 ppm.[28]

Because of varied levels of fluoride in the water supply, the amount of fluoride in infant formulas was reduced in 1979. Components in soy bind fluoride; soy-based formulas usually contain some fluoride. To prevent the possibility of excessive fluoride, the dental hygienist can recommend avoiding the use of fluoridated water (1 ppm) to dilute powdered infant formulas, discontinuing the use of formula by age 1 year, and using a nonfluoridated toothpaste until approximately age 2.[29]

Topical

Topical applications of fluoride include gels, foams, varnishes, dentifrices, prophy paste (polishing paste), and mouth rinses. These high-concentration fluoride sources prevent demineralization when the pH in the mouth decreases. When used in combination with other fluoride sources, a decline in prevalence or severity of dental caries occurs.

HYPER-STATES AND HYPO-STATES

Fluorosis and Bone Health

Mottling of tooth enamel results from overexposure (approximately three to four times the amount necessary to prevent caries) during tooth formation. Ameloblasts are extremely sensitive to excessive fluoride ingestion. Dental **fluorosis** (hypomineralization of enamel) is directly related to fluoride exposure during tooth development and cannot occur after tooth development has been completed. Fluorosed enamel contains a total protein content similar to normal enamel, but it contains a relatively high proportion of immature matrix proteins.

Mild to moderate enamel fluorosis on early-forming enamel surfaces was strongly associated with use of infant formula before 1979. Frequent brushing with fluoridated toothpaste was encouraged, and fluoride supplements were used.

Dental fluorosis varies from very mild cases characterized by whitish opaque flecks, to white or brown staining, to severe dental fluorosis with secondary, extrinsic, brownish discoloration and varying degrees of enamel pitting (Fig. 8-6). When drinking water contains 2 ppm or more of fluoride, teeth appear extremely white; brown stains appear when the fluoride level is greater than 4 ppm. Mild to moderate fluorosis is primarily cosmetic, but teeth are caries-resistant; severe dental fluorosis can result in increased caries rate.

The ingestion of large amounts of fluoride in adults can result in adverse effects on skeletal tissue and kidney func-

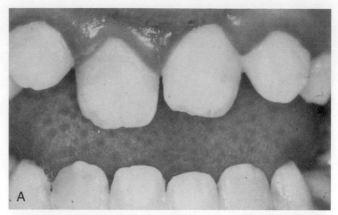
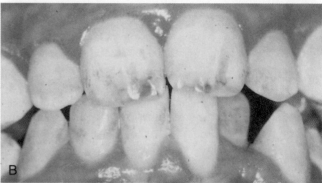
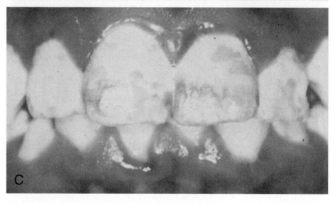

FIGURE 8-6 **A,** Mild fluorosis—white opaque areas in the enamel over less than 50% of the tooth. **B,** Moderate fluorosis—all enamel surfaces of the teeth are affected; brown stain frequently present. **C,** Severe fluorosis—hypoplasia affecting the general shape of the tooth; widespread brown stains, corroded-like appearance of teeth. (Courtesy of Alton McWhorter, DDS, MS; Associate Professor, Department of Pediatric Dentistry; The Texas A&M University System; Baylor College of Dentistry; Dallas, TX.)

tion. These changes may gradually increase in severity, eventually resulting in a general increase in bone density and considerable calcification of ligaments in the neck and vertebral column. Eventually, bones become brittle and break easily.

Dental Caries. A lack of fluoride may result in increased dental caries. The protective effect against caries is greatest during tooth formation. The American Dental Association and the American Academy of Pediatrics recommend exposure of the teeth to fluoride until calcification of all teeth is completed (about age 16). Dosages for fluoride supplements for children are presented in Table 13-2. Various conditions warrant topical fluoride treatment in adults, such as hypersensitivity, exposed root surfaces, white spot lesions, xerostomia, use of smokeless tobacco, and radiation therapy.

Continued use of fluoridated water into adulthood is beneficial in maintaining the integrity of teeth. Posteruption, systemic fluoride is present in saliva and plaque, creating an environment that inhibits demineralization and enhances remineralization of tooth surfaces.

SAFETY

The addition of fluoride in the water supply continues to be opposed by a small but vocal and aggressive minority of people in the United States. Antifluoridation groups have attempted to link water fluoridation to cancer, AIDS, Alzheimer disease, and Down's syndrome, but scientific evidence to support these allegations has not been provided.

Fluoridation is one of the most thoroughly researched health issues in recent history. No trends have been identified that could be attributed to the introduction of or duration of fluoride in drinking water. Fluoridation does not increase the incidence or mortality rate of any chronic condition, including cancer, heart disease, intracranial lesions, nephritis, cirrhosis, or Down syndrome.

In contrast, almost all professional health organizations have concluded that results of numerous long-term community trials of adding fluoride to public water supplies at optimal levels verify the effectiveness, safety, and cost-benefit of this public health measure in reducing the prevalence of dental caries. Fluoridation of water is the most cost-effective method of preventing dental caries and provides the greatest benefit to individuals who can least afford preventive and restorative dentistry.

Dental Hygiene Considerations

- Educate patients about the purpose and value of fluoridation to oral and bone health.
- Contact the state or local health department to determine the fluoride content of the water system in the area. Encourage patients to send samples of well water or home water treatment systems to their state health department to determine fluoride content.
- Long-term use of infant formulas, particularly powdered formulas reconstituted with fluoridated water, can be a factor for mild fluorosis.
- Age-specific fluoride recommendations are listed in Table 8-9.
- Reliably estimate the total amount of fluoride the patient consumes daily in foods and water. Because fluoride is available from multiple sources, the possibility of toxic levels should be considered when recommending fluoride supplements or providing treatment, especially for children. Consider the number of carbonated beverages consumed and consumption of all beverages using fluoridated water. The fluoride content is not listed on the label, making it difficult to approximate the amount of fluoride being consumed.
- Educate patients about the caries process. Encourage patients to practice optimal oral hygiene. Plaque biofilm is the primary factor in caries formation. Appropriate oral hygiene

when using topical fluorides at home also increases their effectiveness.
- Recommend fluoride supplements only when the fluoride level of the home water supply is known to be deficient.
- An adequate fluoride intake is beneficial during development of skeletal tissue and teeth. Encourage fluoride-fortified foods, water, or supplements for breastfed infants, and fluoridated water for children and adolescents, if applicable.
- Growth of cariogenic bacteria is reduced by the presence of fluoride. Suggest use of dentifrices or mouthwashes with fluoride for oral self-care for individuals older than 3 years.
- Caution parents of children younger than 6 years to (1) use only small (pea size) amounts of fluoridated dentifrices, (2) minimize swallowing toothpaste, (3) avoid the use of fluoride mouth rinse, (4) keep fluoride products out of the reach of children, and (5) use a nonfluoridated toothpaste for children 2 years and younger. The fluoride levels in children's toothpastes often equal the levels in adult fluoridated toothpastes.
- If fluoride and calcium supplements are given concurrently, absorption of both is decreased.
- For individuals living in an area where the fluoride content of water is naturally 2 to 4 mg/L, recommend drinking bottled water without fluoride, or use commercially available filters to reduce the fluoride to safer levels.

Nutritional Directions

- Fluoridation of community water supplies is the most effective method of preventing dental caries, including coronal and root caries.
- A 2.2-mg amount of sodium fluoride contains 1 mg of fluoride ion.
- To provide maximum benefits, systemic fluoride is important before tooth eruption, when development of unerupted permanent teeth is occurring.
- Fluoride supplementation is recommended for patients 6 months to 16 years old with less than 0.6 ppm fluoride in their water source (home, child care settings, school, or bottled) if there is no other significant source of fluoride.
- Fluoride supplements are not recommended during pregnancy. There is no known benefit to the developing fetus.[30]
- If a child receives suboptimal levels of fluoride, an increase in dental caries may occur. Exposure to multiple sources of fluoride increases the risk of excess fluoride causing fluorosis.
- Fluoride supplements are inappropriate for individuals living in areas where the fluoride content of drinking water is optimal, unless the bottled or treated water does not contain fluoride.
- Topical availability of fluoride at low concentrations on a daily basis after tooth eruption is important to deter the development of dental caries.
- If caries susceptibility is high, professionally applied and self-applied home fluoride therapies may be a component of the dental hygiene care provided.
- When bottled water is being used, obtain the fluoride content from the distributor or the label.
- Studies have found no association between fluoride supplementation and cancer in humans.
- Aluminum antacids decrease fluoride absorption.

Table 8-9	Age-Specific Guidelines for Fluoride Throughout the Life Cycle	
Age	**Fluoride**	**Comments**
Pregnant women; visit dentist at least once during pregnancy	Fluoride supplementation not indicated Use fluoridated toothpaste/rinse and drink fluoridated water	
Infants, birth–6 mo	Oral supplementation not recommended Use fluoridated water if available	See fluoride supplement schedule in Table 13-2
Infant 6-12 mo (make first dental visit by 12 mo)	Use fluoridated water Oral fluoride supplements only if prescribed by dentist or pediatrician	Fluoride supplements should be used only in accordance with American Dental Association guidelines
Toddler 12-24 mo	Use fluoridated water or oral supplements if prescribed by dentist or pediatrician	Toothpaste should not be used until age 18-24 mo or until the child will spit it out after use Use only a pea-sized amount of toothpaste per day to minimize fluoride ingestion Caregiver supervision is essential
Children 2-3 yr, regular dental visits	Use fluoridated water or supplements as directed Introduce topical fluoride by use of toothpaste	Use pea-sized amount of toothpaste Advise older preschoolers against ingesting toothpaste and rinses Caregiver supervision is essential
Children 3-12 yr	Fluoridated water Fluoridated dentifrice Fluoride supplements only if prescribed by dentist Home fluoride rinses or gels for high-risk children if recommended by dentist	Minimal risk of fluorosis
Adolescents, adults, and elders	Fluoridated water Fluoridated dentifrice Home fluoride rinses or gels for high-risk patients, if recommended by dentist	No risk of fluorosis

From Palmer C, et al: Position of the American Dietetic Association: The impact of fluoride on health. J Am Diet Assoc 2005 Oct; 105(10):1624.

HEALTH APPLICATION Osteoporosis

Osteoporosis is a common and costly disease, increasing in prevalence in men and women. This condition is partly genetically determined. Ten million Americans are affected by osteoporosis, and another 34 million have low bone mass. About 80% of individuals with osteoporosis are women (one in two women older than 50). This condition caused 2 million fractures annually and incurred a financial burden of around $19 billion in medical costs in 2005; this amount is estimated to increase to $25.3 billion by 2025.[1] Fractures resulting from osteoporosis are a significant source of bone pain, disability, and disfigurement.

Osteoporosis is more likely to develop in individuals with at least some of the risk factors listed in Box 8-3. The incidence of osteoporosis is greatest in white, Asian and Hispanic women, especially women who are small and thin. A woman's risk of osteoporosis starts around menopause (age 50 or older). Women can lose 20% of their bone mass within 5 to 7 years after menopause. Bone loss in men increases after age 65. Men who fall and break a hip are twice as likely to die in the year following the incident.[1] For individuals at risk for osteoporosis, an objective of

treatment is to slow or stop the disease progression before irreversible structural changes have occurred. The National Osteoporosis Foundation recommends five steps for preventing osteoporosis:

1. Get the daily recommended amounts of calcium and vitamin D. Dietary modifications for patients at risk of developing osteoporosis should include at least two portions of dairy products daily (to provide 75% of RDAs). For patients who have inadequate intake of milk or milk products (including patients who are lactose intolerant), inclusion of calcium and vitamin D supplements may be indicated.
2. Engage in regular weight-bearing and muscle-strengthening exercise.
3. Avoid smoking and excessive alcohol.
4. Talk to a healthcare provider about bone health.
5. Have a bone mineral density (BMD) test and take medication when appropriate. Specialized tests to

Box 8-3	**Risk Factors for Osteoporosis**

Certain people are more likely to develop osteoporosis than others. Factors that increase the likelihood of developing osteoporosis and broken bones are called "risk factors." Many of these risk factors include:
- Being female
- Older age
- Family history of osteoporosis or broken bones
- Being small and thin
- Certain race/ethnicities such as Caucasian, Asian, or Hispanic/Latino, although African Americans are also at risk
- History of broken bones
- Low sex hormones
  - Low estrogen levels in women, including menopause
  - Missing periods (**amenorrhea**)
  - Low levels of testosterone and estrogen in men
- Diet
  - Low calcium intake
  - Low vitamin D intake
  - Excessive intake of protein, sodium, and caffeine
- Inactive lifestyle
- Smoking
- Alcohol abuse
- Certain medications such as steroid medications, some anticonvulsants, and others
- Certain diseases and conditions such as anorexia nervosa, rheumatoid arthritis, gastrointestinal diseases, and others

From National Osteoporosis Foundation: Fast Facts on Osteoporosis 2008. National Osteoporosis Foundation, Washington, DC. Available at http://www.nof.org/osteoporosis/disease facts.htm. Accessed December 12, 2008.

HEALTH APPLICATION Osteoporosis—cont'd

assess BMD should be conducted on women older than 50, depending on risk factors, and men older than 70 who are at increased risk for osteoporosis.[31]

The oral cavity (teeth, maxilla, and mandible) can be affected by osteoporosis. When identifying periodontal issues, such as tooth mobility or loss, resorption of alveolar bone, temporomandibular disorders, and clinical attachment loss, a relationship to osteoporosis should be considered.[32,33]

To date, there is no cure for osteoporosis, but medications can help prevent or deter bone loss. Medications used to slow bone loss include estrogen hormone, bisphosphonates, calcitonin, estrogen agonists/selective estrogen receptor modulators (SERMs), and PTH. A significant dental consideration for the use of bisphosphonates is the risk for the development of osteonecrosis of the jaw.[34-36]

Commonly used medications for other conditions have a documented effect on bone mineralization. Thiazide diuretics, principally used for blood pressure control, positively affect bone mineralization. Glucocorticoids, used to reduce inflammation, adversely affect bone mineralization. Antiandrogenic drugs for prostate cancer may lead to bone loss.

An adequate calcium intake is important at all stages of life, with a daily intake of a minimum of 1000 mg for all healthy adults and 1200 mg for adults older than 51. Adequate exposure to sunlight and vitamin D intake are also important. The action of these two nutrients is complementary; calcium supports bone formation and repair, and vitamin D helps with calcium absorption. Other nutritional considerations include vitamins B and K, which may reduce fracture risk by increasing bone mineral density. Diets high in fruits and vegetables and whole grains contribute nutrients such as magnesium and may produce an alkaline environment, reducing calcium excretion.[37] High levels of phosphorus, sodium, or caffeine intake may increase calcium loss in urine. High fiber intake (including oxalates and phytates) should be accompanied with increases in calcium. Caffeine should be used in moderation because caffeine increases calcium excretion; however, habitual tea consumption has little effect on bone density.[38,39] Tea contains caffeine, but other nutrients, such as flavonoids, may influence BMD. Plant chemicals or phytochemicals are often a nutritional intervention to prevent bone loss. **Phytochemicals**, natural components of foods, found in soy products and flaxseed, stimulate estrogen secretion, which may boost BMD.[40] A healthcare provider or registered dietitian can tailor the osteoporosis regimen to meet the patient's needs.

CASE APPLICATION FOR THE DENTAL HYGIENIST

During Annie's routine dental examination, her mother asked the dental hygienist whether she should start Annie (age 5) on a fluoride supplement. Annie's examination revealed a caries-free mouth. She brushes her teeth twice a day.

Nutritional Assessment
- Food consumption pattern
- Frequency of carbohydrate intake
- Fluoride content of water consumed; average amount of water/water-based beverages consumed
- Type and amount of toothpaste used

Nutritional Diagnosis
Health-seeking behaviors related to inadequate knowledge about fluoride supplementation.

Nutritional Goals
The patient will practice good oral self-care and receive adequate fluoride to prevent dental caries.

Nutritional Implementation
Intervention: Explain the benefits of fluoride.
Rationale: Fluoride is advantageous to dental health because of its systemic effect before tooth eruption and its topical effects

CASE APPLICATION FOR THE DENTAL HYGIENIST—cont'd

after tooth eruption. The caries-preventive properties of systemic and topical fluoride are additive.

Intervention: Discuss the toxic effects of fluoride.

Rationale: Dental fluorosis is directly related to the level of fluoride exposure during tooth development. It can also have adverse effects on bone structure.

Intervention: Assess current fluoride consumption from (1) food, (2) water supply, (3) carbonated beverages, and (4) fluoridated dentifrices and mouth rinses.

Rationale: (1) All foods contain some fluoride, but the amounts provided in vegetables, meats, cereals, and fruits are insignificant unless large amounts of seafood, tea, or deboned poultry is consumed; (2) water is usually the main source of fluoride, but some municipal water supplies and bottled waters may contain negligible amounts of fluoride; and (3) fluoride is added to 90% of all dentifrices in the United States (many children swallow most of the toothpaste used).

Intervention: Show Annie and her mother how much toothpaste to use, and discuss the importance of not swallowing the toothpaste.

Rationale: Because fluoride in toothpaste can be readily absorbed, toothpaste should not be swallowed to prevent the harmful effects of systemically available fluoride.

Intervention: Encourage the patient and her mother to consume a well-balanced diet with limited amounts of fermentable carbohydrates at snack time.

Rationale: Not only is fluoride important, but also other nutrients are essential for dental health. Snacks, especially carbohydrate-containing foods, increase risk for dental caries.

Intervention: Suggest fluoride supplements only if fluoride intake seems to be low.

Rationale: In many cases, total fluoride exposure seems to be higher than necessary to prevent tooth decay. No more than the amount of fluoride necessary to provide the desired effect should be used.

Intervention: Recommend parental supervision and assistance for Annie's tooth brushing and flossing.

Rationale: Monitoring the child's brushing technique and assisting with flossing will ensure that effective biofilm removal occurs once a day.

Evaluation

If the patient and her mother can demonstrate the toothbrushing procedure, the patient says she will brush her teeth after every meal and will try to eat the foods her mother provides, and the dental caries continue to be minimal, dental hygiene care was effective.

STUDENT READINESS

1. A patient claims that she dislikes milk. How would you advise her to obtain the needed calcium?
2. What are the main physiological roles of calcium, phosphorus, magnesium, and fluoride?
3. How do minerals differ from vitamins?
4. How would you respond to a remark that milk is only for babies?
5. Discuss three dietary factors that affect calcium absorption.
6. Determine the level of fluoride in your community's drinking water.
7. If an adult patient (weight about 75 kg) is drinking only bottled water that does not contain fluoride and dislikes fish and tea, how much topical fluoride would be necessary to furnish the recommendation for fluoride?
8. List five types of over-the-counter calcium supplements available. Evaluate these items for primary sources of calcium and elemental calcium per unit consumed. Find how many tablets or units would have to be consumed daily to receive 1000 mg of elemental calcium.
9. Discuss how to deal with a patient who is opposed to fluoridation.
10. Why would you advise a patient to obtain his or her mineral requirement from food sources rather than mineral supplements (unless ordered by the healthcare provider)?

CASE STUDY

Mrs. J. M., a 69-year-old woman, fell and fractured her hip 6 months ago. She admits she is taking calcium supplements occasionally when she can afford them. She does not like milk and has been unable to walk much since her fall.

1. What additional questions would you ask to clarify the situation?
2. What nutritional advice could you give her about her osteoporosis?
3. What is her RDA for calcium?
4. What foods could you suggest she consume to increase her calcium intake?
5. When should she take her calcium supplement to maximize its absorption?
6. What oral changes might you expect to find in your assessment?
7. What effect would increased vitamin D intake have on her condition?

References

1. National Osteoporosis Foundation: Fast facts. Available at www.nof.org/osteoporosis/diseasefacts.htm. Accessed May 3, 2008.
2. U.S. Department of Health and Human Services: Bone Health and Osteoporosis: A Report of the Surgeon General. Rockville,

MD: U.S. Department of Health and Human Services, Office of the Surgeon General 2004.

3. Moshfegh A, Goldman J, Cleveland L: What we eat in America, NHANES 2001-2002: usual nutrient intakes from food compared to dietary reference intakes. Available at www.ars.usda.gov/SP2UserFiles/Place/12355000/pdf/usual intaketables2001-02.pdf. Accessed May 2, 2008.

4. Wells HF, Buzby JC: Dietary assessment of major trends in U.S. Food consumption, 1970-2005. Economic Information Bulletin, No 33. Economic Research Service, U.S. Department of Agriculture, March 2008.

5. Perez AV, et al: Minireview on regulation of intestinal calcium absorption: emphasis on molecular mechanisms of transcellular pathway. Digestion 2008; 77(1):22-34.

6. Thorpe MP, et al: A diet high in protein, dairy, and calcium attenuates bone loss over twelve months of weight loss and maintenance relative to a conventional high-carbohydrate diet in adults. J Nutr 2008 Jun; 138(6):1096-1100.

7. Napoli N, et al: Effects of dietary calcium with calcium supplements on estrogen metabolism and bone mineral density. Am J Clin Nutr 2007 May; 85(5):1428-1433.

8. Heller L: Calcium and multivitamins drive U.S. market. Nutraingredients—USA 2008 May 5. Available at www. nutraingredients-usa.com/news/printNewsBis.asp?id=85085. Accessed May 9, 2008.

9. Shea B, et al: Meta-analysis of therapies for menopausal osteoporosis, VII: meta-analysis of calcium supplementation for the prevention of postmenopausal osteoporosis. Endocr Rev 2002 Aug; 23(4):552-559.

10. Rafferty K, Walters G, Heaney RP: Calcium forticants: overview and strategies for improving calcium nutriture of the U. S. population. J Food Sci 2007 Nov; 72(9):R152-R158.

11. Nishida M, et al: Calcium and the risk for periodontal disease. J Periodontol 2000 July; 71(7):1057-1066.

12. Fleischer J, et al: The decline in hip bone density following gastric bypass surgery is associated with extent of weight loss. J Clin Endocrinol Metabol 2008 Oct; 93(10):3735-3740.

13. Hind K, Burrows M: Weight-bearing exercise and bone mineral accrual in children and adolescents: a review of controlled trials. Bone 2007 Jan; 40(1):14-27.

14. Wolff I, et al: The effect of exercise training programs on bone mass: a meta-analysis of published controlled trials in pre- and postmenopausal women. Osteoporos Int 1999; 9(1):1-12.

15. Kelley GA, Kelley KS, Tran ZV: Resistance training and bone mineral density in women: a meta-analysis of controlled trials. Am J Phys Med Rehabil 2001 Jan; 80(1):65-77.

16. Chaussain-Miller C, et al: Dentin structure in familial hypophosphatemic rickets: benefits of vitamin D and phosphate treatment. Oral Dis 2007 Sep; 13(5):482-489.

17. Volpe SL: Magnesium, the metabolic syndrome, insulin resistance, and type 2 diabetes mellitus. Crit Rev Food Sci Nur 2008 Mar; 48(3):292-300.

18. Wells IC: Evidence that the etiology of the syndrome containing type 2 diabetes mellitus results from abnormal magnesium metabolism. Can J Physiol Pharmacol 2008 Jan/Feb; 86(1-2):16-24.

19. American Diabetes Association: Nutrition recommendations and interventions for diabetes. Diabetes Care 2008 Jan; 31(Suppl 1):S61-S78.

20. Champagne CM: Magnesium in hypertension, cardiovascular disease, metabolic syndrome, and other conditions: a review. Nutr Clin Pract 2008 Apr; 23(2):142-151.

21. American Academy of Pediatric Dentistry Liaison with Other Groups Committee; American Academy of Pediatric Dentistry Council on Clinical Affairs: Guideline on fluoride therapy. Pediatr Dent 2005-2006; 27(7 Suppl):90-91.

22. Featherstone J: Prevention and reversal of dental caries: role of low-level fluoride. Community Dent Oral Epidemiol 1999; 27:31-40.

23. Sá Roriz Fontelesa C, Zero DT, Moss ME, Fu J: Fluoride concentrations in enamel and dentin of primary teeth after pre- and postnatal fluoride exposure. Caries Res 2005 Nov-Dec; 39(6):505-508.

24. Maupomé G, et al: A comparison of dental treatment utilization and costs by HMO members living in fluoridated and non-fluoridated areas. J Public Health Dent 2007 Fall; 67(4):224-233.

25. U.S. Department of Health and Human Services: Bone health and osteoporosis: a report of the Surgeon General. Available at www.Surgeongeneral.gov/library/oralhealth/. Accessed May 4, 2008.

26. Bailey W, et al: Populations receiving optimally fluoridated public drinking water—United States, 1992-2006. CDC Morb Mortal Wkly Rep 2008 Jul 11; 57(27):737-741. Available at http://www.cdc.gov/mmwr/preview/mmwrhtml/mm5727a1.htm.

27. Gillcrist JA, Brumley DE, Blackford JU: Community fluoridation status and caries experience in children. J Public Health Dent 2001 Summer; 61(3):168-171.

28. Committee on Fluoride in Drinking Water: Fluoride in drinking water: a scientific review of EPA's standards. National Research Council, National Academy of Sciences, Mar 2006. Available at http://dels.nas.edu/dels/rpt_briefs/fluoride_brief_final.pdf. Accessed May 4, 2008.

29. ADA Reports: Position of the American Dietetic Association: the impact of fluoride on health. J Am Diet Assoc 2005 Oct; 105(10):1620-1628.

30. Buzalaf MA, et al: Fluoride content of infant formulas prepared with deionized, bottled mineral and fluoridated drinking water. J Dent Child 2001 Jan-Feb; 68(1):37-41.

31. Centers for Disease Control and Prevention: Recommendations for using fluoride to prevent and control dental caries in the United States. MMWR Morb Mortal Wkly Rep 2001; 50(RR14):1-42.

32. Qaseem A, et al: Screening for osteoporosis in men: a clinical practice guideline from the American College of Physicians. Ann Intern Med 2008 May 6; 148(9):680-684.

33. Dervis E: Oral implications of osteoporosis. Oral Surg Oral Med Oral Pathol Oral Radiol Endod 2005 Sep; 100(3):349-356.

34. Jeffcoat M: The association between osteoporosis and oral bone loss. J Periodontol 2005 Nov; 76(11 Suppl):2125-2132.

35. Edwards BJ, Migliorati CA: Osteoporosis and its implications for dental patients. J Am Dent Assoc 2008 May; 139(5):545-552.

36. Sedghizadeh PP, et al: Oral bisphosphonate use and the prevalence of osteonecrosis of the jaw: an institutional inquiry. J Am Dent Assoc 2009 Jan; 140(1):61-66.

37. Kumar SK, Meru M, Sedghizadeh PP: Osteonecrosis of the jaws secondary to bisphosphonate therapy: a case series. J Contemp Dent Pract 2008 Jan 1; 9(1):63-69.

38. Kitchin B, Morgan SL: Not just calcium and vitamin D: Other nutritional considerations in osteoporosis. Curr Rheumatol Rep 2007 Apr; 9(1):85-92.

39. Chen Z, et al: Habitual tea consumption and risk of osteoporosis: A prospective study in the women's health initiative observational cohort. Am J Epidemiol 2003 Oct 15; 158(8):772-781.

40. Hegarty VM, May HM, Khaw KT: Tea drinking and bone mineral density in older women. Am J Clin Nutr 2000 Apr; 71(4):1003-1007.

Chapter 9

Nutrients Present in Calcified Structures

OUTLINE

LEARNING OBJECTIVES

Upon completion of this chapter, the student will be able to complete the following objectives:

- List physiological roles and how these might apply to oral health along with sources of copper, selenium, chromium, and manganese.
- List ultratrace elements present in the body.

- List reasons why large amounts of one mineral may cause nutritional deficiencies of another.
- Apply dental hygiene considerations for trace elements present in calcified structures.
- Discuss nutritional directions for patients regarding the role of trace elements present in calcified structures.

KEY TERMS

Enteral feedings
Kayser-Fleischer ring
Keshan disease
Manganese madness

Neurotransmitters
Osteodystrophy
Stannous
Total parenteral nutrition (TPN)

Very small amounts of several minerals are essential for optimal growth and development. Many of these ultratrace elements (Table 9-1) are found in enamel and dentin. In a study conducted in India, 18 trace minerals were present in the enamel of healthy and carious primary and permanent teeth. Concentrations of fluoride, strontium, potassium, aluminum, and iron were significantly higher in the enamel of sound permanent teeth than in the carious enamel.[1] The role of minerals may not be obvious as you clinically assess patients; nevertheless, patients with inadequate amounts may exhibit deficiency symptoms.

Tolerable upper intake levels (UL) have not been established for several of these nutrients because of the lack of data. The requirement for these nutrients should be obtained from food sources because even small amounts may be toxic. Evidence has been presented suggesting ultratrace minerals, especially arsenic, boron, nickel, and silicon, may be physiologically essential. Because no human deficiencies have been determined, their importance in humans can only be inferred from results of animal studies. Human requirements have not been quantified. If they are required, the amounts needed are easily met by naturally occurring sources in food, water, and air. Other elements present in calcified structures, such as cadmium, lead, and tin, have no known function and may be contaminants.

COPPER

PHYSIOLOGICAL ROLES

Copper is essential for formation of red blood cells (RBCs) and connective tissue. Its function as a catalyst is important in the formation of collagen from a precollagenous stage. Copper is a component of many enzymes that function in oxidative reactions, and copper-containing enzymes encourage production of **neurotransmitters** (including norepinephrine and dopamine), which transmit messages through the central nervous system.

Copper is readily incorporated into tooth enamel. X-ray fluorescence imaging of teeth shows an increased concentration of copper in carious portions of the tooth. It appears copper is transported and localized mainly in the dentinal tubules; this suggests copper is associated with formation and progression of dental caries.[2] Epidemiological data suggest copper is cariogenic, but in bacteriological studies, copper is cariostatic by reducing acidogenicity of plaque.

REQUIREMENTS

The Institute of Medicine (IOM) established the recommended dietary allowance (RDA) for copper to be 900 μg per day for adults. The UL has been set at 10 g per day for adults (Table 9-2).

ABSORPTION AND EXCRETION

Approximately one-third of dietary copper is absorbed, with absorption occurring in the stomach and duodenum. Absorption is enhanced by a low pH and is decreased with large amounts of calcium and zinc. Copper is principally excreted through bile in feces.

Table 9-1	Trace Element Concentrations in Human Enamel and Dentin	
	Enamel* (ppm)	**Dentin* (ppm)**
Aluminum	1.5-700	10-100
Boron	0.5-39	1-10
Cadmium	0.3-10	
Chromium	<0.1-100	1-100
Copper	0.1-130	0.2-100
Iron	0.8-200	90-1000
Lead	1.3-100	10-100
Lithium	0.23-3.40	
Manganese	0.8-20	0.6-1000
Molybdenum	0.7-39	1-10
Nickel	10-100	10-100
Selenium	0.1-10	10-100
Strontium	26-1000	90-1000
Sulfur	130-530	
Tin	0.03-0.9	
Vanadium	0.01-0.03	1-10
Zinc	60-1800	

Adapted from Gron P: Inorganic chemical and structural aspects of oral mineralized tissues. In Shaw JH, et al (eds): Textbook of Oral Biology. Philadelphia: Saunders, 1978, pp 484-507.*
μg/g dry weight.

Table 9-2	Institute of Medicine Recommendations for Copper				
	EAR (µg/d)*		RDA (µg/d)†		
Life Stage	Male	Female	Male	Female	AI (µg/d)
Birth–6 mo	—	—	—	—	200
7-12 mo	—	—	—	—	220
1-3 yr	260	260	340	340	
4-8 yr	340	340	440	440	
9-13 yr	540	540	700	700	
14-50 yr	685	685	890	890	
>51 yr	700	700	900	900	
Pregnancy					
14-18 yr		785		1000	
19-50 yr		800		1000	
Lactation					
14-18 yr		985		1300	
19-50 yr		1000		1300	

Data from Institute of Medicine (IOM), Food and Nutrition Board: Dietary Reference Intakes for Vitamin A, Vitamin K, Arsenic, Boron, Chromium, Copper, Iodine, Iron, Manganese, Molybdenum, Nickel, Silicon, Vanadium, and Zinc. Washington, DC: National Academy Press, 2001.
*EAR (estimated average requirement)—the intake that meets the estimated nutrient needs of half of the individuals in a group, men and women combined.
†RDA (recommended dietary allowance)—the intake that meets the nutrient needs of almost all (97-98%) individuals in a group.

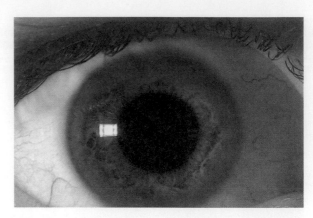

FIGURE 9-I Cornea in Wilson's disease. Copper deposits in the corneal periphery produce the characteristic Kayser-Fleischer ring. This is a complete or incomplete brown-to-green ring near the cornea, best seen in early stages of the disease. (Courtesy of Professor Dame S. Sherlock and J.A. Summerfield. In McLaren DS: A Colour Atlas and Text of Diet-Related Disorders, 2nd ed. London: Mosby-Year Book Europe Limited, 1992.)

Copper deficiency causes a variety of lesions within connective tissues and bone, resulting in failure to grow (in children), spontaneous fractures, osteoporosis, arthritis, arterial disease, and ultimately marked bone deformities with severe deficiency. These lesions have been attributed to abnormal formation of cross-linkages in collagen and elastin. Changes resemble those seen in vitamin C deficiency.

SOURCES

Copper is widely distributed in foods. The richest sources include shellfish, oysters, crabs, liver, nuts, sesame and sunflower seeds, soy products, legumes, and cocoa.

HYPER-STATES AND HYPO-STATES

Copper toxicity is seldom encountered. Copper taken orally is an emetic; 10 mg of oral copper can produce nausea. Serum copper levels are elevated in patients with rheumatoid arthritis, myocardial infarction, conditions requiring administration of estrogen, and pregnancy.

Wilson's disease represents a special metabolic disorder in which large amounts of copper accumulate in the liver, kidney, brain, and cornea. There is also an inability to excrete copper through bile. Copper concentrates in the cornea, causing a characteristic brown or green ring called the **Kayser-Fleischer ring** (Fig. 9-1).

Most copper deficiencies have been detected under unusual conditions, such as with zinc supplementation or in patients receiving **total parenteral nutrition (TPN)** (delivery of all nutritional needs intravenously). Copper deprivation results in profound effects on the bones, brain, arteries, and other connective tissues; decreases hair and skin pigmentation; and causes hematological abnormalities, such as a low white blood cell count. It is reasonable to assume all these effects are ultimately due to an inadequate supply of copper needed for enzyme synthesis and activity.

Dental Hygiene Considerations

- Anemia that cannot be corrected with iron supplements may be due to copper deficiency.
- High doses of zinc supplements decrease copper absorption, possibly leading to anemia-related fatigue.

Nutritional Directions

- High-fiber intakes increase the dietary requirement for copper.
- Large amounts of vitamin C supplements decrease serum bioavailability of copper.

SELENIUM

PHYSIOLOGICAL ROLES

Selenium functions mainly as a cofactor for an antioxidant enzyme that protects membrane lipids, proteins, and nucleic acids from oxidative damage. Selenium works hand in hand with vitamin E; a deficiency of either nutrient increases the requirement for the other. Although selenium has been suspected as a carcinogen, it may actually be an anticarcinogen.

Selenium is present in tooth enamel and dentin. It is probably incorporated into the enamel during amelogenesis. Large amounts during tooth formation may be detrimental to the mineralization process.

REQUIREMENTS

The RDA establishes the adult requirement at 55 µg. The UL is 400 µg per day for adults (Table 9-3). Typical intake in the United States is 60 to 220 µg daily.

SOURCES

Animal products, especially seafood, kidney, liver, and other meats, are rich in selenium. Selenium intake correlates closely with caloric and protein consumption. Selenium in dairy products and eggs is more readily absorbed than selenium from other foods. Whole-grain products and nuts are also good sources.

HYPER-STATES AND HYPO-STATES

Toxicity and deficiency symptoms have occurred in animals from irregular distribution of selenium in soil, but these are rarely seen in humans. Routine ingestion of 2 to 3 mg of selenium can cause toxic symptoms of nausea and vomiting, weakness, dermatitis, hair loss, white blotchy nails, and garlicky breath odor. Cirrhosis of the liver also may develop. Although a moderate intake of selenium has been linked to reduced risks of prostate, lung, and colon cancers and heart disease because of its role as an antioxidant, when blood levels reach a high-normal level, the risk of dying from any cause, specifically cancer, begins to increase.[3]

Animal studies indicate excessive selenium may promote dental caries when given before eruption, whereas moderately high levels seem to have some cariostatic effects. Increased dental caries rates have been observed in areas where the food and water contain higher levels of selenium. Whether this increase in caries is caused by a topical effect on plaque biofilm or by an effect on the structural composition of the tooth is unknown.

Critically ill patients consistently have decreased selenium levels, but selenium administration treatments have not consistently shown improved outcomes.[4] In parts of China, an endemic cardiomyopathy called **Keshan disease** is associated with severe selenium deficiency. Oral selenium prophylaxis is extremely effective in reducing, but not completely eliminating, Keshan disease.

Dental Hygiene Considerations

Decreased selenium levels may cause heart damage, resulting in a heart attack. Selenium is essential for health, but it can also be toxic.

Nutritional Directions

- Because of increased risk of toxicity, selenium supplements should not be taken by patients with cancer, coronary artery disease, arthritis, and HIV, unless recommended by a healthcare provider.
- Gastrointestinal disorders, such as Crohn's disease, can impair selenium absorption.

Table 9-3	Institute of Medicine Recommendations for Selenium		
Life Stage	**EAR (mg/d)***	**RDA (mg/d)†**	**AI (mg/d)‡**
0-6 mo			15
7-12 mo			20
1-3 yr	17	20	
4-8 yr	23	30	
9-13 yr	35	40	
14 ->70 yr	45	55	
Pregnancy ≤18-50 yr	49	60	
Lactation ≤18-50 yr	59	70	

Data from Institute of Medicine (IOM), Food and Nutrition Board: Dietary Reference Intakes for Vitamin C, Vitamin E, Selenium, and Carotenoids. Washington, DC: National Academy Press, 2000.
*EAR (estimated average requirement)—the intake that meets the estimated nutrient needs of half of the individuals in a group, men and women combined.
†RDA (recommended dietary allowance)—the intake that meets the nutrient needs of almost all (97-98%) individuals in a group.
‡AI (adequate intake)—the observed average or experimentally set intake by a defined population or subgroup that seems to sustain a defined nutritional status, such as growth rate, normal circulating nutrient values, or other functional indicators of health. An AI is used if insufficient scientific evidence is available to derive an EAR. For healthy human milk–fed infants, the AI is the mean intake. The AI is not equivalent to an RDA.

CHROMIUM

PHYSIOLOGICAL ROLES

Chromium is involved in carbohydrate and lipid metabolism, especially in the use of glucose. Chromium potentiates the action of insulin. Chromium may facilitate insulin in assisting cells in glucose uptake and energy release. Supplementation may improve systemic insulin sensitivity, but more research is needed. Chromium picolinate improved glycemic control in patients with diabetes in some studies, but other studies have had conflicting results. The American Diabetes Association states: "Benefit from chromium supplementation in people with diabetes or obesity has not been conclusively demonstrated, and therefore, cannot be recommended."[5]

REQUIREMENTS

The adequate intake (AI) of a healthy adult has been estimated to be 20 to 35 µg per day. No UL has been set (Table

Table 9-4	Institute of Medicine Recommendations for Chromium	

Life Stage Group	AI* (µg/d) Male	Female
Birth-6 mo	0.2	0.2
7-12 mo	2.2	2.2
1-3 yr	11	11
4-8 yr	15	15
9-13 yr	25	21
14-18 yr	35	24
19-50 yr	35	25
>51 yr	30	20
Pregnancy		
14-18 yr		29
19-50 yr		30
Lactation		
14-18 yr		44
19-50 yr		45

Data from Institute of Medicine (IOM), Food and Nutrition Board: Dietary Reference Intakes for Vitamin A, Vitamin K, Arsenic, Boron, Chromium, Copper, Iodine, Iron, Manganese, Molybdenum, Nickel, Silicon, Vanadium, and Zinc. Washington, DC: National Academy Press, 2001.
*AI (adequate intake)—the observed average or experimentally determined intake by a defined population or subgroup that seems to sustain a defined nutritional status, such as growth rate, normal circulating nutrient values, or other functional indicators of health. An AI is used if insufficient scientific evidence is available to derive an EAR. For healthy human milk–fed infants, the AI is the mean intake. The AI is not equivalent to an RDA.

9-4). The IOM determined the average chromium content in well-balanced diets was 13.4 µg/1000 kcal. Chromium is poorly absorbed; whether intestinal absorption compensates for increased demand is unclear. Chromium status decreases with age, suggesting that older individuals may be at high risk of deficiency.

SOURCES

Chromium is found in meats, whole-grain cereals, wheat germ, nuts, mushrooms, brewer's yeast, beer, and wine. The refining process depletes grains and cereal of chromium.

Chromium supplements are available as picolinate, nicotinate, or chloride (the form provided in most multivitamin-mineral supplements). The absorption rate of chromium picolinate is superior to the other forms.[6]

HYPER-STATES AND HYPO-STATES

Chromium deficiencies result in decreased insulin sensitivity, glucose intolerance, and an increased risk of diabetes.[7] Chromium toxicity has been caused by use of chromium supplements and by industrial exposure, resulting in liver damage and lung cancer.

Dental Hygiene Considerations

- Assess patients employed in industrial settings or artists using supplies with high chromium content for chromium toxicity.
- Adequate amounts of chromium from food sources may improve glycemic control in individuals with elevated blood glucose levels if their body still secretes insulin. However, it does not replace the need for oral medications or insulin in patients with diabetes mellitus. Currently, supplementation is not recommended.
- Serum chromium levels decline with age.
- More research is needed regarding use of chromium supplements to enhance glycemic control in diabetes and to treat or prevent other health problems.
- Chromium supplements may cause serious renal impairment when taken in excess. This over-the-counter supplement is marketed for weight loss in addition to its role in type 2 diabetes mellitus.

Nutritional Direction

Do not take chromium supplements unless instructed by a healthcare provider. Currently, the evidence is unclear that any type of supplemental chromium can help with fat loss or enhance lean body mass.

MANGANESE

PHYSIOLOGICAL ROLES

Manganese is essential in several enzyme systems and is important for optimal bone matrix development; prevention of osteoporosis; insulin production; and amino acid, cholesterol, and carbohydrate metabolism.

REQUIREMENTS

As shown in Table 9-5, the AI is 1.8 to 2.3 mg per day for adults. The absorption of iron and manganese is inversely proportional, so a large amount of one reduces absorption of the other. The UL has been established at 11 mg per day for adults. Median intake in the United States is 2.1 to 2.3 mg per day for men and 1.6 to 1.8 mg per day for women.

SOURCES

Foods high in manganese are whole-grain cereals, legumes, nuts, tea, leafy vegetables, and infant formula. The bioavailability of manganese from meats, milk, and eggs makes these important sources despite their smaller quantities. It is also a contaminant in the water supply. The U.S. Environmental Protection Agency (EPA) reports the median concentration of ground water in urban areas contains 150 µg/L with some levels reaching 5600 µg/L. The U.S. health reference level is 300 µg/L.[8]

Table 9-5	Institute of Medicine Recommendations for Manganese	
	AI* (µg/d)	
Life Stage Group	**Male**	**Female**
Birth-6 mo	0.003	0.003
7-12 mo	0.6	0.6
1-3 yr	1.2	1.2
4-8 yr	1.5	1.5
9-13 yr	1.9	1.6
14-18 yr	2.2	1.6
≥19 yr	2.3	1.8
Pregnancy		
14-50 yr		2
Lactation		
14-50 yr		2.6

Data from Institute of Medicine (IOM), Food and Nutrition Board: Dietary Reference Intakes for Vitamin A, Vitamin K, Arsenic, Boron, Chromium, Copper, Iodine, Iron, Manganese, Molybdenum, Nickel, Silicon, Vanadium, and Zinc. Washington, DC: National Academy Press, 2001.

*AI (adequate intake)—the observed average or experimentally determined intake by a defined population or subgroup that seems to sustain a defined nutritional status, such as growth rate, normal circulating nutrient values, or other functional indicators of health. The AI is used if insufficient scientific evidence is available to derive an EAR. For healthy infants receiving human milk, AI is the mean intake. The AI is not equivalent to an RDA.

HYPER-STATES AND HYPO-STATES

Manganese dust can be an environmental hazard. Manganese miners and welders have developed a syndrome similar to Parkinson's disease called "**manganese madness.**" Children and especially infants exposed to excessive manganese exhibit neurological symptoms.[9] Manganese miners are exposed to large amounts of manganese fumes, but other groups are at risk for manganese poisoning as well, including workers in factories manufacturing dry alkaline batteries, and workers in facilities making manganese alloys. Symptoms of toxic exposure include ataxia, headache, fatigue, anxiety, and a syndrome similar to Parkinson's disease (memory loss, tremors, and rigid body posture).

Elevated concentrations of manganese in salivary plaque and enamel are associated with increased caries. Studies have not clarified whether this association is due to incorporation of manganese in enamel or its effects on oral bacteria.

Manganese deficiencies have never been reported in individuals consuming a normal diet. Signs of deficiency include abnormal formation of bone and cartilage, growth retardation, congenital malformations, impaired glucose tolerance, and poor reproductive performance.

Dental Hygiene Considerations

Inhaling manganese dust can be toxic. Patients whose occupation exposes them to increased inhalation of manganese (i.e., factory workers, welders, or manganese miners) may exhibit psychotic symptoms or Parkinson-like symptoms.

Nutritional Directions

- Phytate and fiber in bran, tannins in tea, and oxalic acid in spinach inhibit absorption of manganese.
- Consistent low iron intake results in more manganese absorption.
- Manganese should not be confused with magnesium.
- Breast milk contains minimal amounts of manganese, but infant formulas and the water used to mix formula may be 3 to 100 times higher.[9]

MOLYBDENUM

PHYSIOLOGICAL ROLES

Molybdenum functions as an enzyme cofactor. Molybdenum, a trace element present in teeth, may inhibit caries formation. Studies with humans and animals have been inconsistent, however, and molybdenum is not clinically recommended for prevention of dental caries. No mechanism has been proposed for how molybdenum could inhibit caries formation, but rodent studies suggest that molybdenum affects crown morphology.

REQUIREMENTS

The RDA for molybdenum is 45 µg per day for adults. The UL is set at 2000 µg per day for adults (Table 9-6).

SOURCES

Legumes, whole-grain cereals, milk, liver, and many vegetables are good sources.

HYPER-STATES AND HYPO-STATES

Except for deficiency reported during administration of TPN, molybdenum deficiency has not been documented in the United States.

Dental Hygiene Considerations

Consumption of large quantities of molybdenum may result in copper deficiency, making the patient prone to anemia.

Nutritional Directions

Milk and whole grains are good sources of molybdenum.

ULTRATRACE ELEMENTS

Many ultratrace elements have been studied for their potential influence on dental caries. Results of research investigations are complicated by many factors. Nevertheless, some studies suggest relationships between some of these trace elements and the development of caries in humans or animals. Further research is warranted to determine the mechanism of their effects.

Table 9-6	Institute of Medicine Recommendations for Molybdenum				
	EAR (µg/d)*		RDA (µg/d)†		
Life Stage	Male	Female	Male	Female	AI (µg/d)‡
Birth–6 mo	—	—	—	—	2
7-12 mo	—	—	—	—	3
1-3 yr	13	13	17	17	
4-8 yr	17	17	22	22	
9-13 yr	26	26	34	34	
14-18 yr	33	33	43	43	
19-≥31 yr	34	34	45	45	
Pregnancy					
14-50 yr		40		50	
Lactation					
14-18 yr		35		50	
19-50 yr		36		50	

Data from Institute of Medicine (IOM), Food and Nutrition Board: Dietary Reference Intakes for Vitamin A, Vitamin K, Arsenic, Boron, Chromium, Copper, Iodine, Iron, Manganese, Molybdenum, Nickel, Silicon, Vanadium, and Zinc. Washington, DC: National Academy Press, 2001.
*EAR (estimated average requirement)—the intake that meets the estimated nutrient needs of half of the individuals in a group.
†RDA (recommended dietary allowance)—the intake that meets the nutrient needs of almost all (97-98%) individuals in a group.
‡AI (adequate intake)—the observed average or experimentally set intake by a defined population or subgroup that seems to sustain a defined nutritional status, such as growth rate, normal circulating nutrient values, or other functional indicators of health. An AI is used if insufficient scientific evidence is available to derive an EAR. For healthy human milk–fed infants, the AI is the mean intake. The AI is not equivalent to an RDA.

More attention has been given to ultratrace elements as contaminants in the environment and foods. Some are considered to have no harmful effects and are used therapeutically, such as aluminum in antacids.

BORON

Boron may have an effect on the metabolism of calcium, phosphorus, magnesium, or vitamin D, and may be needed to maintain membrane structure. Inadequate amounts of vitamin D increase the boron requirement. Boron is necessary for the development and maintenance of strong, healthy bones. Boron is principally present in foods of plant origin, especially fruits, vegetables, nuts, legumes, and wine.

Boron deficiency affects mineral metabolism. Patients with disturbed mineral metabolic disorders of unknown etiology, such as osteoporosis, may be deficient in boron.

NICKEL

The physiological role of nickel is still unclear. It may be involved in the metabolism of vitamin B_{12} and folic acid. Nickel deficiency results in suboptimal growth in animals. Inadequate nickel alters trace-element composition of bone and impairs iron use. Good sources of nickel include dried beans and peas, grains, nuts, and chocolate.

SILICON

Silicon contributes to the structure and resilience of collagen, elastin, and polysaccharides. Silicon is present in tooth enamel in larger amounts than most other trace elements, but its function, if any, is unknown. Deficiencies in animal studies result in depressed collagen in bone and long bone abnormalities, resulting in malformed joints and defective bone growth. Whole grains and root vegetables are good food sources.

TIN

Tin has no known function in development or maintenance of bone, but it may affect bone metabolism because tin accumulates in bone. The absorption of tin can alter use of calcium and zinc, affecting bone growth and maintenance. Animal studies have shown that a high level of tin in the diet results in decreased collagen synthesis and decreased compressive strength of bones. Although results of studies have been inconsistent, several investigators believe that **stannous** (chemical term for tin) fluoride exhibits more cariostatic activity than other fluoride compounds by reducing plaque biofilm and gingivitis.

Most Americans consume only small amounts of tin daily because most foods contain trace amounts of tin. Foods packed in tin cans that are totally coated with lacquer contain very little tin, but acidic foods, such as pineapple and orange juice and tomato sauce, packed in cans that are not coated with lacquer contain significant amounts of tin. Other sources of tin include stannous chloride, approved for use as a food additive, and stannous fluoride, the active ingredient in some self-applied dentifrices and mouth rinses.

ALUMINUM

Aluminum probably is not an essential nutrient; its presence in the body seems to be harmful. Under normal conditions, very little aluminum is absorbed; the kidneys excrete about the same amount as is absorbed.

Aluminum accumulates in bone and has been observed to cause **osteodystrophy** (defective bone formation) in patients who have received aluminum from routes other than through the gastrointestinal tract. Water used in intravenous solutions and dialysis fluid is sometimes contaminated with aluminum. The kidneys are frequently unable to remove the daily load of aluminum present in these fluids, causing undesirable effects. Aluminum content of these fluids has been reduced, but may still be high because of naturally occurring aluminum in the water used to make the solutions. Aluminum accumulation can occur through oral ingestion of aluminum hydroxide antacids and from the diet.

Aluminum is also present in all dental tissues. Dental caries may be reduced because aluminum enhances the uptake and retention of fluoride and enhances the cariostatic activity of fluoride. Solubility of enamel is decreased, and plaque biofilm formation and acidogenicity are inhibited by aluminum.

LEAD

Much information is available about the harmful effects of lead in the body, but little is known about its beneficial role or its essentiality. As a result of implementation of aggressive public health measures, blood lead levels have decreased markedly since the late 1970s. In the *National Health and Nutrition Examination Survey* (NHANES II) study from 1976-1980, median blood levels were greater than 20 μg/dL, but relatively few adults had levels greater than 20 μg/dL in the NHANES III study conducted from 1988-1994. Based on analysis of mortality data from NHANES III, blood lead levels of 5 to 9 μg/dL were associated with an increased risk of death from all causes, cardiovascular disease, and cancer.[10]

Lead is more readily absorbed from the gastrointestinal tract during infancy and early childhood than in adulthood, meaning children are more susceptible to lead exposure. Lead is ingested from toddlers' normal hand-to-mouth activities; in older children, playing with dirt or lead-contaminated objects may result in lead ingestion. Milk intake results in reduced lead absorption. Nutritional status can influence susceptibility to lead toxicity.

Inorganic lead can have detrimental effects on children. Even low levels of lead exposure may impair intellectual performance. As serum lead levels increase, general cognitive, verbal, and perceptual abilities are increasingly affected by slower learning aptitudes, which seem to be irreversible. Lead toxicity is most pronounced in children and fetuses because it can damage the central nervous system and kidneys. Lead also decreases normal production of RBCs.

A large proportion of absorbed lead is incorporated into the skeleton and teeth. Lead deposited in the enamel matrix has been associated with pitting hypoplasia. The amount of lead in shed deciduous teeth can be used as an index of lead exposure. The effects of lead stored in the bones and teeth are unknown. Elevated levels of lead in the blood have been positively associated with periodontitis for men and women.[11]

LITHIUM

Lithium is another ultratrace element found in calcified structures. As lithium accumulates in animal bones, calcium content decreases. When this substitution is made in apatite of bone and teeth, the structure and solubility properties are changed. A decreased calcium-to-phosphorus ratio of apatite caused by lithium substitution is accompanied by an increase in acid solubility.

VANADIUM

Studies on the essentiality of vanadium have been inconsistent in their findings. Most research has not found vanadium deficiency consistently impairs any biological function in animals. Vanadium is readily incorporated into areas of rapid mineralization of bones and tooth dentin, but its role in bones and teeth is unknown.

The cariostatic effect of vanadium has been studied. Although an inverse correlation between vanadium content in drinking water and caries incidence was observed in one study, animal experiments are inconclusive in their results.

It has been hypothesized that vanadium may exchange for phosphorus in the apatite tooth substance. Shellfish, mushrooms, and parsley contain small amounts of vanadium.

MERCURY

Mercury is not a nutrient, but this toxic substance is often found in the food and water supply either naturally in the environment or emitted by industrial pollution. Even a trace amount of mercury can cause neurological and developmental problems in infants and young children. It is also harmful to the kidney and cardiovascular system. The U.S. Food and Drug Administration (FDA) monitors the presence of contaminants in food and water, issuing warnings as needed. In 2001, the FDA advised women of childbearing age, pregnant and nursing women, and young children to avoid shark, swordfish, mackerel, and tilefish because of the high levels of methyl mercury. In 2004, the FDA and EPA issued a warning to potentially vulnerable consumers (i.e., young children and pregnant and nursing women) to limit their intake of albacore tuna to less than 6 oz per week because of its mercury content.

Dental Hygiene Considerations

- Boron deficiency signs may be related to abnormalities in vitamin D, calcium, phosphorus, or magnesium levels.
- Aluminum is a cariostatic agent, especially in combination with fluoride.
- Dental offices may be a source of methyl mercury in the public water supply. If this contaminated water is consumed by fish, it ends up in the food supply.[12]
- Dental patients in Maine, California, Connecticut, and Vermont, and some European countries must receive informed consent information about the amalgam restorative material being used.[13]
- Seafood is a good source of important nutrients, including omega-3 fats. The American Heart Association recommends at least two servings of fish each week. Encourage fish and shellfish with lower mercury levels, such as salmon, clams, sardines, crabs, tilapia, scallops, catfish, perch, whitefish, canned tuna, cod, and mahi-mahi. (Large, older fish higher up on the food chain such as shark and swordfish, king mackerel, or tilefish are the leading source of mercury in the diet.)

Nutritional Directions

- A diet low in boron increases calcium excretion, so patients with osteoporosis should be encouraged to consume more fresh fruits and vegetables.
- Acidic foods and foods with high nitrate content such as tomatoes can accumulate very high levels of tin if stored in unlaquered opened cans in the refrigerator for more than 3 days. Once opened, these foods should be transferred to glass or plastic containers.
- Consumption of a variety of foods and fluids helps obtain trace minerals and avoid excessive amounts.
- Unrefined foods generally provide more trace minerals than highly refined foods.
- Supplements of these trace elements are not encouraged.
- Some bone meal and oyster shell used for calcium supplementation may contain dangerous amounts of lead.

HEALTH APPLICATION **9** **Alzheimer's Disease**

Alzheimer's disease is the major cause of dementia in individuals older than 65 years old. In 2008, an estimated 5.2 million Americans had Alzheimer's disease; 5 million of those individuals were older than 65. Alzheimer's disease is the seventh leading cause of death. Directly and indirectly, it costs the American society $148 billion annually.[14] The incidence increases with age: 10% of individuals older than 65 and 50% of individuals older than 85 have Alzheimer's disease. It is a slowly progressive disease, characterized by deterioration of judgment, orientation, memory, personality, and intellectual capability, with a usual duration of 8 to 10 years between onset and death.

Known risk factors for developing Alzheimer's disease are age, a family history of Alzheimer's disease, and genes. Currently, there is no treatment available to delay or stop the progressive deterioration of brain cells in Alzheimer's disease. Research suggests the health of the brain is a key to preventing Alzheimer's disease. The Alzheimer's Association has compiled a list of 10 ways to "Maintain Your Brain" because the brain, being one of the body's most highly vascular organs, is closely linked to the overall health of the heart and blood vessels (Box 9-1).

Although much has been learned about the disease, a specific cause has not been determined. Different types of nerve cells of the brain degenerate and die. Similarities observed between aluminum toxicity and Alzheimer's disease led to the hypothesis that dietary or environmental aluminum might be involved. As a result, the public was inaccurately advised that aluminum cookware could be toxic. Chelation therapy was advocated to remove aluminum from the body as an unorthodox treatment for Alzheimer's disease. However, brain lesions and neurotransmitter changes seen in aluminum toxicity and Alzheimer's disease are different. In contrast to the subtle cognitive changes associated with Alzheimer's disease, aluminum toxicity manifests with motor dysfunction.

A key element of disease management is early diagnosis to initiate therapy. Some causes of dementia can be treated, and some of the symptoms can possibly be reversed. A series of evaluations are used to make a clinical diagnosis of Alzheimer's disease, including medical and behavioral assessments. Often, reports from family members and friends provide valuable information regarding mental status of the individual. The Alzheimer's Association has developed "warning signs" for detection of Alzheimer's disease (Box 9-2).

The FDA has approved several medications to treat cognitive symptoms of Alzheimer's disease. Behavioral and psychiatric symptoms, such as physical or verbal outbursts, restlessness, hallucinations, and delusions, are treated with medications specifically to control the symptoms or nondrug treatments. Vitamin E supplementation is sometimes prescribed by the healthcare provider because it is an antioxidant and may protect nerve cells from certain kinds of chemical wear and tear. Although vitamin E may delay slightly the loss of ability to perform daily activities, it should never be used except under the supervision of a healthcare provider.

Many herbal remedies, vitamins, and other nutrition supplements are promoted as memory enhancers or treatments. Studies involving these alternative therapies have been ineffective. Currently, promoters of ginkgo biloba (plant extract), huperzine A (moss extract), coenzyme Q10 (antioxidant naturally occurring in the body), coral calcium, omega-3 fatty acids, and phosphatidylserine (phospholipid) claim these products can cure or prevent Alzheimer's disease.[15] Further scientific studies are required not only to determine the effectiveness of alternative nutritional therapies, but also to observe the performance of these therapies in the body and their reaction with other drugs or nutrients.

Alzheimer's disease has significant effects on nutritional and hydration status. Initially, individuals with Alzheimer's disease may have problems with food purchasing and meal preparation. Appetite and food intake fluctuate with mood swings and increasing confusion. Forgetting when they last ate, they may skip some meals, eat twice, or forget about food cooking on the stove. Changes in food preferences may be tied to decreases in olfactory function. Sweet and salty foods are preferred.

During the middle phase of the illness, individuals with Alzheimer's disease often become agitated and may pace all night, increasing caloric expenditure. Weight loss is common. Energy requirements may increase by 1600 kcal per day, and frequent snacking is necessary to maintain body weight. Because of abnormal sleep patterns, caffeine may need to be discontinued as it stimulates the central nervous system.

Appetite is usually good, but caloric intake is usually inadequate to maintain body weight unless snacks or liquid nutritional supplements or both are provided. Food hoarding (to accumulate or stash food) or failure to chew food sufficiently increases the risk of choking. Ability to use utensils deteriorates. Finger foods may be more appropriate to allow continuation of self-feeding. Foods requiring cutting should be presented already cut. Serving foods one at a time helps decrease confusion. A larger meal at midday, when cognitive abilities are at their peak, is recommended.

During the final stage, which is characterized by severe intellectual impairment, food may not be recognized and may be refused. The individual also may forget how to swallow. **Enteral feedings** (provision of nutrients via tube placed in the nose, stomach, or small intestine) are usually indicated to maintain nutritional status as a result of this impaired cognition.

Box 9-1 Maintain Your Brain

- Head first. Good health starts with your brain. It's one of the most vital body organs, and it needs care and maintenance.
- Take brain health to heart. Heart disease, high blood pressure, diabetes, and stroke can increase your risk of Alzheimer's.
- Your numbers count. Keep your body weight, blood pressure, cholesterol, and blood sugar levels within recommended ranges.
- Feed your brain. Eat a low-fat, low-cholesterol diet that features dark-skinned vegetables and fruits; food rich in antioxidants; vitamins E, C and B_{12}; folate; and omega-3 fatty acids.
- Work your body. Physical exercise keeps the blood flowing and encourages new brain cells. It doesn't have to be a strenuous activity. Do what you can, like walking 30 minutes a day, to keep both body and mind active.
- Jog your mind. Keeping your brain active and engaged increases its vitality and builds reserves of brain cells and connections. Read, write, play games, and do crossword puzzles.
- Connect with others. Leisure activities that combine physical, mental, and social elements may be most likely to prevent dementia. Be social, converse, volunteer, and join.
- Heads up! Protect your brain. Take precautions against injuries. Use your car seat belts; unclutter your house to avoid falls; and wear a helmet when cycling.
- Use your head. Avoid unhealthy habits. Don't smoke, drink excessive alcohol, or use street drugs.
- Think ahead—start today! You can do something today to protect your tomorrow.

From Alzheimer's Association: Brain health. Available at www.alz.org/we_can_help_brain_health_maintain_your_brain.asp. Accessed May 11, 2008.

Box 9-2 Warning Signs of Alzheimer's Disease

- Memory loss of recently learned information
- Difficulty performing familiar tasks
- Problems with language
- Disorientation to time and place
- Poor or decreased judgment
- Problems with abstract thinking
- Misplacing things
- Changes in mood or behavior
- Changes in personality
- Loss of initiative

From Alzheimer's Association: Symptoms of Alzheimer's. Available at http://www.alz.org/alzheimers_disease_symptoms_of_alzheimers.asp. Accessed May 11, 2008.

CASE APPLICATION FOR THE DENTAL HYGIENIST

A young female executive confides in you that she always feels tired and sometimes finds it difficult to get through the day. When you bring up the subject of nutrition, she tells you that she read a book about the importance of minerals and began taking supplements approximately 1 year ago. These self-prescribed supplements include selenium and zinc. She also takes a vitamin C supplement daily. She is concerned about a lack of energy, which she relates to her poor eating habits. Meals are frequently missed or eaten at her desk.

Nutritional Assessment
- Willingness to learn
- Knowledge level regarding food consumption guidelines, such as the MyPyramid and the *Dietary Guidelines for Americans 2005*
- Desire for improving nutritional and general health
- Cultural or religious influences
- Knowledge of the physiological roles of vitamins and minerals
- Recognition of the interactive effects of vitamins and minerals, especially when taken in excess of the RDA

Nutritional Diagnosis
Health-seeking behaviors related to inadequate knowledge of optimal nutrition, healthy eating habits, and the deleterious effects associated with consumption of excess vitamins and minerals.

Nutritional Goals
The patient will use the *Dietary Guidelines for Americans 2005* and MyPyramid to improve her eating pattern and dietary intake of nutrient-dense foods. The patient will recognize the health risks associated with improper supplementation and will decrease reliance on nutritional supplements.

Nutritional Implementation
Intervention: Review the *Dietary Guidelines for Americans 2005*, and discuss how these guidelines support healthy eating habits and disease prevention.
Rationale: Healthy dietary practices can improve energy reserves and overall nutritional status.
Intervention: Encourage consumption of a variety of foods from each of the five main food groups.
Rationale: A nutritious diet is composed of a variety of foods that together supply all the essential nutrients needed for good health.
Intervention: Review serving sizes and emphasize more servings of foods that are nutrient-dense and low in kilocalories. Encourage a meal timetable that is planned according to each day's schedule.
Rationale: Eating an inadequate number of kilocalories from foods that are limited in nutrients can contribute to fatigue and poor nutrition. Scheduled mealtimes throughout the day help

CASE APPLICATION FOR THE DENTAL HYGIENIST—cont'd

to supply an adequate number of kilocalories when appropriate serving sizes of nutritious food are selected.

Intervention: Describe the body's metabolic need for vitamins and minerals. Advise the patient a well-balanced diet can supply all the nutrients needed without supplementation.

Rationale: Vitamins and minerals are required for normal metabolic and physiological functions. When supplements are taken in excess of the DRIs, some nutrients can be harmful.

Intervention: Describe how zinc supplements interact with copper absorption and relate to fatigue. Inform the patient that large amounts of vitamin C in excess of the RDA may decrease the availability of copper in the blood. List the toxic effects of selenium.

Rationale: Because most minerals are supplied by a varied diet, supplementation can result in toxic levels and harmful nutrient interactions.

Intervention: Advise the patient to see her healthcare provider if fatigue persists or worsens.

Rationale: Poor dietary intake may act as a contributing factor to fatigue when the actual cause may be related to a systemic disease or condition.

Evaluation

The patient will improve dietary habits by planning meals and snacks each day. Meal planning will accommodate the patient's work schedule. The patient will use MyPyramid and the Dietary Guidelines to improve the nutritional quality and quantity of her diet. The patient can state the symptoms associated with large quantities of zinc, selenium, and vitamin C, and will stop taking supplements. Persistent or worsening symptoms of fatigue will prompt the patient to seek the advice of a healthcare provider.

STUDENT READINESS

1. List all nutrient interactions indicated in this chapter that decrease absorption of or alter the metabolism of another nutrient. Why would a dental hygienist advise a patient to obtain mineral requirements from food sources rather than mineral supplements (unless ordered by a healthcare provider)?
2. Which trace minerals incorporated into enamel are beneficial? Which weaken the tooth, or make it more susceptible to tooth decay?
3. Which element is involved in insulin metabolism?
4. If a patient is concerned about obtaining adequate amounts of trace elements, what are some suggestions that a dental hygienist can make?
5. Name some minerals that may be useful as well as toxic to patients.

References

1. Shashikiran ND, et al: Estimation of trace elements in sound and carious enamel of primary and permanent teeth by atomic absorption spectrophotometry: an in vitro study. Indian J Dent Res 2007 Oct-Dec; 18(4):157-162.
2. Harris HH, et al: A link between copper and dental caries in human teeth identified by x-ray fluorescence elemental mapping. J Biol Inorg Chem 2008 Feb; 13(2):303-306.
3. Bleys J, Navas-Acien A, Guallar E: Serum selenium levels and all-cause, cancer, and cardiovascular mortality among US adults. Arch Intern Med 2008 Feb 25; 168(4):404-410.
4. Vincent JL, Forceville X: Critically elucidating the role of selenium. Curr Opin Anaesthesiol 2008 Apr; 21(2):148-154.
5. American Diabetes Association: Standards of Medical Care in Diabetes, 2009. Diabetes Care 2009 Jan; 32(Suppl 1): S13-S61.
6. DiSilvestro RA, Dy E: Comparison of acute absorption of commercially available chromium supplements. J Trace Elem Med Biol 2007; 21(2):120-124.
7. Roussel AM, et al: Food chromium content, dietary chromium intake and related biological variables in French free-living elderly. Br J Nutr 2007 Aug; 98(2):326-331.
8. U.S. Environmental Protection Agency: Health effects support document for manganese. EPA 822-R-03-003. Available at www.epa.gov/safewater/ccl/pdf/manganese.pdf. Accessed May 16, 2008.
9. Ljung K, Vahter M: Time to re-evaluate the guideline value for manganese in drinking water? Environ Health Perspect 2007 Nov; 115(11):1533-1538.
10. Schober SE, et al: Blood lead levels and death from all causes, cardiovascular disease, and cancer: results from the NHANES III mortality study. Environ Health Perspect 2006 Oct; 114(10):1538-1541.
11. Saraiva MC, et al: Lead exposure and periodontitis in US adults. J Periodontal Res 2007 Feb; 42(1):45-52.
12. Zhao X, et al: Characterization of methyl mercury in dental wastewater and correlation with sulfate-reducing bacterial DNA. Environ Sci Technol 2008 Apr 15; 42(8):2780-2786.
13. Edlich RF, et al: Need for informed consent for dentists who use mercury amalgam restorative material as well as technical considerations in removal of dental amalgam restorations. J Environ Pathol Toxicol Oncol 2007; 26(4):305-322.
14. Alzheimer's Association: 2008 Alzheimer's disease facts and figures. Alzheimer Dementia 2008; 4(2):110-133. Available at www.alz.org. Accessed May 11, 2008.
15. Alzheimer's Association: Alternative treatments. Available at www.alz.org/alzheimer_disease_alternative_treatments.asp. Accessed May 11, 2008.

Chapter 10

Vitamins Required for Oral Soft Tissues and Salivary Glands

LEARNING OBJECTIVES

Upon completion of this chapter, the student will be able to achieve the following objectives:
- Describe oral soft tissue changes that occur in a B-complex deficiency.

- Differentiate between scientifically based evidence versus food fads concerning vitamins.
- Discuss the role and sources of vitamin B₁₂ for vegetarians.

Test Your NQ

1. **T/F** Milk is a good source of riboflavin.
2. **T/F** Vitamin B$_6$ is the sunshine vitamin.
3. **T/F** Beriberi is caused by niacin deficiency.
4. **T/F** Vegans may be prone to vitamin B$_{12}$ deficiency.
5. **T/F** Complaints of flushing and intestinal disturbances are symptoms of thiamin toxicity.
6. **T/F** A smooth purplish red or magenta tongue may be observed in patients with vitamin B$_6$ deficiency.
7. **T/F** Whole grains are rich in thiamin.
8. **T/F** Carrots are a good source of folate.
9. **T/F** Thiamin requirement is determined by one's caloric requirement.
10. **T/F** The first signs of a nutritional deficiency often occur in the oral cavity.

PHYSIOLOGY OF SOFT TISSUES

The oral cavity can reflect systemic disease before other **signs** (noticeable to the clinician) and **symptoms** (perceived by the patient) become evident; the condition in the oral cavity may also cause systemic problems by affecting the patient's nutrient intake. The oral cavity is the site of a wide variety of systemic disease manifestations for several reasons: (1) it has a rapid cellular turnover rate, (2) it is under constant assault by microorganisms, and (3) it is a trauma-intense environment.

The systemic circulation provides nutrients and removes metabolic waste products from underlying structures and the salivary glands via the blood supply. Figure 10-1 shows healthy gingiva; changes in color, size, shape, texture, and functional integrity of the oral tissues often reflect systemic nutritional disorders. Signs and symptoms in soft oral tissues can be caused by deficiencies of many of the B-complex vitamins, vitamins C and K, iron, and protein (Box 10-1). Nutritional deficiencies result in similar oral signs and symptoms, such as pain, erythema, atrophy of tissues, and infection. **Pyogenic** (producing pus) and **fungating** (skin lesions with ulcerations, necrosis, and foul smell) microorganisms cause local infections in cracked epithelial surfaces. Approximately 90% of the saliva is produced and secreted by three paired sets of major salivary glands: the parotid, submandibular, and sublingual glands (Fig. 10-2). Additionally, the lips and inner lining of the cheeks are equipped with hundreds of minor salivary glands.

Saliva keeps surfaces of the oral cavity healthy and lubricated and is necessary to maintain functional integrity of taste buds. Solid substances first must be dissolved in saliva to be tasted. Healthy adults produce approximately 1 to 1.5 L of saliva per day. **Sympathetic** impulses influence salivary composition; **parasympathetic** stimulation increases the amount of saliva secreted. Sympathetic autonomic nerves stimulate the body in times of stress and crisis. Parasympathetic autonomic nerves balance or slow down impulses from sympathetic nerves.

Compared with plasma, saliva is **hypotonic**, with its main constituent being water. Hypotonic solutions have a lower solute concentration than plasma. Saliva contains more than 20 proteins and glycoproteins, and many electrolytes, including sodium, potassium, calcium, chloride, bicarbonate, inorganic phosphate, magnesium, sulfate, iodide, and fluoride. Saliva functions as a buffer to maintain the oral pH. Buffering substances increase their acid or alkali content to change the pH of the solution. The pH of unstimulated saliva is approximately 6.1, but this can increase to 7.8 at high flow rates. Antimicrobial properties of saliva provide protection and remove toxins, such as tobacco smoke.

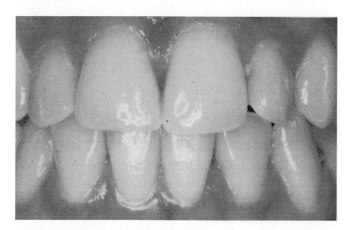

FIGURE 10-1 Normal gingiva. (Courtesy of Barbara D. Altshuler, BSDH, MS, Clinical Assistant Professor, Caruth School of Dental Hygiene, The Texas A&M University System, Baylor College of Dentistry; Dallas, TX.)

Box 10-1	**Vitamins and Minerals Required for Healthy Oral Soft Tissues**

Water-Soluble Vitamins
B Vitamins
Thiamin
Riboflavin
Niacin
Vitamin B$_6$
Folate
Vitamin B$_{12}$
Pantothenic acid
Biotin
Vitamin C

Fat-Soluble Vitamins
Vitamin A
Vitamin K

Minerals
Iron
Zinc
Iodine

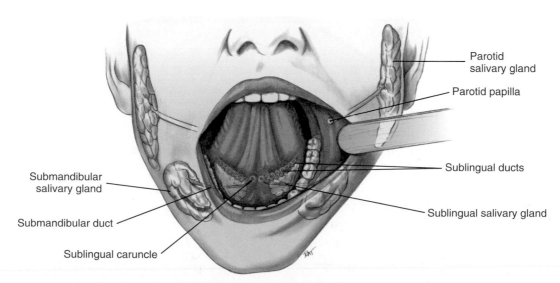

FIGURE 10-2 The major salivary glands and associated structures. (From Fehrenbach MJ, Herring SW: Illustrated Anatomy of the Head and Neck, 3rd ed. Philadelphia: Saunders, 2007.)

The oral cavity is lined with nonkeratinizing mucosa except for the hard palate, dorsum of the tongue, and gingiva surrounding the teeth, which are covered with a keratinized epithelium. The oral cavity may contain **antigenic** (capable of inducing a specific immune response with specific antibodies) substances; the oral mucosa separates a potentially adverse environment from underlying connective tissue.

Mucosal cells have a very rapid turnover rate, resulting in complete turnover in 3 to 5 days. Rapid generation of new cells in the oral epithelia provides replacement tissue for trauma resulting from friction of the teeth and mastication. Additionally, the hundreds of cells in the **filiform papillae** and **fungiform papillae** are in constant transition, from their anabolism until their catabolism (Fig. 10-3). The filiform papillae are smooth, threadlike structures on the dorsum surface of the tongue, whereas the fungiform papillae are red, mushroom-shaped structures scattered throughout the filiform papillae.

Taste buds are located on the **foliate papillae** (vertical grooves located on the lateral borders of the tongue), **circumvallate lingual papillae** (large, mushroom-shaped distinct structures forming a "V") on the dorsal surface, and the fungiform papillae of the tongue. A loss of fungiform and foliate papillae leads to loss of taste buds and changes in taste acuity.

Many filiform papillae cover the anterior two-thirds of the tongue. If the filiform papillae become denuded or atrophied, the tongue appears red and pebbled, or has a strawberry appearance. Fungiform papillae are bright red because of a rich vascular supply. Keratinized cells normally cover the fungiform papillae on the tongue surface. Chronic severe nutrient deficiencies result in loss of fungiform papillae and a smooth red tongue.

Dental Hygiene Considerations

- Because of the rapid turnover rate of oral tissues, the first signs of nutritional deficiency are frequently evident in the oral cavity. The glossal epithelium is usually the first to be affected, followed by areas around the lips. Assess patients for oral signs of nutritional deficiencies.
- The tongue may become edematous as a result of disease or nutritional deficiency.
- Angular cheilitis or **cheilosis** (cracks around the corners of the mouth) and **glossitis** (inflammation of the tongue) are commonly associated with deficiencies of several B-complex vitamins.
- Saliva aids in the ability to speak properly, and taste and swallow foods.
- The composition of saliva affects taste and can be a determining factor in food choices.
- Xerostomia may result in increased incidence of caries, **stomatitis** (inflammation of the oral mucosa), gingival inflammation, and greater susceptibility to oral infections (see Chapter 18).
- Saliva may be used to diagnose some local and systemic diseases and heavy-metal toxicity, such as mercury toxicity.
- Salivary secretion is controlled primarily by cholinergic parasympathetic nerves; patients taking anticholinergic medications (which usually contain atropine) exhibit decreased salivary flow. These medications may be prescribed for bradycardia (low heart rate), diarrhea, peptic ulcers, and occasionally asthma.

Nutritional Directions

- Saliva helps maintain the integrity of the teeth, tongue, and mucous membranes of the oral and oropharyngeal areas.
- Nutritional abnormalities affect oral soft tissues in a variety of ways (e.g., angular cheilitis and glossitis).

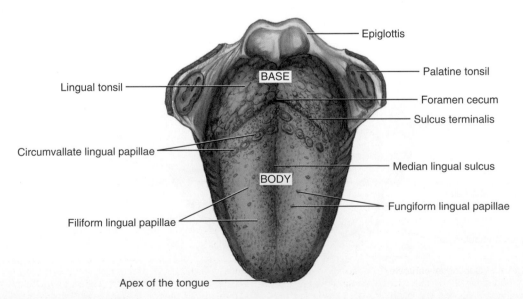

FIGURE 10-3 Papillae on the tongue with its landmarks noted. (From Fehrenbach MJ, Herring SW: Illustrated Anatomy of the Head and Neck, 3rd ed. Philadelphia: Saunders, 2007.)

THIAMIN (VITAMIN B₁)

PHYSIOLOGICAL ROLES

Thiamin functions as a coenzyme in metabolism of energy nutrients via the Krebs cycle or citric acid cycle to produce energy. This role makes it crucial for normal functioning of the brain, nerves, muscles, and heart. However, the main effects of thiamin deficiency are disturbances of carbohydrate metabolism, which is impossible without thiamin. Thiamin is also a necessary component in the synthesis of niacin and helps regulate appetite. It is a constituent of enzymes that degrade sucrose to organic acids that can ultimately dissolve tooth enamel.

REQUIREMENTS

Thiamin is involved in using carbohydrates as kilocalories; the requirement is based on total caloric need. The recommended dietary allowance (RDA) for men (14 years old and older) is 1.2 mg per day and for women (19 years old and older) is 1.1 mg per day (Table 10-1). Participation in rigorous physical activity uses more energy, so more thiamin is required. Also, requirements are increased by pregnancy and lactation, hemodialysis or peritoneal dialysis, fever, hyperthyroidism, cardiac conditions, and alcoholism. No known adverse effects are evident from excessive thiamin intake, including supplements. Care should be taken, however, when consumption is in excess of the RDA because a tolerable upper intake level (UL) was not established for thiamin.

SOURCES

Thiamin is widely distributed in foods, and intake of a variety of foods, including whole grains or enriched grains, can ensure adequate amounts (Table 10-2). Approximately 40% of thiamin intake is provided by whole-grain products and enriched breads, cereals, and pasta. In the meat group, pork is an exceptionally good source. Other good sources include nuts and legumes. Following the guidelines of MyPyramid by eating a variety of foods ensures adequate intake. Thiamin synthesized by intestinal bacteria is absorbed in the large intestine.[1]

HYPO-STATES

Thiamin is required for metabolism of carbohydrates, proteins, and fats; a wide range of symptoms develops with insufficient intake. Primary dietary deficiency usually occurs in developing countries where polished rice is the staple diet. In developed countries, thiamin deficiency is secondary to alcoholism, ingestion of raw fish containing microbial **thiaminase** (an enzyme that inactivates thiamin), chronic febrile states, and total parenteral nutrition (TPN). Cooking deactivates thiaminase.

Thiamin is called the "morale vitamin" because short-term deficiency causes patients to become depressed, irritable, anorexic, fatigued, and unable to concentrate. The brain and central nervous system (CNS), almost entirely dependent on glucose for energy, are seriously impaired when thiamin is unavailable.

Severe thiamin deficiency results in **beriberi**, which causes extensive damage to the nervous and cardiovascular

Table 10-1	Institute of Medicine Recommendations for Thiamin				
	EAR (mg/d)*		RDA (mg/d)†		
Life Stage	Male	Female	Male	Female	AI (mg/d)‡
0-6 mo					0.2
7-12 mo					0.3
1-3 yr	0.4	0.4	0.5	0.5	
4-8 yr	0.5	0.5	0.6	0.6	
9-13 yr	0.7	0.7	0.9	0.9	
14-18 yr	1	1	1.2	1	
19->70 yr	1	0.9	1.2	1.1	
Pregnancy 14-50 yr		1.2		1.4	
Lactation 14-50 yr		1.2		1.4	

Data from Institute of Medicine (IOM), Food and Nutrition Board: Dietary Reference Intakes for Thiamin, Riboflavin, Niacin, Vitamin B₆, Folate, Vitamin B₁₂, Pantothenic Acid, Biotin, and Choline. Washington, DC: National Academy Press, 1998.
*EAR (estimated average requirement)—the intake that meets the estimated nutrient needs of half of the individuals in a group.
†RDA (recommended dietary allowance)—the intake that meets the nutrient needs of almost all (97-98%) individuals in a group.
‡AI (adequate intake)—the observed average or experimentally set intake by a defined population or subgroup that seems to sustain a defined nutritional status, such as growth rate, normal circulating nutrient values, or other functional indicators of health. An AI is used if insufficient scientific evidence is available to derive an EAR. For healthy human milk–fed infants, the AI is the mean intake. *The AI is not equivalent to an RDA.*

Table 10-2	Thiamin Content of Selected Foods	
Food	Portion	Thiamin (mg)
Total Raisin Bran	1 cup	1.50
Wheaties	1 cup	0.75
Trail mix, tropical	1 cup	0.69
Bagel	3½-4 inches	0.56
Lean pork chop, broiled	3 oz	0.46
White rice, cooked	1 cup	0.30
Ham, baked	3 oz	0.30
Green peas, cooked	1 cup	0.28
French toast with butter	1 slice	0.17
Peanuts	¼ cup	0.16
Soy milk	1 cup	0.15
Sweet potato (medium), cooked	1	0.12
Enriched white bread	1	0.11
Whole-wheat bread	1	0.10

Data from U.S. Department of Agriculture, Agricultural Research Service, USDA Nutrient Data Laboratory, USDA National Nutrient Database for Standard Reference, Release 20, 2008. Available at http://www.nal.usda.gov/fnic/foodcomp/search. Accessed Feb 25, 2008.

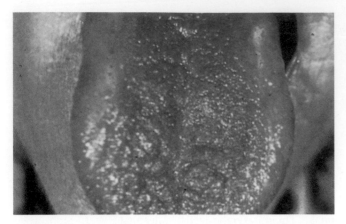

FIGURE 10-4 Glossitis associated with thiamin deficiency. (From American Dental Association Council on Dental Therapeutics: Oral Manifestations of Metabolic and Deficiency Changes. Chicago, IL.)

systems. *Beriberi* means "I cannot"; patients with this severe thiamin deficiency cannot move easily. The classic chronic form of beriberi manifests with impairment of sensory and motor function without involvement of the CNS. Other symptoms include muscular wasting (dry beriberi), edema (wet beriberi), deep muscle pain in the calves, peripheral paralysis, tachycardia, and an enlarged heart.

Whether or not a thiamin deficiency is evident in oral tissues is controversial. Some clinicians have associated a flabby, red, and edematous tongue with thiamin deficiency (Fig. 10-4). The fungiform papillae enlarge and become hyperemic.

Dental Hygiene Considerations

- A careful medical, social, and dietary history, including a clinical assessment of the oral cavity, alcohol consumption, and activity level, helps identify early stages of thiamin deficiency.
- Risk of alcohol abuse or dependence is based on how much and how often an individual drinks. Moderation is considered 4 to 14 drinks per week for men and 3 to 7 drinks per week for women.[2]
- Vitamin deficiencies seldom occur in isolation. If a deficiency is suspected, symptoms of other vitamin B deficiencies also may be present.
- Because thiamin is essential for carbohydrate metabolism, a thiamin deficiency is closely linked to aberrations of brain function. For patients who are confused or have altered thought processes, assess nutrient intake.
- Carbohydrate loading or a very-high-carbohydrate diet and high physical activity slightly increase the thiamin requirement. (Generally, increased intake results in increased thiamin consumption.)
- Thiamin deficiency has been reported in patients after gastrectomy[3] and bariatric surgery.[4,5]
- Although immediate clinical response to thiamin therapy is often dramatic, ultimate recovery may be incomplete, and relapses may occur, especially if precipitating factors persist.

Nutritional Directions

- Raw fish contain an active enzyme, thiaminase, which destroys thiamin.
- Baking soda added to cooking water to enhance the color of vegetables destroys thiamin.
- Overcooking and high temperatures destroy thiamin.
- Antacids reduce use of thiamin.
- Some diuretics can increase thiamin excretion.

Wernicke-Korsakoff syndrome is another thiamin deficiency disease typically associated with alcoholism, which is characterized by mental confusion, **nystagmus** (involuntary rapid movement of the eyeball), and **ataxia** (a gait disorder characterized by uncoordinated muscle movements). These symptoms occur most frequently in malnourished alcoholics. Alcohol intake increases thiamin requirement; also, total nutrient intake is usually poor in alcoholics. Early diagnosis is essential to initiate thiamin therapy early in the course of the disease and to prevent permanent damage and death.

RIBOFLAVIN (VITAMIN B₂)

PHYSIOLOGICAL ROLES

Riboflavin functions as a coenzyme in the metabolism of carbohydrate, protein, and fat to release cellular energy. Closely related to the metabolism of protein, all conditions requiring increases in protein (e.g., growth spurts or burns) lead to additional riboflavin requirements. Riboflavin is also essential for healthy eyes and maintenance of mucous membranes. Along with thiamin, riboflavin is necessary for synthesis of niacin.

REQUIREMENTS

As shown in Table 10-3, the Institute of Medicine (IOM) recommends an intake of 1.3 mg per day for men (14 years old and older) and 1.1 mg per day for women (19 years old and older). This level is influenced by individual energy requirements. Additionally, when nitrogen balance is positive, more riboflavin is retained. No UL has been established.

SOURCES

Although milk and milk products are excellent sources of riboflavin, approximately 30% of the dietary intake is furnished by foods in the grain group (Table 10-4). Meat, poultry, and fish also provide about one-fourth of the dietary requirement. As with thiamin, riboflavin synthesized by intestinal bacteria is absorbed in the large intestine.[1]

HYPO-STATES

The body carefully guards its limited riboflavin stores. Even in severe deficiency, one-third of the normal amount is

Table 10-3	Institute of Medicine Recommendations for Riboflavin				
	EAR (mg/d)*		RDA (mg/d)†		
Life Stage	*Male*	*Female*	*Male*	*Female*	AI (mg/d)‡
0-6 mo					0.3
7-12 mo					0.4
1-3 yr	0.4	0.4	0.5	0.5	
4-8 yr	0.5	0.5	0.6	0.6	
9-13 yr	0.8	0.8	0.9	0.9	
14-18 yr	1.1	0.9	1.3	1	
19->70 yr	1.1	0.9	1.3	1.1	
Pregnancy 14-50 yr		1.2		1.4	
Lactation 14-50 yr		1.3		1.6	

Data from Institute of Medicine (IOM), Food and Nutrition Board: Dietary Reference Intakes for Thiamin, Riboflavin, Niacin, Vitamin B_6, Folate, Vitamin B_{12}, Pantothenic Acid, Biotin, and Choline. Washington, DC: National Academy Press, 1998.
*EAR (estimated average requirement)—the intake that meets the estimated nutrient needs of half of the individuals in a group.
†RDA (recommended dietary allowance)—the intake that meets the nutrient needs of almost all (97-98%) individuals in a group.
‡AI (adequate intake)—the observed average or experimentally set intake by a defined population or subgroup that seems to sustain a defined nutritional status, such as growth rate, normal circulating nutrient values, or other functional indicators of health. An AI is used if insufficient scientific evidence is available to derive an EAR. For healthy human milk–fed infants, the AI is the mean intake. *The AI is not equivalent to an RDA.*

Table 10-4	Riboflavin Content of Selected Foods	
Food	Portion	Riboflavin (mg)
Beef liver	3 oz	3.08
Total, whole grain	1 cup	2.13
Soybeans	1 cup	1.3
Wheaties	1 cup	0.85
Chocolate milkshake, thick	11 oz	0.61
Yogurt, plain	8 oz	0.53
Eggnog	1 cup	0.48
Milk	1 cup	0.45
Low-fat cottage cheese	1 cup	0.37
Spinach, cooked	½ cup	0.21
Lean pork loin, baked	3 oz	0.19
Cornbread	1 piece	0.16
Cheddar cheese	1 cup	0.11

Data from U.S. Department of Agriculture, Agricultural Research Service, USDA Nutrient Data Laboratory, USDA National Nutrient Database for Standard Reference, Release 20, 2008. Available at http://www.nal.usda.gov/fnic/foodcomp/search. Accessed Feb 25, 2008.

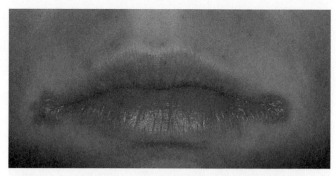

FIGURE 10-5 Angular cheilitis. (From Ibsen OAC, Phelan JA: Oral Pathology for the Dental Hygienist, 5th ed. St. Louis: Elsevier Saunders, 2009.)

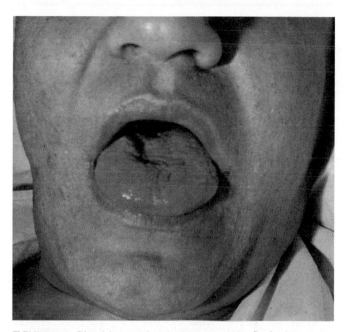

FIGURE 10-6 Glossitis associated with severe riboflavin deficiency. (From McLaren DS: A Colour Atlas and Text of Diet-Related Disorders, 2nd ed. London: Mosby-YearBook Europe Limited, 1992.)

present in the liver, kidney, and heart. Primary riboflavin deficiency is uncommon, but is encountered in patients with multiple nutrient deficiencies as a result of poor nutrient absorption or use. Because riboflavin is essential to the functioning of vitamin B_6 and niacin, riboflavin deficiency leads to symptoms related to secondary deficiency of these nutrients.

Symptoms associated with riboflavin deficiency, or ariboflavinosis, include angular cheilitis (Fig. 10-5), glossitis (Fig. 10-6), dermatitis, and anemia. With consistently inadequate intake, these symptoms may be observed within 8 weeks. Along with angular cheilosis, the lips may become extremely red and smooth. Fungiform papillae become swollen and slightly flattened and mushroom-shaped during early stages of riboflavin deficiency; the tongue has a pebbly or granular appearance. Severe chronic deficiencies lead to progressive papillary atrophy and patchy, irregular denudation of the tongue. The tongue may become purplish red or magenta in color because of vascular proliferation and decreased circulation. In more advanced cases, the entire tongue may become atrophic and smooth (see Fig. 10-6). These symptoms, especially glossitis and dermatitis, may be secondary to vitamin B_6 deficiency.

Dental Hygiene Considerations

- Hyperthyroidism, fevers, the added stress of injuries or surgery, excessive alcohol consumption, and malabsorption syndromes increase riboflavin requirements. Assess patients with these conditions for signs of deficiency: cheilitis, papillary atrophy, glossitis, and dermatitis.
- Congenital facial abnormalities may occur if the mother is deficient in riboflavin at the time of conception.
- Bilateral cheilosis may not be riboflavin deficiency; consider improperly constructed dentures, fungal (candidiasis) or yeast infection, and aging that may contribute to cheilosis.
- Phenothiazines and antibiotics increase excretion of riboflavin, so monitor for a deficiency in patients on long-term therapy.

Nutritional Directions

- Enriched products provide more riboflavin than their whole-grain counterparts.
- Lighted display cases have the potential to cause decomposition of riboflavin when milk is marketed in translucent plastic containers.
- A mixed diet that contains a pint of low-fat milk and 4 to 6 oz of meat daily ensures adequate riboflavin intake.
- Vegans and other individuals who do not consume milk or milk products are at risk of developing riboflavin deficiency.
- Toxicity symptoms are not observed with oral consumption of riboflavin.

NIACIN (VITAMIN B₃)

PHYSIOLOGICAL ROLES

The term *niacin* is loosely used to refer to two compounds, nicotinic acid and nicotinamide. Both compounds are used by the body. Niacin is crucial as a coenzyme in energy (ATP) production. It functions with riboflavin in glucose production and metabolism and is involved in lipid and protein metabolism. Niacin also functions in enzymes involved in the microbial degradation of sucrose to produce organic acids.

REQUIREMENTS

The body obtains niacin not only directly from the diet, but also indirectly from conversion of an amino acid, tryptophan, and from synthesis by intestinal microorganisms. RDAs are given in terms of niacin equivalents (NE), which include dietary sources of niacin plus its precursor, tryptophan. Approximately 1 mg of niacin may be formed from 60 mg of dietary tryptophan. Niacin requirements are related to caloric intake. The RDA NE for adults is 14 to 16 mg daily (Table 10-5). The UL for adults is 35 mg daily. There is no known adverse effect related to dietary intake of niacin occurring naturally in foods.

SOURCES

Niacin is widely distributed in plant and animal foods. Good sources include meats, cereals, legumes, seeds, and nuts

Table 10-5   Institute of Medicine Recommendations for Niacin

Life Stage	EAR (mg/d)*† Male	EAR (mg/d)*† Female	RDA (mg/d)‡§ Male	RDA (mg/d)‡§ Female	AI (mg/d)¶	UL (mg/d)
0-6 mo					2	ND¶
7-12 mo					4	ND
1-3 yr	5	5	6	6		10
4-8 yr	6	6	8	8		15
9-13 yr	9	9	12	12		20
14-18 yr	12	11	16	14		30
≥19 yr	12	11	16	14		35
Pregnancy						
14-18 yr		14		18		30
≥19 yr		14		18		35
Lactation						
14-18 yr		13		17		30
≥19 yr		13		17		35

Data from Institute of Medicine (IOM), Food and Nutrition Board: Dietary Reference Intakes for Thiamin, Riboflavin, Niacin, Vitamin B₆, Folate, Vitamin B₁₂, Pantothenic Acid, Biotin, and Choline. Washington, DC: National Academy Press, 1998.
*EAR (estimated average requirement)—the intake that meets the estimated nutrient needs of half of the individuals in a group.
†Niacin equivalents.
‡RDA (recommended dietary allowance)—the intake that meets the nutrient needs of almost all (97-98%) individuals in a group.
§AI (adequate intake)—the observed average or experimentally set intake by a defined population or subgroup that seems to sustain a defined nutritional status, such as growth rate, normal circulating nutrient values, or other functional indicators of health. An AI is used if insufficient scientific evidence is available to derive an EAR. For healthy human milk–fed infants, the AI is the mean intake. *The AI is not equivalent to an RDA.*
¶Preformed niacin.
¶ND—not determinable because of lack of data of adverse effects in this age group and concern with regard to lack of ability to handle excess amounts. Source of intake should be from food and formula to prevent high levels of intake.

(Table 10-6). Approximately 65% of the niacin in the U.S. diet is provided from meat and milk. Tryptophan is found mainly in milk, eggs, and meats. The RDA for NE is easily met with foods high in niacin plus foods having tryptophan.

HYPER-STATES AND HYPO-STATES

Supplemental doses of nicotinic acid (3 to 6 g per day) are effective in reducing LDL cholesterol and triglycerides, while increasing HDL cholesterol. (Nicotinamide does not function in this role.) Niacin-induced changes in serum lipid levels produce significant improvements in coronary heart disease. The use of 250 mg of nicotinic acid daily results in the vitamin functioning as a vasodilator, producing flushing of the skin, nausea, itching, tachycardia, fainting, and blurred vision. To avoid these problems, long-acting or extended-release niacin is taken once a day. Because the body is able to store some niacin, larger doses associated with supple-

ments may lead to serious problems, including abnormal liver function and gout. The extended-release form of niacin is associated with few gastrointestinal symptoms without increasing liver damage.

Niacin deficiency is usually associated with a maize (corn) diet because corn products contain all the essential amino acids except tryptophan. This diet increases the body's requirements for tryptophan and niacin. The deficiency is also seen in alcoholics, but is unlikely in individuals who consume adequate protein. Niacin deficiency results in degeneration of the skin, gastrointestinal tract, and nervous system, a condition known as **pellagra**. Symptoms of pellagra have been referred to as "the 3 Ds"—dermatitis, diarrhea, and depression or dementia. The term *pellagra* is derived from the Latin word for animal hide; the skin may be rough and look like goose flesh. The most striking and characteristic sign of pellagra is a reddish skin rash, especially on the face, hands, or feet, which is always bilaterally symmetrical (i.e., it appears on both sides of the body at the same time) (Fig. 10-7A). It flares up when the skin is exposed to strong sunlight. Neurological symptoms include depression, apathy, headache, fatigue, and loss of memory. If untreated, death may occur.

Deficiency also affects mucous membranes: (1) painful stomatitis causes diminished food intake, and (2) lesions in the gastrointestinal tract result in diarrhea and less vitamin absorption. Pellagrous glossitis begins with swelling of the papillae at the tip and lateral borders of the tongue. The tongue becomes painful, scarlet, and edematous (Fig. 10-7B). Atrophic changes involve loss of the filiform and fungiform papillae, and the tongue becomes smooth and shiny. The mucosa is also reddened. Fissures occur in the epithelium and along the sides of the tongue; these become infected rapidly. The gingiva may become inflamed, resembling ulcerative gingivitis. The corners of the lips are initially pale; fanlike fissuring occurs that radiates into the perioral epithelium and may leave permanent scars.

Table 10-6	Niacin Content of Selected Foods	
Food	**Portion**	**Niacin (mg)**
Beef liver	3 oz	15.8
Chicken breast, baked	3 oz	12.3
Tuna, canned	3 oz	11.3
Salmon, cooked	3 oz	8.5
Halibut, broiled	3 oz	6.4
Wheaties	1 cup	6.2
Peanuts	¼ cup	4.9
Turkey, dark meat, cooked	1 cup	3.3
Potato, baked	1	2.4
Milk, protein fortified	1 cup	0.3
Milk, skim	1 cup	0.3

Data from U.S. Department of Agriculture, Agricultural Research Service, USDA Nutrient Data Laboratory, USDA National Nutrient Database for Standard Reference, Release 20, 2008. Available at http://www.nal.usda.gov/fnic/foodcomp/search. Accessed Feb 25, 2008.

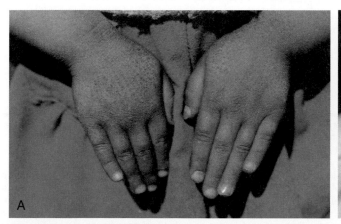 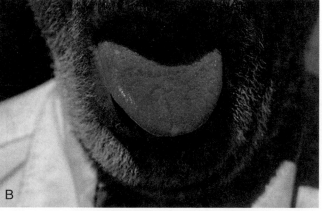

FIGURE 10-7 A, Symmetrical chapping of dorsum of hands. This is a common site for the skin changes of pellagra to occur. A careful history and full examination permit the diagnosis to be made. **B,** Scarlet tongue. The tongue in pellagra is frequently scarlet in appearance and extremely painful. However, this may occur in many non-nutritional conditions, and other signs, especially those in the skin, have to be present to make the clinical diagnosis. Fissuring of the tongue alone is not significant. (From McLaren DS: A Colour Atlas and Text of Diet-Related Disorders, 2nd ed. London: Mosby-YearBook Europe Limited, 1992.)

Dental Hygiene Considerations

- Assess patients, especially alcoholics and immigrants from areas with a heavy dependence on corn or maize, for oral signs of niacin deficiency. Symptoms to watch for include complaints of a nonspecific burning sensation through the oral cavity; smooth, shiny, bright red tongue swollen at the tip and lateral margins; stomatitis; and red and inflamed marginal and attached gingiva.
- Prolonged treatment with isoniazid for tuberculosis may lead to niacin deficiency. Niacin supplements may be prescribed by the healthcare provider to prevent deficiency.

Nutritional Directions

- Patients should understand a frequent side effect of a therapeutic dose of nicotinic acid is flushing. This should be discussed with the healthcare provider.
- Nicotinic acid, nicotinamide, and niacinamide are correct terms for niacin and should not be confused with nicotine.

VITAMIN B₆ (PYRIDOXINE)

Vitamin B_6 is the term commonly used for a group of three compounds, pyridoxine, pyridoxal, and pyridoxamine. All three forms can be used by the body in their role as coenzymes.

PHYSIOLOGICAL ROLES

Several essential roles for vitamin B_6 have been identified. In addition to (1) its role as a coenzyme in protein metabolism, vitamin B_6 plays a part in (2) conversion of tryptophan to niacin, (3) hemoglobin synthesis, (4) synthesis of unsaturated fatty acids from essential fatty acids, (5) energy production from glycogen, and (6) proper functioning of the nervous system including synthesis of neurotransmitters.

REQUIREMENTS

The current RDA for vitamin B_6 ranges from 1.1 to 1.7 mg daily for adults (Table 10-7). The requirement for vitamin B_6 increases with protein intake because of its major role in amino acid metabolism. Limited amounts of vitamin B_6 are produced by microorganisms in the digestive tract. The UL has been determined to be 100 mg per day for adults. Four groups in the U.S. population are frequently deficient in vitamin B_6: women of childbearing age, especially current and former users of oral contraceptives; male smokers; non-Hispanic African-American men; and individuals older than 65 years.[6]

Table 10-7	Institute of Medicine Recommendations for Pyridoxine/Vitamin B₆					
	EAR (mg/d)*		**RDA (mg/d)†**			
Life Stage	*Male*	*Female*	*Male*	*Female*	**AI (mg/d)‡**	**UL (mg/d)§¶**
0-6 mo					0.1	ND¶
7-12 mo					0.3	ND¶
1-3 yr	0.4	0.4	0.5	0.5		30
4-8 yr	0.5	0.5	0.6	0.6		40
9-13 yr	0.8	0.8	1	1		60
14-18 yr	1.1	1	1.3	1.2		80
19-50 yr	1.1	0.9	1.3	1.1		100
51->70 yr	1.4	1.3	1.7	1.5		100
Pregnancy						
14-18 yr		1.6		1.9		80
>19 yr		1.6		1.9		100
Lactation						
14-18 yr		1.7		2		80
>19 yr		1.7		2		100

Data from Institute of Medicine (IOM), Food and Nutrition Board: Dietary Reference Intakes for Thiamin, Riboflavin, Niacin, Vitamin B₆, Folate, Vitamin B₁₂, Pantothenic Acid, Biotin, and Choline. Washington, DC: National Academy Press, 1998.
*EAR (estimated average requirement)—the intake that meets the estimated nutrient needs of half of the individuals in a group.
†RDA (recommended dietary allowance)—the intake that meets the nutrient needs of almost all (97-98%) individuals in a group.
‡AI (adequate intake)—the observed average or experimentally set intake by a defined population or subgroup that seems to sustain a defined nutritional status, such as growth rate, normal circulating nutrient values, or other functional indicators of health. An AI is used if insufficient scientific evidence is available to derive an EAR. For healthy human milk–fed infants, the AI is the mean intake. *The AI is not equivalent to an RDA.*
§UL (tolerable upper intake level)—the highest level of daily nutrient intake that is likely to pose no risk of adverse health effects to almost all individuals in the general population. As intake increases above the UL, the risk of adverse effects increases. Unless specified otherwise, the UL represents total nutrient intake from food, water, and supplements.
¶Vitamin B₆ as pyridoxine.
¶ND—not determinable because of lack of data of adverse effects in this age group and concern with regard to lack of ability to handle excess amounts. Source of intake should be from food and formula to prevent high levels of intake.

SOURCES

Meat, poultry, and fish are good sources of vitamin B_6. Other good sources include some fruits, nuts, fortified cereals, whole-grain products, and vegetables (Table 10-8). Foods from animal and plant sources provide 48% and 52% of the total vitamin B_6 intake. Canning, roasting, boiling, or stewing meat and various food-processing techniques can reduce pyridoxine content of the food as the vitamin is lost in the water.

ABSORPTION AND EXCRETION

Absorption of vitamin B_6 differs from other B-complex vitamins. All three forms of the vitamin are converted to an absorbable form by an intestinal enzyme. Body stores are small, and repletion is gradual.

HYPER-STATES AND HYPO-STATES

Numerous studies have suggested possible benefits of supplemental amounts of vitamin B_6 in coronary heart disease, sickness during pregnancy, premenstrual syndrome, carpal tunnel syndrome, and neuropathies. Because of inconsistent findings, supplemental amounts beyond the UL are not currently recommended. Acute pyridoxine toxicity is uncommon; however, routine consumption of megadoses has documented side effects, including ataxia and **severe sensory neuropathy** (impairment of the ability to sense touch, vibration, temperature, and pinprick) and, in some instances, bone pain and muscle weakness. In most cases, complete recovery occurs with discontinuation of megadose supplementation.

Deficiency rarely occurs alone; vitamin B_6 deficiency is most commonly observed along with deficiency of several other B vitamins. Individuals with poor-quality diets in addition to overall low nutrient intake (e.g., alcoholics and elderly individuals) may experience a deficiency. Clinical signs include CNS abnormalities or convulsions, dermatitis with cheilosis and glossitis, impaired immune responses, and anemia. Pyridoxine deficiency–induced glossitis is denoted by pain, edema, and papillary changes. Initially, the tongue has a scalded sensation, followed by reddening and hypertrophy of the filiform papillae at the tip, margins, and dorsum (Fig. 10-8).

🦷 Dental Hygiene Considerations

- Patients may present with pain of the tongue, which precedes redness and swelling of the tip of the tongue. Eventually, atrophy of papillae results in a smooth, purplish tongue. Angular cheilitis, oral ulcers, and stomatitis also may be noted.
- Intake of this vitamin may be decreased in patients with advanced age, poor education, and lower income status. Encourage foods high in vitamin B_6, and monitor for deficiency signs and symptoms, especially in older patients.
- In animal studies, the presence of pyridoxine alters oral flora and reduces incidence of dental caries.
- Use of drugs affecting vitamin B_6 metabolism warrants supplementation to avoid secondary vitamin B_6 deficiency. These drugs include isoniazid and cycloserine (for tuberculosis), penicillamine (for Wilson's disease, lead poisoning, kidney stones, and arthritis), theophylline (for asthma), and OCAs.
- Excessive pyridoxine can reduce clinical benefits of levodopa therapy in patients with Parkinson's disease or other neurological problems. Encourage these patients to limit intake of foods fortified with vitamin B_6 and to avoid vitamin B_6 supplements. If the desired effects of the drug are not seen, or if over-the-counter supplements are being taken, refer the patient to the healthcare provider.

Table 10-8	Pyridoxine (Vitamin B_6) Content of Selected Foods	
Food	**Portion**	**Pyridoxine (mg)**
Total, whole grain	1 cup	2
Beef liver	3 oz	0.9
Prune juice	1 cup	0.6
Potato, baked	1	0.5
Banana	1	0.4
Peanut butter	2 Tbsp	0.3
Halibut, cooked	3 oz	0.3
Turkey, cooked	3 oz	0.3
Chicken breast, baked	3 oz	0.3
Tuna, canned	3 oz	0.3
Sunflower seeds	1 oz	0.2
Spinach, cooked	½ cup	0.2
Pinto beans	½ cup	0.2
Tomato juice	6 oz	0.2
Lima beans, cooked	½ cup	0.2
Cantaloupe	1 cup	0.1

Data from U.S. Department of Agriculture, Agricultural Research Service, USDA Nutrient Data Laboratory, USDA National Nutrient Database for Standard Reference, Release 20, 2008. Available at http://www.nal.usda.gov/fnic/foodcomp/search. Accessed Feb 25, 2008.

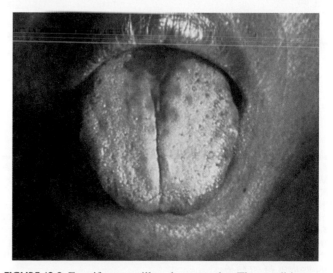

FIGURE 10-8 Fungiform papillary hypertrophy. The condition can be seen and felt as a tongue blade is drawn lightly over the anterior two-thirds of the tongue. The tongue may have a berry-like appearance. (Courtesy of Dr. H.H. Sandstead. From McLaren DS: A Colour Atlas and Text of Diet-Related Disorders, 2nd ed. London: Mosby-YearBook Europe Limited, 1992.)

Nutritional Directions

- Vitamin B_6 supplements should not be taken unless ordered by a healthcare provider.
- If supplements are needed, signs and symptoms improve within 1 week.
- Adequate daily intake of vitamin B_6 is important.
- Vitamin B_6 is removed during grain processing and not replaced during enrichment; whole-grain breads and cereals are better choices.

Stores of vitamin B_6 in a mother's body are critical to the well-being of her newborn infant. Oral contraceptive agents (OCAs) taken before conception may reduce maternal vitamin B_6 levels during pregnancy and in breast milk. An increase in dietary intake of vitamin B_6 may be recommended for women taking OCAs, especially if a pregnancy is planned in the near future.

FOLATE/FOLIC ACID

The generic term *folate* encompasses several compounds that have nutritional properties similar to those of folic acid. Several different metabolically active forms have been identified. The terms *folate, folic acid,* and *folacin* are used interchangeably. Folate is the natural form found in foods, whereas folic acid is a synthetic form used in vitamin supplements and food fortification. Natural folates are chemically unstable.

PHYSIOLOGICAL ROLES

Folate functions as a coenzyme for approximately 20 enzymes. As such, it has an important role in synthesis of RNA and DNA. It functions in conjunction with vitamins B_{12} and C in maintaining normal levels of mature red blood cells (RBCs). It has an important role in proper formation of neural tubes during fetal development.

REQUIREMENTS

As shown in Table 10-9, the RDA is 400 µg for adults. Folate can be expressed as dietary folate equivalents (DFEs), which are equivalent to 1 µg of folate. Requirements for folate are increased during periods of growth and development, such as adolescence, pregnancy, and lactation, because of its role in DNA formulation.

SOURCES

Rich sources of folate include liver, green leafy vegetables, fortified cereals and grain products, legumes, and some fruits (grapefruit and oranges) (Table 10-10). Folate pro-

Table 10-9	Institute of Medicine Recommendations for Folate*					
	EAR (µg/d)†		**RDA (µg/d)‡**			
Life Stage	*Male*	*Female*	*Male*	*Female*	AI (µg/d)§	UL (µg/d)¶¶
0-6 mo					65	ND**
7-12 mo					80	ND
1-3 yr	120	120	150	150		300
4-8 yr	160	160	200	200		400
9-13 yr	250	250	300	300		600
14-18 yr	330	330	400	400		800
19->70 yr	320	320	400	400		1000
Pregnancy						
14-18 yr		520		600		800
≥19 yr		520		600		1000
Lactation						
14-18 yr		450		500		800
≥19 yr		450		500		1000

Data from Institute of Medicine (IOM), Food and Nutrition Board: Dietary Reference Intakes for Thiamin, Riboflavin, Niacin, Vitamin B_6, Folate, Vitamin B_{12}, Pantothenic Acid, Biotin, and Choline. Washington, DC: National Academy Press, 1998.
*Dietary folate equivalents.
†EAR (estimated average requirement)—the intake that meets the estimated nutrient needs of half of the individuals in a group.
‡RDA (recommended dietary allowance)—the intake that meets the nutrient needs of almost all (97-98%) individuals in a group.
§AI (adequate intake)—the observed average or experimentally set intake by a defined population or subgroup that seems to sustain a defined nutritional status, such as growth rate, normal circulating nutrient values, or other functional indicators of health. An AI is used if insufficient scientific evidence is available to derive an EAR. For healthy human milk–fed infants, the AI is the mean intake. *The AI is not equivalent to an RDA.*
¶UL (tolerable upper intake level)—the highest level of daily nutrient intake that is likely to pose no risk of adverse health effects to almost all individuals in the general population. As intake increases above the UL, the risk of adverse effects increases. Unless specified otherwise, the UL represents total nutrient intake from food, water, and supplements.
¶Folate from fortified foods or supplements.
**ND—not determinable because of lack of data of adverse effects in this age group and concern with regard to lack of ability to handle excess amounts. Source of intake should be from food and formula to prevent high levels of intake.

Table 10-10	Folate Content of Selected Foods	
Food	**Portion**	**Folate (μg)**
Total, whole grain	1 cup	400
Beef liver	3 oz	228
Pinto beans	½ cup	147
Asparagus, cooked	½ cup	134
Spinach, cooked	½ cup	131
Enriched white rice	½ cup	131
Navy beans	½ cup	127
Turnip greens, cooked	½ cup	85
Broccoli	½ cup	84
Orange juice	1 cup	72
Romaine lettuce	1 cup	64
Tomato juice	6 oz	51
Navel orange	1	48
Enriched macaroni	½ cup	46
Dry roasted peanuts	1 oz	36
Cantaloupe	1 cup	33

Data from U.S. Department of Agriculture, Agricultural Research Service, USDA Nutrient Data Laboratory, USDA National Nutrient Database for Standard Reference, Release 20, 2008. Available at http://www.nal.usda.gov/fnic/foodcomp/search.

duced by intestinal bacteria can be absorbed in the large intestine.[1]

In 1996 the U.S. Food and Drug Administration (FDA) mandated the addition of specific amounts of folic acid to all enriched cereals and grain products.[1] Since then, folate intake and serum folate levels have been closely monitored because of potential risks of some individuals consuming excessive amounts. Blood folate concentrations first increased substantially after the fortification of cereal products, and then decreased slightly.[7,8] The reason for the decline may be attributed to the popularity of low carbohydrate weight loss diets. In Canada, where folate fortification is also mandatory, grains contribute approximately 41% of total folate intake, followed by fruits and vegetables, which contribute approximately 21%.[9] Women of childbearing age in the United States and Canada are achieving positive folate status, but it may not be enough to achieve folate concentration associated with a significant reduction in neural tube defects.[10,11]

ABSORPTION AND EXCRETION

Dietary folate must undergo some changes to be absorbed. The intestinal enzyme that accomplishes this requires a slightly acidic pH and is activated by the presence of zinc. Naturally occurring folate is not as well absorbed as supplements, and individuals needing larger amounts, especially menstruating women who may become pregnant, may need a supplement in addition to fortified folate-rich foods.

HYPER-STATES AND HYPO-STATES

In large doses, folate may cause kidney damage and mask symptoms of vitamin B_{12} deficiency. It also has been reported

Box 10-2	Drugs That May Negatively Affect Folate Status*

Anticonvulsants
Oral contraceptives
Analgesics
Metformin (antihyperglycemic)
Sulfasalazine (anti-inflammatory, antiarthritic)
H_2-receptor blockers (decreased gastric acid secretion)
Antacids
Triamterene (diuretic)
Methotrexate (antiarthritic, antineoplastic)
Alcohol

*Nutritional status may be negatively affected because of interference with folate absorption or metabolism or both.

to affect natural killer cells in postmenopausal women.[12] **Natural killer cells** are a part of the nonspecific immune response that can kill tumor cells and viral-infected cells. Folate protects against cancer initiation, but facilitates progression and growth of preneoplastic cells and subclinical cancers.[13] Additionally, an increased risk of cognitive decline has been reported in elderly individuals taking folic acid supplements.[14,15] A high folic acid intake may be harmful for some people. The UL of 1000 μg per day for adults is applicable to supplements and fortified foods, not to naturally occurring folate in food.

Folate deficiency, the most common vitamin deficiency among the B-complex vitamins, may occur secondary to excessive alcohol consumption, pregnancy and lactation, kidney dialysis, liver disease, inadequate dietary intake, gastrointestinal disease, or medications that interfere with folate absorption or metabolism or both (Box 10-2).

Deficiency symptoms first appear in rapidly dividing cells, such as in the gastrointestinal tract, RBCs, and white blood cells (WBCs). RBCs do not develop normally; they become pale and extremely large (megaloblastic), but cannot transport oxygen to cells, a condition known as **megaloblastic anemia**.

Folic acid deficiency during pregnancy is associated with an increased risk of spina bifida and other **neural tube defects (NTDs)** (birth defects of the skull, brain, and spinal cord), cleft palate and lip, and low birth weight and premature infants. NTDs decreased by 19% after folic acid fortification in the U.S. food supply.[16]

Glossitis is usually present in individuals with folic acid deficiency. The tongue becomes fiery red, and papillae are absent (Fig. 10-9). Folic acid deficiency impairs immune responses and resistance of the oral mucosa to penetration by pathogenic organisms such as *Candida*.

VITAMIN B_{12} (COBALAMIN)

Vitamin B_{12}, or cobalamin, represents a complex group of compounds that contain cobalt. (The only known physiological function of cobalt is as an integral component of vitamin B_{12}.) It is the only vitamin that contains a mineral.

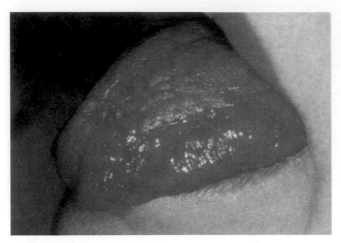

FIGURE 10-9 Folic acid deficiency. Fiery red tongue completely devoid of papillae. (Courtesy of Dr. W.R. Tyldesley. From McLaren DS: A Colour Atlas and Text of Diet-Related Disorders, 2nd ed. London: Mosby-YearBook Europe Limited, 1992.)

Nutritional Directions

- Folate may be called folic acid or folacin.
- Prolonged cooking destroys folate.
- More recent research indicates folic acid supplements should not be used to prevent cardiovascular events.[19]
- Folate is easily destroyed by food processing; raw vegetables provide more folate than cooked ones.
- Adequate folic acid is important in the periconceptual period (400 μg per day before conception and 600 μg per day for pregnant women) because the critical time for neural tube formation is the first month of pregnancy.
- Long-term use of folic acid and other B vitamin supplements do not lower a woman's risk or cancer, but they do not increase it either.[20]
- Orange juice is a good source of folate because vitamin C protects it from deterioration. Choosing fortified cereals and crackers also enhances folate intake.

Dental Hygiene Considerations

- Evaluate oral status for folate deficiency. Observe for swelling and pallor or reddening of the tip of the tongue (depending on the degree of anemia) with atrophy of filiform papillae, reddening of the fungiform papillae at the tip and lateral border, and formation of small ulcers. Posterior progression eventually leads to complete atrophy of the filiform papillae and formation of bright red spots (fungiform papillae). Angular cheilitis (see Fig. 10-5) and painful ulcerations of the buccal mucosa and palatal and gingival epithelia may also occur.
- Factors increasing the metabolic rate, such as infection and hyperthyroidism, or the cellular turnover rate, such as a malignancy, increase folate requirement. Assess folate intake by questioning about dietary intake.
- Folic acid supplementation may improve resistance to the development of periodontal inflammation in patients deficient in folate.
- Among patients with periodontal disease (**periodontitis**), serum folic acid concentration is lower in those who smoke than in nonsmokers.[17]
- Folate is one of the most common nutrient deficiencies after bariatric surgery.[18] Encourage patients who have had this procedure to adhere to strict eating behavior guidelines and supplement prescriptions.
- Folate absorption is lower when folate is given to individuals taking anticonvulsants and OCAs.
- Increased gingival inflammation has been associated with OCAs. Encourage women taking OCAs to increase their consumption of folate-rich foods.
- Phenytoin (Dilantin) is associated with gingival overgrowth (see Fig. 16-12). Certain studies have shown folate supplementation reduces the severity and incidence of this overgrowth. However, patients taking anticonvulsants should be closely monitored if folate supplements are prescribed because high intakes can decrease effectiveness of the medication.

PHYSIOLOGICAL ROLES

Vitamin B_{12} functions as a coenzyme in conjunction with folate metabolism in nucleic acid synthesis. It also functions in the metabolism of certain amino acids, fatty acids, carbohydrates, and folate. Vitamin B_{12} is essential in formation and regeneration of RBCs and for myelin synthesis. **Myelin** is the lipid substance that insulates nerve fibers and affects transmission of nerve impulses. It is also essential for a normal functioning nervous system.

REQUIREMENTS

The RDA for adults is 2.4 μg daily (Table 10-11). A high vitamin B_{12} intake results in accumulation in the liver with increasing age, but this may be desirable because serum vitamin B_{12} levels decline in elderly individuals because of lower absorption rates. No UL has been established, but caution of excessive intake is warranted.

SOURCES

Microorganisms (bacteria, fungi, and algae) can synthesize vitamin B_{12}. Vitamin B_{12} is not found in plants unless they are fortified or contaminated by microorganisms (legumes and root vegetables). More than 80% of dietary vitamin B_{12} is provided by meat and animal products (Table 10-12). Gastrointestinal flora produce small amounts of absorbable vitamin B_{12}.

ABSORPTION AND EXCRETION

Vitamin B_{12} from food is released from its protein bond by hydrochloric acid and enzymes in the stomach and intestine. Free vitamin B_{12} combines with salivary **R-binder** (protein produced by the salivary glands) in the stomach. In the small intestine, trypsin (pancreatic enzyme) removes the R-binder, and vitamin B_{12} combines with **intrinsic factor**, a glycoprotein secreted by the parietal cells in the stomach. Absorption of vitamin B_{12} occurs at specific receptor sites in the ileum and is possible only if it is bound to intrinsic factor. The vitamin is recycled from bile and other intestinal secretions.

Table 10-11	Institute of Medicine Recommendations for Vitamin B_{12}				
	EAR (µg/d)*		RDA (µg/d)†		
Life Stage	*Male*	*Female*	*Male*	*Female*	AI (µg/d)‡
0-6 mo					0.4
7-12 mo					0.5
1-3 yr	0.7	0.7	0.9	0.9	
4-8 yr	1	1	1.8	2.4	
9-13 yr	1.5	1.5	1.8	1.8	
14->70 yr	2	2	2.4	2.4	
Pregnancy 14-50 yr		2.2		2.6	
Lactation 14-50 yr		2.4		2.8	

Data from Institute of Medicine (IOM), Food and Nutrition Board: Dietary Reference Intakes for Thiamin, Riboflavin, Niacin, Vitamin B_6, Folate, Vitamin B_{12}, Pantothenic Acid, Biotin, and Choline. Washington, DC. National Academy Press, 1998.
*EAR (estimated average requirement)—the intake that meets the estimated nutrient needs of half of the individuals in a group.
†RDA (recommended dietary allowance)—the intake that meets the nutrient needs of almost all (97-98%) individuals in a group.
‡AI (adequate intake)—the observed average or experimentally set intake by a defined population or subgroup that seems to sustain a defined nutritional status, such as growth rate, normal circulating nutrient values, or other functional indicators of health. An AI is used if insufficient scientific evidence is available to derive an EAR. For healthy human milk–fed infants, the AI is the mean intake. *The AI is not equivalent to an RDA.*

Table 10-12	Vitamin B_{12} Content of Selected Foods	
Food	Portion	Vitamin B_{12} (µg)
Beef liver	3 oz	63.5
New England clam chowder with milk	1 cup	12.1
Special K cereal	1 cup	6
Lean beef, cooked	3 oz	3
Salmon, cooked	3 oz	2.4
Yogurt, plain, skim milk	8 oz	1.4
Shrimp, cooked	3 oz	1.3
Low-fat milk	1 cup	1.3
Lean pork chop, broiled	3 oz	0.6
Whole egg	1	0.6
Chicken breast, baked	3 oz	0.3

Data from U.S. Department of Agriculture, Agricultural Research Service, USDA Nutrient Data Laboratory, USDA National Nutrient Database for Standard Reference, Release 20, 2008. Available at http://www.nal.usda.gov/fnic/foodcomp/search. Accessed Feb 25, 2008.

Excessive amounts are bound to a protein and stored for 3 to 4 years in the liver, or they are excreted.

HYPER-STATES AND HYPO-STATES

No benefits are seen from large quantities of vitamin B_{12}, but no harmful effects have been observed either. Approximately 5% to 20% of older adults have marginal or frank vitamin B_{12} deficiency.[21] An excessive intake of folic acid from supplements delays the diagnosis of, or exacerbates the effects of, vitamin B_{12} deficiency, causing anemia and cognitive impairment.[22,23] Injections of vitamin B_{12} are popular treatments for fatigue and weakness, but few individuals meet accepted medical criteria for its use. A deficiency of vitamin B_{12} is rarely caused by insufficient dietary sources,

unless strict vegan diets are followed. Lack of intrinsic factor, R-binder, or an enzyme needed for absorption of vitamin B_{12}, is the primary cause of deficiency. **Pernicious anemia**, which is characterized by abnormally large RBCs, glossitis, gastrointestinal disturbances, weakness, and neurologic manifestations, occurs frequently in elderly patients relative to **achlorhydria** (decreased production of hydrochloric acid in the stomach) and decreased synthesis of intrinsic factor by the parietal cells.

Cobalamin malabsorption is caused by inability to release vitamin B_{12} from food.[24] Patients develop a lemon-yellow tint of the skin and eyes as a result of concurrent anemia and jaundice from inability to produce RBCs; a smooth, beefy red tongue; and neurologic disorders. Deficiency symptoms develop very slowly.

Initial oral symptoms of vitamin B_{12} deficiency include **glossopyrosis** (unexplained pain of the tongue), followed by swelling and pallor with eventual disappearance of the filiform and fungiform papillae. The tongue may be completely smooth, shiny, and deeply reddened with a loss or distortion of taste (Fig. 10-10). Bright red, diffuse, excruciatingly painful lesions may occur in the buccal and pharyngeal mucosa and undersurface of the tongue. An oral examination may reveal stomatitis or a pale or yellowish mucosa, xerostomia, cheilosis, hemorrhagic gingiva, and bone loss.

Neurological symptoms, such as numbness or tingling, occur as a consequence of demyelination of the nerves. Deficiency symptoms are rapidly corrected with vitamin B_{12} injections. Oral cobalamin is also an efficacious, cost-efficient, and safe method of treating vitamin B_{12} deficiency, but it is not commonly used by most healthcare providers.[25] A crystalline form of vitamin B_{12} does not require gastric acid or enzymes for initial digestion, and large oral doses (containing more than 200 times the RDA) can reverse biochemical signs of vitamin B_{12} deficiency in older adults.[26,27]

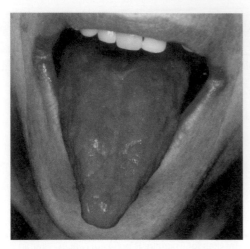

FIGURE 10-10 Pernicious anemia. (From Ibsen OAC, Phelan JA: Oral Pathology for the Dental Hygienist, 5th ed. St. Louis, Elsevier Saunders, 2009.)

Dental Hygiene Considerations

- Assess for oral signs of deficiency; signs and symptoms of vitamin B_{12} deficiency are similar to those of folic acid deficiency except that burning tongue pain precedes physical signs of vitamin B_{12} deficiency.
- Without R-binder, absorption of vitamin B_{12} is drastically reduced. Patients with xerostomia may have poor absorption of vitamin B_{12}.
- Patients older than 50 are encouraged to choose fortified sources of vitamin B_{12} to meet their needs because the synthetic form is better absorbed than naturally occurring vitamin B_{12} in foods.
- Concomitant ingestion of megadoses of ascorbic acid via foods or supplements can destroy substantial amounts of vitamin B_{12} and produce vitamin B_{12} deficiency. If the patient is prone to or has vitamin B_{12} deficiency and takes large amounts of vitamin C supplements, advise the patient to decrease vitamin C intake gradually to approximately the RDA level.
- Patients who have had permanent gastric surgery or ileal damage require other forms of vitamin B_{12} for life. Vitamin B_{12} injections and nasal gel do not require intrinsic factor.
- Because of the profound changes in digestive physiology after gastric bypass surgery, vitamin B_{12} is one of the nutrients of concern.[29]
- Some antiulcer medications decrease the production of acid by the parietal cells, inhibiting vitamin B_{12} absorption. Histamine receptor antagonists (H_2 blockers) (ranitidine [Zantac EFFERdose], famotidine [Pepcid], and cimetidine [Tagamet]) do not affect vitamin B_{12} status, but prolonged use of proton-pump inhibitors (esomeprazole [Nexium], lansoprazole [Prevacid], omeprazole [Prilosec OTC], pantoprazole [Protonix], and rabeprazole [Aciphex]) by older adults negatively affects vitamin B_{12} status. Oral supplementation with recommended amounts of vitamin B_{12} does not prevent this decline.[30] Encourage patients taking these medications to consult their healthcare provider if vitamin B_{12} is not being addressed.

Nutritional Directions

- Because vitamin B_{12} is found only in meat products, vegans (i.e., strict vegetarians) require vitamin B_{12}–fortified foods or a daily supplement.
- Vitamin B_{12} shots are not a panacea for "tired blood."

Children with vitamin B_{12} deficiency (e.g. vegans) may have stunted growth. Other symptoms include anorexia (loss of appetite), altered taste sensation, abdominal pain, and general weakness. A vitamin B_{12} deficiency is also associated with poor cognitive performance.[28]

PANTOTHENIC ACID

PHYSIOLOGICAL ROLES

Pantothenic acid is similar to other B vitamins in its metabolic roles. Pantothenic acid plays a key role in carbohydrate, fat, and protein metabolism. Additionally, it is important in synthesis and degradation of triglycerides, phospholipids, and sterols, and in formation of certain hormones and nerve-regulating substances.

REQUIREMENTS

The estimated average requirement (EAR), RDA, or UL has not been determined for pantothenic acid for any age group. The adequate intake (AI) for adults is 5 mg per day (Table 10-13).

SOURCES

Pantothenic acid is synthesized by most microorganisms and plants. It is particularly abundant in animal foods and whole-grain cereals (Table 10-14). Bacteria in the digestive tract also produce pantothenic acid. The usual intake of pantothenic acid in the United States is reported to be 5 to 10 mg per day.

HYPO-STATES

Naturally occurring dietary deficiency of pantothenic acid has not been documented.

Dental Hygiene Considerations

- Pantothenic acid deficiency rarely occurs alone, but may occur along with other B vitamin deficiencies.
- Pantothenic acid may help in wound healing, so ensure that patients undergoing oral or periodontal surgery are eating a well-balanced diet.

Table 10-13	Institute of Medicine Recommendations for Pantothenic Acid	
Life Stage		**AI (mg/d)***
0-6 mo		1.7
7-12 mo		1.8
1-3 yr		2
4-8 yr		3
9-13 yr		4
14-18 yr		5
19->70 yr		5
Pregnancy 14-50 yr		6
Lactation 14-50 yr		7

Data from Institute of Medicine (IOM), Food and Nutrition Board: Dietary Reference Intakes for Thiamin, Riboflavin, Niacin, Vitamin B6, Folate, Vitamin B12, Pantothenic Acid, Biotin, and Choline. Washington, DC: National Academy Press, 1998.
*AI (adequate intake)—the observed average or experimentally set intake by a defined population or subgroup that seems to sustain a defined nutritional status, such as growth rate, normal circulating nutrient values, or other functional indicators of health. An AI is used if insufficient scientific evidence is unavailable to derive an EAR. For healthy human milk–fed infants, the AI is the mean intake. *The AI is not equivalent to an RDA.*

Table 10-14	Pantothenic Acid Content of Selected Foods	
Food	**Portion**	**Pantothenic Acid (mg)**
Total, whole grain	1 cup	12.5
Liver	3 oz	6.4
Mushrooms, shiitake, cooked	1 cup	5.2
Sunflower seeds	1/4 cup	2
Tuna salad submarine	6-inch roll	1.9
Yogurt, skim milk	8 oz	1.5
Mushrooms, canned	1 cup	1.3
Trail mix	1 cup	1.3
Milk, skim	1 cup	0.9
Corn, canned	1/2 cup	0.7
Lean beef, cooked	3 oz	0.5
Baked beans	1/2 cup	0.3
Broccoli	1/2 cup	0.3

Data from U.S. Department of Agriculture, Agricultural Research Service, USDA Nutrient Data Laboratory, USDA National Nutrient Database for Standard Reference, Release 20, 2008. Available at http://www.nal.usda.gov/fnic/foodcomp/search. Accessed Feb 25, 2008.

Nutritional Directions

- Distribution of this vitamin is widespread.
- Diets including whole-grain unprocessed foods contain more pantothenic acid.

Table 10-15	Institute of Medicine Recommendations for Biotin
Life Stage	**AI (μg/d)***
0-6 mo	5
7-12 mo	6
1-3 yr	8
4-8 yr	12
9-13 yr	20
14-18 yr	25
19->70 yr	30
Pregnancy 14-50 yr	30
Lactation 14-50 yr	35

Data from Institute of Medicine (IOM), Food and Nutrition Board: Dietary Reference Intakes for Thiamin, Riboflavin, Niacin, Vitamin B6, Folate, Vitamin B12, Pantothenic Acid, Biotin, and Choline. Washington, DC: National Academy Press, 1998.
*AI (adequate intake)—the observed average or experimentally set intake by a defined population or subgroup that seems to sustain a defined nutritional status, such as growth rate, normal circulating nutrient values, or other functional indicators of health. An AI is used if insufficient scientific evidence is unavailable to derive an EAR. For healthy human milk–fed infants, the AI is the mean intake. *The AI is not equivalent to an RDA.*

BIOTIN

PHYSIOLOGICAL ROLES

Biotin functions as a coenzyme in metabolism of carbohydrates, proteins, and fats. It has an important biochemical role in every living cell in maintaining metabolic homeostasis. Biotin also plays an important role in regulating gene transcription,[31] and aids in use of protein, folic acid, pantothenic acid, and vitamin B12.

REQUIREMENTS

Because of insufficient data, only an AI for biotin has been established for all age groups (Table 10-15). Intakes of 10 to 200 μg per day are considered safe and adequate.[32]

SOURCES

Although biotin is widely distributed in foods, its availability is low compared with that of other water-soluble vitamins. Rich sources of biotin include egg yolk, liver, and cereals. Microflora in the gastrointestinal tract probably provide part of the body's needs. Biotin is included in many dietary supplements, infant formulas, and baby foods. Food composition tables usually do not report biotin content of food.

HYPO-STATES

Biotin deficiency can be produced by the ingestion of **avidin**, the protein found in raw egg whites. Avidin is denatured by heat; cooked egg white does not present a problem. Twelve to 24 raw egg whites per day can produce anorexia, nausea, vomiting, glossitis, pallor, depression, and dry scaly dermatitis.

Oral signs of biotin deficiency are pallor of the tongue and patchy atrophy of the lingual papillae. Although the pattern resembles geographic tongue, it is confined to the lateral margins or is generalized to the entire dorsum.

Dental Hygiene Considerations

- Assess patients for signs of deficiency: glossitis, lingual and mucous pallor, and papillary atrophy.
- Antibiotics reduce the production of biotin by intestinal bacteria.

Nutritional Directions

- Drinking or eating large amounts of raw egg whites over a long period may lead to biotin deficiency.
- Eggs should be cooked to decrease avidin's binding capacity and to minimize the danger of *Salmonella* poisoning.
- A balanced diet that includes a variety of foods contains adequate amounts of biotin.

OTHER VITAMINS

As you have already learned, most nutrients perform more than one physiological function. Although one nutrient may appear to be more important in calcified structures and of lesser importance in oral soft structures, its roles actually are equally important. The following nutrients have been discussed in previous chapters, but they have important functions in soft oral tissues that the dental hygienist should not overlook.

VITAMIN C

Vitamin C is involved in improving the host defense mechanism by ensuring optimal activity of WBCs. It has an important role in protecting soft oral tissues from infections caused by bacterial toxins and antigens and protecting tooth enamel from plaque microorganisms.

The role of vitamin C in collagen formation is well known. Vitamin C deficiency causes weakened collagen, leading to gingivitis and poor wound healing (see Fig. 7-10).

VITAMIN A

Vitamin A, necessary for maintaining the integrity of epithelial tissues, is a significant factor in the development and maintenance of salivary glands. Large amounts of vitamin A have an antikeratinizing effect on epithelial cells. Vitamin A increases synthesis of cellular proteins that stimulate growth and influence metabolism.

Vitamin A deficiency produces squamous metaplasia with keratin production in the duct cells of salivary glands. This results in decreased salivary secretion and xerostomia. Oral and oropharyngeal cancers have been associated with vitamin A deficiency in humans.

VITAMIN E

As discussed in Chapter 7, cell membranes contain polyunsaturated fatty acids that are susceptible to peroxidation. Vitamin E plays a major role as an antioxidant to neutralize free radicals, especially in membranes that contain a large proportion of unsaturated fatty acids. Not only does it prevent inflammation of the periodontium, but also it promotes the integrity of cell membranes of the mucosa.

Dental Hygiene Considerations

- One of the first signs of vitamin C deficiency is increased susceptibility to infections. During later stages, the gingiva becomes reddened and swollen, and bleeds easily with an increased risk of candidiasis and petechiae; also, the collagenous structure is weakened, and wound healing is slow.
- When a deficiency exists, vitamin C supplementation has been shown to decrease permeability of the sulcular epithelium and to increase collagen synthesis.
- Parotid gland enlargement has been associated with deficiencies of vitamins A and C and protein malnutrition.
- Vitamin A deficiency may result in retarded epithelialization, impaired wound healing and tissue regeneration, and increased risk of candidiasis.

Nutritional Directions

- Foods rich in antioxidants (vitamins A and E, and carotene) may suppress chemically induced neoplasias in the mouth, esophagus, and stomach. However, a meta-analysis indicated an increased risk of mortality owing to supplementation of these nutrients, and so they should not be recommended until further research indicates their use is beneficial.
- Vitamin C functions in maintaining the health of the gingiva, maintaining periodontal health. A varied and adequate diet including at least one vitamin C–rich food daily provides adequate amounts.

HEALTH APPLICATION **10** Supplements

Many people, motivated by general health concerns, take vitamin and mineral supplements. More than half of the people who take multivitamins say they do so to prevent disease, and 38% say they take them to feel better.[33] A daily multivitamin-mineral (MVM) tablet is frequently considered nutritional "insurance" to cover dietary indiscretions. These supplements usually contain 100% of the recommended intake for 10 vitamins and 10 minerals except for calcium (100% reference daily intake [RDI] for calcium makes the pill too large). There is no standard or regulation indicating which vitamins and minerals or how much are included in an MVM supplement. An estimated $22.1 billion was spent on dietary supplements in 2006 with $7.2 billion of that for vitamins.[34] These supplements are subject to misrepresentation and misuse because they are misunderstood by most consumers.

The Dietary Supplement Health and Education Act of 1994 defines dietary supplements as vitamins, minerals, amino acids, sports nutrition and weight loss supplements, homeopathic medicines, herbs and botanicals, and other products containing a dietary substance to supplement intake. In other words, a dietary supplement is any product intended for consumption in tablet, capsule, powder, softgel, gelcap, or liquid form, not meant for use as a conventional food or as a sole item of a meal or the diet.[35] Dietary supplements include more than 29,000 different products.

In 2007, the FDA implemented good manufacturing practices to ensure that supplements are produced in a quality manner, do not contain contaminants or impurities, and are labeled accurately. Guidelines are provided regarding claims food manufacturers can indicate on the label about the physiological effects of the product. Manufacturers must notify the FDA if they want to make a claim on the product along with evidence of the product's effectiveness and safety. This new rule became effective in June 2008; smaller manufacturers have 3 years to comply. Manufacturers of vitamins, herbal pills, and other dietary supplements have to test all of their products' ingredients. The new mandate is needed to ensure that products are free of contamination and impurities.

More than 1200 supplements have been tested for 15 nutrients.[36] These studies indicated 10% of the supplements contained none of the vitamins or minerals that were indicated on the label. For three nutrients (thiamin, vitamin B_6, and iron), the levels in some of the products were 10 times higher than listed. Some supplements contained undeclared active ingredients normally used in prescription drugs; some supplements contained significantly less of the vitamin than listed on the label. ConsumerLab.com, a watchdog of the supplement industry, found that more than half of the 21 MVM supplements tested had too much (or too little) of certain vitamins, or were contaminated with dangerous substances such as lead or selenium. If the FDA finds that supplements do not contain the ingredients they claim, the agency would consider the products adulterated or misbranded. In minor cases, the FDA could ask the manufacturer to remove an ingredient or revise its label. In more serious cases, it could seize the product, file a lawsuit, or seek criminal charges. All supplements cannot

be assumed to be safe. Because there are no uniform manufacturing rules for these products, a MVM supplement may not contain what the bottle claims, could be contaminated with something from the manufacturing plant, or might have tainted ingredients.

The United States Pharmacopeia (USP), the National Sanitation Foundation International (NSF), and ConsumerLab.com (CL) are nonprofit groups that verify whether companies offer contamination-free products and use good manufacturing practices. The presence of the USP, NSF, or CL symbol on the label helps to ensure the quality of the product because the symbols mean that the product has been tested to disintegrate and dissolve in the gastrointestinal tract, contains uniform quality (potency and purity), and contains the ingredients listed on the packaging. These organizations require an expiration date on the packaging. These symbols do not indicate that the supplement is safe for everyone or has any benefits. Not every brand has the seals; some manufacturers may not submit their products for testing.

In the preliminary State of the Science report, the National Institutes of Health indicated that in most instances, the evidence does not indicate the need for most MVM supplements, but the use of supplementation is endorsed when there is a demonstrated vitamin or mineral deficiency based on laboratory tests.[32] According to the American Dietetic Association, some nutrients are more likely to be inadequate during particular phases of life, as follows:[37]

- Iron and folic acid—for adolescent girls and women during childbearing years
- Vitamin B_{12}—for people who are older than 50 years
- Vitamin D—for older adults, people with heavily pigmented skin, and people exposed to inadequate ultraviolet-B radiation

In addition, the American Dietetic Association recognizes that during specific circumstances, typical nutritional needs or eating patterns change, so healthcare professionals should explore more closely to determine whether a nutrient supplement is appropriate.[37] (1) Food intake patterns less than 1600 kcal are typically inadequate in vitamins and minerals. (2) Certain stages during the life cycle result in increased nutrient needs or poor use. During pregnancy, a MVM supplement (specially formulated with higher levels of folic acid and iron and a complement of other vitamins and minerals) is recommended, and vitamins B_{12} and D are recommended for older adults, who are more at risk for suboptimal nutrition because of lower caloric intake and poor absorption of vitamin B_{12} and lack of exposure to the sun and poor conversion of vitamin D into the form needed. (3) Supplements may be used to prevent, treat, or manage disease or other conditions. This would include supplementation with calcium and vitamin D for osteoporosis, and electrolyte replacement to treat acute diarrhea. (4) Supplementation is recommended as a public health measure for large subpopulation groups, such as folic acid supplementation for all women of childbearing age to prevent NTDs. (5) Individuals who limit the variety of foods in their diet may need a MVM supplement, especially if they omit whole food groups. Examples include vegans (because of difficulty in consuming adequate amounts of calcium, iron, and zinc, and vitamins D and B_{12}); people who eliminate all dairy foods (because of lack of calcium and vitamin D); and patients who severely restrict food choices because of allergies and food intolerances, such as celiac disease (because of malabsorption and elimination of grain-based foods).

Homeopathic medicine is very popular; this medical philosophy, dating back to the late 1700s, endorses the idea that bodies have a self-healing response. Theoretically, if a certain substance causes a symptom in a healthy person, a *very small amount* of the same substance may cure the symptoms. However, the website from the National Center for Complementary and Alternative Medicine of the National Institutes of Health notes that studies on homeopathy have been contradictory.[38] Some studies suggest the results are similar to a placebo effect, whereas others have found positive effects not readily explained in scientific terms. Homeopathics are benign in general because they are so dilute it is unlikely they cause harm if used properly.

Patients may also be taking amino acid and folic acid supplements or unconventional items or herbal products described as "natural." These supplements may be deemed safe and desirable, but may adversely affect an existing medical condition or interact with other supplements or prescribed medications. Heroin, cocaine, and tobacco also can be considered "natural" plant-based substances, but lead to obvious health issues and are unsafe.

Megadoses of vitamins with intakes of 20 to 600 times the RDAs are sometimes advocated. Vitamin megadosage is defined as a dosage more than 10 times greater than the RDA. A megadose of a vitamin is actually a misnomer because at these levels, the vitamin is functioning as a drug rather than as a nutrient. This practice is dangerous and should be supervised by a healthcare provider to ensure toxicities do not occur. A well-established principle of pharmacological therapy is that all substances are potentially toxic at large enough doses. The body processes vitamins differently from food than in pill form, probably because foods interact with each other in a way that may help nutrient absorption.

Patients become their own diagnosticians by self-prescribing MVM supplements. They usually do not consult a healthcare provider. Consumers use dietary supplements to help them achieve their self-care goals, which develop out of a sense of alienation from the established healthcare system. Dietary supplements are, in their opinion, an easy means to ensure good health; treat and prevent serious illnesses, colds, and the flu; increase mental acuity; and alleviate depression. These individuals may delay seeking medical attention for various health problems. Many patients consider vitamins safe to take in any amount, but each year thousands of cases of supplement toxicity occur, especially in children. The potencies of these self-prescribed supplements vary widely, containing insignificant amounts to more than 5000% of the RDI.

Dietary supplements are not intended to treat disease, but to improve the nutrient intake that may help prevent disease. Currently, there may be no evidence of harm, but there is inconsistent evidence of effectiveness in the prevention of these chronic diseases.

Public health nutrition would be served best by insisting on a scientifically sound basis for dietary supplementation. Despite the consensus of popular opinion, healthy patients do not need dietary supplements if they eat a well-balanced diet using a variety of foods. Foods are the best source of nutrients. Folate supplementation exceeding the UL can alter how cancer cells are formed, and studies suggest that it may promote tumor growth. Obtaining nutrients from dietary sources rather than by supplementation reduces the potential for nutrient deficiencies, excesses, and potential interactions with other drugs or medical conditions. A vast body of observational and epidemiological studies has associated an increased dietary intake of antioxidants from fruits and vegetables with reduced risks of a range of diseases, including cancer. Despite this, when such antioxidants have been extracted and put into supplements, according to randomized clinical trials, the results do not produce the same benefits and may even be harmful.

One of the biggest dangers is the effect supplements may have on people's attitudes: "I'm taking vitamins; I don't have to exercise, I can continue to smoke, and I can eat however I like." For patients who choose to self-prescribe supplements, low levels of nutrients that do not exceed the RDA are recommended. Amounts greater than 100% of the RDA should be limited to the treatment of specific circumstances under medical supervision.

Store brands of vitamins are often identical to name brands; expensive supplements are no better than less costly supplements. Except for vitamin E, "natural" vitamins are no more beneficial than synthetic vitamins. (An all-natural vitamin E should contain only d-α-tocopherol.) Also, food folate is not as well absorbed as synthetic folic acid. Other components in foods, however, may help with the absorption and use of some nutrients.

Daily MVM supplements are most effective when taken with a meal. It takes longer for the stomach to empty when it is full, allowing more time for the supplement to dissolve and be absorbed. Some nutrients may compete or block the action or absorption of another nutrient; it may be necessary to take single supplements at different meals to avoid potential interactions. Chelated supplements are marketed to have superior absorption ability, but they are broken down by gastric acids and absorbed similar to other supplements. Most supplements marked "time release" also have no value. The body does not need to maintain a constant level of vitamins as for some medications, such as antibiotics.

In addition, herbs or supplements can be found in many oral health products (Box 10-3) that may cause adverse reactions when taken with over-the-counter or prescription medications. The dental professional should be cognizant of products containing herbs or supplements when recommending them to patients. Look for the American Dental Association Seal of Acceptance on the product.

A medical history should include specific queries about dietary and herbal supplements because many patients typically do not inform healthcare professionals of their usage. Document the type of supplement, amount, poten-

Box 10-3	"ABCD" Approach to Asking Patients about Use of Dietary Supplements

Ask
- What do you take: what form, what brand, what dose, and what else?
- How long have you been taking it, how much do you take, and how often?
- Why do you take it, why was it recommended and by whom?
- Does it do what you thought it would?

Be
- Wary of any single nutrient used (e.g., vitamin C, E, or B_{12}) not recommended by a healthcare provider or registered dietitian, and doses exceeding the National Academy of Sciences, Institute of Medicine, Food and Nutrition Board dietary reference intakes.
- Sure to look up supplements used in a reliable resource.

Communicate
- Any concerns or risks about safety, drug-nutrient interactions, toxicity to the patient

Document
- Supplements used, risks of concern, communication with patient, interaction

Do
- Not get into the supplement business; when in doubt or wanting to refer a patient, contact the credentialed nutrition professional, a registered dietitian.

From Touger-Decker R: Vitamin and mineral supplements: what is the dentist to do? J Am Dent Assoc 2007 Sep; 138(9):1222-1226.

Box 10-4	Selected Ingredients Used in Oral Healthcare Products

- Bloodroot
- Calendula
- Cayenne
- Chamomile
- Clove oil
- Coenzyme Q10
- Echinacea
- Eucalyptus
- Fennel
- Garlic
- Ginger
- Goldenseal
- Grape seed extract
- *Lactobacillus acidophilus*
- Lemon balm
- Licorice root
- Lycopene
- Lysine
- Myrrh
- Nettle leaves
- Prickly ash
- Rhatany
- Sage
- Soy
- Tea
- Tea tree oil (*Melaleuca alternifolia*)
- Vitamin C
- Watercress
- Witch hazel
- Zinc

From Goldie MP: Dietary supplements and herbs: implications for client care. Access 2002, 16:28-35.

HEALTH APPLICATION 10   Supplements—cont'd

tial interactions, and dental implications (Box 10-4). By asking additional questions to determine why the patient is taking the supplement, the dental hygienist can discuss the benefits of a balanced diet, fluids, exercise, and smoking cessation. More importantly, a careful investigation of peer-reviewed literature and use of scientifically based, current, quality research with valid clinical trials would provide dental hygienists with accurate information to help assess a patient's intake and provide advice.

All health professionals are responsible for reporting any damaging effects or illness resulting from nutritional sup-

plements to the FDA (http://www.fda.gov/medwatch), and submitting complaints to the Federal Trade Commission (FTC) regarding misleading advertising (http://www.ftc.gov/ftc/complaint.htm). Dental hygienists must consider whether or not their academic training and scope of practice qualifies them to provide advice regarding dietary supplement usage. Promoting healthy eating patterns and lifestyles according to national guidelines is the appropriate advice to provide patients. A complete nutritional assessment of the patient needs to be conducted to validate the use of a supplement.

CASE APPLICATION FOR THE DENTAL HYGIENIST

A young mother of a 3-year-old says she has heard that she should be taking folate supplements because she is considering discontinuing her birth control pills. She is concerned about the effects of the birth control pills on her nutritional status and their effect on a fetus should she become pregnant.

Nutritional Assessment
- Types of foods consumed
- Knowledge base of foods rich in folate
- Current use of any dietary supplements
- Motivation to change eating habits
- Knowledge of physiological values and absorption of folate

CASE APPLICATION FOR THE DENTAL HYGIENIST—cont'd

Nutritional Diagnosis

Health-seeking behavior related to nutritional status and effects on fetus.

Nutritional Goals

The patient will consume foods rich in folate and ask her healthcare provider about the need to take a multivitamin supplement or a folate supplement.

Nutritional Implementation

Intervention: Evaluate the oral area for symptoms of folate or other nutrient deficiencies.

Rationale: This will help determine whether or not she is currently deficient and help determine whether or not she should consult her healthcare provider immediately.

Intervention: Teach the following about folate: (1) different names used, (2) functions, (3) requirements, and (4) sources.

Rationale: This provides the patient with a sound base of knowledge about folic acid.

Intervention: Discuss symptoms of folate deficiency and harmful effects of too much folic acid.

Rationale: Although it is important that the patient obtain adequate amounts of folic acid to prevent NTDs, too much can also be harmful.

Intervention: Discuss the stability of folate during cooking and processing.

Rationale: Knowing folate can easily be destroyed during food preparation allows the patient to make decisions based on her eating habits determine whether or not her diet provides adequate amounts of folate.

Intervention: Explain her requirement for folic acid is increased because of the birth control pills, and because of the needs of the fetus and other physiological changes occurring early during pregnancy.

Rationale: This knowledge will help her realize the importance of changing dietary patterns consistently.

Evaluation

The patient should increase her intake of folate-rich foods (cereal products that are fortified with folate; oranges; liver; raw, green, leafy vegetables). Additionally, she should consult her healthcare provider before she discontinues the OCA and begins taking a multivitamin. She can state why she has an increased requirement for folic acid and why it is important not to take excessive amounts.

STUDENT READINESS

1. Name the two water-soluble vitamins most involved in the metabolism of fats, proteins, and carbohydrates to form energy (ATP) through the citric acid or Krebs cycle.

2. Match the conditions associated with the appropriate vitamin deficiency:

Thiamin	Cheilosis
Riboflavin	Scurvy
Iodine	Pellagra
Niacin	Megaloblastic anemia
Vitamin B_{12}	Beriberi
Ascorbic acid	Graves' disease

3. Why is it important that water-soluble vitamins be consumed daily?

4. Define "vitamin megadose." What are the disadvantages of taking vitamin megadoses?

5. Name three foods that are good sources of each of the following nutrients: thiamin, riboflavin, vitamin B_{12}, and folate.

6. What would you teach a vegan about vitamin B_{12}?

7. Discuss why signs and symptoms of deficiencies of water-soluble vitamins appear periorally. List signs and symptoms of deficiencies you should be alert for, and list vitamins that might be implicated.

8. What recommendations could you offer to a patient to ensure the availability of folate? Why is folate so important before and during pregnancy?

9. Evaluate five of the stress or megavitamin supplement preparations in a drugstore or health food store. List the amounts of vitamin C, niacin, and vitamin B_6 (pyridoxine) in them, and compare those amounts with the RDAs for children younger than 10 years old, men 19 to 24 years old, and women 25 to 50 years old.

CASE STUDY

A 32-year-old man presents with the following symptoms: swollen tongue with reddening at the tip, small oral ulcerations, and gingival hyperplasia. The patient is being treated with long-term anticonvulsant medication.

1. Is a dietary assessment indicated? Explain your answer.

2. What are the possible effects of the patient's medication on his nutritional and oral status?

3. If a deficiency exists, which vitamins/minerals are most likely lacking? Why?

4. Which types of foods and food preparation methods should be suggested? Why?

5. What advice should you give regarding oral care?

References

1. Said HM, Mohammed ZM: Intestinal absorption of water-soluble vitamins: an update. Curr Opin Gastroenterol 2006 Mar; 22(2):140-146.

2. American Psychiatric Association: Diagnostic and Statistical Manual of Mental Disorders, 4th ed, Text Revision. Washington, DC: American Psychiatric Association, 2004.

3. Sekiyama S, Takagi S, Kondo Y: Peripheral neuropathy due to thiamine deficiency after inappropriate diet and total gastrectomy. Tokai J Exp Clin Med 2005 Sep; 30(3):137-140.

4. Worden RW, Allen HM: Wernicke's encephalopathy after gastric bypass that masqueraded as acute psychosis: a case report. Curr Surg 2006 Mar-Apr; 63(2):114-116.

5. Parkes E: Nutritional management of patients after bariatric surgery. Am J Med Sci 2006 Apr; 331(4):207-213.

6. Morris MS, et al: Trends of vitamin B_6 status in US population sample. Am J Clin Nutr 2008 May; 87(5):1446-1454.

7. Bailey LB: The rise and fall of blood folate in the United States emphasizes the need to identify all sources of folic acid. Am J Clin Nutr 2007 Sep; 86(3):528-530.

8. Pfeiffer CM, et al: Trends in blood folate and vitamin B_{12} concentrations in the United States, 1988-2004. Am J Clin Nutr 2007 Sep; 86(3):718-727.

9. Sherwood KL, et al: One-third of pregnant and lactating women may not be meeting their folate requirements from diet alone based on mandated levels of folic acid fortification. J Nutr 2006 Nov; 136(11):2820-2826.

10. Shuaibi AM, et al: Folate status of young Canadian women after folic acid fortification of grain products. J Am Diet Assoc 2008 Dec; 108(12):2090-2094.

11. Dowd JB, Aiello A: Did national folic acid fortification reduce socioeconomic and racial disparities in folate status in the US? Int J Epidemiol 2008 Oct; 37(5):1059-1066.

12. Troen AM, et al: Unmetabolized folic acid in plasma is associated with reduced natural killer cell cytotoxicity among post-menopausal women. J Nutr 2006; 136:189-194.

13. Smith AD, Kim YI, Refsum H: Is folic acid good for everyone? Am J Clin Nutr 2008 Mar; 87(3):517-533.

14. Morris MS, et al: Folate and vitamin B_{12} status in relation to anemia, macrocytosis, and cognitive impairment in older Americans in the age of folic acid fortification. Am J Clin Nutr 2007 Jan; 85(1):193-200.

15. Morris MC, et al: Dietary folate and vitamin B_{12} intake and cognitive decline among community dwelling older persons. Arch Neurol 2005; 62:641-645.

16. Centers for Disease Control and Prevention: Spina bifida and anencephaly before and after folic acid mandate—United States, 1995-96 and 1999-2002. MMWR Morb Mortal Wkly Rep 2004; 53:362-365.

17. Erdemir EO, Bergstrom J: Relationship between smoking and folic acid, vitamin B_{12} and some haematological variables in patients with chronic periodontal disease. J Clin Periodontol 2006 Dec; 33(12):878-884.

18. Parkes E: Nutritional management of patients after bariatric surgery. Am J Med Sci 2006 Apr; 331(4):207-213.

19. Albert CM, et al: Effect of folic acid and B vitamins on risk of cardiovascular events and total mortality among women at high risk for cardiovascular disease. JAMA 2008 May 7; 299(17):2027-2036.

20. Zhang SM, et al: Effect of combined folic acid, vitamin B_6, and vitamin B_{12} on cancer risk in women: A randomized trial. JAMA 2008 Nov 5; 300(17):2012-2021.

21. Park S, Johnson MA: What is an adequate dose of oral vitamin B_{12} in older people with poor vitamin B_{12} status? Nutr Rev 2006 Aug; 64(8):373-378.

22. Morris MS, et al: Folate and vitamin B_{12} status in relation to anemia, macrocytosis, and cognitive impairment in older Americans in the age of folic acid fortification. Am J Clin Nutr 2007 Jan; 85(1):193-200.

23. Johnson MA: If high folic acid aggravates vitamin B_{12} deficiency what should be done about it? Nutr Rev 2007 Oct; 65(10):451-458.

24. Andres E, et al: Vitamin B_{12} (cobalamin) deficiency in elderly patients. Can Med Assoc J 2004 Aug 3; 171(3):251-259.

25. Graham ID, et al: Oral cobalamin remains medicine's best kept secret. Arch Gerontol Geriatr 2007 Jan-Feb; 44(1):49-59.

26. Eussen SJ, et al: Oral cyanocobalamin supplementation in older people with vitamin B_{12} deficiency: a dose-finding trial. Arch Intern Med 2005 May 23; 165(10):1167-1172.

27. Park S, Johnson MA: What is an adequate dose of oral vitamin B_{12} in older people with poor vitamin B_{12} status? Nutr Rev 2006 Aug; 64(8):373-378.

28. Fanjiang G, Kleinman RE: Nutrition and performance in children. Curr Opin Clin Nutr Metab Care 2007 May; 10(3):342-347.

29. Poitou BC, et al: Nutritional deficiency after gastric bypass: diagnosis, prevention and treatment. Diabetes Metab 2007 Feb; 33(1):13-24.

30. Dharmarajan TS, et al: Do acid-lowering agents affect vitamin B_{12} status in older adults? J Am Med Dir Assoc 2008 Mar; 9(3):162-167.

31. Halsted CH: Absorption of water-soluble vitamins. Curr Opin Gastroenterol 2003; 19(2):113-117.

32. Thompson J: Vitamins, minerals and supplements: part three. Community Pract 2005 Nov; 78(11):407-408.

33. Rock CL: Multivitamin-multimineral supplements: who uses them? Am J Clin Nutr 2007 Jan; 85(1):2277S-2279S.

34. Zelman KM: The truth behind the top 10 dietary supplements. WebMD September 1, 2007. Available at webmd.com/diet/features/truth-behind-top-10-dietary-supplements?ecd=wnl_day_083107. Accessed May 26, 2008.

35. Dietary Supplement Health and Education Act of 1994, Pub. L. No 103-417; §784, 108 Stat. Appendix A, 1994. Available at http://www.health.gov/dietsupp/ch.1.htm. Accessed May 26, 2008.

36. Dwyer J: State of the science: multivitamin-mineral supplements and chronic disease risk. May 17, 2006. Available at http://ods.od.nih.gov/pubs/fnce2006/Multivitamin-Mineral-SupplementsAndChronicDiseaseRisk_Dwyer.pdf. Accessed June 2, 2008.

37. Position of the American Dietetic Association: fortification and nutritional supplements. J Am Diet Assoc 2005 Aug; 105(8):1300-1311.

38. NIH National Center for Complementary and Alternative Medicine. Research report: questions and answers about homeopathy. Available at http://nccam.nih.gov/health/homeopathy/#q8. Accessed June 2, 2008.

Chapter 11

Water and Minerals Required for Oral Soft Tissues and Salivary Glands

OUTLINE

WATER
Physiological Roles
Requirements and Regulation
Absorption
Sources
Hyper-States and Hypo-States

ELECTROLYTES

SODIUM
Physiological Roles
Requirements and Regulation
Sources
Hyper-States and Hypo-States

CHLORIDE
Physiological Roles
Requirements and Regulation
Sources
Hyper-States and Hypo-States

POTASSIUM
Physiological Roles
Requirements and Regulation

Sources
Hyper-States and Hypo-States

IRON
Physiological Roles
Requirements
Absorption and Excretion
Sources
Hyper-States and Hypo-States

ZINC
Physiological Roles
Requirements
Absorption and Excretion
Sources
Hyper-States and Hypo-States

IODINE
Physiological Role
Requirements
Sources
Hyper-States and Hypo-States

LEARNING OBJECTIVES

Upon completion of this chapter, the student will be able to achieve the following objectives:
- Describe the process of osmosis.
- Explain fluid and electrolyte balance.
- Identify normal fluid requirements and factors that may affect these requirements.
- Discuss the roles, imbalances, and sources of water, sodium, potassium, iron, zinc, and iodine.

- Describe oral signs and symptoms of fluid and electrolyte imbalances.
- Identify nutritional directions for patients with fluid and electrolyte imbalances.
- Identify diseases and medications that may require patients to restrict sodium intake.
- Identify the most prominent oral symptoms or signs of iron, zinc, and iodine deficiency.

KEY TERMS

Aldosterone
Anions
Antidiuretic hormone (ADH)
Cations
Cretinism
Diaphoresis
Essential hypertension
Extracellular fluid (ECF)
Fluid volume deficit (FVD)
Fluid volume excess (FVE)
Goiter
Goitrogens
Heme iron
Hemochromatosis
Hyperkalemia

Hypernatremia
Hypodipsia
Hypokalemia
Hyponatremia
Intracellular fluid (ICF)
Longitudinal fissures
Myxedema
Nonheme iron
Osmoreceptors
Peripheral
Renin
Solutes
Solvent
Transferrin

Test Your NQ

1. **T/F** Thirst is the primary regulator of fluid intake.
2. **T/F** Meats are more than half water.
3. **T/F** Water is the most abundant component in the body.
4. **T/F** Heme iron is provided by meat sources and is more readily absorbed than iron from vegetable or grain products.
5. **T/F** Normal fluid requirements are eight 8-oz cups of total water daily.

6. **T/F** The RDA for sodium is 5000 mg per day.
7. **T/F** Taste alteration is a symptom of zinc deficiency.
8. **T/F** Potassium is principally found in extracellular fluid.
9. **T/F** Broccoli is a good source of potassium.
10. **T/F** Oral pallor is associated with iodine deficiency.

Water and several mineral elements are essential for maintenance of healthy oral tissues, including tooth enamel. Visual signs of deficiencies in the gingiva, mucous membranes, and salivary glands are less obvious than the signs observed with the B-vitamin complex and vitamin C deficiencies previously discussed. Nevertheless, water and several minerals have a significant effect on the integrity of the oral cavity and, ultimately, nutritional status. Oral problems associated with hyper-states or hypo-states are slow to develop and may not be critical immediately. Chronically decreased salivary flow attributable to inadequate body fluids may lead to rampant tooth decay and eventually loss of teeth.

WATER

Water is the most abundant component in the body. At birth, water constitutes approximately 75% to 80% of body weight. Because such a large percentage of the infant's body weight consists of water, fluid loss is more significant in infants than in adults. Total body water decreases with age, representing 50% to 60% of the total body weight of an adult. Adipose tissue contains less water than muscle; a person with a large amount of fat has a lower percentage of total body water.

Women's bodies, with inherently larger fat stores, contain less water compared with men's bodies, which have a higher percentage of lean muscle tissue.

Body fluids are distributed intracellularly and extracellularly. **Intracellular fluid (ICF)**, which constitutes 60% of the body's fluid weight, includes all the fluid within cells (chiefly the cells of muscle tissue). **Extracellular fluid (ECF)** consists of fluid outside the cells. Fluid compartments are separated from one another by the presence of semipermeable membranes. These membranes serve as barriers by preventing movement of certain substances; however, they do not completely isolate the compartments. Water is essentially unrestricted in its movement from compartment to compartment. Certain dissolved substances, or **solutes**, such as glucose, amino acids, and oxygen, also cross membranes freely. The cellular membranes allow the maintenance of solute concentration by their selectivity.

When two compartments are separated by semipermeable membranes, and the movement of some solutes is restricted, osmosis occurs. Osmosis is the movement of water from an area of lower solute concentration to one of a higher solute concentration. Osmotic pressure within the body equalizes the solute concentration of intracellular and extracellular fluids by shifting small amounts of water in the direction of the higher concentration of solute, as shown in Figure 11-1.

PHYSIOLOGICAL ROLES

Water has several important physiological roles: (1) It acts as a **solvent** (fluid in which substances are dissolved), enabling chemical reactions to occur by entering into some reactions, such as hydrolysis; (2) it maintains the stability of all body fluids, as the principal component and medium for fluids (blood and lymph), secretions (saliva and gastrointestinal fluids), and excretions (urine and perspiration); (3) it enables the transport of nutrients to the cells and provides a medium for excretion of waste products; (4) it acts as a lubricant between cells to permit movement without friction; and (5) it regulates body temperature by evaporating as perspiration from the skin and vapor from the mouth and nose. Negative fluid balance has serious detrimental effects on many physiological functions. A few days without water can be fatal.

REQUIREMENTS AND REGULATION

To maintain normal hydration, the Institute of Medicine (IOM) established an adequate intake (AI) for total fluid (beverages, water, and food). As shown in Table 11-1, men require 3.7 L (15 to 16 cups) per day, and women require 2.7 L (11 to 12 cups) per day. No tolerable upper intake level (UL) is established for water.

Overconsumption and underconsumption of fluids can occur over short periods. However, if adequate amounts of fluids are available, consumption matches physiological needs over an extended period. Individuals who consume a high-protein or high-fiber diet, have diarrhea or vomiting, or are physically active or exposed to warm or hot weather require more fluids.

Water is lost by a variety of routes: (1) urination, (2) perspiration, (3) expiration, and (4) defecation. Urine production depends on the amount of fluid intake and the type of diet eaten. However, waste products must be kept in solution; minimum urine output to eliminate waste products is 400 to 600 mL per day.

Water losses in the form of sweat can vary greatly. An increase in body temperature is accompanied by increased sweating and respiration. Strenuous exercise can greatly affect the amount of water lost through the skin. Vapor in expired air varies with the rate of respiration. The presence of respiratory inflammation also elevates the respiration rate. Approximately 100 to 200 mL of water is lost each day in feces; this is dramatically increased in individuals with diarrhea.

Water losses result in stimulation of water intake, via thirst, and decreased kidney output to maintain fluid balance. Saliva also may help maintain water balance because saliva flow is reduced in dehydration, leading to drying of the mucosa and the sensation of thirst.

Normal fluid requirements (Fig. 11-2) can be drastically changed in different climatic environments, with various exercise levels, diet, and social activities, and with illnesses resulting in (or are accompanied by) diarrhea or vomiting. The body cannot store water, so the amount lost must be replaced.

In healthy individuals, thirst is an early sign of the body's need for fluids.[1-3] Older patients often have a reduced sensation of thirst. When 2% of body water is lost, osmoreceptors are stimulated, creating a physiological desire to ingest liquids. **Osmoreceptors** are neurons in the hypothalamus that are sensitive to changes in serum osmolality levels. Stimulation of osmoreceptors not only causes thirst, but also increases the release of **antidiuretic hormone (ADH)** from the pituitary gland (Fig. 11-3). ADH causes the body to retain fluid by decreasing urinary output. Conversely, if there is too much water in the body, ADH secretion is inhibited, and excess water is eliminated.

Decreased blood pressure also stimulates the release of the enzyme **renin**, which ultimately leads to increased

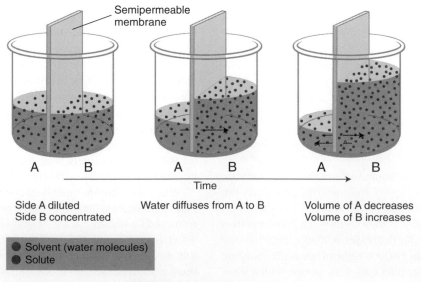

FIGURE 11-1 Osmotic pressure.

Table 11-1 | Institute of Medicine Recommendations for Water

Life Stage	AI[a] Male (L/d)[b]	Female (L/d)[b]
0-6 mo	0.7[c]	0.7[c]
7-12 mo	0.8[d]	0.8[d]
1-3 yr	1.3[e]	1.3[e]
4-8 yr	1.7[f]	1.7[f]
9-13 yr	2.4[g]	2.1[h]
14-18 yr	3.3[i]	2.3[g]
>18 yr	3.7[j]	2.7[k]
Pregnancy 14-50 yr		3[l]
Lactation 14-50 yr		3.8[m]

Data from Institute of Medicine (IOM), Food and Nutrition Board: Dietary Reference Intakes for Water, Potassium, Sodium, Chloride, Chloride, and Sulfate. Washington, DC: National Academies Press, 2005.

[a]AI (adequate intake)—the observed average or experimentally set intake by a defined population or subgroup that seems to sustain a defined nutritional status, such as growth rate, normal circulating nutrient values, or other functional indicators of health. An AI is used if insufficient scientific evidence is available to derive an EAR. For healthy human milk–fed infants, the AI is the mean intake. The AI is not equivalent to an RDA.

[b]L = liter. 1 L = 4¼ cups.

[c]Assumed to be from human milk.

[d]Assumed to be from human milk, complementary foods, and beverages. This includes ~0.6 L (~3 cups) as total fluid, including formula or human milk, juices, and drinking water.

[e]Total water. This includes ~0.9 L (~4 cups) as total beverages, including drinking water.

[f]Total water. This includes ~1.7 L (~5 cups) as total beverages, including drinking water.

[g]Total water. This includes ~1.8 L (~8 cups) as total beverages, including drinking water.

[h]Total water. This includes ~1.6 L (~7 cups) as total beverages, including drinking water.

[i]Total water. This includes ~2.6 L (~11 cups) as total beverages, including drinking water.

[j]Total water. This includes ~3 L (~13 cups) as total beverages, including drinking water.

[k]Total water. This includes ~2.7 L (~9 cups) as total beverages, including drinking water.

[l]Total water. This includes ~3 L (~10 cups) as total beverages, including drinking water.

[m]Total water. This includes ~3.1 L (~13 cups) as total beverages, including drinking water.

release of the hormone **aldosterone** by the adrenal cortex. This release of aldosterone results in retention of sodium and water by the kidneys, and excretion of potassium and hydrogen ions, causing blood pressure to increase.

ABSORPTION

No digestion is necessary for water absorption; it is transported easily in both directions across the intestinal mucosa by osmosis. In 1 hour, 1 liter can be absorbed from the small intestine. Normally, almost all the fluid is absorbed with a small amount excreted with the feces.

SOURCES

During the process of metabolism, liquids and solid foods provide water. Some fruits and vegetables have a higher percentage of water than does milk, and meats are more than half water (Table 11-2). Regardless of its source, fluids act the same physiologically. Water liberated in the process of metabolism is also available to the body. Metabolism of fat produces approximately twice as much water as the metabolism of protein or carbohydrate; this process supplies about 300 to 350 mL per day.

Plain tap water is the most natural source of fluids, best for quenching thirst, most economical, and healthiest. Many Americans have become disenchanted with tap water. Although not perfect, the United States has one of the safest public water supplies in the world. During the past century, many improvements in Americans' health can be attributed to improvements in the drinking water, such as community fluoridation and controlling infectious diseases. When ground water becomes polluted, it is no longer safe to drink. Arsenic and radon can occur naturally in the environment and contaminate the water. Other water contaminants result from the use of fertilizers and pesticides, microbial contamination, and manufacturing processes. Drugs have been detected in the drinking water of several major metropolitan areas. These drugs could be from medications not absorbed by individuals and eliminated through physiological discharges or numerous other reasons. Many pharmaceuticals pass through sewage and drinking water treatment plants. Many cases of gastrointestinal illness from water are from small or individual water systems.

The U.S. Environmental Protection Agency (EPA) regulates the levels of contaminants allowed in drinking water in public water systems. Water utility companies are required to provide Consumer Confidence Reports to their customers annually. Private well owners are responsible for ensuring their water is safe from contaminants of high concern. Wastewater is treated, but most treatments do not remove all drug residue. The EPA is concerned and is looking at methods to detect and quantify pharmaceuticals in wastewater.

Because of mistrust of the water supply, and a desire for a safer and more convenient form of fluid intake, consumers frequently choose bottled water. In 2006, the bottled water market was $10.8 billion and growing. These waters come with many labels: mineral water, Artesian water, purified water, and spring water. Although this trend has resulted in increased fluid intake, numerous problems are associated with this practice. Many consumers think bottled water is healthier, but the quality of these waters has been questioned, and in some cases tap water is purer than bottled water. Some brands of bottled water come from pristine, underground rural sources; other brands are actually tap water. Bottlers claim their products are safe, and they clean the water with advanced treatments, but they do not routinely test or treat for pharmaceuticals. Most bottled waters do not contain fluoride. Bottled water is regulated by the U.S. Food and Drug Administration (FDA), but fluoride

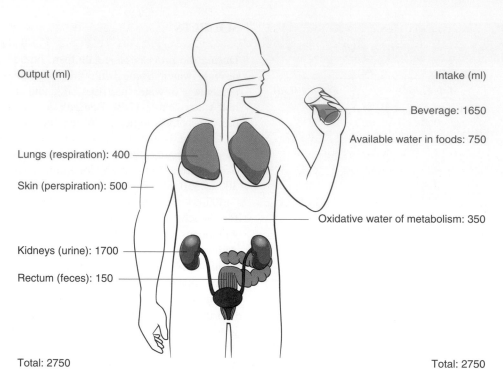

<table>
<tr><td>Output (ml)</td><td></td><td>Intake (ml)</td></tr>
</table>

Beverage: 1650

Available water in foods: 750

Lungs (respiration): 400

Skin (perspiration): 500

Oxidative water of metabolism: 350

Kidneys (urine): 1700

Rectum (feces): 150

Total: 2750   Total: 2750

FIGURE 11-2 Fluid intake and output. (Adapted from Davis JR, Sherer K: Applied Nutrition and Diet Therapy for Nurses, 2nd ed. Philadelphia: Saunders, 1994.)

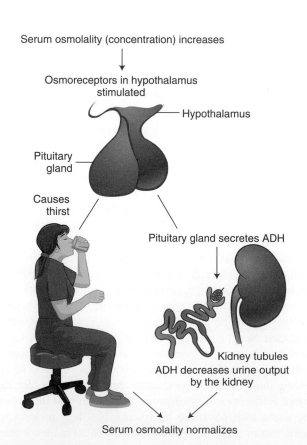

Serum osmolality (concentration) increases

Osmoreceptors in hypothalamus stimulated

Hypothalamus

Pituitary gland

Causes thirst

Pituitary gland secretes ADH

Kidney tubules ADH decreases urine output by the kidney

Serum osmolality normalizes

FIGURE 11-3 The role of osmoreceptors and antidiuretic hormone (ADH) in fluid balance.

Table 11-2	Percentage of Water in Foods
Food Item	**% Water**
Beer and wine	90-95
Milk, fruit juice, fruit drinks	85-90
Cooked cereals	85-90
Fruits (strawberries, melons, grapefruit, peaches, pears, oranges, apples, grapes, cucumbers, tomatoes)	80-85
Vegetables (lettuce, celery, cabbage, broccoli, onions, carrots)	80-85
Cottage cheese and yogurt	75-80
Vegetables (potatoes, corn)	70-75
Fish and seafood	70-80
Liquid drinks for weight loss, muscle gain, meal replacement	70-85
Fish and seafood	70-80
Rice and pasta	65-80
Eggs	65-80
Stew, pasta and meat dishes, casseroles (with meat and meatless), meatloaf, tacos, enchiladas, macaroni and cheese	60-80
Sauces and gravies	50-85
Ice cream	50-60
Beef, chicken, lamb, pork, turkey, veal	45-65
Cheese	40-50
Breads, bagels, biscuits	30-45
Ready-to-eat breakfast cereals	2-5
Chips, pretzels, candies, crackers, dried fruit, popcorn	1-5

Adapted from Grandjean A, Campbell S: Hydration: Fluids for Life. Washington, DC: ILSI North America, 2004.

does not have to be listed on the label unless it is added. Another concern is the amount of energy required to produce the plastic bottles that are not biodegradable.

In addition to plain bottled water, manufacturers are adding other ingredients; many of these are nutrients. Supermarket shelves are filled with sports and energy drinks; vitamin water; and drinks containing amino acids, B vitamins, caffeine, green tea, vitamin C, ginger, cranberry extracts, or ginkgo (*Ginkgo biloba*). These drinks are often expensive. Many of these flavored beverages contain additional kilocalories, which are consumed in overabundant amounts by most Americans. When people consume high-kilocalorie beverages, they eat approximately the same amount of food, not reducing their caloric intake as a result of the beverage intake.[4] So these beverages are especially dangerous for individuals trying to control their energy intake and weight.

One popular liquid supplement contains 8333% of the recommended dietary allowance (RDA) for vitamin B_{12} and 2000% of the RDA for vitamin B_6. Contrary to what the commercial advertisements would have us believe, B vitamins are not little packets of energy. The vitamins help the body use the energy in foods, but extra B vitamins do not provide additional energy bursts. Almost all Americans get adequate amounts of B vitamins in their diets.

Energy drinks (Red Bull, Rush Energy, Monster Energy), containing high kilocalories and high caffeine levels, are the fastest growing beverage category in the United States. Between June 2006 and June 2007, Americans spent $744 million on energy drinks.[5] Energy drinks usually contain 140 kcal per 8 oz, which is all from carbohydrates. These beverages may include some nutrients, but few include the principal nutrients lacking in Americans' diets—calcium, potassium, folate, and vitamin D. Energy drinks are inappropriate for athletic activities because of the transient dehydrating effect of the caffeine.

Although caffeine is beneficial for physical and mental performance in some cases, very little research has been conducted to validate the benefits of very high caffeine intake. Caffeine significantly increases a person's metabolic rate and may be associated with increased wakefulness. Very high caffeine intake has been associated with nervousness, restlessness, anxiety, insomnia, gastrointestinal upset, tremors, and psychomotor agitation. Moderate amounts of caffeine do not cause these effects in most individuals. Energy drinks have contributed to increases in emergency department visits owing to excessive caffeine intake and combining these drinks with alcohol. In the medical community, many are concerned about potential negative problems associated with the stimulant's use in beverages and the fact caffeine content is not indicated on the product.[6] Use of energy drinks may increase the risk for caffeine overdose in caffeine abstainers, as well as habitual consumers of caffeine from coffee, soft drinks, and tea, and could contribute to caffeine withdrawal symptoms.

Sports drinks (Gatorade, POWERade) are popular among children and sports enthusiasts. They may contain fewer kilocalories than soda and some fruit juices. They are designed to restore fluid balance and provide energy for use during exercise. Research suggests enamel erosion with various beverages occurs in the following order: energy drinks, sports drinks, regular soda, and diet soda.[7] Calcium added to sports drinks lessens the erosive potential to teeth.[8]

Americans consume 21% of their daily kilocalories from all beverages, an increase from 13% to 15% in the 1970s. Approximately 50% of the increase in energy intake occurring over the past 20 years is contributed by the consumption of sweetened beverages.[9] Most people are unaware of how many kilocalories are in the beverages they drink, but these kilocalories are a major contributor to the alarming increase in obesity. Although water is the only fluid truly needed by the body, many other liquids are acceptable, and some, such as low-fat milk, contribute significant amounts of protein, calcium, and vitamin D. Figure 11-4A depicts the beverage intake pattern of adults in the United States from the 1999-2002 *National Health and Nutrition Examination Survey* (NHANES); the beverages in these amounts and proportions represent almost 500 kcal daily. Figure 11-4B is a suggested beverage consumption pattern that would provide slightly more than 200 kcal (or 10% of a 2200-kcal diet).[9]

HYPER-STATES AND HYPO-STATES

Regulation of fluid intake and excretion by the kidneys usually maintains fluid balance in the body despite a wide range of fluid intake. Imbalances may occur, however. **Fluid volume excess (FVE)** is the relatively equal gain of water and sodium in relation to their losses; **fluid volume deficit (FVD)** results from relatively equal losses of sodium and water.

Fluid Volume Excess

Fluid volume excess mainly occurs in ECF compartments secondary to an increase in total body sodium content (Fig. 11-5). Because water follows sodium, an excess of sodium leads to an increase in total body water. Excess fluid moves into the interstitial compartments, located between cells and in body cavities such as the joints, pleura, and gastrointestinal tract, causing edema.

Congestive heart failure, chronic renal failure, chronic liver disease, and high levels of steroids may predispose an individual to FVE because of sodium retention. Diseases causing a loss of protein and reduced serum albumin levels (e.g., malnutrition and renal diseases) may contribute to FVE because the osmotic forces ordinarily exhibited by proteins and albumin are lacking. Common manifestations of FVE include rapid weight gain, puffy eyelids, distended neck veins, and elevated blood pressure. **Peripheral** edema is observed, such as in the legs and feet. Treatment involves correction of the underlying problems, or therapy for the specific disease. Treatment may involve fluid or sodium restriction or both, or the use of diuretics.

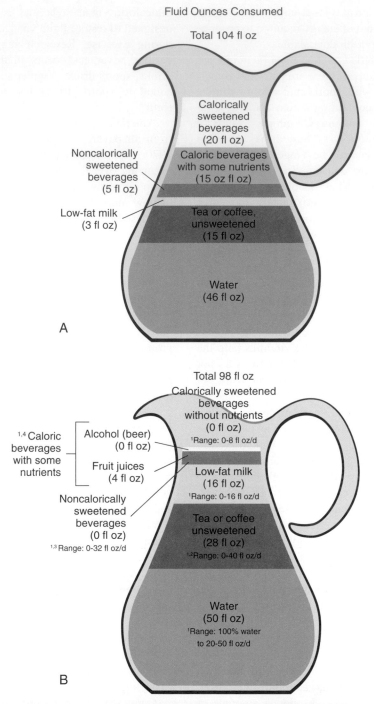

FIGURE II-4 **A,** Average daily beverage intake patterns for U.S. adults 19 years old and older, 1999-2002. **B,** Suggested beverage consumption patterns (10% of energy from beverages) for a person with a 2200-kcal daily energy requirement. The values 50 fl oz, 28 fl oz, 16 fl oz, and 4 fl oz are shown for illustrative purposes only; the total should sum to 98 fl oz, as shown at the top of the figure. [1]The Beverage Guidance Panel's suggested range for each beverage. [2]Range: caffeine is a limiting factor up to 400 mg per day or ~32 fl oz coffee per day (can replace water). [3]Can substitute for tea and coffee with the same limitations regarding caffeine. [4]100% fruit juices, 0-8 fl oz per day; alcoholic beverages, 0-1 drink per day for women and 0-2 drinks per day for men; whole milk, 0 fl oz per day. 1 fl oz = 29.57 mL. (Redrawn from Popkin BM, et al: A new proposed guidance system for beverage consumption in the United States. Am J Clin Nutr 2006 Mar; 83[3]:529-542.)

Fluid Volume Deficit

In FVD, the sodium-to-water ratio remains relatively equal; ADH and aldosterone secretions are not activated. Prolonged inadequate fluid intake can result in FVD. However, FVD is usually associated with excessive loss of fluids from the gastrointestinal tract (vomiting, diarrhea, drainage tubes), urinary tract (diuretics, polyuria, or excessive urination), or skin (sweating). Fever increases the need for electrolytes, increases fluid losses in dehumidified air (e.g., in an airplane), and causes **diaphoresis** or excessive sweating.

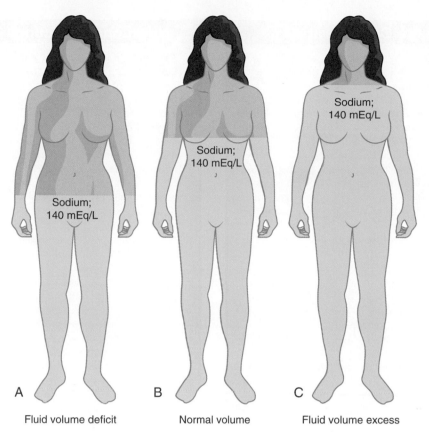

FIGURE 11-5 **A-C,** Fluid-volume disturbances. Compared with normal body fluids (**B**), in fluid volume deficit (FVD) (**A**), equal percentages of water and sodium losses occur, producing an isotonic depletion. In fluid volume excess (**C**), water and sodium are retained, producing an isotonic expansion. (Adapted from Davis JR, Sherer K: Applied Nutrition and Diet Therapy for Nurses, 2nd ed. Philadelphia: Saunders, 1994.)

Dehydration adversely influences cognitive function and motor control. Decreased food and fluid intake can result from dementia, anorexia, nausea, or fatigue. Other, less obvious reasons are an inability to (1) obtain water, such as with impaired movement; (2) activate the thirst mechanism, as in **hypodipsia** (diminished thirst); or (3) swallow, as in neuromuscular problems or unconsciousness. Excessive fluid losses occasionally occur with prolonged exercise.

Common characteristics of FVD include weight loss, confusion and fatigue, sunken eyes, hypotension, and orthostatic hypotension. Classic signs are dry tongue with **longitudinal fissures** (slits or wrinkles that extend lengthwise on the tongue) (Fig. 11-6), xerostomia, shrinkage of oral mucous membranes, decreased skin turgor, dry skin, and decreased urinary output. A diminished salivary flow is associated with inadequate fluid intake. Pale yellow or almost colorless urine indicates adequate hydration. Dark yellow urine with a strong odor, advancing to painful urination, and (eventually) cessation of urine formation are progressive signs of inadequate water intake and dehydration. Treatment involves replacing lost fluid. If FVD is mild, oral fluids are likely to be sufficient. Intravenous solutions are needed with significant FVD.

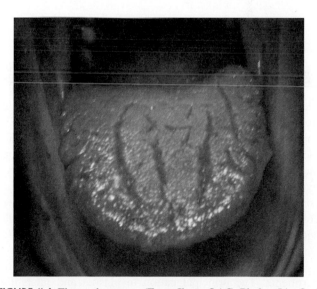

FIGURE 11-6 Fissured tongue. (From Ibsen OAC, Phelan JA: Oral Pathology for the Dental Hygienist, 5th ed. St Louis, Saunders, 2009.)

Dental Hygiene Considerations

- Direct measurement of the total amount of body water is impossible. Evaluation of physical signs of fluid deficit or excess is vital to diagnosis and treatment.
- Assess patients for puffy eyelids or distended neck veins; ask if they have observed recent unintentional weight changes, check their blood pressure, and refer to a healthcare provider if necessary. A rapid weight loss or gain of 3% or greater of total body weight is significant.
- Observe for dry tongue with longitudinal fissures, xerostomia, or shrinkage of oral mucous membranes; adequacy of salivary flow; decreased skin turgor; and dry skin. Inquire about frequency and amount of urine output and fluid intake.
- Salivary flow measurements may be indicated for patients who present with FVD.
- Reduced total body water, decreased renal function, decreased renin activity, and aldosterone secretion in geriatric patients place them at risk for dehydration. In addition, this population may drink less fluid because of dementia, immobility, or fear of incontinence.
- The greater surface area-to-body mass ratio in infants places this group at risk for FVD.
- Rapid weight changes generally indicate loss or gain of water rather than fatty tissue; a loss or gain of 480 mL (2 cups) of fluid is equivalent to a loss or gain of 1 lb.
- Because of the sensitivity of the oral mucosa to the body's fluid volume, increases and decreases in body fluid affect the fit of a denture. FVD generates a loose-fitting prosthesis, whereas FVE may create a tight-fitting prosthesis. Patients may present with ulcerations in each situation and find the prosthesis uncomfortable to wear.
- Question patients regarding use of herbal supplements. Ma-huang (ephedra) and products containing this herb can cause xerostomia.

Nutritional Directions

- To help with conversion of total water intake: 1 L = 33.8 fluid oz, and 1 cup = 8 fluid oz.
- Encourage patients experiencing a "dry mouth" to increase fluid intake and salivary production by chewing sugarless gum, preferably gum containing xylitol.
- Habitual intake of caffeinated beverages (coffee, tea, soft drinks, and other caffeinated beverages) contributes to the daily total water intake similar to that contributed by noncaffeinated beverages.[10]
- Most experts consider moderate caffeine consumption to be about 300 mg, or about 3 cups of coffee for all populations, including sensitive subpopulations such as pregnant women.[11]
- Based on limited data, moderate amounts of alcohol ingestion increase fluid excretion and do not result in appreciable fluid losses.
- High-protein diets, such as diets in which protein foods are principally eaten with minimal fruit and vegetable intake, require larger amounts of water to eliminate the higher levels of urinary waste products.
- Because of fluid loss through perspiration, patients need to drink fluid during exercise. (Loss of 1 lb of body weight during exercise means that at least 2 cups of water have been lost.) In most cases, water is the most appropriate choice.
- To make wise beverage choices, read labels on bottled waters to see what ingredients they contain.
- Most tap water is safe and economical and tastes good.
- Water is the preferred beverage to fulfill daily fluid needs. Beverages with no or few kilocalories should take precedence over the consumption of beverages with more kilocalories.[9]

ELECTROLYTES

Electrolytes are compounds or ions that dissociate in solution; they are also known as **cations** if they have a positive charge, and **anions** if they have a negative charge. Cations include sodium, potassium, calcium, and magnesium; anions include chloride, bicarbonate, and phosphate. The body's hydration status depends on an electrolyte balance of equal concentrations of cations to anions. Because the electrolyte concentration in plasma is so low, it is expressed as milliequivalents per liter (mEq/L). Electrolytes are important in water balance and acid-base (pH) balance.

Electrolyte distribution is different in ICF and ECF compartments. The principal cation in plasma and interstitial fluid is sodium; the principal anion is chloride. The principal cation in ICF is potassium; the principal anion is phosphate. The major difference between intravascular fluid and interstitial fluid is the large amount of protein in the former. Because sodium and potassium are the major cations, these are discussed in more detail.

SODIUM

PHYSIOLOGICAL ROLES

The important physiological roles of sodium include (1) maintaining normal ECF concentration by affecting the concentration, excretion, and absorption of potassium and chloride, and water distribution; (2) regulating acid-base balance; and (3) facilitating impulse transmission in nerve and muscle fibers. Sodium is present in calcified structures in the body; its function in bones and teeth is unclear. It is also present in saliva. Sodium concentration in saliva determines one's recognition of salt in food.

REQUIREMENTS AND REGULATION

Because sodium is so readily available in foods, no RDA has been established. The IOM estimates a safe minimum intake might be set at 500 mg per day. This amount is increased in the face of abnormal losses. Sodium regulation involves several mechanisms. To keep the ECF concentration normal, the sodium-potassium pump is constantly moving sodium from the cell to the ECF. Aldosterone released by the adrenal cortex results in sodium reabsorption or excretion by the kidneys depending on the body's need

(Fig. 11-7). The kidneys can adjust sodium excretion to match sodium intake despite large variations in intake. If serum sodium is high, aldosterone is inhibited, and sodium is excreted; the opposite is true for depressed serum sodium levels.

For most adults, the AI for sodium is 1500 mg per day with the upper limit being 2300 mg per day (Table 11-3). This AI does not apply to highly active individuals, such as endurance athletes, who lose large amounts of sodium through sweat. Currently, the American Heart Association dietary guidelines and the daily values (DV) on food labels are based on a recommended intake of no more than 2400 mg daily.

Average consumption of salt is approximately 4000 mg per day for men and 2900 mg per day for women.[12] MyPyramid encourages decreasing salt intake to 2300 mg per day. However, further research is needed to determine the optimal amount that is safe and efficacious in reducing cardiovascular events for the entire population.[13-15]

SOURCES

About 10% of the sodium consumed by people comes from the natural content of foods and fluids regularly ingested. Sodium is a natural constituent of most foods (Table 11-4); animal foods such as meat, saltwater fish, and eggs and dairy products, and some vegetables (beets, carrots, celery,

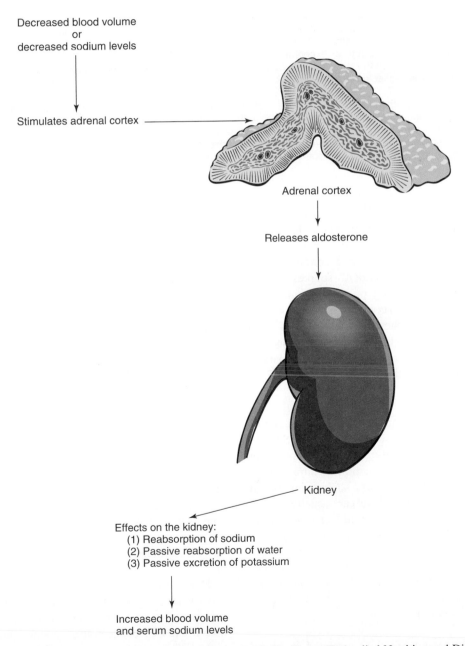

Decreased blood volume
or
decreased sodium levels

Stimulates adrenal cortex

Adrenal cortex

Releases aldosterone

Kidney

Effects on the kidney:
(1) Reabsorption of sodium
(2) Passive reabsorption of water
(3) Passive excretion of potassium

Increased blood volume
and serum sodium levels

FIGURE 11-7 Effects of aldosterone on sodium levels. (Adapted from Davis JR, Sherer K: Applied Nutrition and Diet Therapy for Nurses, 2nd ed. Philadelphia: Saunders, 1994.)

Table 11-3 Institute of Medicine Recommendations for Sodium and Chloride

Life Stage	AI* for Sodium Male (g/d)	AI* for Sodium Female (g/d)	UL† for Sodium Male (g/d)	UL† for Sodium Female (g/d)	AI for Chloride Male (g/d)	AI for Chloride Female (g/d)	UL for Chloride Male (g/d)	UL for Chloride Female (g/d)
0-6 mo	0.12	0.12	ND‡	ND‡	0.18	0.18	ND‡	ND‡
7-12 mo	0.37	0.37	ND‡	ND‡	0.57	0.57	ND‡	ND‡
1-3 yr	1	1	1.5	1.5	1.5	1.5	2.3	2.3
4-8 yr	1.2	1.2	1.9	1.9	1.9	1.9	2.9	2.9
9-14 yr	1.5	1.5	2.2	2.2	2.3	2.3	3.4	3.4
14-50 yr	1.5	1.5	2.3	2.3	2.3	2.3	3.6	3.6
51-70 yr	1.3	1.3	2.3	2.3	2	2	2.3	2.3
>70 yr	1.2	1.2	2.3	2.3	1.8	1.8	2.3	2.3
Pregnancy 14-50 yr		1.5		2.3		2.3		3.6
Lactation 14-50 yr		1.5		2.3		2.3		3.6

Data from Institute of Medicine (IOM), Food and Nutrition Board: Dietary Reference Intakes for Water, Potassium, Sodium, Chloride, Chloride, and Sulfate. Washington, DC: National Academies Press, 2005.

*AI (adequate intake)—the observed average or experimentally set intake by a defined population or subgroup that seems to sustain a defined nutritional status, such as growth rate, normal circulating nutrient values, or other functional indicators of health. An AI is used if insufficient scientific evidence is available to derive an EAR. For healthy human milk–fed infants, the AI is the mean intake. The AI is not equivalent to an RDA.

†UL (tolerable upper intake level)—the highest level of daily nutrient intake that is likely to pose no risk of adverse health effects to almost all individuals in the general population. As intake increases above the UL, the risk of adverse effects increases. Unless specified otherwise, the UL represents total nutrient intake from food, water, and supplements.

‡ND—not determinable because of lack of data of adverse effects in this age group and concern with regard to lack of ability to handle excess amounts. Source of intake should be from food and formula to prevent high levels of intake.

spinach, and other dark green leafy vegetables) contain measurable amounts of sodium. Processed, cured, canned, pickled, convenience, and fast foods, and condiments are significant sources of sodium. "Hidden" sources include softened and bottled water, baking powder, baking soda, dentifrices (including toothpastes containing baking soda or sodium fluoride), antibiotics, chewing tobacco, and over-the-counter medications (e.g., antacids, cough medicines, or laxatives). Food manufacturers are developing and marketing products containing less sodium.

HYPER-STATES AND HYPO-STATES

Serum sodium concentration is an index of water deficit or excess, not an index of sodium levels of the body. Sodium levels in the blood are significantly higher than potassium levels because sodium is the major cation in intravascular fluid. **Hypernatremia** (elevated serum sodium level) and **hyponatremia** (low serum sodium level) are usually a result of hormonal imbalances or increased fluid loss or retention. "True" hypernatremia or hyponatremia, or imbalances caused by too much or too little sodium intake, rarely occur in adults. If renal and hormonal mechanisms for sodium retention and excretion function efficiently, and water intake is adequate, the amount of dietary sodium causes little change in total body sodium; sodium fluctuations do affect plasma volume.

Because water and sodium are closely related, a change in one causes a change in the other. Hypernatremia can be associated with FVD or FVE. A very high sodium intake can be toxic, especially if accompanied with insufficient fluids (Box 11-1).

Water deprivation (as occurs in unconscious, debilitated individuals or infants), insensible water loss (as a result of exposure to dry heat, sweating, hyperventilation), and watery diarrhea lead to a loss of water in excess of sodium. Infants are more prone to watery diarrhea, whereas older patients are susceptible to water deprivation. If polyuria is not balanced with increased water intake, hypernatremia may occur.

Symptoms of hypernatremia are a result of fluid moving from the ICF to the ECF in an attempt to equalize sodium and water balance. This movement of fluid causes atrophy of tissue cells. Cells in the central nervous system shrink, producing hallucinations, disorientation, lethargy, and possibly coma. Other signs are extreme thirst; dry, "sticky" tongue and oral mucous membranes; fever; and convulsions. A sticky tongue can be identified by slowly rolling a tongue depressor over the lateral side of the tongue; tacky filiform papillae stick to the tongue depressor and rise up.

Hyponatremia may develop when sodium losses exceed water losses, or when fluids are retained, leading to a greater concentration of water than of sodium. Because of the decrease in ECF concentration, sodium moves from the ECF to the ICF, and water enters the ICF, causing cellular edema. This can cause problems, especially in the cranium where

Table 11-4	Sodium Content of Food*
Foods	**Approximate Sodium Content (mg)**
Breads, Cereals, and Grain Products	
Cereal, pasta, rice (unsalted), cooked	<5 per ½ cup
Cereal, ready-to-eat	Trace per ¾-1 cup
Bread, whole grain or enriched	90-210 per slice
Biscuits and muffins	170-590 each
Saltines	312 per 8 crackers
French fries	168 per small order
Vegetables	
Fresh or frozen vegetables (cooked without added salt)	<70 per ½ cup
Vegetables, canned or frozen with sauce	140-780 per ½ cup
Tomato juice, canned	438 per ½ cup
Fruit	
Fruits (fresh, frozen, or canned)	<10 per ½ cup
Milk, Cheese, and Yogurt	
Milk and yogurt	120-170 per 1 cup
Buttermilk	260 per 1 cup
Natural cheeses	110-460 per 1 oz
Cottage cheese (regular and low-fat)	460 per ½ cup
Processed cheese and cheese spreads	350-450 per 1 oz
Meat, Poultry, and Fish	
Fresh meat, poultry, fish	<90 per 3 oz
Cured ham, sausages, luncheon meat, frankfurters, canned meats	750-1350 per 3 oz
Fats and Dressings	
Oil	None
Vinegar	<6 per 1 Tbsp
Prepared salad dressings	80-250 per 1 Tbsp
Butter or margarine, unsalted	1 per 1 tsp
Salt pork, cooked	360 per 1 oz
Miscellaneous	
Catsup, mustard, chili sauce, tartar sauce, steak sauce, teriyaki sauce, Worcestershire sauce	125-690 per 1 Tbsp
Soy sauce	871 per 1 Tbsp
Salt	2000 per 1 tsp
Baking soda	1260 per 1 tsp
Dill pickles (3¾ inches long)	833 per whole
Spaghetti/marinara/pasta sauce	515 per ½ cup
Baking powder	488 per 1 tsp
Green olives	408 per 5 medium
Sports drinks	50-125 per 8 oz
Meal replacement beverages	190-290 per 8 oz
Snack and Convenience Foods	
Canned and dehydrated soups	630-1100 per 1 cup
Canned and frozen main dishes	800-1400 per 8 oz serving
Nuts and popcorn, unsalted	<5 per 1 oz
Nuts, potato chips, corn chips, nacho chips, salted	150-300 per 1 oz
Pork rind, deep-fried	520 per 1 oz

Data from U.S. Department of Agriculture, Agricultural Research Service, USDA Nutrient Data Laboratory, USDA National Nutrient Database for Standard Reference, Release 20, 2008. Available at http://www.nal.usda.gov/fnic/foodcomp. Accessed February 28, 2008.
*The ranges are rough guides: Individual food items may be higher or lower in sodium.

Box 11-1	Guidelines for Implementing the *Dietary Guidelines for Americans* for Sodium Intake (2300 mg)

- Avoid foods with concentrated sources of sodium, and do not add salt to foods.
- Avoid adding salt to food at the table or in recipes. Flavor foods with herbs, spices, wine, lemon, lime, or vinegar (see Table 11-5 for additional ideas).
- Salt substitutes can contain sodium, potassium, and other minerals. Salt substitutes should not be used unless approved by a healthcare provider or dietitian.
- Sodium is found naturally in most foods. Animal products such as meat, fish, poultry, milk, and eggs are naturally higher in sodium than fruits and vegetables.
- Restaurant meals should be selected carefully because of their high sodium content.
- Limit the following high-sodium processed foods:
  Meats: Smoked, cured, salted, or canned meats, fish, or poultry, including bacon, cold cuts, ham, frankfurters, and sausages; sardines, anchovies, and marinated herring; pickled meats or pickled eggs
  Dairy products: Processed cheese, blue cheese, buttermilk
  Vegetables: Sauerkraut, pickled vegetables prepared in brine, commercially frozen vegetable mixes with sauces
  Breads and cereals: Breads, rolls, and crackers with salted tops
  Soups: Canned soups, dried soup mixes, broth, bouillon (except salt-free)
  Fats: Salad dressings containing bacon bits, salt pork, dips made with instant soup mixes and processed cheese
  Beverages: Commercially softened water, cocoa mixes, club soda, sports drinks, tomato or vegetable juice
  Miscellaneous: Casserole and pasta mixes; salted chips, popcorn, and nuts; olives; commercial stuffing; gravy mixes; seasoning salts (garlic, celery, onion), light salt, monosodium glutamate (MSG); meat tenderizer; catsup, prepared mustard, prepared horseradish, soy sauce
- Read food labels. Compare the sodium content of products.
- Use reduced sodium or no-salt-added products. Read the ingredient list on food labels to identify and avoid sources of sodium additives such as salt, sodium chloride (NaCl), sodium caseinate, MSG, trisodium phosphate, sodium ascorbate, and sodium bicarbonate.
- Foods making nutrient claims must meet certain labeling guides (see Box 1-4).

Table 11-5	Herbs and Spices to Complement Foods

Food	Herbs/Spices
Soups	Bay, tarragon, marjoram, parsley, rosemary
Poultry	Garlic, ginger, oregano, rosemary, sage, tarragon
Beef	Onion, bay, chives, cloves, cumin, garlic, pepper, marjoram, rosemary, thyme, ginger
Lamb	Garlic, marjoram, oregano, rosemary, thyme
Pork	Onion, coriander, cumin, garlic, ginger, hot pepper, pepper, sage, thyme, ginger
Cheese	Basil, chives, curry, dill, fennel, garlic, marjoram, oregano, parsley, sage, thyme
Fish	Dill, curry powder, paprika, fennel, tarragon, garlic, parsley, thyme
Fruit	Cinnamon, coriander, cloves, ginger, mint
Bread	Caraway, marjoram, oregano, poppy seed, rosemary, thyme
Carrots	Cinnamon, cloves, nutmeg, marjoram, sage
Green beans	Dill, oregano, tarragon, thyme
Potatoes, rutabaga	Dill, garlic, paprika, parsley, sage
Winter squash/ sweet potatoes	Cloves, nutmeg, cinnamon, ginger
Other vegetables	Basil, chives, dill, tarragon, marjoram, mint, parsley, pepper, thyme
Salads	Basil, chives, French tarragon, garlic, parsley, arugula, sorrel (best if fresh or added to salad dressing, or use herbs and vinegars for extra flavor.)

there is no room for expansion. Sodium deficiency may lead to a decrease in salivary flow or a decrease in the sodium concentration of saliva.

Water intoxication or hyponatremia can occur when individuals drink too much water (many liters a day). The blood sodium level decreases to a dangerously low level, causing headaches, blurred vision, cramps, swelling of the brain, coma, and possibly death.

Heat exhaustion in unacclimated individuals may result in a sodium deficit. Hyponatremia also may occur in individuals who drink excessive quantities of water as part of a psychiatric disorder, or when excessive amounts of diuretics are given. Hyperglycemia may precipitate hyponatremia because the elevated blood glucose level draws water into the vascular space (edema), causing a dilutional effect. Excessive vomiting and diarrhea, especially in infants, can also lead to a sodium deficit.

Early symptoms of hyponatremia are nausea and abdominal cramps. Other symptoms—headache, confusion, lethargy, and coma—are the result of cellular edema. Even though there is cellular edema, peripheral edema is not present. This is because the water is primarily retained within cells rather than in the interstitial compartment. Chronic hyponatremia is usually well tolerated. It may or may not be treated, depending on the precipitating cause and severity.

Dental Hygiene Considerations

- Assess patients for signs and symptoms of hypernatremia (thirst; dry, sticky tongue; xerostomia) and hyponatremia.
- The salt recognition threshold is determined by sodium concentration of saliva (i.e., the lower the level of sodium in the saliva, the easier it is for one to detect a small amount of salt in food).
- Patients with hypertension who are salt sensitive need to consume 2300 mg or less of sodium daily. Encourage these patients to use herbs and spices to flavor food instead of high-sodium seasonings.
- A low salt recognition threshold is desirable for patients who need to curtail salt intake for health reasons, but in a hyponatremic patient, diminished salt consumption could contribute further to sodium depletion.
- Sodium deficiency may lead to a decreased salivary flow rate.
- High levels of sodium (greater than 2 g per day) cause loss of calcium in the urine.
- Identify "hidden" sources of sodium in a patient's diet. Educate the patient regarding sodium intake reduction.

Nutritional Directions

- Stress the importance of appropriate sodium intake, as recommended by the healthcare provider.
- Dietary sodium restriction is rarely the cause of hyponatremia. Sodium depletion may occur in combination with excessive losses as a result of vomiting, diarrhea, surgery, or profuse perspiration from exercise or fever.
- To convert milligrams of sodium to milliequivalents, divide the number by 23 (the atomic weight of sodium). For example, 1000 mg of sodium ÷ 23 = 43 mEq of sodium.
- Table salt contains sodium and chloride (40% sodium and 60% chloride), 1 tsp of salt is equivalent to 2000 mg of sodium.
- Many low-sodium or reduced-sodium foods are available as alternatives to foods processed with salt and other sodium-containing ingredients. Compare labels for the sodium content of these foods to find the lowest value.
- The water supply and use of water softeners are "hidden" sources of sodium.

CHLORIDE

PHYSIOLOGICAL ROLES

Chlorine is the primary anion connected with sodium in ECF to help maintain ECF balance, osmotic equilibrium, and electrolyte balance. Large concentrations of chloride are present in gastric secretions, which are important for protein digestion and creating an acidic environment to inhibit bacterial growth and enhance iron, calcium, and vitamin B_{12} absorption.

REQUIREMENTS AND REGULATION

The AI for chloride has been set by the IOM at 2300 mg per day (see Table 11-3). Chloride intake and losses parallel those of sodium.

SOURCES

Most chloride intake is from salt (sodium chloride). Sources of chloride are the same as those for sodium, including processed foods. Water is an additional source of chloride.

HYPER-STATES AND HYPO-STATES

Toxicity from chloride can be caused by excessive intakes of salt (NaCl), dehydration, renal failure, diarrhea, and Cushing's syndrome. Conditions associated with sodium depletion, such as persistent heavy sweating, chronic diarrhea, vomiting, or chronic renal failure, may precipitate hypochloremia and an acid-base imbalance.

POTASSIUM

PHYSIOLOGICAL ROLES

Potassium has the following important physiological roles: (1) maintains cellular (ICF) concentration, (2) directly affects muscle contraction (especially cardiac) and electrical conductivity of the heart, (3) facilitates transmission of nerve impulses, and (4) regulates acid-base balance. Potassium is important to sustain good muscle function for physically active individuals.

REQUIREMENTS AND REGULATION

Similar to sodium, there is no RDA for potassium. As shown in Table 11-6, the AI for potassium has been established by the IOM at 4700 mg per day for all adults. This is equivalent to approximately 10 servings of fruits and vegetables each day. No UL has been set for healthy adults.

Poor food choices result in diets deficient in potassium. Additionally, high intake of meats and other animal proteins cause further depletion of this mineral. Based on the NHANES III study, average potassium intake is significantly lower than the AI, averaging slightly above 3000 mg per day for men and 2300 mg per day for women.[14] Low potassium consumption can cause sensitivity to salt, further increasing the risk of hypertension.[16]

The sodium-potassium pump regulates potassium levels. Depending on cellular needs, potassium is constantly moving either into or out of cells. Aldosterone indirectly affects serum potassium levels. If aldosterone is released, sodium is reabsorbed, but potassium is excreted. Subsequently, if aldosterone is inhibited, potassium is retained in the body (see Fig. 11-7). Approximately 92% of ingested potassium is excreted in the urine.[17] Some is lost through feces or sweat.

SOURCES

Sources of potassium are naturally available from foods and fluids regularly ingested (Table 11-7). Dairy, meat, and

Table 11-6	Institute of Medicine Recommendations for Potassium	
	AI*	
Life Stage	Male (g/d)	Female (g/d)
0-6 mo	0.4	0.4
7-12 mo	0.7	0.7
1-3 yr	3	3
4-8 yr	3.8	3.8
9-13 yr	4.5	4.5
≥14 yr	4.7	4.7
Pregnancy		
≥18 yr		4.7
Lactation		
≥18 yr		5.1

Data from Institute of Medicine (IOM), Food and Nutrition Board: Dietary Reference Intakes for Water, Potassium, Sodium, Chloride, Chloride, and Sulfate. Washington, DC: National Academies Press, 2005.

*AI (adequate intake)—the observed average or experimentally set intake by a defined population or subgroup that seems to sustain a defined nutritional status, such as growth rate, normal circulating nutrient values, or other functional indicators of health. An AI is used if insufficient scientific evidence is unavailable to derive an EAR. For healthy human milk–fed infants, the AI is the mean intake. The AI is not equivalent to an RDA.

Table 11-7	Potassium Content of Selected Foods	
Food	Portion	Potassium (mg)
Potato, baked	1	926
Acorn squash, baked	½ cup	486
Lima beans	½ cup	478
Cantaloupe	1 cup	473
Fruited yogurt	8 oz	440
Banana	1	422
Spinach, cooked	½ cup	419
Apricots, dried	10 halves	410
Ensure	8 oz	410
Peaches, dried	3 halves	388
Milk	1 cup	382
Pinto beans	½ cup	373
Sirloin steak, broiled	3 oz	371
Kidney beans	½ cup	303
Tomatoes, stewed	½ cup	264
Beets, cooked	½ cup	259
Orange juice	½ cup	236
Fresh broccoli, cooked	½ cup	229
Zucchini, cooked	½ cup	228
Asparagus, cooked	½ cup	202
Oatmeal	1 cup	164
Wheat germ bread	1 slice	71
Wheat bran bread	1 slice	67
Gatorade sports beverage	8 oz	37

Data from U.S. Department of Agriculture, Agricultural Research Service, USDA Nutrient Data Laboratory, USDA National Nutrient Database for Standard Reference, Release 20, 2008. Available at http://www.nal.usda.gov/fnic/foodcomp. Accessed February 28, 2008.

grains contribute 56%, and fruits and vegetables contribute 44% of total dietary potassium. Milk is the number one single food source of potassium for all age groups in the United States.[17] Processed foods usually contain less potassium than fresh products. Potassium supplements and salt substitutes are another source; salt substitutes (potassium chloride [KCl]) often replace sodium with potassium.

HYPER-STATES AND HYPO-STATES

Minor deviations in serum potassium levels can be life-threatening. Abnormal levels are referred to as either **hyperkalemia** (elevated serum potassium level) or **hypokalemia** (low serum potassium level).

Hyperkalemia has three causes: (1) impaired renal excretion, (2) increased shift of potassium out of cells, and (3) increased potassium intake. Acute or chronic renal failure impairs potassium excretion, resulting in potassium being retained in the body. This is logical because 80% is excreted through the kidneys. Increased serum potassium levels can result from an increased dietary intake, excessive administration of potassium supplements orally or intravenously, or excessive use of potassium-containing salt substitutes. Burns, trauma, crushing injuries, myocardial infarction, Addison's disease, insulin deficiency, hypoaldosteronism, increased catabolism, and acidosis can allow for secretion of potassium by the distal nephron.

Hyperkalemia is life-threatening because cardiac arrest may occur. Elevated potassium levels are irritating to the body; symptoms include muscle weakness (the first sign), tingling and numbness in the extremities, diarrhea, brady-cardia, abdominal cramps, confusion, and electrocardiographic changes. Treatment for hyperkalemia involves potassium restriction or using medications to remove potassium.

Potential consequences of chronic potassium deficiency are often unrecognized. Problems include hypertension, heart attacks, strokes, kidney stones, and a loss of bone minerals that can lead to osteoporosis. Potassium deficiency can cause individuals to feel tired, weak, and irritable, while unable to pinpoint a cause.

Excessive loss or inadequate intake of potassium can result in hypokalemia. Potassium loss occurs through the gastrointestinal and renal tracts and by excessive sweating. Because potassium is contained in gastric and intestinal secretions, vomiting and diarrhea may cause hypokalemia. Some potassium is lost through sweat; excessive perspiration can lead to hypokalemia. Drugs, such as the diuretics furosemide and hydrochlorothiazide and the antibiotics carbenicillin and amphotericin B, are the major offenders. Cushing's syndrome, hyperaldosteronism, an excess of insulin, hypomagnesemia, alcoholism, and alkalosis also cause hypokalemia.

Potassium is the major ICF cation; deficits can affect every body system. Death from cardiac or respiratory arrest can occur. Clinical manifestations are anorexia, absence of bowel sounds, muscle weakness in the legs, leg cramps, and electrocardiographic changes.

Dental Hygiene Considerations

- Be aware of factors that can cause potassium to increase or decrease. Refer the patient to the healthcare provider or dietitian as needed.
- Patients consuming a potassium supplement should avoid gastrointestinal irritants, such as pepper, caffeine, and alcohol.

Nutritional Directions

- Stress the importance of appropriate potassium intake.
- Read labels; salt substitutes may be high in potassium. Consult a healthcare provider or dietitian before using potassium-containing salt substitutes.
- Encourage patients taking potassium-wasting diuretics to consume high-potassium foods if they are not taking a potassium supplement.
- Medical conditions that can interfere with excretion of potassium include diabetes, renal failure, severe heart events, and adrenal insufficiency.
- Medications that can interfere with excretion of potassium are angiotensin-converting enzyme inhibitors, angiotensin receptor blockers, and potassium-sparing diuretics.

IRON

PHYSIOLOGICAL ROLES

Every cell contains iron; approximately 4 g (less than 1 tsp) is present in the entire body. Iron is a major component of hemoglobin, which transports oxygen from the lungs to the tissues, including the oral soft and hard tissues. It also catalyzes many oxidative reactions within cells and participates in the final steps of energy metabolism. Other roles include (1) conversion of beta carotene to vitamin A, (2) synthesis of collagen, (3) formation of purines as part of nucleic acid, (4) removal of lipids from the blood, (5) detoxification of drugs in the liver, and (6) production of antibodies.

Lactoferrin, a salivary glycoprotein, is capable of binding iron. It has an antibacterial action by competing with iron-requiring organisms in the mouth for limited amounts of available iron.

REQUIREMENTS

The IOM recommends 18 mg per day for women 19 to 50 years old, 8 mg per day for women 51 years old and older, and 8 mg per day for men 19 years old and older (Table 11-8). The RDA is higher for premenopausal women than for men or postmenopausal women because of blood loss during menstruation. During the reproductive phase of a woman's life, iron loss is at least twice that of a man or of a postmenopausal woman. Despite the fact that premenopausal women need more iron, dietary consumption tends to be less than that of men. Iron requirements also increase during times of impaired absorption (diarrhea), periods of rapid growth, and heavy physical activity because of the increased need for oxygen transport and energy production.

The RDA is based on the approximation that 10% of dietary iron is absorbed. The demand for iron replenishment is constant because cells are continually being replaced; the life of a red blood cell is 120 days. When a cell dies, iron is recycled, being released and transported to various storage sites to be used again. A UL for iron was established at 45 mg per day for adults.

ABSORPTION AND EXCRETION

Similar to calcium, iron is poorly absorbed. Most of the iron in food is in the oxidized form of ferric iron (Fe^{3+}). Gastric acid in the stomach helps promote iron absorption. By binding to the serum protein **transferrin**, iron is continuously transported through the body because transferrin functions to recycle the iron.

Absorption of **heme iron** parallels the body's need; absorption of **nonheme iron** depends on intraluminal and meal composition and physiological need. Heme iron is provided by meat sources containing hemoglobin from red blood cells and myoglobin from muscle molecules. The recommendation is based on consumption of at least 75% of iron intake from heme sources. Nonheme iron is present in eggs, milk, and plants. Acidic conditions enhance iron absorption, but calcium and manganese interfere with its absorption. Factors affecting iron absorption are listed in Figure 11-8.

Combinations of food can enhance iron absorption. A meal of roast beef (rich in iron) with potatoes (rich in vitamin C) increases iron absorption.

SOURCES

Iron is probably the most difficult mineral to obtain in adequate amounts in the American diet. Although liver is often considered the best source of iron, meats (especially beef), egg yolk, dark green vegetables, and enriched breads and cereals all contribute significant amounts (Table 11-9). Iron supplements come in two forms; the ferrous form is better absorbed than the ferric form.

HYPER-STATES AND HYPO-STATES

The body cannot easily eliminate excess iron; this may explain why iron absorption rates are poor. The body seldom overcomes its regulation of intestinal absorption. Iron overload may occur, however, if ingestion of iron is extremely elevated. **Hemochromatosis** is an uncommon disorder in which iron is absorbed at a high rate despite elevated iron

Table 11-8	Institute of Medicine Recommendations for Iron						
	EAR (mg/d)*		**RDA (mg/d)†**		**AI (mg/d)‡**		
Life Stage	*Male*	*Female*	*Male*	*Female*	*Male*	*Female*	**UL (mg/d)§**
0-6 mo					0.27	0.27	40
7-12 mo	6.9	6.9	11	11			40
1-3 yr	3	3	7	7			40
4-8 yr	4.1	4.1	10	10			40
9-13 yr	5.9	5.7	8	8			40
14-18 yr	7.7	7.9	11	15			45
19-50 yr	6	8.1	8	18			45
≥51 yr	6	5	8	8			45
Pregnancy							
14-18 yr		23		27			45
19-50 yr		22		27			45
Lactation							
14-18 yr		7		10			45
19-50 yr		6.5		9			45

Data from Institute of Medicine (IOM), Food and Nutrition Board: Dietary Reference Intakes for Vitamin A, Vitamin K, Arsenic, Boron, Chromium, Copper, Iodine, Iron, Manganese, Molybdenum, Nickel, Silicon, Vanadium, and Zinc. Washington, DC: National Academy Press, 2001.
*EAR (estimated average requirement)—the intake that meets the estimated nutrient needs of half of the individuals in a group.
†RDA (recommended dietary allowance)—the intake that meets the nutrient needs of almost all (97-98%) individuals in a group.
‡AI (adequate intake)—the observed average or experimentally set intake by a defined population or subgroup that seems to sustain a defined nutritional status, such as growth rate, normal circulating nutrient values, or other functional indicators of health. An AI is used if insufficient scientific evidence is available to derive an EAR. For healthy human milk–fed infants, the AI is the mean intake. The AI is not equivalent to an RDA.
§UL (tolerable upper intake level)—the highest level of daily nutrient intake that is likely to pose no risk of adverse health effects to almost all individuals in the general population. As intake increases above the UL, the risk of adverse effects increases. Unless specified otherwise, the UL represents total nutrient intake from food, water, and supplements.

stores in the liver. Accumulation of iron throughout the body may develop with excessive iron intake or multiple blood transfusions. Inexpensive red wines contain wide variations in iron content (10 to 350 mg/L) and have been associated with hemochromatosis. Initially, it is difficult to diagnose because of its resemblance to other conditions in which fatigue and general weakness are symptoms.

Elevated iron stores have been associated with increased risk of coronary heart disease and liver disease. Iron supplements should not be taken indiscriminately and without a comprehensive laboratory workup.

Iron-deficiency anemia continues to be a worldwide problem. A deficiency can lead to various symptoms, such as microcytic anemia, fatigue, faulty digestion, blue sclerae, pale conjunctivae, and tachycardia. Iron-deficiency anemia may be caused by inadequate dietary intake of iron; accelerated iron demand; increased iron losses; and inadequate absorption secondary to diarrhea, decreased acid secretions, or antacid therapy. Iron deficiency is frequently the result of postnatal feeding practices and has a serious impact on growth and on mental and psychomotor development in infants and children.

The most prominent oral signs of iron deficiency include pallor of the lips and oral mucosa, angular cheilitis, atrophy of filiform papillae, and glossitis (see Figs. 16-1 and 16-2). Oral candidiasis and a reduced resistance to infection are frequently associated with iron deficiency.

Dental Hygiene Considerations

- Despite the prevalence of iron-deficiency anemia, supplements are not recommended without laboratory testing to indicate a deficiency.
- The most prominent sign of iron deficiency in the oral cavity is pallor and swelling of the tongue. The patient also may complain of soreness and burning of the tongue. Atrophic changes progress from a patchy denudation of papillae to a smooth, reddened tongue.
- Hemochromatosis is common among chronic alcoholics, usually men, who may drink more than 1 L of inexpensive wine daily. Do not recommend iron-rich and iron-fortified foods to patients with this condition.
- Iron-containing supplements are the leading cause of poisoning deaths in children younger than 6 years old in the United States. Encourage storing iron supplements in a place inaccessible to children.
- Assess patients with renal failure, individuals experiencing periods of rapid growth (pregnant women, infants, toddlers, teenage girls), and vegans for adequate intake of iron-rich foods.
- Maintain good oral hygiene practices when iron supplements are taken to prevent extrinsic staining of teeth. The abrasive effect of baking soda can help reduce staining. Liquid forms of iron can be taken through a straw.
- Because older adults may have a reduced production of gastric acid, this can interfere with and reduce iron absorption, increasing the risk of an iron deficiency. A referral to the healthcare provider may be necessary.

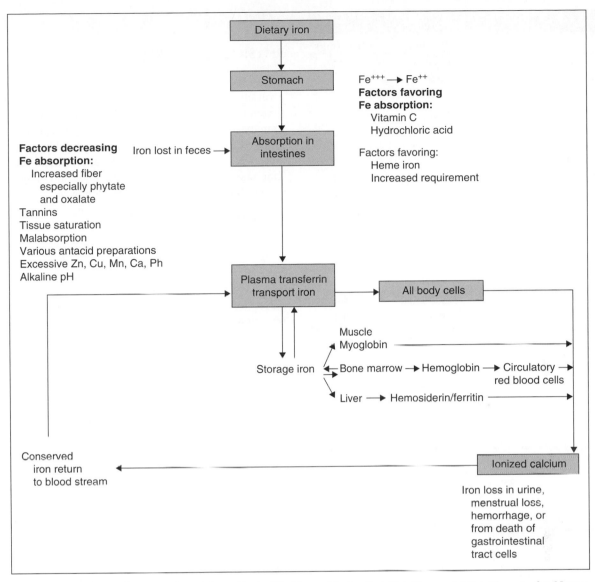

FIGURE 11-8 Iron absorption and use. (Adapted from Davis JR, Sherer K: Applied Nutrition and Diet Therapy for Nurses, 2nd ed. Philadelphia: Saunders, 1994.)

Nutritional Directions

- A food rich in vitamin C with supplements or meals increases iron absorption, especially nonheme iron. Take iron with orange juice, tomato juice, or vitamin C–enriched juices such as apple juice.
- If nonheme-containing grains or vegetables are consumed with small amounts of heme iron, absorption of the nonheme iron doubles.
- Because the iron provided in a vegan diet is the nonheme form, iron absorption is lower than for individuals consuming animal foods. Iron requirements may double for vegans.
- Chemicals (not caffeine) intrinsic to tea and coffee decrease iron absorption. No decrease in iron absorption occurs when tea or coffee is drunk 1 hour before a meal.

- Vitamin A deficiency can cause iron deficiency because vitamin A helps to transport iron from the storage sites.
- Taking iron supplements with food and in divided doses reduces the gastrointestinal symptoms associated with these supplements.
- A common treatment of hemochromatosis or iron overload is to donate blood regularly.
- Avoid taking iron supplements with milk and calcium supplements because calcium interferes with iron absorption. (Only calcium carbonate does not affect absorption of iron.)

Table 11-9 Iron Content of Selected Foods

Food	Portion	Iron (mg)
Total, whole grain	1 cup	22.5
Total Raisin Bran	1 cup	18
Multi Bran Chex	1 cup	15.6
Chicken liver	3 oz	10.5
Instant oatmeal, fortified	½ cup	7
Beef liver	3 oz	5.9
Spinach, cooked	½ cup	3.2
Lean beef sirloin	3 oz	3.1
Ground beef	3 oz	2.6
Shrimp, breaded and fried	3 oz	2.6
Navy beans	½ cup	2.2
Lean rib lamb chop	3 oz	2.1
Tofu, firm	½ cup	2
Kidney beans	½ cup	1.5
Prune juice	½ cup	1.5
Bologna	3 oz	1.1
Wheat bran bread	1 slice	1.1
Sauerkraut	½ cup	1
Apricots, dried	10 halves	0.9
Raisins	½ cup	0.8
Green peas	½ cup	0.8
Chicken breast	3 oz	0.9
Broccoli	½ cup	0.5

Data from U.S. Department of Agriculture, Agricultural Research Service, USDA Nutrient Data Laboratory, USDA National Nutrient Database for Standard Reference, Release 20, 2008. Available at http://www.nal.usda.gov/fnic/foodcomp. Accessed Feb 25, 2008.

ZINC

PHYSIOLOGICAL ROLES

Zinc is a component in more than 200 enzymes that perform a variety of functions affecting cell growth and replication; sexual maturation, fertility, and reproduction; night vision; immune defenses; and taste, smell, and appetite. Zinc is required for DNA, RNA, and protein synthesis. In this role, zinc is essential for bone growth and mineral metabolism. Zinc-containing enzymes are important in collagen synthesis and bone resorption and remodeling.

REQUIREMENTS

The IOM recommends a daily intake of 11 mg for men and 8 mg for women (Table 11-10). Although some concerns have been expressed about marginal intakes, zinc deficiencies have not been reported in Americans consuming a variety of foods. Vegans absorb less zinc than individuals who consume animal foods. The zinc requirement for vegans is definitely higher, and may be twice the RDA for individuals consuming meats. (The RDA is based on the traditional American diet in which most people consume meat.) The UL for zinc is 40 mg per day.

ABSORPTION AND EXCRETION

Bioavailability of zinc varies widely; approximately 25% to 40% of dietary zinc is absorbed. Absorption depends on several factors, including body size; total dietary zinc; and the presence of other potentially interfering substances, such as calcium, fiber, and phosphate salts. Higher quality protein

Table 11-10 Institute of Medicine Recommendations for Zinc

Life Stage	EAR (mg/d)*		RDA (mg/d)†		AI (mg/d)‡		UL (mg/d)§
	Male	Female	Male	Female	Male	Female	
0-6 mo					2	2	4
7-12 mo	2.5	2.5	3	3			5
1-3 yr	2.5	2.5	3	3			7
4-8 yr	4	4	5	5			12
9-13 yr	7	7	8	8			23
14-18 yr	8.5	7.5	11	9			34
≥19 yr	9.4	6.8	11	8			40
Pregnancy							
14-18 yr		10		12			34
19-50 yr		9.5		11			40
Lactation							
14-18 yr		10.9		13			34
19-50 yr		10.4		12			40

Data from Institute of Medicine (IOM), Food and Nutrition Board: Dietary Reference Intakes for Vitamin A, Vitamin K, Arsenic, Boron, Chromium, Copper, Iodine, Iron, Manganese, Molybdenum, Nickel, Silicon, Vanadium, and Zinc. Washington, DC: National Academy Press, 2001.
*EAR (estimated average requirement)—the intake that meets the estimated nutrient needs of half of the individuals in a group.
†RDA (recommended dietary allowance)—the intake that meets the nutrient needs of almost all (97-98%) individuals in a group.
‡AI (adequate intake)—the observed average or experimentally set intake by a defined population or subgroup that seems to sustain a defined nutritional status, such as growth rate, normal circulating nutrient values, or other functional indicators of health. An AI is used if insufficient scientific evidence is unavailable to derive an EAR. For healthy human milk–fed infants, the AI is the mean intake. The AI is not equivalent to an RDA.
§UL (tolerable upper intake level)—the highest level of daily nutrient intake that is likely to pose no risk of adverse health effects to almost all individuals in the general population. As intake increases above the UL, the risk of adverse effects increases. Unless specified otherwise, the UL represents total nutrient intake from food, water, and supplements.

improves zinc absorption. Many substances in plant products (e.g., fiber and phytate) interfere with zinc absorption.

Zinc is lost in the feces. Abnormal losses from diarrhea increase zinc requirements.

SOURCES

Protein-rich foods are good sources of zinc. Lamb, beef, crustaceans (especially oysters), eggs, and peanuts contain significant amounts of zinc (Table 11-11).

HYPER-STATES AND HYPO-STATES

Consumption of high levels of zinc normally causes vomiting and diarrhea, epigastric pain, lethargy, and fatigue, and can result in renal damage, pancreatitis, and death. There is a connection with an excess of zinc and reduced copper status, altered iron function, decreased immune function, and decrease in high-density lipoproteins (HDL). Supplementation is recommended only under medical supervision.

In developing countries, severe zinc deprivation has been related to excessive consumption of inhibitors, which adversely affect zinc absorption, rather than inadequate zinc intake. Individuals at particular risk of zinc deficiency include individuals whose zinc requirements are high (e.g.,

during periods of rapid growth), older adults, total vegetarians whose diet consists primarily of cereal protein or is generally nutrient deficient, and individuals with severe malabsorption (diarrhea) or other chronic health problems (Box 11-2).

Oral manifestations of zinc deficiency include changes in the epithelium of the tongue, such as thickening of epithelium; increased cell numbers; impaired keratinization of epithelial cells; increased susceptibility to periodontal disease; and flattened filiform papillae. Zinc deficiency in humans is associated with loss of taste and smell acuity, poor appetite, and impaired wound healing. Decreased linear growth and hypogonadism in adolescent boys are principal manifestations of zinc deficiency. Zinc deficiency also results in congenital defects, such as skeletal abnormalities, especially cleft palate and lip. Collagen synthesis defects are seen in zinc-deficient animals. Even when adequate amounts of zinc are provided for an extended time, abnormalities in mineral metabolism are not completely reversed. When zinc deficiency is diagnosed, zinc supplementation is vital.

Table 11-11	Zinc Content of Selected Foods	
Food	**Portion**	**Zinc (mg)**
Total, whole grain	1 cup	18.8
Oysters, breaded and fried	6	16
Total Raisin Bran	1 cup	15
Lobster	3 oz	6.2
Lean sirloin, broiled	3 oz	6
Taco (large)	1	6
Lean hamburger patty	3 oz	5.8
Beef liver	3 oz	4.8
Lamb chop	3 oz	4.4
Lean veal chop	3 oz	4.3
Crab, cooked	3 oz	3.6
Peanuts	½ cup	2.4
Yogurt, plain	8 oz	2.4
Pecans	1 oz	1.3
Milk	1 cup	1
Chicken breast	3 oz	0.9
Cheddar cheese	1 oz	0.9
Navy beans	½ cup	0.9
Pinto beans	½ cup	0.8
Spinach, cooked	½ cup	0.7
Kidney beans	½ cup	0.6
Whole egg	1	0.5

Data from U.S. Department of Agriculture, Agricultural Research Service, USDA Nutrient Data Laboratory, USDA National Nutrient Database for Standard Reference, Release 20, 2008. Available at http://www.nal.usda.gov/fnic/foodcomp. Accessed Feb 25, 2008.

Box 11-2	**Causes of Zinc Deficiency**

- Dietary deficiency
- Poor food selection
- Edentulism
- Inadequate zinc intake
- Vegan diet
- Very-low-kilocalorie diets
- Eating disorders
- Low income
- Periods of rapid growth
- Poor appetite
- Total parenteral nutrition (TPN)
- Decreased absorption
- High fiber
- High phytate
- High dietary iron-to-zinc ratio
- High calcium
- Pica
- Malabsorption syndromes
- Alcoholic cirrhosis
- Pancreatic insufficiency
- Chronic renal disease
- Advanced age
- Increased loss
- Thiazide diuretics
- Alcoholism
- Oral penicillamine therapy
- Disease states/conditions
- Acrodermatitis enteropathica
- Down syndrome
- Sickle-cell disease
- Leukemia
- Hemolytic anemia
- Cancer
- Diabetes
- Thalassemia

From Davis JR, Sherer K: Applied Nutrition and Diet Therapy for Nurses, 2nd ed. Philadelphia: Saunders, 1994.

Dental Hygiene Considerations

- Patients with abnormalities of taste because of zinc deficiency may respond to supplementation, but additional zinc is ineffective in reversing abnormal taste acuity associated with other conditions.
- Supplementation in zinc-depleted patients is beneficial for wound healing, but unnecessary for healthy individuals.
- Zinc supplementation interferes with use of iron and copper and adversely affects HDL levels. Do not advocate indiscriminate use of zinc.
- Zinc lozenges and zinc supplements are marketed to treat cold symptoms. Use beyond 1 week is potentially harmful. Research indicates zinc is ineffective for treating the common cold.
- Reduced food intake associated with zinc deficiency may impair growth of the parotid gland.

Nutritional Directions

- Small amounts of animal protein can significantly improve bioavailability of zinc from a legume-based meal.
- Fruits and vegetables are low in zinc, whereas peanuts and peanut butter have higher amounts.
- Meat, fish, and poultry are the preferred sources of zinc because of its bioavailability from plant foods.
- If a well-balanced diet is consumed, zinc supplements are rarely needed, and may be harmful.
- Large amounts of iron can decrease zinc absorption from food. Iron supplements between meals allow greater zinc absorption.

IODINE

PHYSIOLOGICAL ROLE

Iodine is required for the production of thyroxine, the hormone secreted by the thyroid gland. Thyroxine regulates the basal metabolic rate; an altered metabolic rate affects other nutrient requirements. Thyroid hormones are essential for normal brain development.

REQUIREMENTS

The adult RDA for iodine is 150 µg daily. Because iodine is related to the metabolic rate, needs are increased during periods of accelerated growth, especially during pregnancy and lactation. As shown in Table 11-12, the RDA for pregnant and lactating women is higher because of critical needs of the fetus and infant during this period. The UL for iodine is 1100 µg per day.

Based on the NHANES III survey, iodine intake has decreased since the first NHANES study in the 1970s, but average intake is currently considered to be adequate. Pregnant and breastfeeding women need to be aware of the importance of adequate intake.

SOURCES

A major source of iodine is seafood and plants grown near the ocean. Other natural sources include molasses, yogurt, and milk. The iodine content of common foods varies significantly. The iodine content of foods is not reflected on package labeling.

Table 11-12 Institute of Medicine Recommendations for Iodine

Life Stage	EAR (µg/d)* Male	Female	RDA (µg/d)† Male	Female	AI (µg/d)‡ Male	Female	UL (µg/d)§
0-6 mo					110	110	ND¶
7-12 mo					130	130	ND¶
1-3 yr	65	65	90	90			200
4-8 yr	65	65	90	90			300
9-13 yr	73	73	120	120			600
14-18 yr	95	95	150	150			900
≥19 yr	95	95	150	150			1100
Pregnancy ≥14 yr		160		220			900
Lactation ≥14 yr		209		290			900

Data from Institute of Medicine (IOM), Food and Nutrition Board: Dietary Reference Intakes for Vitamin A, Vitamin K, Arsenic, Boron, Chromium, Copper, Iodine, Iron, Manganese, Molybdenum, Nickel, Silicon, Vanadium, and Zinc. Washington, DC: National Academy Press, 2001.
*EAR (estimated average requirement)—the intake that meets the estimated nutrient needs of half of the individuals in a group.
†RDA (recommended dietary allowance)—the intake that meets the nutrient needs of almost all (97-98%) individuals in a group.
‡AI (adequate intake)—the observed average or experimentally set intake by a defined population or subgroup that seems to sustain a defined nutritional status, such as growth rate, normal circulating nutrient values, or other functional indicators of health. An AI is used if insufficient scientific evidence is available to derive an EAR. For healthy human milk–fed infants, the AI is the mean intake. The AI is not equivalent to an RDA.
§UL (tolerable upper intake level)—the highest level of daily nutrient intake that is likely to pose no risk of adverse health effects to almost all individuals in the general population. As intake increases above the UL, the risk of adverse effects increases. Unless specified otherwise, the UL represents total nutrient intake from food, water, and supplements.
¶ND—not determinable because of lack of data of adverse effects in this age group and concern with regard to lack of ability to handle excess amounts. Source of intake should be from food and formula to prevent high levels of intake.

The best safeguard for an adequate intake is the use of iodized salt. Until the 1920s, endemic iodine deficiency disorders were prevalent in the Great Lakes, Appalachian, and Northwestern regions of the United States. Iodized salt virtually eliminated endemic goiter in the United States and remains the mainstay of iodine deficiency disorder eradication in the United States and worldwide. When stored under high humidity conditions, significant amounts of iodine are lost, but light or dry heat has little effect.[18]

HYPER-STATES AND HYPO-STATES

Very high levels of iodine may cause adverse effects in some individuals. Excessive amounts of iodine can result in enlargement of the thyroid gland similar to the condition produced by deficiency. Thyroiditis, hypothyroidism, hyperthyroidism, **goiter** (enlargement of the thyroid gland), and sensitivity reactions have occurred in relation to excessive iodine intake through foods, dietary supplements, topical medications, and iodinated contrast media.

An iodine deficiency may cause profound metabolic and emotional influences ranging from a mild deceleration of catabolic functions, with sensitivity to cold, dry skin, and mildly elevated blood lipids, to mild depression of mental functions. Endemic goiter occurs where the soil or water is low in iodine content (Fig. 11-9). Fetuses, newborns, and young children are particularly vulnerable to iodine deficiency. A deficiency of iodine remains the most frequent cause worldwide, after starvation, of preventable mental retardation in children.[19] Even a mild deficiency during pregnancy may lower intelligence by 10 to 15 IQ points and increases the risk of neurodevelopmental abnormalities.[20] Iodine repletion in moderately iodine-deficient school-age children is beneficial by improving cognitive and motor function, increasing concentrations of growth factors, and improving somatic growth.[21] Because of the prevalence of marginal iodine nutrition status of pregnant women in the United States, the Public Health Committee of the American Thyroid Association has recommended daily iodine supplementation for all pregnant and lactating women in the United States and Canada.[22]

With insufficient iodine intake, the thyroid cannot produce adequate amounts of thyroxine. The pituitary gland continues to secrete thyroid-stimulating hormone (TSH), resulting in further hypertrophy and engorgement of the thyroid gland. Goiter is usually associated with iodine deficiency, but may be caused by excessively large intake of **goitrogens** contained in cabbage, cauliflower, Brussels sprouts, broccoli, kale, raw turnips, and rutabagas.

Goiter is the main disorder resulting from low iodine intake. Other iodine-deficiency disorders include stillbirths, abortions, and congenital anomalies; endemic **cretinism**, usually characterized by impaired mental development and deaf mutism related to fetal iodine deficiency; and impaired mental function. Children born to mothers with severe iodine deficiency have delayed eruption of primary and secondary teeth and an enlarged tongue. Craniofacial growth and development are altered; malocclusion is common.

Dental Hygiene Considerations

- Assess patients for possible thyroid problems.
- Enlargement of the thyroid gland can indicate hyperthyroidism or hypothyroidism. Refer these patients to a healthcare provider.
- The American Thyroid Association recommends a supplement of 150 μg of iodine per day during pregnancy and lactation.[19]
- For women who are pregnant or breastfeeding, stress the importance of an adequate iodine intake.
- Severe hypothyroidism is termed **myxedema**; hyperthyroidism is also called Graves' disease.

Nutritional Directions

- Sea salt has been advocated by health food promoters, but its iodine content is negligible. Purchase salt that is fortified with iodine, which is indicated on the label.
- Individuals consuming large amounts of seaweed, a rich source of iodine, may be at risk for iodine toxicity.

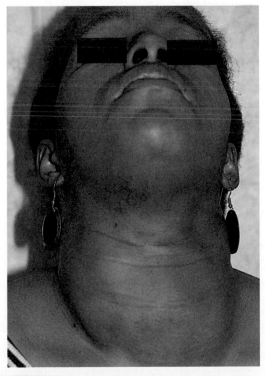

FIGURE 11-9 Goiter resulting from iodine deficiency. (From Swartz M: Textbook of Physical Diagnosis: History and Examination, 5th ed. Philadelphia: Saunders, 2006.)

Of the more than 50 million Americans who have hypertension warranting some form of treatment, only 34 million are aware of it, and 27 million seek treatment. Hypertension has been called mankind's most common disease. Approximately one in four adult Americans has hypertension. Hypertension is common in African Americans, individuals 60 years old and older, individuals with a family history, individuals with sedentary lifestyles, individuals with high alcohol intakes, patients with dyslipidemia, patients with diabetes, and obese individuals. Individuals who are normotensive at age 55 years have a 90% lifetime risk of developing hypertension.

Hypertension is defined as a persistent elevation of systolic blood pressure greater than 140 mm Hg and diastolic pressure greater than 90 mm Hg (Table 11-13). For patients with diabetes and chronic kidney disease, the goal is 130/80 mm Hg or less. For every increment of blood pressure above normal levels, there is a commensurate increase in risk of cardiovascular complications, stroke, peripheral vascular disease, and renal insufficiency. Hypertension may result in myocardial infarction, cerebrovascular accident, or heart failure. Uncontrolled hypertension can affect blood vessels in the eyes, kidneys, and nervous system. Hypertension cannot be cured, but it can be controlled. One of the goals of *Healthy People 2010* is to reduce the proportion of adults with hypertension from 28% to 16%.[23] Significant progress has been made toward meeting this goal, mainly by Americans taking action to control their blood pressure.[24]

Causes
Several important causal factors for hypertension have been identified, including excess body weight, excess sodium intake, minimal physical activity, inadequate intake of fruits and vegetables and potassium, and excess alcohol intake. Body fat deposited in the trunk increases the risk of developing essential hypertension independent of the overall level of obesity, whereas peripherally deposited fat does not. **Essential hypertension** is elevated blood pressure of unknown cause.

A weight loss of 10% is as effective at reducing blood pressure as pharmacological treatment. Despite the fact that sodium restriction alone does not always result in lower blood pressure for all patients with hypertension, sodium reduction is effective in lowering the mean blood pressure in salt-sensitive adults. There is no precise method of identifying salt sensitivity. Sodium restriction enhances effectiveness of diuretics and other pharmacological treatments (see Box 11-1). The American Heart Association recommendations are consistent with the *Dietary Guidelines for Americans* in reducing sodium. Generally, when sodium must be restricted, hidden sources of sodium should be considered: (1) sodium bicarbonate and other sodium products used as leavening agents; (2) sodium benzoate, used as a preservative in margarine and relishes; (3) sodium citrate and monosodium glutamate, used to enhance flavors in gelatin desserts, beverages, and meats; (4) sodium bicarbonate or sodium fluoride added to dentifrices or used in place of commercial dentifrices and mouth rinses; (5) some medications, particularly when taken regularly and

frequently, such as antacids, laxatives, and cough medicines; and (6) chewing tobacco.

High potassium intake has a protective effect against hypertension. Potassium increases urinary sodium excretion. A customary high sodium-to-low potassium ratio consumed when most foods are highly processed may be detrimental to normal blood pressure regulation. Increasing dietary potassium intake from natural foods is a factor in reducing blood pressure and in the development of cardiovascular disease (CVD)[25] and subsequent CVD.[26] Overall, a diet rich in potassium, magnesium, and calcium; whole grains; fruits and vegetables; and low-fat and nonfat foods, and low in sodium can lead to a 15% decrease in heart disease and 27% fewer strokes.

Drug therapy is effective, but for prehypertensive and treated hypertensive individuals, lifestyle changes are also important. Dietary modifications reduce blood pressure for many individuals with mild to moderate hypertension. Health-promoting lifestyle modifications are recommended to prevent the progressive increase in blood pressure and cardiovascular disease. Looking at the overall dietary pattern instead of one single nutrient is the key for assessing risk. The dental hygienist can continue to monitor blood pressure, and educate and support the patient's efforts toward reducing blood pressure values. The DASH (Dietary Approaches to Stop Hypertension) approach to prevention and treatment of hypertension combines all the dietary factors related to hypertension.

DASH (Dietary Approaches to Stop Hypertension)
The DASH study measured the effects of eating patterns on blood pressure in Americans. By combining an eating plan with lifestyle modifications designed to prevent and treat hypertension, this approach is effective in reducing high blood pressure and other chronic health conditions. DASH focuses on a dietary pattern instead of decreasing kilocalories or restricting specific nutrients. It emphasizes fruits, vegetables, low-fat or nonfat dairy products, whole grains, nuts, fish, and poultry, and it reduces and limits saturated fat, total fat, cholesterol, red meats, and sweets. The dietary pattern is rich in nutrients commonly lacking in American diets—fiber, potassium, magnesium, and calcium (Box 11-3 and Table 11-14). Participants in the study had an average reduction of 6 mm Hg for systolic pressure and 3 mm Hg for diastolic pressure. Participants with hypertension had greater decreases in blood pressure than nonhypertensive participants. Improvement in blood pressure occurred within 2 weeks after beginning the study. Adherence to the DASH diet is associated with a reduced risk of coronary heart disease and stroke among middle-aged women during 24 years of follow-up.[27]

To reduce sodium intake, patients need to retrain their taste buds by gradually reducing salt intake. For example, patients should remove the salt shaker from the table or refrain from using the salt packet included with fast foods. In a study of 354 adults with prehypertension or stage I hypertension, participants rated the saltiness and palatability of a pattern containing 2300 mg sodium daily as being acceptable.[28]

DASH recommendations are consistent with diets for the prevention of cancer, osteoporosis, heart disease, and dia-

HEALTH APPLICATION Hypertension—cont'd

betes. The National High Blood Pressure Education Program recommends the DASH diet for preventing and managing hypertension. In addition, the DASH diet is a dietary pattern–based template for all healthy individuals to implement the *Dietary Guidelines for Americans* and meet their nutrient recommendations. Individuals following the DASH diet achieve at least two-thirds of the dietary reference intake (DRI) recommendations for most nutrients despite their reduced energy intake.[29] The pattern offers individualization and flexibility in food choices.

Nonpharmacological treatment of hypertension can work if supported by the healthcare provider, and the patient is strongly motivated. When applied together, salt restriction (less than 6 g per day), moderate alcohol intake (less than two servings per day in men and less than one serving peer day in women), weight loss for individuals whose body mass index (BMI) is greater than 25, regular exercise, and following a DASH diet (providing 2500 mg of potassium) can achieve decreases of approximately 10 to 15 mm Hg systolic blood pressure.[30]

Table 11-13	Classification of Blood Pressure for Adults	
Category	**Systolic Pressure (mm Hg)**	**Diastolic Pressure (mm Hg)**
Normal	<120	<80
Prehypertension	120-139	*or* 80-89
Stage 1 hypertension	140-159	*or* 90-99
Stage 2 hypertension	>160	*or* ≥100

Data from the National Heart Lung and Blood Institute: Prevention, detection, evaluation and treatment of high blood pressure (JNC 7). Hypertension 2003; 42:1206-1252. Available at http://www.nhlbi.nih.gov/guidelines/hypertension/index.htm.

Table 11-14	DASH Food Plan*
Food Group	**Daily Servings**
Grains and grain products	6-8
Vegetables	4-5
Fruits	4-5
Low-fat or fat-free dairy foods	2-3
Meats, poultry, and fish	≤6 oz
Nuts, seeds, and dry beans	4-5 per week
Fats and oils†	2-3 tsp
Sweets	5 Tbsp per week
Nutrient Target Totals/2000-kcal Dietary Pattern‡	
3932 mg potassium	28 g dietary fiber
450 mg magnesium	27% fat
1131 mg calcium	6% saturated fat
18% protein	150 mg cholesterol
55% carbohydrates	

Adapted from U.S. Department of Health and Human Services, National Institutes of Health, National Heart Lung and Blood Institute: Facts about the DASH eating plan. NIH Publication 01-4082; May 2003.
*The DASH (Dietary Approaches to Stop Hypertension) Eating Plan is based on 2000 kcal/d. The number of daily servings per food group may vary depending on caloric needs. It closely follows the Food Guide Pyramid with a few modifications.
†Fat content changes serving counts for fats and oils. For example, 1 Tbsp of regular salad dressing equals 1 serving; 1Tbsp of a low-fat dressing equals ½ serving; 1 Tbsp of a nonfat dressing equals 0 servings.
‡Lin PH, et al: The PREMIER intervention helps participants follow the Dietary Approaches to Stop Hypertension dietary pattern and the current Dietary Reference Intakes recommendations. J Am Diet Assoc 2007 Sep; 107(9):1541-1551.

Box 11-3	Dietary Approaches to Stop Hypertension (DASH)

- Make gradual changes (i.e., make changes to one food group at a time).
- Attain and maintain a healthy weight (BMI 18.5 to 24.9).
- Reduce sodium intake.
- Maintain recommended calcium, potassium, and magnesium intake.
- Increase intake of fresh fruits, vegetables, and low-fat or nonfat dairy foods.
- Reduce total fat intake to 27% of total kilocalories, with 6% from saturated fats, and 300 mg of cholesterol. Use reduced-fat and fat-free condiments; choose low-fat meats, fish, and poultry (6 oz per day); and select low-fat sweets.
- Consume edible skins on fruits, vegetables, and whole grains to increase dietary fiber. Gradually increase these foods, and increase fluids to avoid gastrointestinal distress associated with increased fiber intake.
- Consume fatty fish (e.g., mackerel, herring, salmon) several times a week to provide omega-3 fatty acids and help reduce saturated fat intake.
- Restrict alcohol intake to one drink or less per day for women and two drinks or less per day for men.
- Do not use potassium, calcium, or magnesium supplements unless recommended by the healthcare provider or dietitian.
- Begin a smoking cessation program.
- Participate in some type of relaxation or stress reduction therapy.
- Participate in a regular aerobic exercise program for at least 30 minutes per day, most days of the week. Initiate an exercise program gradually.

Adapted from U.S. Department of Health and Human Services, National Institutes of Health, National Heart, Lung, and Blood Institute: Facts about the DASH eating plan. NIH Publication 01-4082; May 2003.

CASE APPLICATION FOR THE DENTAL HYGIENIST

An older gentleman is your patient and complains of a dry mouth and sore tongue. He states that he has not been thirsty, and his intake of fluids has been poor for 4 days. His healthcare provider recently prescribed a diuretic for hypertension and told him to eliminate salt and add more fruits and vegetables to his diet. He complains that "nothing tastes good."

Nutritional Assessment
- Blood pressure value
- Oral mucous membranes, tongue characteristics
- Fluid likes and dislikes
- Mental changes

Nutritional Diagnosis
Fluid volume deficit related to diuretic and poor fluid or food intake.

Nutritional Goals
Patient will have good skin turgor and moist oral mucous membranes and will increase his intake of liquids and food.

Nutritional Implementation
Intervention: Explain the need for fluid intake.
Rationale: Knowledge and involvement in care increase compliance.
Intervention: Encourage the patient to drink his favorite fluids, preferably water, on a regular schedule.
Rationale: The patient is more apt to drink his favorite fluid, and, in doing so, he will replace fluids lost because of the diuretic.
Intervention: Identify methods to increase salivary flow and oral lubrication.
Rationale: The patient's degree of oral comfort will improve, and soft tissue will heal.
Intervention: Explain the importance of oral hygiene and how to perform oral self-care procedures.

Rationale: Less saliva allows more food debris to remain on the teeth, which may increase caries risk. Because the oral mucosa and gingival tissues are more susceptible to trauma, an extra-soft bristle brush may be appropriate for plaque removal, and the patient should be cautioned against aggressive oral hygiene. Other oral physiotherapy aids may be warranted for optimal plaque biofilm removal.
Intervention: Explore challenges the patient will encounter with foods low in salt and discuss ways to enhance the flavor of food without using sodium (see Box 11-1 and Table 11-5). Explain that as his salt intake decreases, the salt in the saliva will also decrease so that after about 3 months of moderately low intake, his preferred salt level for foods will decrease, and his taste for food will gradually improve.
Rationale: Most Americans consume about four to seven times the recommended amount of sodium. The sodium concentration in saliva determines a patient's recognition of salt in food; higher levels of sodium in saliva means higher levels of sodium are needed for the sodium to be detected.
Intervention: Discuss types of dentifrices consistent with the healthcare provider's order to eliminate salt.
Rationale: Sodium bicarbonate or sodium fluoride is added to some dentifrices and mouth rinses; these would increase his sodium intake, especially if oral hygiene is practiced several times a day, and the patient ingests the dentifrice or mouth rinse.
Intervention: Have the patient record his dietary intake for 1 to 3 days. Compare this record with the DASH diet.
Rationale: Suggestions can be tailored to the patient's needs. The patient can set a goal based on the information presented.

Evaluation
Desired outcomes include the patient's adequate consumption of preferred beverages each day, moist oral mucous membranes, and no dental caries.

STUDENT READINESS

1. Define intracellular fluid and extracellular fluid. What are the principal electrolytes found in each?
2. Record your daily fluid intake. How does this record compare with the required intake?
3. Fluid is essential for survival. Discuss the advantages and disadvantages of water intake versus other fluids, such as milk, carbonated beverages, tea, and coffee.
4. List five clinical observations indicating fluid volume deficit. What type of medication is frequently prescribed that affects hydration status?
5. What can cause hypernatremia and hyponatremia? Why is altering the salt intake of patients with these conditions not usually the mode of treatment?
6. What can cause FVD or FVE?
7. What is the general effect of food processing on the sodium and potassium content of foods?
8. Explain the physiological change that occurs when salt intake is decreased, and why adding large amounts

of salt to foods is unwise. Would you consider salt addictive?
9. Discuss dental hygiene interventions for iron-deficiency anemia. Discuss factors affecting iron absorption.
10. A patient asks you why he has to take zinc when his iron stores are depressed. How would you respond?
11. Which two nutrients that were discussed are important for collagen formation?
12. Name the electrolyte(s) or mineral(s) discussed in this chapter associated with the following symptoms:
    - Shrinkage of mucous membranes
    - Thirst
    - Oral pallor
    - Taste abnormalities
    - Lethargy
    - Enlargement of thyroid
    - Poor wound healing
    - Swollen tongue
    - Loss of appetite
13. The *Dietary Guidelines for Americans* and the American Heart Association recommend restricting

red meat in the diet. Their recommendations also include increasing intake of fiber from cereal and vegetable sources to help reduce blood lipid levels. Discuss how these two recommendations affect the known deficiency of iron stores in the U.S. population in general. Would you anticipate that long periods of compliance with cholesterol-reducing protocols might necessitate the use of iron supplements in affected individuals?

14. Identify the guidelines in the DASH diet that would be beneficial to the older adult in the Case Application box in this chapter.

CASE STUDY

A 17-year-old boy complains of a dry mouth; difficulty in swallowing food; dry, sticky tongue; and dry skin. The patient reports he has just recovered from the flu, which was accompanied by diarrhea and vomiting. He also informs you he is currently training for an athletic competition and exercises 3 to 4 hours a day. A 24-hour diet recall reveals the patient's fluid intake includes 48 to 72 oz of caffeinated soft drinks without any other beverages and a high protein intake.

1. What other information should you obtain about the patient's dietary intake?
2. Could the patient's oral symptoms be attributed to his current fluid intake?
3. Is salivary analysis indicated for this patient?
4. What suggestions could you make that would decrease his symptoms of xerostomia? Identify ideas to increase his fluid intake.
5. What oral self-care practices would you recommend to relieve his oral discomfort and facilitate swallowing?

CASE STUDY

A 15-year-old girl comes into the dental office reporting a history of iron-deficiency anemia. She has clinical symptoms typical of this anemia: glossitis; smooth, shiny, red tongue; and painful cracks at the corners of her mouth. Her healthcare provider has prescribed ferrous sulfate and zinc to correct this deficiency.

1. When evaluating dietary intake, what are some foods you would need to watch for to assess iron intake?
2. If the patient is having problems with ferrous sulfate (e.g., constipation, nausea), would it be advisable to resolve the anemia by just increasing iron intake? Why or why not?
3. Why has the healthcare provider ordered zinc supplements?
4. What should you tell her about iron from plant or animal foods?
5. What can she do to help increase absorption of iron?

References

1. Vreeman R: Medical myths. BMJ. 2007 Dec 22; 335(7633): 1288-1289.
2. Valtin H: "Drink at least eight glasses of water a day." Really? Is there scientific evidence for "8 × 8"? Am J Physiol Regul Integr Comp Physiol 2002 Nov; 283(5):R993-R1004.
3. Institute of Medicine (IOM), Food and Nutrition Board: Dietary Reference Intakes for Water, Potassium, Sodium, Chloride, and Sulfate. Washington, DC: National Academy Press, 2004.
4. Flood JE, et al: The effect of increased beverage portion size on energy intake at a meal. J Am Diet Assoc 2006 Dec; 106(12):1984-1990.
5. Energy drinks behind the buzz. Consumer Reports 2007 Sep; 72(9):6-7.
6. Reissig CJ, Strain EC, Griffiths RR: Caffeinated energy drinks—A growing problem. Drug Alcohol Depend 2009 Jan 1; 9(1-3):1-10.
7. Oliver MM, Drause PR: Powering up with sports and energy drinks. J Pediatr Health Care 2007 Jun; 21(6):413-416.
8. Hooper S, et al: A comparison of enamel erosion by a new sports drink compared to two proprietary products: a controlled, crossover study in situ. J Dent 2004 Sep; 32(7): 541-545.
9. Popkin BM, et al: A new proposed guidance system for beverage consumption in the United States. Am J Clin Nutr 2006 Mar; 83(3):529-542.
10. Grandjean AC, et al: The effect of caffeinated, non-caffeinated, caloric and non-caloric beverages on hydration. J Am Coll Nutr 2000 Oct; 19(5):591-600.
11. International Food Information Council Foundation: Fact Sheet: Caffeine and Health, 2007. Available at www.ific.org. Accessed Jan 24, 2009.
12. Moshfegh A, Goldman J, Cleveland L: What We Eat in America, NHANES 2001-2002: Usual Nutrient Intakes from Food Compared to Dietary Reference Intakes. U.S. Department of Agriculture, Agricultural Research Service, September, 2005.
13. Cohen HW, Hailpern SM, Alderman MH: Sodium intake and mortality in the NHANES II follow-up study. Am J Med 2006 Mar; 119(3):275.e.7-275.e.14.
14. Cohen HW, Hailpern SM, Alderman MH: Sodium intake and mortality follow-up in the Third National Health and National Examination Survey (NHANES III). J Gen Intern Med 2008 Sept; 23(9):1297-1302.
15. Cook NR, et al: Long term effects of dietary sodium reduction on cardiovascular disease outcomes: observational follow-up of the Trials of Hypertension Prevention (TOHP) BMJ 2007 Apr; 334(7599):885.
16. Houston MC, Harger KJ: Potassium, magnesium, and calcium: their role in both the cause and treatment of hypertension. J Clin Hypertens (Greenwich). 2008 Jul; 10(7 Suppl 2):3-11.
17. Rafferty K, Heaney RP: Nutrient effects on the calcium economy: emphasizing the potassium controversy. J Nutr 2008 Jan; 138(1):166S-171S.
18. Dasgupta PK, Liu Y, Dyke JV: Iodine nutrition: iodine content of iodized salt in the United States. Environ Sci Technol 2008 Feb 15; 42(4):1315-1323.
19. Berbel P, et al: Iodine supplementation during pregnancy: a public health challenge. Trends Endocrinol Metab 2007 Nov; 18(9):338-343.
20. International Council for the Control of Iodine Deficiency Disorders: Iodine and the brain. Available at www.iccidd.org/. Accessed September 16, 2008.
21. Zimmermann MB: The adverse effects of mild-to-moderate iodine deficiency during pregnancy and childhood: a review. Thyroid 2007 Sep; 17(9):829-835.

22. The Public Health Committee of the American Thyroid Association: Iodine supplementation for pregnancy and lactation—United States and Canada: recommendations of the American Thyroid Association. Thyroid 2006 Oct; 16(10):949-951.

23. U.S. Department of Health and Human Services: Healthy People 2010. Washington, DC: USDHHS, January 2000.

24. U.S. Department of Health and Human Services. Progress toward Healthy People 2010 targets: heart disease and stroke. Available at http://www.healthypeople.gov/Data/midcourse/html/focusareas/FA12ProgressHP.htm. Accessed September 18, 2008.

25. Adrogue HJ, Madias NE: Sodium and potassium in the pathogenesis of hypertension. N Engl J Med 2007; 356(19): 1966-1978.

26. Cook NR, et al: Joint effects of sodium and potassium intake on subsequent cardiovascular disease. Arch Intern Med 2009 Jan 12; 169(1):32-40.

27. Fung TT, et al: Adherence to a DASH-style diet and risk of coronary heart disease and stroke in women. Arch Intern Med 2008 Apr 14; 168(7):713-720.

28. Karanja N, et al: Acceptability of sodium-reduced research diets, including the Dietary Approaches to Stop Hypertension diet, among adults with prehypertension and stage 1 hypertension. J Am Diet Assoc 2007 Sep; 107(9):1530-1538.

29. Lin PH, et al: The PREMIER intervention helps participants follow the Dietary Approaches to Stop Hypertension dietary pattern and the current Dietary Reference Intakes recommendations. J Am Diet Assoc 2007 Sep; 107(9):1541-1551.

30. O'Shaughnessy KM: Role of diet in hypertension management. Curr Hypertens Rep 2006 Aug; 8(4):292-297.

PART II

Considerations of Clinical Nutrition

Chapter 12

Nutritional Requirements Affecting Oral Health in Women

OUTLINE

HEALTHY PREGNANCY
Factors Affecting Fetal Development
Factors Affecting Oral Development
Nutritional Requirements for Pregnancy
Dietary Intake and Counseling

LACTATION
Nutritional Recommendations for Breastfeeding
Dietary Patterns for Lactating Women

ORAL CONTRACEPTIVE AGENTS

MENOPAUSE

LEARNING OBJECTIVES

Upon completion of this chapter, the student will be able to achieve the following objectives:

- Assess nutrients commonly supplemented during pregnancy and lactation.
- Use national guidelines to recommend food intake during pregnancy and lactation to provide adequate nutrients.

- List factors affecting fetal development.
- Implement nutrition and oral health considerations for patients who are pregnant or breastfeeding.
- Apply nutritional directions for patients who are pregnant or breastfeeding.

KEY TERMS

Anencephaly
Atrophic gingivitis
Dysesthesia
Erythropoiesis
Gravida
Hormone replacement therapy (HRT)
Low birth weight (LBW)
Menopause

Menopausal gingivostomatitis
Nutritional insult
Perimenopause
Pica
Preeclampsia
Premature
Thromboembolism

Test Your NQ

1. **T/F** All efforts should be made to satisfy a pregnant woman's food cravings because cravings reflect an innate need for certain nutrients.
2. **T/F** The fetus is nourished from the mother's nutrient stores.
3. **T/F** After pregnancy, most mothers have at least one carious lesion because calcium was pulled from teeth for use by the developing fetus.
4. **T/F** A woman should eat twice as much food when she is pregnant because she is eating for two.
5. **T/F** Most women should gain 25 to 35 lb during a pregnancy.

6. **T/F** Vitamin A is the only nutrient warranting global supplementation during pregnancy.
7. **T/F** Virtually all women can produce enough milk to support the nutritional needs of the infant.
8. **T/F** Breast milk that is too thin must be nutritionally inadequate.
9. **T/F** If the breast milk supply is inadequate, a feeding should be omitted to have more milk available later.
10. **T/F** WIC is a governmental program that provides supplemental foods for women, infants, and children.

HEALTHY PREGNANCY

Although there is no specific definition of a healthy pregnancy, the health of the mother and the infant is important. In addition to continued preservation of the mother's physical health, her emotional and psychological well-being are important. Goals for the infant include being (1) full term (born between the 39th and 41st week of gestation) and (2) mature (weighing more than 6 lb). Infants with a **low birth weight (LBW)** (weighing less than $5\frac{1}{2}$ lb) or who are **premature** (gestational age less than 37 weeks) have more abnormalities and increased morbidity (infections and illnesses) and mortality, and decreased mental performance. The rate of mortality among infants born before 37 weeks of gestation has been increasing; at least 75% of deaths in infants occur in infants who were born premature.[1] Primary factors for a successful pregnancy are nutritional status before conception, appropriate weight gain, and adequate intake of essential nutrients during pregnancy. If the mother's nutritional status is poor, the placenta apparently does not perform its function well.

A classic report published in 1970 by the National Academy of Sciences established a basis for increased nutritional requirements during pregnancy. This report was followed by further recommendations regarding weight gain and nutrient supplements published in *Nutrition during Pregnancy*.[2] This information was compiled by separate subcommittees of the Institute of Medicine (IOM) that evaluated available scientific information to establish guidelines for optimal outcomes. A more recent report suggests *Nutrition during Pregnancy* was written when undernutrition and inadequate weight gain were the main concerns, whereas the primary concern now has shifted to obesity and excess weight gain.[3]

FACTORS AFFECTING FETAL DEVELOPMENT
Preconceptional Nutritional Status
"Getting healthy" before pregnancy is important. One of the most important times for prenatal care is before a pregnancy

begins. Ideally, weight adjustments of overweight or underweight women should be achieved before conception. Losing 15 to 20 lb before conception may be enough to avoid some weight-related pregnancy complications (e.g., preeclampsia, cesarean delivery, and large-for-gestational-age infants). **Preeclampsia** is a potentially serious complication of pregnancy involving high blood pressure that often leads to premature delivery. Preconceptual obesity or underweight not only hampers fertility, but also can set the stage for metabolic problems in pregnancy. Infant deaths are 23% more likely to occur when the mother is obese, and 70% more likely when the mother is morbidly obese.[4]

Maternal health and fetal growth and development are affected by nutrient intake, not only during the pregnancy, but also before conception. By the time a woman has her first prenatal visit, fetal development has already progressed beyond a critical period during which a lack of folic acid or certain exposures may have already compromised the health and well-being of the mother and fetus. In addition to eating a well-balanced diet, prenatal vitamins are encouraged in anticipation of a pregnancy to ensure a good environment for the fetus from the beginning. Low levels of iron and folic acid before the pregnancy have been linked to premature births and stunted growth.

When a pregnancy occurs less than 1 year after a previous pregnancy, the woman may not have adequate maternal nutritional reserves; this may contribute to increased incidence of preterm births and fetal growth retardation, and increased risk of maternal mortality and morbidity. Because of the rapid development of body parts and organs during the first trimester, birth defects are likely to occur if usual dietary habits are poor, or if drugs are used during this critical period. Infant birth weights are affected more by nutrient intake during the second and third trimesters.

Although poor nutrient intake can result in an infant with a low birth weight, it is commonly believed the fetus is protected at the mother's expense. In some instances, such as with calcium and iron, higher requirements are met by more efficient maternal absorption to meet fetal needs. For other nutrients, such as iron and calcium, inadequate maternal intake may deplete the mother's stores, and the infant's stores may be suboptimal at birth as well.[5]

Unusual Dietary Patterns

Pica, or an abnormal consumption of specific food and nonfood substances, such as dirt, clay, baking soda, paint chips, stones, cloth, baby powder, starch (laundry and corn), large quantities of ice, or other inedible items, affects 20% to 30% of women considered to be at high risk of having premature or LBW infants.[6] Women practicing pica behaviors are usually from lower socioeconomic groups or have less than a high school education; are in poor nutritional health; may be an adolescent having clinical problems, such as pregnancy-induced hypertension; or are affected by behavioral/environmental factors, such as alcohol or substance abuse. Pica is more likely to be practiced by African-American women living in rural areas with a positive childhood and family history of pica. Nutrient deficiencies, especially iron-deficiency anemia, may result from these abnormal behaviors; however, the scientific literature does not support a causal relationship with pica.[7] Pica may result in lead poisoning, and, depending on the snack, the substance consumed can cause teeth to wear down quickly.

Beliefs about cravings and folklore that could influence dietary selections are cultural and regional. These beliefs may not be supported by scientific information and may be detrimental. Familiarity with local beliefs is needed to counsel **gravidas** (pregnant women) about beliefs that are potentially detrimental to good nutrition during pregnancy. Special dietary restrictions may be practiced based on food fads, or ethnic, cultural, or religious customs. In addition to assessing the effects of these on nutritional status, an awareness of these practices allows the dental hygienist to provide guidance about desirable food choices that are within these constraints.

Health Care

Availability and use of healthcare services are related to problems in pregnancy. Inadequate prenatal care leads to problems for the mother and the fetus. Prenatal care is important to protect the embryo from the effects of chronic health problems later in life, such as diabetes and hypertension.

Age

Maternal age can be a factor in the increased number of LBW infants among gravidas younger than 18 years old. Most adolescent girls do not complete linear growth and achieve gynecological maturity until age 17. Nutritional requirements are quite high to meet the growth needs for both the adolescent and the fetus. Not only are many of these girls still growing and storing nutrients in their own bodies, but also most have an inadequate intake of calcium, iron, vitamins A and D, niacin, and kilocalories. About one of every three teenage mothers shows signs of significant bone loss after giving birth, but greater calcium and vitamin D

consumption during pregnancy may protect against bone loss.

Intake of calorie-dense foods and erratic eating may preclude adequate intake of required nutrients. The socioeconomic disadvantages of these young mothers may affect their diet as a result of the amount of food available and their uninformed selections. Increased energy requirements are usually met without concentrated effort as a result of the increased appetite.

Pregnancy after age 35 is influenced by the woman's overall health. Maternal risks involve medical conditions, such as diabetes, hypertension, and cardiovascular problems. These conditions are closely supervised to lessen their impact on the fetus. However, as more women older than 35 are choosing to become pregnant, the number of myocardial infarctions during pregnancy seems to have increased.[8] A woman needs to be particularly aware of maintaining her nutritional health if a pregnancy after age 35 is anticipated.

Weight Gain

Successful pregnancies depend on ideal preconceptional weight plus appropriate weight gain during gestation. However, weight gain during pregnancy influences the birth weight more than the prepregnancy weight.

In 1990, the IOM recommended that women with a body mass index (BMI) in the desirable range should gain 1 lb weekly during the second and third trimesters, with a total weight gain of 25 to 35 lb; women weighing less than their ideal weight before pregnancy should gain 30 to 40 lb; and overweight women should gain 15 to 25 lb during pregnancy.[2] Pregnancy weight gains within the IOM recommendations are associated with better outcomes. The possible exception is very obese women, who may benefit from weight gains less than the 15 lb recommended.[9] Only about 33% to 40% of U.S. women gain within IOM recommendations.

Too little or too much weight gain during pregnancy can harm the mother and fetus. Some women are concerned about gaining too much weight during pregnancy, whereas others, recognizing the need to eat for two, consume excessive amounts of food. LBW, which is associated with health problems for the infant, can occur with an inadequate amount of maternal weight gain.

Excessive weight gain during pregnancy can increase the risk of gestational diabetes, pregnancy-induced high blood pressure, miscarriage or stillbirth, and difficulties during delivery. The goal for women who are overweight before pregnancy is to avoid excessive weight gain, but to consume adequate kilocalories to allow optimal fetal growth. Excess weight gain increases postpartum weight retention and may contribute to development of maternal obesity.

A more recent study indicated children are more likely to be overweight at 3 years of age if their mother gained adequate or excessive amounts (according to the 25-year-old IOM guidelines) compared with children whose mothers did not gain enough weight.[10] Additionally, women who gain excessive weight during pregnancy (more than 22 lb) were more likely to retain the weight and gain additional weight over time.[11] The IOM is reviewing the pregnancy weight guidelines to consider revising them; the results are expected by summer 2009.

Oral Health

Studies indicate only 49% to 58% of women receive dental care during their pregnancy.[12,13] Women who do not receive routine dental care either before or during pregnancy are at markedly increased risk of receiving no counseling regarding the importance of oral health care during this period. Even though a gravida may not be having dental problems, it is very important she maintain proper oral hygiene care. Attitudes and behaviors about dental care during pregnancy may be influenced by fear of harm to the woman or fetus or patient safety concerns. Routine dental care received during the second trimester (gestational weeks 13 to 21) was not associated with an increased risk of serious medical events, preterm deliveries, spontaneous abortions, or fetal deaths or anomalies.[14]

Numerous factors contribute to increased incidence of oral changes observed in most pregnant women. Pregnancy gingivitis (Fig. 12-1A) usually becomes evident in the

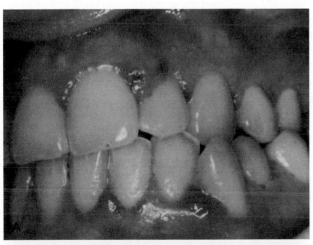

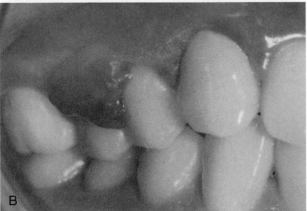

FIGURE 12-1 A, Pregnancy gingivitis. **B,** Pregnancy tumor. (From Perry DA, Beemsterboer PL: Periodontology for the Dental Hygienist, 3rd ed. St. Louis: Saunders, 2007.)

second month of pregnancy. Hormonal changes (estrogen and progesterone) associated with pregnancy contribute to an increased susceptibility to gingivitis and periodontitis. If irritating plaque biofilm is allowed to accumulate, gingivitis (red, swollen, tender gums that are likely to bleed) occurs and may result in large lumps called "pregnancy tumors" (Fig. 12-1B). Numerous studies indicate periodontal disease during pregnancy is a significant risk factor for preeclampsia or delivering a premature or LBW infant, or both.[15-17]

Nausea is common during pregnancy; the resultant recurring vomiting increases oral exposure to gastric acid secretions, which may cause erosion of the tooth enamel. In addition to nausea and vomiting, gastroesophageal reflux disease (GERD) is common during pregnancy because of normal physiologic changes that affect the lower esophageal sphincter.[18] Evidence shows a strong association between GERD and dental erosion.[19] The acid from vomiting should be neutralized using a paste of baking soda and water, rubbing it on the teeth, and rinsing after 30 seconds. This is followed by brushing and flossing.

Drugs and Medications

The use of tobacco, alcohol, caffeine, some medications, megadoses of nutrients, and illegal drugs may detrimentally affect the fetus. A large amount of caffeine (e.g., more than 7 cups per day of coffee) is associated with LBW and may be associated with increased risk of miscarriage.[20-22] The American Dietetic Association maintains pregnant women should not consume more than 300 mg of caffeine (less than 2 cups of coffee) per day.[22,23] Brewed coffee can contain 150 to 500 mg caffeine per 16-oz cup, so minimizing caffeine intake may be challenging for some pregnant women.

Alcohol is a folic acid antagonist. Alcohol can cross the placenta, and alcohol intake during pregnancy may lead to fetal alcohol syndrome (discussed in Health Application 12). Alcohol consumption near the time of conception may increase the risk of cleft lip or palate; however, the risk is decreased if the woman is taking folic acid.[24] Pregnant women should consult their healthcare provider before taking any drug, including nonprescription, over-the-counter drugs and herbal products.

Artificial Sweeteners

Non-nutritive sweeteners classified as generally recognized as safe (GRAS) can be used during pregnancy. Saccharin, acesulfame, aspartame, sucralose, and neotame are considered safe if consumed within acceptable daily intakes.[23] However, pregnant women with the genetic disorder phenylketonuria should not use aspartame during any period of their life span.

Food Safety

During pregnancy, women are at high risk for foodborne illness because of physiological changes that may increase exposure of the mother and fetus to hazardous substances. Pregnant women should avoid unpasteurized juices, milk, and milk products; raw sprouts; and meat, poultry, eggs, fish, and shellfish that are raw or undercooked. Certain foodborne illnesses can be especially dangerous; for example, listeriosis can cause miscarriage, premature birth, stillbirth, or acute illness in the newborn. To reduce the risk of listeriosis, pregnant women should heat leftovers and ready-to-eat foods (e.g., deli meats, hot dogs, luncheon meats, refrigerated smoked fish, refrigerated pâtés, and meat spreads) until steaming hot (165° F), and avoid soft cheeses (Brie, feta, blue, Camembert, and Mexican-style) and homemade cheese.[23] Other food-handling precautions as discussed in Chapter 15 should be heeded.

Pregnant women should avoid raw fish and any seafood that may be contaminated with mercury and polychlorinated biphenyls (PCBs). The U.S. Food and Drug Administration (FDA) has advised pregnant women to avoid consuming large fish, including shark, swordfish, king mackerel, and tilefish, because they may contain large amounts of methyl mercury. Moderate amounts (12 oz or less weekly) of other fish lower in mercury, such as shrimp, salmon, catfish, and pollock, should be limited to 12 oz per week. Tuna should be limited to 6 oz per week. State and local health departments have information relevant to fish caught locally or sold in a particular location. If the information is unavailable, pregnant women should limit consumption of fish from local water to 6 oz per week.[23,25]

Lead, available in tap water leached from plumbing and in dust from deteriorating lead-based paint, can negatively affect socialization and behaviors. Absorbed lead accumulates and is stored in the bones. Much later, it can be released from maternal bones into the bloodstream. Regardless of the source, lead is absorbed by fetal brain cells in place of the calcium needed for thought processes. This results in lifelong developmental problems, such as reduced attention span, increased impulsive behavior, and lower intelligence.

FACTORS AFFECTING ORAL DEVELOPMENT

In general, the potential arrangement of teeth, their eruption time, and pits and fissures on the enamel are attributed to heredity. However, the availability of nutrients in utero is closely associated with whether teeth achieve their optimum genetic potential.

Tooth development begins by the sixth week of gestation. Calcification of deciduous teeth begins about the fourth month; development of more than 60% of the 52 deciduous and permanent teeth is initiated during gestation (Table 12-1). By the fourth month of pregnancy, the mandible is calcified. All the primary teeth and many permanent teeth are at various stages of development when the infant is born. Critical periods for various stages of tooth development occur at different times. Nutrients supplied by the mother must be available for development of pre-eruptive teeth and soft tissues in proper sequence.

Severe and irreversible damage results if **nutritional insult** (deficiency or excessive amounts of specific nutrients) or infection occurs during critical stages, especially in dentin or enamel formation (Table 12-2). After eruption, the tooth has no mechanism to repair itself. Severe nutrient

deficiencies can result in malformations such as cleft palate, cleft lip, and shortened mandible. Less severe nutrient deficiencies can reduce the size of the tooth, interfere with tooth formation, delay time of tooth eruption, and increase susceptibility of teeth to caries. Almost all nutrient deficiencies that occur in utero affecting developing teeth result in increased susceptibility to dental caries for the child.

When a gravida develops a fever during an infection, the resultant disruption of calcium and phosphorus balance affects the developing fetal tooth structure. This disruption in tooth structure formation continues for as long as it takes to regain this balance.

The dentin and enamel of the tooth depend on many nutrients: vitamin C for formation of collagen matrix, and calcium, magnesium, phosphorus, and vitamin D for mineralization. Infants whose mother had low levels of vitamin D during pregnancy may be at increased risk for tooth enamel defects and early childhood tooth decay.[26] Keratin in enamel depends on vitamin A for its synthesis. An inadequate amount of any of these nutrients during tooth development results in an imperfect matrix, with subsequent imperfection of the mineralization (see Table 12-2). Folate deficiency, known to cause neural tube defects, can result in incomplete formation of cranial bones.

The benefits of fluoride supplements during pregnancy in preventing dental caries in infants are uncertain. Fluoride passes through the placenta to the fetus and is incorporated into fetal bones and teeth. Whether the placenta can filter excess fluoride is unknown. Although fluoride supplements are considered safe for the mother and fetus, oral fluoride supplements during pregnancy seem to have minimal benefits on the developing fetus.

NUTRITIONAL REQUIREMENTS FOR PREGNANCY

The dietary reference intakes (DRIs) for pregnancy indicate advisable nutrient intake for optimal health of the mother and fetus. Accelerated growth and metabolism increases most nutrient requirements to some extent. Each vitamin and mineral is not separately discussed; Table 12-3 shows the increased amounts recommended for each of the nutrients. Based on several national studies, the following mean nutrient intakes are commonly below recommended intakes for pregnant women: fiber; vitamins D, E, B_6, and folate; and the minerals iron, zinc, calcium, and magnesium.[27] In addition to low intake of these nutrients, gravidas on vegan diets frequently consume inadequate amounts of vitamin B_{12} and are at increased risk of inadequate intake of iron and vitamin D.

Energy and Kilocalories

During pregnancy, kilocalorie requirements increase slightly to ensure nutrient and energy needs. The estimated energy requirement (EER) does not increase for the first trimester of pregnancy, allows an additional 340 kcal per day during the second, and an additional 452 kcal during the third trimester. This additional energy is needed (1) to build new

Table 12-1   Chronology of Development of the Human Dentition

Tooth	Hard Tissue Formation Begins	Amount of Enamel Formed at Birth	Enamel Completed	Eruption	Root Completed
Primary Dentition					
Maxillary					
Central incisor	4 mo in utero	Five-sixths	1½ mo	7½ mo	1½ yr
Lateral incisor	4½ mo in utero	Two-thirds	2½ mo	9 mo	2 yr
Cuspid	5 mo in utero	One-third	9 mo	18 mo	3¼ yr
First molar	5 mo in utero	Cusps united	6 mo	14 mo	2½ yr
Second molar	6 mo in utero	Cusp tips still isolated	11 mo	24 mo	3 yr
Mandibular					
Central incisor	4½ mo in utero	Three-fifths	2½ mo	6 mo	1½ yr
Lateral incisor	4½ mo in utero	Three-fifths	3 mo	7 mo	1½ yr
Cuspid	5 mo in utero	One-third	9 mo	16 mo	3¼ yr
First molar	5 mo in utero	Cusps united	5½ mo	12 mo	2¼ yr
Second molar	6 mo in utero	Cusp tips still isolated	10 mo	20 mo	3 yr
Permanent Dentition					
Maxillary					
Central incisor	3-4 mo	—	4-5 yr	7-8 yr	10 yr
Lateral incisor	10-12 mo	—	4-5 yr	8-9 yr	11 yr
Cuspid	4-5 mo	—	6-7 yr	11-12 yr	13-15 yr
First bicuspid	1½-1¾ yr	—	5-6 yr	10-11 yr	12-13 yr
Second bicuspid	2-2¼ yr	—	6-7 yr	10-12 yr	12-14 yr
First molar	At birth	Sometimes a trace	2½-3 yr	6-7 yr	9-10 yr
Second molar	2½-3 yr	—	7-8 yr	12-13 yr	14-16 yr
Mandibular					
Central incisor	3-4 mo	—	4-5 yr	6-7 yr	9 yr
Lateral incisor	3-4 mo	—	4-5 yr	7-8 yr	10 yr
Cuspid	4-5 mo	—	6-7 yr	9-10 yr	12-14 yr
First bicuspid	1¾-2 yr	—	5-6 yr	10-12 yr	12-13 yr
Second bicuspid	2¼-2½ yr	—	6-7 yr	11-12 yr	13-14 yr
First molar	At birth	Sometimes a trace	2½-3 yr	6-7 yr	9-10 yr
Second molar	2½-3 yr	—	7-8 yr	11-13 yr	14-15 yr

Adapted and slightly modified by Massler and Shour from Logan WAG, Kronfeld R. J Am Dent Assoc 1933; 20:420. From DePaola DP, et al: Nutrition and dental medicine. In Shils ME, et al (eds): Modern Nutrition in Health and Disease, 10th ed. Philadelphia: Lea & Febiger, 2005, pp 1152-1178.

Table 12-2   Nutrient Deficiencies and Tooth Development

Nutrient	Effect on Tissue
Protein	Delayed tooth eruption; increased caries susceptibility; dysfunctional salivary glands
Vitamin A	Disturbed keratin matrix of enamel; increased enamel hypoplasia; increased caries susceptibility; decreased epithelial tissue development; dysfunction of tooth morphogenesis
Vitamin D	Poor calcification; pitting
Calcium/phosphorus	Decreased calcium concentration; hypomineralization (hypoplastic defects)
Ascorbic acid	Disturbed collagen matrix of dentin; alterations of dental pulp
Fluoride/iron/zinc	Increased caries susceptibility
Iodine	Delayed tooth eruption
Magnesium	Hypoplasia of enamel

Compiled from information in DePaola DP, et al: Nutrition and dental medicine. In Shils ME, et al (eds): Modern Nutrition in Health and Disease, 9th ed. Philadelphia: Lea & Febiger, 2005, pp 1152-1178; Nizel AE: Preventing dental caries: the nutritional factors. Pediatr Clin North Am 1977; 24:144-155; and Shaw JH, Sweeney EA: Oral health. In Schneider HA, et al (eds): Nutritional Support of Medical Practice. Philadelphia: Harper & Row, 1983.

Table 12-3	Vitamin-Mineral Recommended Dietary Allowances and Supplements				
	Nonpregnant Women	**Pregnant (19-30 years old)**		**Lactating (19-30 years old)**	
Nutrient	**(19-30 years old)**	**Amount of Nutrient**	**Percent Increase**[a]	**Amount of Nutrient**	**Percent Increase**[a]
Vitamin A	**700 μg RE**	**770 μg RE**	10	**1200 μg RE**	71
Vitamin D	5 μg*	5 μg*	0	5 μg*	0
Vitamin E	**15 α-TE**	**15 α-TE**	0	**19 α-TE**	27
Vitamin K	90 μg*	90 μg*	0	90 μg*	0
Vitamin C	**75 mg**	**85 mg**	13	**120 mg**	60
Thiamin	**1.1 mg**	**1.4 mg**	27	**1.4 mg**	27
Riboflavin	**1.1 mg**	**1.4 mg**	27	**1.6 mg**	45
Niacin	**14 mg NE**	**18 mg NE**	28	**17 mg NE**	21
Vitamin B_6	**1.3 mg**	**1.9 mg**	46	**2 mg**	54
Folate	**400 μg**	**600 μg**	50	**500 μg**	25
Vitamin B_{12}	**2.4 μg**	**2.6 μg**	8	**2.8 μg**	17
Calcium	1000 mg*	1000 mg*	0	1000 mg*	0
Phosphorus	**700 mg**	**700 mg**	0	**700 mg**	0
Magnesium	**310 mg**	**350 mg**	9	**310 mg**	0
Fluoride	3 mg*	3 mg*	0	3 mg*	0
Iron	**18 mg**	**27 mg**	50	**9 mg**	[−50%]
Zinc	**8 mg**	**11 mg**	38	**12 mg**	50
Iodine	**150 μg**	**220 μg**	47	**290 μg**	93
Selenium	**55 μg**	**60 μg**	9	**70 μg**	27
Copper	**900 μg**	**1000 μg**	11	**1300 μg**	44

Data from Institute of Medicine, Food and Nutrition Board: Dietary Reference Intakes for: (1) Vitamin C, Vitamin E, Selenium, and Carotenoids. (2000); (2) Calcium, Phosphorus, Magnesium, Vitamin D, and Fluoride (1997); (3) Vitamin A, Vitamin K, Arsenic, Boron, Chromium, Copper, Iodine, Iron, Manganese, Molybdenum, Nickel, Silicon, Vanadium, and Zinc (2001). Washington, DC: National Academy Press.
Note: This table presents recommended dietary allowances (RDAs) in **bold type** and adequate intakes (AIs) in regular type followed by an asterisk (*).
[a]Percent increase for pregnant women above nonpregnancy recommendation.

tissues (including added maternal tissues and growth of the fetus and placenta), (2) to support increased metabolic expenditure, and (3) to enable physical movement of the additional weight.

Dieting for weight loss is never recommended during pregnancy, and severe dietary restrictions are inappropriate when a woman is trying to conceive. Avoidance of carbohydrate-rich foods from whole grains to reduce kilocalories, either preconceptionally or during pregnancy, negatively affects folic acid consumption from foods; this situation may be detrimental to the fetus.

Unless the gravida is significantly underweight before conception, additional kilocalories are not needed during the first trimester. Because requirements for many nutrients are increased, it is more important foods be chosen wisely, using principally nutrient-dense foods. Animal studies have shown that making poor food choices (junk food) during pregnancy and lactation predisposes the offspring to obesity and the early onset of hyperglycemia, hyperinsulinemia, and hyperlipidemia.[28] Appropriate weight gain reflects adequacy of energy intake and influences birth weight. When caloric intake is slightly inadequate, physiological adaptations spare energy for fetal growth. With adequate or generous kilocalories, energy balance is achieved in different ways depending on individual behavioral changes in food intake or energy expenditures and on adjustments in basal metabolism or fat stores.

Fat

The requirement for vitamins and minerals increases proportionately higher than caloric needs; therefore fats should be limited because of their minimal nutrient contribution. Hormonal changes result in significant elevations of serum cholesterol and triglycerides during the second trimester of pregnancy. Polyunsaturated fatty acids reduce serum lipids, and omega-3 fatty acids may improve some obstetrical complications. Omega-3 fatty acids (docosahexaenoic acid) and omega-6 fatty acids (arachidonic acid) are important for mental and visual development of infants.[29] Docosahexaenoic acid accumulates rapidly in the fetal brain and retina during the latter part of gestation and early postnatal life.

Protein

Protein is the basic nutrient for growth; an additional 21 g of protein, or a total of 67 g daily, is recommended. This can be accomplished with an additional 3 oz of meat or meat substitute (21 g protein), or by adding 2 oz of meat and 8 oz of milk (24 g protein). Because Americans consume more than 65 g of protein daily, additional amounts are not required.

Calcium and Vitamin D

Calcium and vitamin D work together in the formation of skeletal tissue and teeth. During pregnancy, hormonal and physiological adjustments promote increased calcium absorption and retention. This extra calcium is thought to be stored in maternal bone for fetal availability in the third trimester when fetal bone growth is rapid. Because of the enhanced calcium absorption and use, additional calcium supplementation is believed to be unnecessary. Pregnant women should consume the same amount of calcium as others in their age group.

The recommended 1000 mg per day of calcium for women older than 19 years of age can be met by three servings of milk or dairy products. Pregnant women younger 19 may need 4 cups of milk to provide the necessary 1300 mg per day. Dairy products may be incorporated into cooking or eaten in different forms, such as cheese, ice cream, or yogurt, for variety (see Table 8-2 and Box 8-2). A commonly reiterated myth is that a fetus removes calcium from the mother's teeth. This is a false statement. If the gravida has sufficient calcium in her diet, problems do not develop. If the diet is deficient in calcium, the embryo's requirements are met first; some of the calcium may come from the mother's bones, not from her teeth.

Vitamin D intake during pregnancy is associated with infant growth, bone ossification, tooth enamel formation, and neonatal calcium homeostasis. Suboptimal vitamin D status has been documented in many urban populations, including those with adequate sunlight, which suggests maternal vitamin D insufficiency during pregnancy is more common than previously realized. Vitamin D status must be assessed and may require supplementation to ensure adequate bone mass in the infant.[30] However, a more recent study indicated maternal and fetal adaptations during pregnancy provide the necessary calcium relatively independently of vitamin D status.[31]

B Vitamins

Several of the B-vitamin requirements are based on energy or caloric intake; usually, their intake increases automatically with intake of additional kilocalories. However, adequate intake of some B vitamins is difficult to achieve without careful selection of foods or supplementation.

The recommended dietary allowance (RDA) for folate (600 μg) during pregnancy is significantly more than the nonpregnant RDA. The role of folate as coenzyme is essential for nucleic acid synthesis. A folate deficiency that impairs cell growth and replication may cause fetal anomalies. Folate also is required for red blood cell (RBC) formation, which is increased in pregnancy. Orofacial clefts and neural tube defects, such as spina bifida and **anencephaly** (absence of a major portion of the brain and skull), have been attributed to inadequate folate intake before conception and during the first trimester. Ideally, attention should be focused on folate intake when a woman is considering a pregnancy because 50% to 70% of neural tube defects can be prevented if the woman consumes sufficient folic acid before conception and throughout the first trimester of the pregnancy.

Because of the crucial effects of folic acid during pregnancy, the FDA requires supplementation of all grain products with specific amounts of folic acid. Since the implementation of folic acid fortification, neural tube defects have declined 46% to 50% in countries that have adopted a folic acid fortification program.[32,33] In an effort to promote increased consumption of folic acid, the March of Dimes and the Grain Foods Foundation have created a new Folic Acid for a Healthy Pregnancy seal to help women quickly and easily identify products fortified with folic acid.

Meeting the requirement for folate solely from food intake is difficult for most women. Conscientious daily selections of raw fruits and vegetables, especially green leafy vegetables, can help ensure adequate intake. Whole-grain products and folic acid–fortified grains and cereals may also contribute significant amounts (see Tables 1-4 and 10-10). Absorption from supplements is better than from natural folate in foods. In 2007, approximately 60% of women of childbearing age were still not consuming a daily supplement containing folic acid.[34] Folic acid education promoting consumption of the vitamin from foods rich in folate, supplements, and fortified foods containing folic acid can increase the possibility of all women of childbearing age consuming adequate amounts and preventing neural tube defects.

Although folate intake is essential, some women take supplements providing eight times the RDA. High intakes may be transferred to the fetus; however, other nutrients (especially vitamin B$_{12}$) may be adversely affected by excess supplementation.

Iron

A common problem among nonpregnant women is iron-deficiency anemia, so many women begin pregnancy with diminished iron stores. Increased iron during gestation is needed for production of RBCs and the placenta, and to compensate for cord and blood loss at delivery.

The fetus acts as a parasite in that fetal **erythropoiesis**, the formation of RBCs, occurs at the expense of maternal iron stores. Iron-deficiency anemia is seldom seen in full-term infants. During the last half of pregnancy, iron absorption increases from the normal 10% to 20% to approximately 25% if adequate iron is available. Fetal accumulation of iron occurs principally in the last trimester. Premature infants, having a shortened gestation, have insufficient time to acquire adequate iron and may be born with iron-deficiency anemia; however, premature infants absorb iron very efficiently.

When maternal iron-deficiency anemia is diagnosed on initiation of prenatal care, it is associated with low caloric and iron intake; inadequate gestational gain; and increased risks of preterm delivery, LBW, and impaired intellectual development.[35] Maternal iron deficiency requires increased cardiac output to maintain adequate oxygen for maternal and fetal cells; if hemorrhage occurs at delivery, prognosis is poor.

Approximately 27 mg of iron is needed daily during pregnancy. Because the average American diet does not provide this amount within the normal caloric requirements, daily iron supplements (30 mg elemental iron) are usually recommended. Initiation of supplements before gestational week 24 prevents iron deficiency. Low-dose iron supplementation during pregnancy, even if the gravida is not anemic, improves the woman's iron status and seems to protect the infant from iron-deficiency anemia.[36] If iron supplements are not provided, it may take 2 years after delivery before maternal serum iron levels are normal.[2]

Zinc

Zinc is crucial early in pregnancy during the formation of fetal organs, but requirements are highest in late pregnancy for fetal growth and development. The RDA for zinc is 12 mg during pregnancy. An increase in high-protein foods, especially meats, improves zinc intake.

Iodine

In the United States, iodine nutrition status has declined among women of childbearing age over the last 3 decades. Laboratory indices do not indicate an iodine deficiency.[37] Because of the marginal iodine nutritional status of pregnant women, however, the Public Health Committee of the American Thyroid Association recommends daily iodine supplementation for all pregnant and lactating women in the United States and Canada.[38]

Vitamin-Mineral Supplements

In the United States, vitamin-mineral supplementation is commonly recommended during pregnancy. Supplementation should be based on evidence of a benefit and a lack of harmful effects. Food is considered to be the optimal vehicle for providing nutrients, but supplements may be warranted during this period. Supplement composition should be based on the nature of an identified nutritional need. Excessive amounts of many nutrients may have detrimental effects on the fetus (Table 12-4). Even if recommended by a healthcare provider, a supplement should not reduce the woman's motivation to maintain or improve the quality of her diet because, in most instances, nutrients in foods are better absorbed than those available in pills.

The IOM subcommittee concluded that iron is the only known nutrient warranting global supplementation during pregnancy. Based on findings from the Centers for Disease Control and Prevention (CDC), 27% of women in their third trimester of pregnancy have iron-deficiency anemia.[39] Consequently, 30 mg of ferrous iron is recommended to provide adequate amounts of iron during the second and third trimesters of pregnancy.

Dietary folate intake does not usually meet the RDA recommendations, but since folate enrichment of cereal products began in 1998, maternal folate status has improved significantly. A folate supplement may be prudent if adequacy of intake is questionable. It should be initiated before conception because birth defects from lack of folate intake may occur before the woman realizes she is pregnant. Because of the number of unintentional pregnancies in women 15 to 24 years old, a multivitamin supplement is recommended for all young women.

As a result of several studies showing a relationship between high doses of vitamin A supplements and birth defects, the FDA issued recommendations for women of childbearing age. Early during pregnancy, 10,000 IU of vitamin A (preformed from animal sources) may increase the risk of birth defects. Ordinary multivitamins typically contain 5000 IU, but some brands can contain much more—sometimes 25,000 IU. Excess vitamin A during the first trimester can result in severe craniofacial and oral clefts and limb defects. Intake of preformed vitamin A should be limited to about 100% of the daily value (DV) (5000 IU). Liver and other animal products and fortified foods and vitamin supplements listing retinyl palmitate and retinyl acetate as ingredients contain preformed vitamin A. Beta carotene, which the body converts to vitamin A, is much less toxic. Fortified foods containing beta carotene and fruits and vegetables that contain natural beta carotene should be chosen whenever possible.

Nutritional supplementation may be warranted in high-risk pregnancies, including adolescent pregnancies; multiple gestations (carrying more than one fetus); and pregnancies in women who use cigarettes, alcohol, or other drugs. Women who are younger than 25 or do not routinely consume

Table 12-4	Nutrient Supplementation Associated with Deleterious Fetal Outcomes
Nutrient	**Effects on Fetus**
Vitamin A	Pharmacologic use of vitamin A analogues has resulted in major congenital defects (malformation of cranium, face, heart, thymus, and central nervous system) and spontaneous abortion, especially during first trimester
Vitamin D	Excessive intake of vitamin D can result in hyperabsorption of calcium, hypercalcemia, calcification of soft tissues, and mental retardation
Vitamin E	Associated with higher incidence of spontaneous abortions
Vitamin K	Menadione administered parenterally has been associated with hemolytic anemia, hyperbilirubinemia, and kernicterus in the newborn
Vitamin C	Megadoses of vitamin C have been reported to cause vitamin C dependency with symptoms of conditional scurvy observed postpartum
Iodine	Large amounts of iodides have resulted in infants with congenital goiter, hypothyroidism, and mental retardation
Zinc	Large amounts of zinc supplements during third trimester were implicated in premature delivery and stillbirth
Fluoride	Well water containing 12-18 ppm fluoride produced offspring with significant mottling of deciduous teeth

Data from Worthington-Roberts B: Nutrition deficiencies and excesses: impact on pregnancy, part 2. J Perinatol 1985; 5(4):12. Reprinted by permission from Macmillan Publishers Ltd.

milk, dairy products, or foods fortified with calcium and vitamin D should take a calcium supplement. Supplementation of vitamin D may be required for some women living in Northern latitudes with limited regular exposure to sunlight. Research suggests higher intakes of vitamin D may be required, but more study is needed to determine the most effective dosage. If the iron supplement contains more than 30 mg of iron, supplemental amounts of zinc and copper are also needed.[2]

If supplementation is warranted for a gravida of any age, the specific nutrient amounts for a daily multivitamin-mineral preparation are shown in Table 12-5. Compliance with taking the nutrition supplement is poor; only about 50% of the vitamins are taken.[40] Many women stop taking the supplement because of nausea and vomiting, whereas others indicate the size of the pill is a factor. Patients should be encouraged to take the prescribed supplement and informed of the importance and reasons why it is needed. Positive effects from use of prenatal supplements, convenient supply, affordability, and reinforcement by healthcare providers enhance adherence.[41]

DIETARY INTAKE AND COUNSELING

Prenatal nutritional care improves outcome by saving lives, averting LBW, and decreasing the costs of care that are consequences of LBW. Although adequate weight gain is the most reliable measurable tool for assessing adequacy of caloric intake, food choices can provide adequate kilocalories, yet be deficient in vital nutrients. Nutrient intake warrants more attention than weight gain. For this reason, the IOM subcommittee recommends routine assessment of dietary practices for all gravidas in the United States to determine the need for improved diet or vitamin-mineral supplementation. Most women are highly motivated to make dietary changes during their pregnancy.

Because of the importance of nutrition information for expectant mothers, the MyPyramid website now has a link to a pyramid and information for pregnant and breastfeeding mothers. Dental hygienists can use this tool to obtain nutrition guidance for their patients or to help women personalize their own nutrition information. MyPyramid for Moms can be personalized by entering a woman's age, height, prepregnancy weight, physical activity level, and due date (Fig. 12-2). Through links on this website, other information available for the gravida include issues such as nutritional needs, weight gain, dietary supplements, food safety, and special health needs.

Pregnant women may have little or no nutritional knowledge. Although knowledge is the key to wise food choices, nutrition counseling is often unavailable or ignored during pregnancy. In many cases, low-income expectant mothers have more opportunities to receive nutritional information through established programs such as the Supplemental Nutrition Program for Women, Infants, and Children (WIC) than do more affluent women through the private sector.

Identification of poor and desirable food habits and dietary patterns can serve as the foundation for appropriate nutrition counseling and intervention. Identified nutritional problems, such as pica or fad dieting, or risk factors, such as alcohol abuse, may require special attention. Breastfeeding should also be promoted. Most importantly, it must be determined whether the gravida understands what foods she should be eating.

LACTATION

Exclusive breastfeeding for 4 to 6 months with the addition of complementary foods beginning at least by 6 months and continuing until 12 months is the ideal method of feeding infants. Breastfeeding is gaining in popularity. In 2005-2006, 77% of mothers breastfed newborns, with 41% still breastfeeding 6 months later.[43] For the first time, the percentage of infants initially breastfed exceeded the *Healthy People 2010* target of 75%.[44] This increase in breastfeeding rates shows outstanding gains, particularly for groups less likely to breastfeed—women who are African American, are younger than 20, have less than a high school education, are in their first pregnancy, are employed, and participated in WIC. Increased "baby friendly" hospital practices improve the chances of breastfeeding beyond 6 weeks.[45]

The Subcommittee on Nutrition during Lactation published *Nutrition during Lactation* to help healthcare providers understand how nutrition relates to the outcome of lactation and aids in formulating guidelines for clinical application in the United States.[46] The subcommittee concluded virtually all women are able to produce enough breast milk providing essential nutrients to support the growth and health of infants. Breastfeeding has many advantages for the infant and mother (Box 12-1); some are discussed in Chapter 13.

Breast milk is all the infant needs for about the first 6 months of life for optimal growth and development, with rare exceptions. The principal reason given by mothers for stopping breastfeeding is they perceive the infant is not satisfied by breast milk alone.[46] Breastfeeding continues to provide important nutrition and protection from illness and infection beyond the first 6 months of life. There is no specific age when breastfeeding should be terminated, and

Table 12-5	Nutrient Supplementation during Pregnancy	
Nutrient	**Amount of Supplement Recommended**
Vitamin C	50 mg
Vitamin B$_6$	2 mg
Folate	300 µg
Iron	30 mg
Zinc	15 mg
Copper	2 mg

Data from Institute of Medicine, Food and Nutrition Board: Nutrition during Pregnancy. Washington, DC: National Academy Press, 1990.

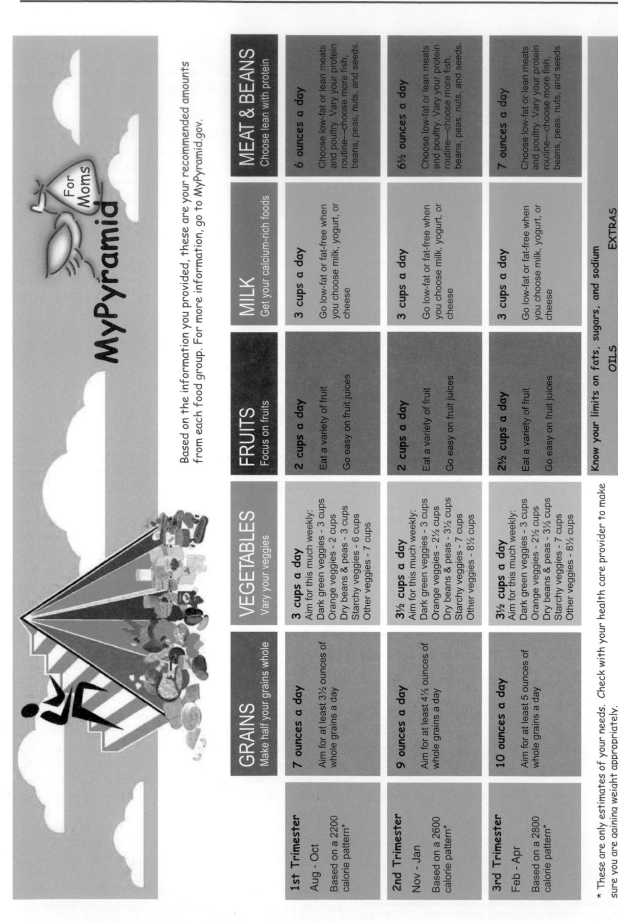

FIGURE I2-2 MyPyramid for Moms. Based on information provided by the mother (pregnant in the first trimester; age 32; height 5 feet, 7 inches; prepregnancy weight 150 lb; and moderately active [30 to 60 minutes of physical activity 5 days a week]), these are the recommended amounts from each food group. (From U.S. Department of Agriculture, Center for Nutrition Policy and Promotion, cnpp-16. Available at www.MyPyramid.gov.)

🦷 Dental Hygiene Considerations

Assessments

- *Physical*: level of education, income status, culture, religion, prenatal health care, medical history (including drugs taken), dental history, oral examination, feelings about weight gain.
- *Dietary*: health and nutritional knowledge and skills; adequacy of intake based on a well-balanced diet using a variety of foods, including enriched grain products; vegetarianism; food budget; food cravings and aversions; fad diets; beliefs about nutrition during pregnancy; pica, alcohol use, and caffeine intake.

Interventions

- Become familiar with local nutritional practices and beliefs about pregnancy; these beliefs are regional and may be affected by cultural beliefs.
- Refer patients at risk of inadequate intakes of specific nutrients to a registered dietitian or healthcare provider.
- Emphasize consumption of a well-balanced diet with three to six meals throughout the day to ensure optimal intake of nutrients.
- Patients who might become pregnant should have a high folate intake. If a woman of childbearing age is not taking a multivitamin supplement and is following a carbohydrate-restricted diet, refer her to a healthcare provider or a registered dietitian.
- Ask pregnant patients whether they are taking a prenatal supplement. If not, refer them to a healthcare provider.
- Seize pregnancy as the ideal opportunity to discuss good nutritional and oral hygiene habits needed during this period and for the newborn infant. Proper oral tissue development of the fetus depends on adequate nutrition of the mother.
- Encourage foods high in calcium. Low calcium intake may impair bone mineral deposition, especially in women younger than 25. Consuming the recommended 1300 mg of calcium daily is particularly important for pregnant teens to meet calcium demands. The use of dietary calcium is preferred because these foods also provide other valuable nutrients—protein, riboflavin, and vitamin D.
- Snacking is acceptable for pregnant women. Provide information on avoidance of acid attacks and resultant tooth decay by recommending appropriate oral hygiene techniques after snacking and encouraging foods such as nuts, raw vegetables, yogurt, and popcorn.
- If the mother has a strong preference for sweets, the infant's diet is also likely to be high in sugar. Review the gravida's diet for the form and frequency of sugar-containing foods, and suggest modifications or substitutions as indicated. This could create a healthier pattern for the patient and alleviate potential dental problems for the infant.
- Encourage pregnant patients to use iodized salt.
- Because of the increased risk of preterm or LBW infants associated with pregnancy gingivitis and other periodontal issues, encourage excellent oral hygiene habits throughout the day.
- Encourage pregnant women to enroll in educational breastfeeding classes that address benefits, techniques, common problems, myths, and skills training.

📎 Nutritional Directions

- Preventive oral care, including limiting frequency of fermentable carbohydrate intake and adequate oral hygiene care, is important for the mother and the fetus.
- Nutrient needs must be met by deliberate preplanning and informed food choices.
- Encourage sexually active women of childbearing age who drink alcohol to use reliable methods to prevent pregnancy, plan their pregnancies, and stop drinking before becoming pregnant.[42]
- A dentist or healthcare provider may recommend fluoride supplements in areas with a nonfluoridated water supply, but supplementation is generally not recommended in areas where the water is fluoridated (see Chapter 8). A complete assessment of fluoride intake is essential before prescribing fluoride supplements to avoid the risk of fluorosis.
- Low-fat or skim milk may be used to control weight, decrease saturated fat intake, and provide equivalent nutrients.
- Although the pregnant patient is "eating for two," her energy requirements are not double.
- Moderate increases in whole grains, milk, and legumes can provide additional protein and other important nutrients.
- Calcium, vitamin D, and vitamin B_{12} supplements are advisable for vegans, who exclude all animal products. Pregnant vegans should be referred to a registered dietitian.
- Vitamin D may be a special concern for women with minimal exposure to sunlight or routine use of sunscreens. Regular exposure to sunlight and foods fortified with vitamin D (e.g., milk and cheese) are recommended.
- Powdered milk ($\frac{1}{3}$ cup) can be added to soups, cooked cereals, mashed potatoes, or casseroles if the gravida has an aversion to milk.
- Adverse symptoms, such as nausea or constipation, frequently occur from iron supplementation. Rather than discontinuing the supplement, take it with meals, or consult the healthcare provider about possibly decreasing the dosage.
- Absorption of iron from supplements or foods is enhanced if taken between meals with vitamin C–rich foods, such as orange juice, while avoiding milk, tea, or coffee.
- Moderately intensive exercise during pregnancy is beneficial if medical reasons do not prevent it. Exercise at this time enhances blood flow, which delivers nutrients to the fetus, improves mood and energy level, and increases cardiovascular fitness and endurance.

mothers are encouraged to continue breastfeeding beyond the minimum of 6 months as long as they feel it is needed.

NUTRITIONAL RECOMMENDATIONS FOR BREASTFEEDING

For most nutrients, recommendations for lactating women are similar to the recommendations for pregnant women. Energy requirements are proportional to the quantity of milk produced. Approximately 85 kcal are needed for every 100 mL of milk produced, requiring approximately a 500-

---

Box 12-1 | Advantages of Breastfeeding

For the Mother

- Maternal hormones produced as a result of lactation facilitate contractions of the uterus and control postpartum bleeding.
- Prepregnancy weight is achieved sooner because breastfeeding burns kilocalories.[a]
- Breastfeeding is less expensive than formula feeding.
- Mother-infant bonding is enhanced with breastfeeding.
- Breastfeeding saves time because there are no bottles to clean, prepare, warm, or sterilize.
- Working mothers who breastfeed miss less work because of a sick infant.
- Prolactin, the hormone that helps the milk "come down," relaxes the mother.
- The mother is at reduced risk of premenopausal breast and ovarian cancer.

For the Infant

- Human milk is nutritionally balanced with maximum bioavailability for infants. It is easy for the infant to digest.
- Breast milk has immunological properties that help reduce infant morbidity (especially certain infectious gastrointestinal[b] and respiratory diseases, and earaches) and mortality. Within 4 hours after exposure to germs, antibodies in the milk change to meet the needs of the infant.
- Breast milk constantly changes in composition to meet the changing needs of the infant, especially a premature infant.

- Human milk reduces the risk of food allergies and prevents or delays the occurrence of atopic dermatitis, cow's milk allergy, and asthma (wheezing) in early childhood.[c]
- Breastfeeding promotes infant oral-motor and structural development; this can mean fewer dental bills or a decreased need for orthodontic work.
- Incidence of thumb sucking and tongue thrusting is lower in breastfed infants.
- Breastfed infants are exposed to a variety of tastes through the mother's milk.
- Breast milk reduces a child's risk for diabetes.
- Breast milk provides better brain development. Longer periods of exclusive breastfeeding during an infant's first year increases some measures of a child's cognitive development; this may lead to a smarter child and adult.[d]
- Prolonged breastfeeding may reduce the risk of overweight in childhood. Breastfeeding for more than 4 months is associated with lower adolescent BMI, independent of race or parental education.[e,f]
- Breastfeeding longer than 6 months provides health benefits well beyond the breastfeeding period. A quantitative review of the evidence indicates that exclusively breastfed infants may have lower blood cholesterol concentrations in later life.[g]
- Breastfeeding is associated with a reduction in risk for post-neonatal death.[h]

[a]Haksu IE, McDougald DM, Anderson AK: Effect of infant feeding on maternal body composition. Int Breastfeed J 2008 Aug 6; 3:18.
[b]Monterrosa EC, et al: Predominant breast-feeding from birth to six months is associated with fewer gastrointestinal infections and increased risk for iron deficiency among infants. J Nutr 2008 Aug; 138(8):1499-1504.
[c]Greer FR, et al: Effects of early nutritional interventions on the development of atopic disease in infants and children: the role of maternal dietary restriction, breastfeeding, timing of introduction of complementary foods, and hydrolyzed formulas. Pediatrics 2008 Jan; 121(1):183-191.
[d]Kramer M, et al: Breastfeeding and child cognitive development: new evidence from a large randomized trial. Arch Gen Psychiatry 2008 May; 65(5):578-584.
[e]Woo JG, et al: Breastfeeding helps explain racial and socioeconomic status disparities in adolescent adiposity. Pediatrics 2008 Mar; 121(3):e458-e465.
[f]Harder T, et al: Duration of breastfeeding and risk of overweight: a meta-analysis. Am J Epidemiol 2005 Sep 1; 163(5):397-403.
[g]Owen CG, et al: Does initial breastfeeding lead to lower blood cholesterol in adult life? A quantitative review of the evidence. Am J Clin Nutr 2008 Aug; 88(2):305-314.
[h]Chen A, Rogan WJ: Breastfeeding and the risk of post-neonatal death in the United States. Pediatrics 2004 May; 113(5):e435-e439.

---

kcal daily increase. Although this increase may not be fully adequate to cover the needs for milk production, the 2 to 4 kg of fat accumulated during pregnancy is available to supply additional kilocalories. Return to prepregnancy weight is accelerated. The major determinant of milk production is the infant's demand for milk, not maternal energy intake. Weight loss during lactation has no apparent deleterious effects on milk production.

Carbohydrate intake from whole grains, dairy, fruits, and vegetables is important for maintaining lactose synthesis and milk volume. The amount of protein recommended is slightly higher than for pregnancy—an additional 25 g or a total of 70 g daily. Other nutrients needed in larger quantities than during pregnancy include vitamins A, E, C, riboflavin, B_6, and B_{12}, and the minerals copper, zinc, iodine, and selenium. Maternal vitamin B_6 status affects amounts found in breast milk, and this adequacy affects infant growth. A source of vitamin B_{12} intake, from either foods or supplements, is crucial for optimal infant nurture. Neurological impairments have occurred in children of breastfeeding vegan mothers who were eating no or very limited foods of animal origin, which is the source of vitamin B_{12}. A lactating woman also requires additional fluids to replace those secreted in the milk. An additional 1000 mL per day (4 cups) of fluids is needed.

DIETARY PATTERNS FOR LACTATING WOMEN

The dietary pattern of a lactating woman is similar to that of a pregnant woman. Consumption of 3 cups of milk or dairy products fortified with vitamin D daily provides approximately 1000 mg of calcium and 300 IU of vitamin D, which are adequate amounts for women older than 19 years. Much higher doses would be needed to achieve adequate concentrations in exclusively breastfed infants of mothers younger than 19, so vitamin D supplementation in these infants is recommended.[31] Other high-calcium foods may also be used. High-protein foods may include 6 to 8 oz of meat daily, depending on the quantity of milk consumed. Adequate servings of fresh fruits, vegetables, and whole-grain products help provide the added caloric requirement.

Repletion of iron stores is important, and a prenatal vitamin is encouraged for postpartum women for its iron and folate content. Women who have mild iron deficiency are less sensitive to their infants' cues and have more difficulty bonding with their infants.[48,49] Women who are anemic are more likely to experience postpartum depression.[50]

Many substances consumed by the mother have been thought to affect breast milk. Certain foods, especially strongly flavored foods such as raw onion, garlic, curry, chili peppers, and chocolate, may cause gastrointestinal distress, rash, or irritability in the infant. These foods need to be omitted only if the infant is affected.

Many non-nutritive substances and drugs may be secreted in breast milk. Alcohol may impair milk flow and is transmitted in breast milk in approximately the same proportions as in the mother's blood. Intake should be limited to less than 0.5 g/kg daily. Large amounts of coffee and tea intake may adversely affect the iron content of human milk. Caffeine can be transferred to the infant in the breast milk, so caffeine intake should be moderate (300 mg).

Because of the risk of medications being passed into breast milk, all drugs, including over-the-counter medications and herbal remedies, should be used cautiously and only if essential. Medications that are less likely to be secreted into the milk can be prescribed by the healthcare provider.

MyPyramid for Moms provides individualized nutrition guidance to meet the needs of the breastfeeding mother that is consistent with the *Dietary Guidelines for Americans 2005* (Fig. 12-3). A fact sheet for breastfeeding mothers can be downloaded from the website (www.MyPyramid.gov). This fact sheet provides tips for eating a balanced diet, healthy weight maintenance, physical activity, and use of dietary supplements.

Dietary assessment of routine food intake by a registered dietitian is suggested, followed by nutrition counseling regarding foods rich in nutrients deficient in the diet. Continued use of the prenatal vitamin or a multivitamin supplement is recommended to ensure an adequate supply of folate if the woman may become pregnant again.

ORAL CONTRACEPTIVE AGENTS

Many nutrients (especially folate, vitamin B_6, zinc, and magnesium) are affected by oral contraceptive agents (OCAs). Low-estrogen preparations now being used do not adversely affect the woman's vitamin levels as much as earlier preparations. Lower levels of water-soluble vitamins are due to decreased intestinal absorption and increased metabolism. However, vitamin deficiencies have been identified only when the diet was marginal.

Low levels of vitamins B_6 and B_{12} have been noted in women using OCAs. Increased amounts of pyridoxine may

Dental Hygiene Considerations

Assessments
- *Physical*: socioeconomic status, types of drugs, over-the-counter medications, supplements, and herbals used.
- *Dietary*: adequacy of kilocalories, nutrients, and fluid intake; alcohol and caffeine intake.

Interventions
- For a postpartum patient, encourage a gradual return to pre-pregnancy weight (maximum weight loss of 4 lb per month for lactating women) through a balanced diet and moderate exercise.
- Encourage lactating women to obtain their nutrients from a well-balanced diet.
- Stress the importance of nutrients from fruits and vegetables, whole-grain breads and cereals, calcium-rich dairy products, and protein-rich and carbohydrate-rich foods.
- Encourage intake of at least 10 to 12 cups of fluid each day.
- Encourage increased intake of nutrient-dense foods to achieve a caloric intake of at least 1800 kcal daily.
- Discourage the use of strict weight loss diets and appetite suppressants.
- Emphasize the importance of milk, cheese, or other calcium-rich dairy products.
- Encourage intake of vitamin D–fortified foods, such as fortified milk or cereal, for women with limited exposure to ultraviolet light.
- For vegans who are breastfeeding, stress the importance of a balanced diet with appropriate supplements, especially vitamin B_{12}, in sufficient quantities. Offer a referral to a registered dietitian.

Nutritional Directions

- Breastfeeding helps with weight loss.
- Intake of coffee (regular and decaffeinated), other caffeine-containing beverages, and medications should be limited. Encourage fluids such as juice, milk, and water.

be indicated because estrogen increases the production of tryptophan, which uses pyridoxine in its metabolism. Low levels of vitamin B_6 also are independently associated with the risk for thromboembolism, so supplementation may be indicated.[51] A **thromboembolism** is an obstruction of a blood vessel with a clot-type substance carried in the blood from the site of origin to plug another vessel. Depression and impaired glucose tolerance attributed to OCAs may be alleviated with pyridoxine supplementation. Megaloblastic anemia reported in women taking OCAs may be related to decreased folate absorption or to low levels of vitamin B_{12}.

Progestins can cause weight gain related to increased appetite and altered carbohydrate metabolism. Estrogens may lead to an increase in subcutaneous fat and fluid retention.

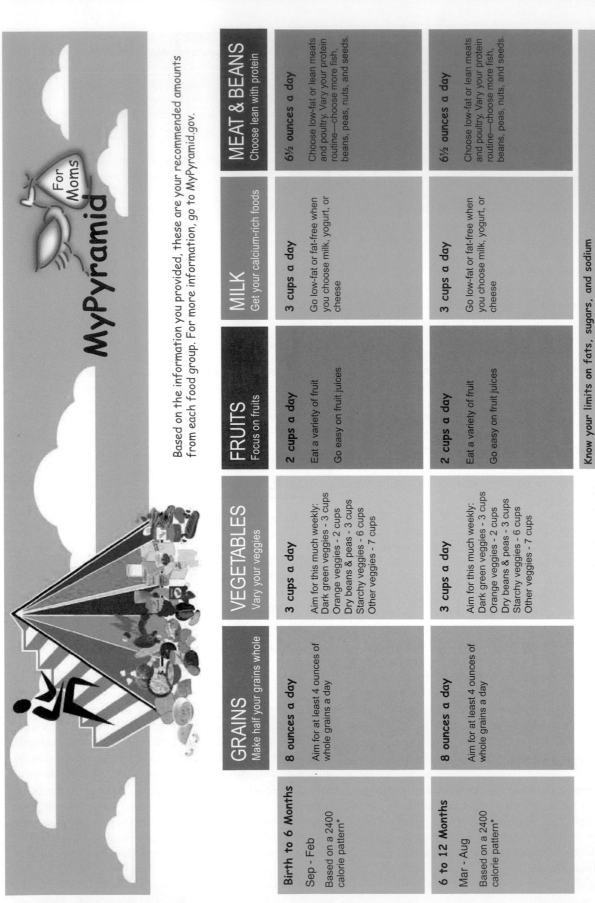

MyPyramid

For Moms

Based on the information you provided, these are your recommended amounts from each food group. For more information, go to MyPyramid.gov.

	GRAINS Make half your grains whole	VEGETABLES Vary your veggies	FRUITS Focus on fruits	MILK Get your calcium-rich foods	MEAT & BEANS Choose lean with protein
Birth to 6 Months Sep - Feb Based on a 2400 calorie pattern*	**8 ounces a day** Aim for at least 4 ounces of whole grains a day	**3 cups a day** Aim for this much weekly: Dark green veggies - 3 cups Orange veggies - 2 cups Dry beans & peas - 3 cups Starchy veggies - 6 cups Other veggies - 7 cups	**2 cups a day** Eat a variety of fruit Go easy on fruit juices	**3 cups a day** Go low-fat or fat-free when you choose milk, yogurt, or cheese	**6½ ounces a day** Choose low-fat or lean meats and poultry. Vary your protein routine—choose more fish, beans, peas, nuts, and seeds.
6 to 12 Months Mar - Aug Based on a 2400 calorie pattern*	**8 ounces a day** Aim for at least 4 ounces of whole grains a day	**3 cups a day** Aim for this much weekly: Dark green veggies - 3 cups Orange veggies - 2 cups Dry beans & peas - 3 cups Starchy veggies - 6 cups Other veggies - 7 cups	**2 cups a day** Eat a variety of fruit Go easy on fruit juices	**3 cups a day** Go low-fat or fat-free when you choose milk, yogurt, or cheese	**6½ ounces a day** Choose low-fat or lean meats and poultry. Vary your protein routine—choose more fish, beans, peas, nuts, and seeds.

Know your limits on fats, sugars, and sodium

	OILS Aim for this much:	EXTRAS Limit extras (solid fats and sugars) to this much:
Birth to 6 Months	7 teaspoons a day	360 calories a day
6 to 12 Months	7 teaspoons a day	360 calories a day

* These are only estimates of your needs while you breastfeed. Check with your health care provider to make sure you are losing the weight gained during pregnancy.

The calories and amounts of food you need change over time while you are breastfeeding. Your Plan may show different amounts of food for different months, to meet your changing nutritional needs.

FIGURE 12-3 MyPyramid for Moms. Based on information provided by the mother (breastfeeding; age 32; height 5 feet, 7 inches; prepregnancy weight 150 lb; and moderately active [30 to 60 minutes of physical activity, 5 days a week]), these are the recommended amounts from each food group. (From U.S. Department of Agriculture, Center for Nutrition Policy and Promotion, cnpp-16. Available at www.MyPyramid.gov.)

Use of OCAs is associated with increased risk of heart disease owing to changes in serum lipids. Progestin seems to cause an undesirable decrease in high-density lipoprotein (HDL) cholesterol levels and elevation of low-density lipoprotein (LDL) and total cholesterol levels (discussed in Chapter 5). The net effect on serum lipids depends on the amount and ratio of progestin and estrogens. OCAs containing progestin and estrogen have been shown to have little or no effect on HDL cholesterol levels, but may increase fasting triglyceride levels.

Various drugs and herbal medications can either increase or decrease the effect of OCAs. Grapefruit juice increases the bioavailability of estradiol in OCAs; avoidance within 1 to 2 hours of taking the OCA is recommended.[52]

MENOPAUSE

During the different stages of life, hormonal changes have many repercussions on general health. Female hormonal changes seem to be related to increased incidence of osteoporosis, which may be accompanied by some oral conditions, heart disease, and some cancers that occur later in life.

Perimenopause and **menopause** usually begin in the late 40s, but genetics, general health, and the age of menarche influence when it actually occurs in a particular woman. For several years before menopause, a range of symptoms may be experienced, including changes in menstruation, fatigue, night sweats, hot flashes, insomnia, loss of bone density, and mood swings. This cluster of symptoms is called perimenopause. Menopause (decreased production of estrogen and progesterone by the ovaries resulting in termination of menses) occurs between the ages of 35 and 58. Estrogen production decreases approximately 60%. Loss of the beneficial effects of estrogen causes health and nutrition issues.

Less estrogen affects the natural process of bone turnover, resulting in a decrease of bone mass. Estrogen receptors on the bone-resorbing osteoclasts increase activity in response to the estrogen level, whereas estrogen receptors on the bone-forming osteoblasts decrease their activity. Bone resorption exceeds bone formation, sometimes resulting in a 30% to 50% trabecular bone loss and 25% to 35% cortical bone loss.[53] The rate of bone loss is rapid in early menopause, then slows and gradually decreases for 8 to 10 years after menstruation.[54] This bone loss may result in osteopenia or osteoporosis (discussed in Chapter 8). The alveolar bone provides a potential labile source of calcium; changes in the alveolar process may be used for early diagnosis of osteoporosis.[55] A referral to the healthcare provider should be offered.

Reduced salivary gland secretion is a possible cause for increased dental caries and may lead to increased prevalence of oral **dysesthesia** (impairment of the sense of touch) and taste alterations. Senile **atrophic gingivitis** (abnormally pale gingival tissues) may develop concurrently. **Menopausal gingivostomatitis** (dry and shiny gingivae and edematous mucosa) results in easily bleeding gingiva that may be abnormally pale to quite erythematous. Postmenopausal women with osteoporosis exhibit an exaggerated response to dental plaque biofilm, including increased bleeding on probing, loss of dentoalveolar bone height, and decreased bone mineral density of the alveolar crestal and subcrestal bone. Uncontrolled osteoporosis may lead to edentulism; markedly resorbed residual alveolar ridges may be unsuitable for conventional dentures or dental implants.[54]

Declines in estrogen and progesterone production are accompanied by increased body fat and decreased lean tissue. Weight gain is frequently observed, and weight loss becomes more difficult because body metabolism is lower, and physical activity may be reduced. Also, blood lipid levels are negatively affected. Total and LDL cholesterol levels may increase with a concurrent decrease in HDL cholesterol levels.

Medically, symptoms of perimenopause and menopause may be treated with **hormone replacement therapy (HRT)**, which consists of low levels of estrogen and progesterone. This treatment is controversial, but when HRT treatment is initiated at the onset of menopause, increased osteoblastic activity reduces risk of osteoporosis and promotes oral health by inhibiting gingival inflammation, periodontitis, and the consequent loss of teeth. If the symptoms significantly affect the quality of life, decisions regarding HRT should involve the woman's genetic and medical history.

Plant-based foods, especially phytoestrogens and soluble fiber, may help decrease symptoms and regulate blood cholesterol levels. Foods containing phytoestrogens include soy products or isoflavone extracts. Herbal supplements also used to decrease menopausal symptoms include *Ginkgo biloba,* black cohosh, and flaxseed. The potential benefits, risks, and combination of supplements with food or medications or both remain uncertain.[56]

Nutritional approaches to reduce menopausal symptoms continue to focus on quality of dietary choices and healthy weight maintenance. Adequate amounts of calcium, vitamins D and K, and magnesium are important for protecting bone health. Intake of adequate amounts of fruits, vegetables, and grains, following the *Dietary Guidelines for Americans,* are effective in possibly reducing risk of cancer and coronary heart disease. The need to restrict energy intake may result in inadequate protein intake, which leads to loss of muscle mass.[57] Physical exercise, including aerobic activity and resistance and weight-bearing exercise, is beneficial for bone and cardiovascular health and weight control.

Dental Hygiene Considerations

Assessments
- *Physical*: age, medical history (including drugs taken), dental history, oral examination, physical activity, oral radiographic findings.
- *Dietary*: health and nutritional knowledge and skills, adequacy of calcium and vitamin D intake from food and supplements, caffeine intake.

Interventions
- Maintain meticulous daily oral self-care to reduce the risk for periodontal disease resulting from an exaggerated response to plaque biofilm.
- For patients with xerostomia, provide counseling on preventive strategies, such as home and office fluoride applications; use of xylitol gum or mints; and minimizing choice of cariogenic snacks and beverages, to reduce caries risk.
- Patients not prescribed HRT or other medications to deter progressive bone loss may exhibit increased alveolar bone loss, and their periodontal condition should be carefully monitored at regular intervals with the use of oral radiographs.

Nutritional Directions

- Encourage a minimum of 3 servings of low-fat dairy products or foods fortified with calcium and vitamin D (e.g., orange juice) to maintain bone mass. Consumption of greater than 90 mg per day of isoflavones in soy products may be effective in increasing the bone mass of menopausal women.
- Calcium and vitamin D supplementation beyond the tolerable upper intake level (UL) should be discouraged unless taken under the supervision of a healthcare provider.
- Encourage good sources of lean protein and regular exercise to maintain muscle mass.
- Choose whole grains, vegetables, fruit, low-fat dairy products, and lean meat or soy substitutes to minimize the risk of cardiovascular disease and to maximize bone health.
- If xerostomia is present, recommend avoidance of alcohol and alcohol-containing products to minimize burning and discomfort in the oral tissues.
- Provide nutritional counseling about noncariogenic snack choices.

HEALTH APPLICATION 12 Fetal Alcohol Spectrum Disorder

The CDC, American College of Obstetricians and Gynecologists, American Academy of Pediatrics, and March of Dimes all recommend no alcohol intake during pregnancy. No prenatal period has been shown to be safe from the deleterious effects of alcohol.

Fetal alcohol syndrome (FAS) is a cluster of birth defects resulting from prenatal alcohol exposure. An infant with FAS is born exhibiting full effects of the alcohol (Box 12-2), characterized by a pattern of minor facial anomalies, prenatal and postnatal growth retardation, and functional or structural central nervous system abnormalities. Fetal alcohol spectrum disorder (FASD) is a combination of irreversible birth defects and behavioral challenges in infants and children whose mothers consumed some alcohol during the pregnancy. Based on more recent studies, the prevalence of FAS in the general population of the United States is estimated to be 0.33 to 3 per 1000 births, and the prevalence of FASD is at least 10 per 1000, or 1% of all births.[58,59]

Nearly 40,000 infants are born each year bearing some features typical of FASD.[60] FASD can result from 2 oz per day of alcohol. Smaller amounts of alcohol consumption may be associated with adverse effects such as spontaneous abortion, growth retardation, cleft palate, or some of the neurological and behavioral effects of FASD without the physical abnormalities. Prenatal alcohol exposure can cause damage to the brain that results in significant problems with regulating behavior and optimal thinking and learning.[61] This condition, called fetal alcohol effects, is difficult to diagnose.

FASD is totally preventable by abstaining from the use of alcohol. The first trimester, especially the first month, is the most vulnerable time for the fetus because the woman may not even be aware of the pregnancy. Four to five drinks a day, or at least 45 drinks per month, can produce the full FAS syndrome (see Box 12-2). Despite the risk for FASD, the 2002 Behavior Risk Factor Surveillance System (BRFSS) reported that 10% of pregnant women reported using alcohol with nearly 2% engaging in binge drinking.[62]

The FAS child has specific physiological deformities (Fig. 12-4), but how alcohol affects the fetus is not fully understood. Accumulation of toxic levels of alcohol may interfere with cell formation. Several nutrients, especially folic acid, magnesium, and zinc, may be involved. The mental and physical abnormalities cannot be reversed.

Even with adequate nutrition, normal development of fetal organs is jeopardized. Other habits that usually accompany alcohol consumption (e.g., smoking, excessive amounts of coffee the "morning after," poor eating habits with little attention to needed nutrients, and perhaps use of tranquilizers) may also adversely affect the unborn child. Ethanol is a source of energy; chronic alcoholics may have a relatively low intake of protein, essential fats, vitamins, and minerals. Alcohol may impair placental transport of amino acids, calcium, and some vitamins.

Because the brain has a special affinity for alcohol, it is one of the first organs affected. Intellectual impairment is frequently reported in children with FAS. Even at birth, the circumference of the head is small (microcephaly), indicating abnormal brain capacity (i.e., weight of 140 g in an infant with FAS compared with a normal brain weighing 400 g). Fewer brain cells exist, with damaged cells preventing normal functioning; fewer neurons result in disorganized thought. The thinking ability of the brain is permanently disturbed. The average IQ is 68; maladaptive behaviors are common. Additionally, as a result of fewer total body cells, abnormal weight gain affects normal cell development and growth.

Because of the global adverse effects of alcohol intake, healthcare providers should advise pregnant women and women who might become pregnant to abstain from alcohol. Nutritional counseling and other efforts to improve food intake, such as referral to a social worker for food or monetary resources, are warranted. The subcommittee recommended the use of multivitamin-mineral supplements for heavy substance abusers who have difficulty changing their habits to improve nutrient intake.

Box 12-2   Signs of Fetal Alcohol Syndrome

Fetal alcohol syndrome is a cluster or pattern of related problems, not just a single birth defect. The severity of symptoms varies, but the symptoms are irreversible. Facial features are more difficult to identify in preschool-age children. Signs of fetal alcohol syndrome may include the following:

- Small head circumference and brain size (microcephaly)
- Distinctive facial features: small eyelid openings; eyes close together; a sunken nasal bridge; a short, upturned, undefined nose; an exceptionally thin upper lip; and a smooth skin surface between the nose and upper lip
- Oral cavity: small teeth with faulty enamel, prominent ridges in palate, cleft lip or palate, and small jaws
- Ears poorly formed and incorrectly positioned
- Heart defects
- Deformities of joints, limbs, and fingers
- Weak skeletal muscles (hypotonia) and poor coordination
- Slow physical growth before and after birth
- Vision difficulties, including nearsightedness (myopia)
- Intellectual disabilities and delayed development
- Abnormal behavior such as poor judgment, distractibility and short attention span, hyperactivity, poor impulse control, extreme nervousness and anxiety, and social interaction problems

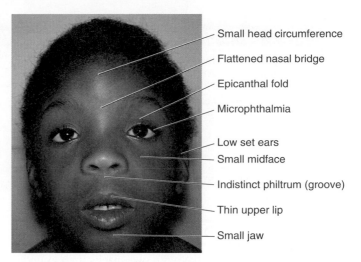

FIGURE 12-4 Facial anomalies of a child with fetal alcohol syndrome. (From Zitelli BJ, Davis HW: Atlas of Pediatric Physical Diagnosis, 4th ed. St Louis: Mosby, 2002.)

CASE APPLICATION FOR THE DENTAL HYGIENIST

Your regular patient, Betty, a 16-year-old, confides to you on her 6-month recall appointment she is 3 months pregnant. Even though she and her parents have decided to keep the infant, she has not seen a healthcare provider yet. Betty indicates that her mother lost a tooth with each child so she expects the same thing will happen to her.

Nutritional Assessment

- Knowledge about nutrition during pregnancy
- Special dietary restrictions; food fad practices; ethnic, cultural, or religious customs
- Adequacy of diet, especially kilocalories, protein, calcium, vitamin D, iron, and folate
- Medications (including vitamin supplements), drug, and tobacco use
- Support of parents, living arrangements, and social support
- Psychological status

Nutritional Diagnosis

Altered nutrition: less than body requirements related to lack of nutritional information and weight concerns.

Nutritional Goals

The patient will consume a well-balanced diet (based on MyPyramid for Moms) with additional kilocalories during the second and third trimesters, and verbalize ways to increase protein, iron, calcium, and folate intake.

Nutritional Implementation

Intervention: Encourage Betty to visit an healthcare provider as soon as possible.
Rationale: Fetal outcome is affected by nutrient intake during pregnancy; birth defects are likely to occur if dietary habits are poor, or if drug use occurs early in the pregnancy. Inadequate prenatal care leads to poor outcomes for the mother and fetus.

Intervention: Clarify nutritional misconceptions by providing written material and discussing the principal nutrients needing to be increased. Provide the name of a registered dietitian with whom she can discuss these concerns.
Rationale: Nutritional requirements are quite high to meet the growth needs of the adolescent and the fetus because Betty is still growing and storing nutrients in her own body.
Intervention: Teach Betty about the importance of consuming enough calcium and vitamin D during the pregnancy.
Rationale: Calcium and vitamin D are important in the formation of skeletal tissue and teeth.
Intervention: Discuss fermentable carbohydrates, and determine how frequently Betty consumes them.
Rationale: Fermentable carbohydrates, especially soft foods stick to the teeth, enhance plaque formation and increase severity of periodontal issues. Parental food selections reflect the foods a child is exposed to and accepts.
Intervention: Talk to Betty about gingivitis during pregnancy, why it occurs, and the risks associated with it.
Rationale: Hormonal changes during pregnancy lead to an increased risk of oral problems affecting pregnancy outcome.
Intervention: Discuss nutrients needing to be increased during pregnancy. Provide snack ideas (cheese, nuts, yogurt, milkshakes, popcorn, raw vegetables, and fruits) that contain these nutrients.
Rationale: Most teenagers have an inadequate intake of kilocalories, calcium, iron, vitamins A and D, and niacin. Adequate intake of kilocalories, protein, calcium, iron, B vitamins, and zinc is essential for a healthy infant and to protect fetal stores.
Intervention: Explain the effects of her nutritional status on oral development of her infant.
Rationale: Nutrition can determine whether teeth achieve their optimum genetic potential.

CASE APPLICATION FOR THE DENTAL HYGIENIST—cont'd

Intervention: Explain why she should limit her intake of coffee, tea, and especially carbonated beverages containing caffeine. Explain why she should abstain from alcohol use.

Rationale: Large amounts of caffeine could be responsible for malformations and increased susceptibility to decay of the primary first molars. Alcohol consumption may cause FASD.

Evaluation

Betty should improve eating habits to consume at least the number of food groups recommended in MyPyramid for Pregnancy and Breastfeeding. Other behaviors, such as decreasing sugar intake, consuming milk and dairy products (for calcium and vitamin D intake), and consuming raw fruits and green leafy vegetables (for folate intake), will increase intake of nutrients needed during pregnancy. Betty has been taking appropriate action toward oral hygiene self-care to prevent or minimize periodontal problems.

STUDENT READINESS

1. Plan food intake for 1 day with two snacks for a gravida who has four new carious lesions. What reasons would you give her for restricting sugar intake?
2. Explain what pica is, and the type of individuals who may be practicing this behavior.
3. Why is it undesirable to lose weight during pregnancy?
4. List five effects on oral development of the fetus when maternal nutrient intake is inadequate.
5. Why is oral health care especially important during pregnancy?
6. Which nutrients may be needed if dietary assessment indicates deficient intake that cannot be corrected by changing eating habits?
7. List advantages of breastfeeding, especially on oral-motor development.

CASE STUDY

A 32-year-old mother of two children (3 years old and 6 months old) who is breastfeeding complains of bleeding and sore gums and tongue. She has not returned to the healthcare provider since the birth of her younger child because of lack of time. She has returned to her job as a clerk at a local department store. When questioned about her diet, she reports she drinks a cup of coffee on her way to work; she usually takes a peanut butter and jelly sandwich and soft drink for lunch; and during the evening, she grabs something fast and easy to eat such as hot dogs, canned soup, crackers, cookies, chips, or soft drinks. She complains she is tired and irritable and feels this is because of the stress imposed on her by the two children and her work.

1. List probable causes of the mother's symptoms.
2. Discuss the added stress of pregnancy and lactation on her nutritional needs.
3. Determine other foods that should be readily available for her to consume, such as cottage cheese, yogurt, nuts, fresh fruit, and raw vegetables.
4. Discuss possible nutrition-related causes of the "bleeding and sore gums and tongue."
5. As a dental hygienist, outline the steps to take to reach your recommendations.

References

1. MacDorman MF, et al: Trends in preterm-related infant mortality by race and ethnicity: United States, 1999-2004. Hyattsville, MD: U.S. Department of Health and Human Services, CDC, National Center for Health Statistics, 2007. Available at http://www.cdc.gov/nchs/products/pubs/pubd/hestats/infantmort99-04/infantmort99-04.htm. Accessed July 13, 2008.
2. Institute of Medicine (IOM), Subcommittee on Nutritional Status and Weight Gain during Pregnancy: Nutrition during Pregnancy. Washington, DC: National Academy Press, 1990.
3. Board on Children, Youth and Families, Food and Nutrition Board: Influence of Pregnancy Weight on Maternal and Child Health: Workshop Report. Washington, DC: National Academies Press, 2007.
4. Thompson DR, et al: Maternal obesity and risk of infant death based on Florida birth records for 2004. Public Health Rep 2008 Apr; 123(4):487-493. Available at www.publichealthreports.org/userfiles/123_4/487-493.pdf. Accessed July 13, 2008.
5. Institute of Medicine (IOM), Food and Nutrition Board: Dietary Reference Intakes for Vitamin A, Vitamin K, Arsenic, Boron, Chromium, Copper, Iodine, Iron, Manganese, Molybdenum, Nickel, Silicon, Vanadium, and Zinc. Washington, DC: National Academy Press, 2000.
6. Institute of Medicine (IOM): WIC Nutrition Risk Criteria: A Scientific Assessment. Washington, DC: National Academy Press, 1996.
7. Shelton J: Are food cravings the body's way of telling us that we are lacking certain nutrients? Available at ScientificAmerican.com. Accessed June 3, 2005.
8. Roth A, Elkayam U: Acute myocardial infarction associated with pregnancy. J Am Coll Cardiol 2008 Jul 15; 52(3): 171-180.
9. Olson CM: Achieving a healthy weight gain during pregnancy. Annu Rev Nutr 2008; 28:411-423.
10. Oken E, et al: Gestational weight gain and child adiposity at age 3 years. Am J Obstet Gynecol 2007 Apr; 196(4):322.e1-322.e8.
11. Amorim AR, et al: Does excess pregnancy weight gain constitute a major risk for increasing long-term BMI? Obesity 2007 May; 15(5):1278-1286.
12. Habashneh A, et al: Factors related to utilization of dental services during pregnancy. J Clin Periodontol 2005 Jul; 32(7):815-821.
13. Lydon-Rochelle MT, et al: Dental care use and self-reported dental problems in relation to pregnancy. Am J Public Health 2004 May; 94(5):765-771.
14. Michalowics BS, et al: Examining the safety of dental treatment in pregnant women. J Am Dent Assoc 2008 Jun; 139(6):685-695.

15. Ruma M, et al: Maternal periodontal disease, systemic inflammation and risk for preeclampsia. Am J Obstet Gynecol 2008 Apr; 198(4):389.e1-e5. Epub 2008 Mar 4.

16. Boggess KA, et al: Maternal periodontal disease in early pregnancy and risk for a small-for-gestational-age infant. Am J Obstet Gynecol 2008 May; 194(5):1316-1322.

17. Vergnes JN: Studies suggest an association between maternal periodontal disease and preeclampsia. Evid Based Dent 2008; 9(2):46-47.

18. Ali RA, Egan LJ: Gastroesophageal reflux disease in pregnancy. Best Pract Res Clin Gastroenterol 2007; 21(5): 793-806.

19. Milosevic A: Gastro-oesophageal reflux and dental erosion. Evid Based Dent 2008; 9(2):54.

20. Bech BH, et al: Effect of reducing caffeine intake on birth weight and length of gestation: Randomized controlled trial. BMJ 2007 Feb 24; 334(7590):409.

21. Higdon JV, Frei B: Coffee and health: A review of recent human research. Crit Rev Food Sci Nutr 2006; 46(2): 101-123.

22. Weng X, Odouli R, Li DK: Maternal caffeine consumption during pregnancy and the risk of miscarriage: A prospective cohort study. Am J Obstet Gynecol 2008 Mar; 198(3):279.e1-279.e8.

23. Position of the American Dietetic Association: Nutrition and lifestyle for a healthy pregnancy outcome. J Am Diet Assoc 2008 Mar; 108(3):553-561.

24. Romitti PA, et al: Maternal periconceptional alcohol consumption and risk of orofacial clefts. Am J Epidemiol 2007 Oct 1; 166(7):775-785.

25. U.S. Food and Drug Administration and U.S. Environmental Protection Agency: What you need to know about mercury in fish and shellfish. EPA-823-F-04-009. March 2004. Available at www.cfsan.fda.gov/~dms/admehg3b.html. Accessed July 13, 2008.

26. Preidt R: Mom's vitamin D levels affect baby's dental health. HealthDay Available at www.nlm.nih.gov/medlineplus/print/news/fullstory_66609.html. Accessed July 12, 2008.

27. Giddens JB, et al: Pregnant adolescent and adult women have similarly low intakes of selected nutrients. J Am Diet Assoc 2000 Nov; 100(11):1334-1340.

28. Bayol SA, et al: Offspring from mothers fed a "junk food" diet in pregnancy and lactation exhibit exacerbated adiposity which is more pronounced in females. J Physiol 2008 Jul 1; 586(13):3219-3230.

29. Eilander A, et al: Effects of n-3 long chain polyunsaturated fatty acid supplementation on visual and cognitive development throughout childhood: a review of human studies. Prostaglandins Leukot Essent Fatty Acids 2007 Apr; 76(4): 189-203.

30. Javaid MK, et al; Princess Anne Hospital Study Group: Maternal vitamin D status during pregnancy and childhood bone mass at age 9 years: a longitudinal study. Lancet 2006 Jan 7; 367(9504):36-43.

31. Kovacs CS: Vitamin D in pregnancy and lactation: maternal, fetal, and neonatal outcomes from human and animal studies. Am J Clin Nutr 2008 Aug; 88(Suppl):520S-528S.

32. U.S. Department of Health and Human Services: Reduce the occurrence of spina bifida and other neural tube defects, 16-15. In Healthy People 2010. Available at http://www.healthypeople.gov/document/html/volume2/16mich.htm#_Toc494699666. Accessed on July 20, 2008.

33. DeWals P, et al: Reduction in neural-tube defects after folic acid fortification in Canada. N Engl J Med 2007 Jul 12; 357:135-142.

34. Centers for Disease Control and Prevention (CDC): Use of supplements containing folic acid among women of childbearing age-United States, 2007. MMWR Morb Mortal Wkly Rep 2008 Jan 11; 57(01):5-8. Available at www.cdc.gov/mmwr. Accessed January 11, 2008.

35. Schümann K, et al: On risks and benefits of iron supplementation recommendations for iron intake revisited. J Trace Elem Med Biol 2007; 31(3):147-168.

36. Rioux FM, LeBlanc CP: Iron supplementation during pregnancy: what are the risks and benefits of current practices? Appl Physiol Nutr Metab 2007 Apr; 32(2):282-288.

37. Hollowell JG, Haddow JE: The prevalence of iodine deficiency in women of reproductive age in the United States of America. Public Health Nutr 2007 Dec; 10(12A): 1532-1539.

38. Public Health Committee of the American Thyroid Association: Iodine supplementation for pregnancy and lactation—United States and Canada: recommendations of the American Thyroid Association. Thyroid 2006 Oct; 16(10): 949-951.

39. Centers for Disease Control and Prevention (CDC): Iron deficiency—United States, 1999-2000. MMWR Morb Mortal Wkly Rep 2002; 51:897-899.

40. Nguyen P, et al: Effect of iron content on the tolerability of prenatal multivitamins in pregnancy. BMC Pregnancy Childbirth 2008 May 15; 8:17.

41. Tessema J, et al: Motivators and barriers to prenatal supplement use among minority women in the United States. J Am Diet Assoc 2009 Jan; 109(1):102-108.

42. Ethen MK, et al: Alcohol consumption by women before and during pregnancy. Matern Child Health J 2008 Mar 4 [Epub ahead of print].

43. McDowell MM, Wang CY, Kennedy-Stephenson J: Breastfeeding in the United States: findings from the National Health and Nutrition Examination Survey, 1999-2006. NCHS Data Brief; no. 5. Hyattsville, MD: National Center for Health Statistics, 2008. www.cdc.gov/nchs/data/databriefs/db05.htm Accessed May 1, 2008.

44. U.S. Department of Health and Human Services: Healthy People 2010. Washington, DC: U.S. Department of Health and Human Services. 2000. Available at www.healthypeople.gov/document/html/objectives/160119.htm. Accessed July 25, 2008.

45. DiGirolamo AM, Grummer-Strawn LM, Fein SB: Effect of maternity-care practices on breastfeeding. Pediatrics 2008 Oct; 122(suppl).S43-S49.

46. Institute of Medicine (IOM), Subcommittee on Nutritional Status and Weight Gain during Pregnancy: Nutrition during Lactation. Washington, DC: National Academy Press, 1991.

47. Li R, et al: Why mothers stop breastfeeding: mothers' self-reported reasons for stopping during the first year. Pediatrics 2008 Oct; 122(suppl): S69-S76.

48. Perez EM, et al: Mother-infant interactions and infant development are altered by maternal iron deficiency anemia. J Nutr 2005 Apr; 135(4):850-855.

49. Beard JL, et al: Maternal iron deficiency anemia affects postpartum emotions and cognition. J Nutr 2005 Feb; 135(2):267-272.

50. Corwin EJ, et al: Low hemoglobin level is a risk factor for postpartum depression. J Nutr 2003 Dec; 133(12): 4139-4142.

51. Lussana F, et al: Blood levels of homocysteine, folate, vitamin B_6 and B_{12} in women using oral contraceptives compared to non-users. Thromb Res 2003; 112(1-2):37-41.

52. Voiles KM, Kelly WN: Potential interactions between oral contraceptives and other medications and natural substances. US Pharmacist 2004; 29(1). Available at www.uspharmacist.com/index.asp?show=article&page=8_1193.htm. Accessed June 29, 2008.

53. Ma DF, et al: Soy isoflavone intake inhibits bone resorption and stimulates bone formation in menopausal women: meta-analysis of randomized controlled trials. Eur J Clin Nutr 2008 Feb; 62(2):155-161.

54. Friedlander AH: The physiology, medical management and oral implications of menopause. J Am Dent Assoc 2002 Jan; 133(1):73-81.

55. DePaola DP, et al: Nutrition and dental medicine. In Shils ME, et al (eds): Modern Nutrition in Health and Disease, 10th ed. Philadelphia: Lippincott Williams & Wilkins, 2005.

56. Position of the American Dietetic Association and Dietitians of Canada: Nutrition and women's health. J Am Diet Assoc 2004 Jun; 104(6):984-1001.

57. Bopp MJ, et al: Lean mass loss is associated with low protein intake during dietary-induced weight loss in postmenopausal women. J Am Diet Assoc 2008 Jul; 108(7):1216-1220.

58. Sampson PD, et al: Incidence of fetal alcohol syndrome and prevalence of alcohol-related neurodevelopmental disorder. Teratology 1997 Nov; 56(5):317-326.

59. May PA, Gossage JP: Estimating the prevalence of fetal alcohol syndrome: a summary. National Institutes of Health, National Institute on Alcohol Abuse and Alcoholism. Available at http://pubs.niaaa.nih.gov/publications/arh25-3/159-167.htm. Accessed July 26, 2008.

60. May PA, Gossage JP: Estimating the prevalence of fetal alcohol syndrome: A summary. Alcohol Res Health 2001; 25(3):159-167.

61. Fryer SL, et al: Prenatal alcohol exposure affects frontal-striatal BOLD response during inhibitory control. Alcohol Clin Exp Res 2007 Aug; 31(8):1415-1424.

62. Centers for Disease Control and Prevention (CDC): Alcohol consumption among women who are pregnant or who might become pregnant—United States, 2002. MMWR Morb Mortal Wkly Rep 2004; 53(50):1178-1181.

Chapter 13

Nutritional Requirements during Growth and Development and Eating Habits Affecting Oral Health

LEARNING OBJECTIVES

Upon completion of this chapter, the student will be able to achieve the following objectives:

• Describe the procedure for introducing solid foods after the initial stage of feeding by bottle or breast.
• Discuss ways to handle typical nutritional problems that occur in infants, young children, school-age children, and adolescents.

• Apply dental hygiene aspects related to nutritional needs during infancy, early childhood, elementary school years, and adolescence to patient care.
• Assess nutrition education needs for patients during infancy, early childhood, elementary school years, and adolescence.
• Discuss physiological changes that alter the nutritional status of infants and adolescents.

KEY TERMS

Baby bottle tooth decay (BBTD)
Bruxism
Cleft lip
Cleft palate

Food jags
Innate
Non-nutritive sucking
Sealants

Test Your NQ

1. **T/F**   Commercial infant formulas are standard in their nutrient content.
2. **T/F**   Fluoride should be provided to all infants from birth if the water supply is not fluoridated.
3. **T/F**   Solid foods should be introduced at 6 weeks of age.
4. **T/F**   Orange juice is the first fruit juice to offer an infant.
5. **T/F**   More nutrients are required during adolescence than during any other stage of life.

6. **T/F**   Toddlers may refuse to eat anything except one food for several days.
7. **T/F**   Breastfed infants do not need any supplements during the first 4 months.
8. **T/F**   Bottle-fed infants are less likely to develop malocclusion.
9. **T/F**   The energy needs of children and adolescents are high to support growth and development and physical activity level.
10. **T/F**   To reduce the risk of plaque biofilm, toddlers and children should not be given snacks.

Many of the nutritional objectives established by the federal government in *Healthy People 2010* (see Chapter 1) are targeted to specific age groups and stages throughout the life span. Achievement of these goals improves the optimal health of infants and children, affecting their long-term health status and life span.

INFANTS

An infant's health status at birth and future lifelong health depend on feeding and nurturing the newborn by the mother or caretaker. Infancy is a time of rapid transition from virtually nothing but milk to a varied diet consisting of some foods from each of the food groups being consumed on a daily basis. The infant is normally able to thrive on human milk or commercially available artificial infant milk, but many of the physiological systems are immature at birth. Because of the small stomach capacity, frequent feedings are needed.

Pregnant patients expect the dental hygienist to provide information concerning infant feeding methods affecting the oral cavity. The practitioner should be prepared to address these issues and base counseling on evidence-based information. Feeding patterns present during the child's first 2 years create an environment for optimal development of genetically determined factors contributing to orofacial development and swallowing patterns.

GROWTH

Growth is the definitive test of health and is used as the most sensitive and specific indicator of nutritional status. Increased size results in greater nutritional requirements, but the need for kilocalories per kilogram decreases as one grows. Dental hygienists working with new parents, infants, and children should be familiar with normal growth and developmental patterns that reflect adequacy of nutritional intake. The birth weight of an infant doubles in 4 months (from 7½ to 15 lb), and by 1 year, it has usually tripled. Length or height increases 50% by 1 year of age. The Centers for Disease Control and Prevention (CDC) growth charts for determining appropriate growth rates are available in Appendix B.

NUTRITIONAL REQUIREMENTS

Adequate nutrition is more important during infancy and childhood than any other stage of the life cycle. As might be expected from the rapid growth rate, energy requirements are much higher per pound or kilogram of weight than for an adult: 95 to 83 kcal/kg per day between 3 and 12 months of age versus 29 to 37 kcal/kg per day for adults. Infants have a higher resting metabolic rate, and intestinal absorption is relatively inefficient.

The adequate intake (AI) for protein is 1.52 g/kg daily from birth to 6 months of age, and the recommended dietary allowance (RDA) for older infants is 1.2 g/kg; this translates to about 9.1 to 11 g per day (Table 13-1). Recommended protein intakes are based on mean protein intake of breastfed infants. As a result of immature renal function, total protein should not exceed 20% of the kilocalories. Breast milk and artificial breast milk (commercial formula) provide about 50% of kilocalories from fat to supply the high energy needs.

BREAST MILK

Human milk is the optimal source of nutrients for infants and contains all the right nutrients to help infants reach their maximum potential (Fig. 13-1). Human milk is very complex, and its exact chemical makeup is unknown. It contains living cells, hormones, active enzymes, and antibodies. Specific protein fractions synthesized in breast tissue help protect against infections by destroying bacteria, viruses, and parasites. Because the infant's immune system is not fully developed, human milk provides distinct advantages over formula. Regardless of the nutritional status of the mother, the overall composition of breast milk is constant.

Breast milk is normally thin with a slightly bluish color. Compared with cow's milk, human milk is high in lactose and relatively low in protein. Breast milk contains substantial amounts of long-chain fatty acids. Arachidonic acid and doxosahexaenoic acid (DHA) are important in development of brain and retinal tissue. Human milk is relatively high in cholesterol. Lipase enzyme inherent in breast milk improves

Table 13-1	Dietary Reference Intakes for Infants Compared with Nutrient Content of Human Breast Milk, Cow's Milk, and Artificial Breast Milk				
	Dietary Reference Intake[a]				Average Artificial
Nutrient	0-6 months old	7-12 months old	Human Breast Milk (per liter)	Cow's Milk[b] (per liter)	Breast Milk (per liter)
Kilocalorie	95/kg (3 mo)*[c]	83/kg[c]	650	670	680
	85/kg (6 mo)*[c]				
Protein	9.1 g/d*	**11 g/d**	11	20	15
Fat	31 g/d*	30 g/d*	40-45	36	36
Cholesterol	ND	ND	100-200	119	10-30
Calcium	210 mg/d*	270 mg/d*	264-210	1220	500
Phosphorus	100 mg/d*	275 mg/d*	121-158	935	300
Iron	0.27 mg/d*	**11 mg/d**	0.35	0.5	12[d]
Sodium	12 g/d	0.27 g/d	6.6	21	10
Potassium	0.4 g/d	0.7 g/d	13	11	20
Renal solute load (mOsm/L)	N/A	N/A	79	221	150

Note: Recommended dietary allowances (RDAs) are presented in bold type, and adequate intakes (AIs) are followed with an asterisk (*).
[a]Data from Institute of Medicine, Food and Nutrition Board: Dietary Reference Intakes for: Vitamin A, Vitamin K, Arsenic, Boron, Chromium, Copper, Iodine, Iron, Manganese, Molybdenum, Nickel, Silicon, Vanadium, and Zinc (2001); Calcium, Phosphorus, Magnesium, Vitamin D, and Fluoride (1997); Energy, Carbohydrate, Fiber, Fat, Fatty Acids, Cholesterol, Protein, and Amino Acids (2002); Water, Potassium, Sodium Chloride, and Sulfate (2004). Washington, DC: National Academies Press.
[b]Whole milk (3.5% fat content).
[c]TEE (total energy expenditure).
[d]Iron fortified.

N/A, Not applicable; *ND*, Not determined.

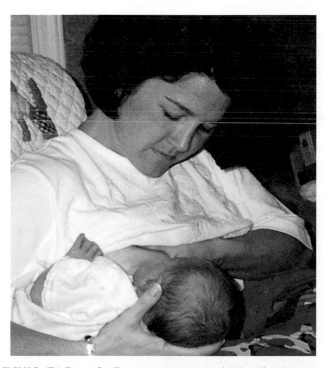

FIGURE 13-1 Breastfeeding promotes a special bonding between mother and infant. (From Lowdermilk DL, Perry SE: Maternity Nursing, 7th ed. St. Louis: Mosby, 2006.)

fat digestion. Results of studies to determine the relationship of early breastfeeding and formula feeding with later lipoprotein levels are conflicting regarding the effect of human milk on development of heart disease.[1]

The low mineral content of human milk is ideal for the infant's immature kidneys. Although the iron content is low, inherent compounds in human milk promote iron use.[2] Iron deficiency in breastfed infants is rare.[3] Because of the high bioavailability of iron, additional sources of iron are unnecessary during the first 4 to 6 months for breastfed infants. Supplemental foods during that time may reduce iron absorption. At 4 to 6 months, iron-rich foods or a daily low-dose oral iron supplement should be initiated.

Breast milk provides about 0.01 mg per day of fluoride regardless of drinking water and maternal plasma levels. Despite the low levels of fluoride breastfed infants receive during this period of life, risk of dental caries does not seem to increase. As shown in Table 13-2, the American Dental Association (ADA) and American Academy of Pediatric Dentistry (AAPD) recommend delaying fluoride supplements for all infants until 6 months of age.

ARTIFICIAL INFANT MILK

Although nutrients differ slightly for various brands, all commercial formulas comply with standards set by the Infant Formula Act established in 1980 (see Table 13-1). The

Table 13-2   Fluoride Supplementation*

Age of Child	Parts per Million (ppm) of Fluoride in Water Supply†		
	<0.3	0.3-0.6	>0.6
Birth–6 mo	0	0	0
6 mo–3 yr	0.25	0	0
3-6 yr	0.50	0.25	0
6-16 yr	1.00	0.50	0

From American Academy of Pediatric Dentistry: Guideline on fluoride therapy. Pediatr Dent 2002 Suppl; 24(7 Suppl):66-67.
*Approved by the American Dental Association, American Academy of Pediatrics, and American Academy of Pediatric Dentistry.
†0.1 part per million (ppm) = 1 mg/L.

U.S. Food and Drug Administration (FDA) requires that these products meet strict standards. Artificial infant milk formulas duplicate breast milk as close as technology allows, but the exact composition of breast milk cannot be duplicated. No artificial infant milk can match the benefits of breast milk. Commercial artificial infant milk formulas are continually being modified to duplicate more closely components of human milk and to meet nutrient needs of various groups of infants. Adequate nutrients are provided in an appropriate caloric concentration (about 20 kcal/oz) for full-term infants. Nonfat cow's milk is the basis for most infant formulas, modified to ensure that the performance of formula-fed infants (i.e., growth, absorption of nutrients, gastrointestinal tolerance, and reactions in blood) matches that of breastfed infants. Infants given artificial infant milk tend to weigh more than breastfed infants, which may put them at greater risk for obesity as adults; however, more research is needed to confirm this association.

Almost all commercial formulas have been modified to contain DHA, which is a natural ingredient of breast milk. Brain growth relative to body weight is highest during the last trimester of a pregnancy. Decreased accumulation of DHA during brain and retinal development results in a variety of behavioral, cognitive, and visual delays, so it is crucial that infants born during the last trimester (premature) receive an infant formula containing DHA (or breast milk).

As established by the guidelines of the American Academy of Pediatrics (AAP), electrolyte, mineral, and vitamin contents are similar (see Table 13-1). Adequate amounts of these nutrients (except for fluoride and iron) are furnished if the infant receives 150 to 180 mL/kg per day of a commercial formula with iron.

Because of increasing cases of fluorosis reported, no fluoride is added to formulas; they contain a small amount of inherent fluoride as a result of some of the ingredients and processing. The ADA, concerned about the risk of fluorosis in infants receiving artificial infant milk, recommend the use of ready-to-feed (RTF) formula, or using fluoride-free water or water that contains minimal levels of fluoride.[4,5] RTF is expensive and requires extra packaging and transportation for distribution. Alternative acceptable waters that contain no or minimal amounts of fluoride—purified, demineralized,

deionized, distilled, or reverse osmosis filtered water[4]—can be regionally produced and are readily available in local stores.

Infant formulas containing probiotics and prebiotics have been developed, which should be beneficial for the gastrointestinal health of infants. Infants receiving these formulas tolerate them well and show a similar rate of weight gain compared with infants fed a conventional formula.[6]

Commercial artificial infant milk is more appropriate for infants than cow's or goat's milk. Malnutrition has been reported in infants fed home-recipe formulas. This may be related to variations in nutrient composition or unsanitary handling practices that may result in frequent infections or gastrointestinal disorders. In other countries, infants become malnourished and die when food manufacturers fail to include required nutrients or prevent contaminants, or when water mixed with the formula was dirty or contaminated.

Many different formulas are available to substitute when an infant does not tolerate a cow's milk protein–based formula. Cow's milk allergy, the most common allergy, affects 2% to 3% of infants and young children.[7] Soy protein–based formulas are the most commonly used substitute, accounting for nearly 25% of the formula market. Studies using soy formulas raise no clinical concerns with respect to nutritional adequacy, sexual development, thyroid disease, immune function, or neurodevelopment.[8] These formulas are not recommended for preterm infants, however, because of their different nutritional requirements.

The most common reason for using soy-based formulas is for relief of perceived formula intolerance (spitting, vomiting, fussiness) or symptoms of colic. Controlled trial studies comparing cow's milk protein–based and soy protein–based formulas have not shown a significant benefit from soy-based formulas in prevention or management of infantile colic, fussiness, or prevention of atopic disease in healthy or high-risk infants.[9] Lactose-free and reduced lactose–containing cow's milk formulas are also available and could be used for circumstances in which elimination or a reduction in lactose is required. Soy protein–based formulas are appropriate for infants with galactosemia and hereditary lactase deficiency and in situations in which a vegetarian diet is preferred. For infants with cow's milk protein allergy, hydrolyzed protein formula should be considered.[10] Numerous specialized formulas are available for infants with special metabolic problems, such as Phenyl-Free (Mead Johnson Nutrition) for phenylketonuria.

Infant formulas should be discontinued at about 1 year of age, and vitamin D–fortified whole milk should be provided until age 2. Low-fat milk is not recommended for children younger than 2 years. Special toddler formulas are nutritionally beneficial and do not need refrigeration, but they are unnecessary.

FEEDING PRACTICES

Contrary to rigid feeding schedules enforced in the past, infants today are generally fed on demand (when they are hungry). A pattern usually develops within about 2 weeks, with the infant eating six times daily at 4-hour intervals. Gradually, a pattern of feeding evolves, allowing the infant and the parents to sleep through the night. Touching helps to strengthen feelings of love, security, and trust, and is as important as the nutrients in the formula. The infant should never be left alone with the bottle propped during feedings.

Oral and Neuromuscular Development

Sucking is more difficult from the breast than from a bottle. Breastfeeding requires the infant to open the mouth wide, move the jaws back and forth, and squeeze with the gingiva to extract the milk, a process called suckling. Suckling encourages maximum development of the genetically defined jaw and chin. Breastfed infants are less likely to develop malocclusion—high premaxilla, abnormal alveolar ridges, and palate and posterior crossbite.[11-13] Infants breastfed for 1 year require 40% less orthodontia than bottle-fed infants.[14] Sucking from a bottle or on a pacifier, thumb, or fingers may result in narrower upper and lower dental arches.[15] **Non-nutritive sucking** (sucking on thumb, fingers, or a pacifier), which begins in utero, is normal. Use of a pacifier does not seem to interfere with successful breastfeeding.[16] Non-nutritive sucking is important in development of self-regulation and the ability to control emotions. However, if it continues too long, problems with tooth alignment and jaw development may occur.

Eating is not instinctive, but is a combination of instinctive behaviors during the first month, followed by primitive motor reflexes and learned behaviors. Eating is the most complex physical task humans do—using all the body's organ systems and requiring the simultaneous coordination of all the sensory systems.

A successful feeding regimen is based on the developmental stage of the infant or child. Nutrition is related to neuromuscular maturation, especially for infants. Suckling is replaced with sucking by 4 months of age, when orofacial muscles are used with the mouth more pursed, and the tongue moving back and forth. This backward movement of the tongue makes the smacking noises that occur. A forward motion of the tongue and dropping the mandible is typical during the first 3 months. If semisolid foods are offered at this time, the tongue forces the food out; no discriminating taste is occurring, just reflex action.

The sucking motion becomes developed enough for the infant to eat and handle semisolid foods from a spoon around 4 to 6 months of age. Development of fine, gross, and oral motor skills to consume foods correlates with the need for additional caloric and nutrient needs. If foods are not added by 6 months of age, growth may decline below normal growth curves.

At about 6 to 8 months old, infants develop the ability to receive food and pass it to the gingiva in a chewing motion. Eight teeth normally erupt between 6 and 12 months of age. When the infant can chew, pureed foods are not required; some variety of texture is mandatory if infants are going to accept unfamiliar foods later in life. Unless textured foods are offered, the development of oral musculature may be slow or delayed, affecting the child's speech.

Introduction of Foods

Good nutrition is essential for rapid growth and development that occurs during an infant's first year. As foods are added to the infant's selections to include most food groups, the timing of the transition, how the infant is fed, and the quality of the foods offered can have important health implications.[17]

An infant's developmental readiness determines which foods should be fed and the texture of foods to be fed. Infants are mature enough to begin eating from a spoon when they are able to hold their necks steady and sit with support, draw in their lower lip as a spoon is removed from the mouth, and retain and swallow food. At 4 to 6 months of age, infants are usually ready to eat solid foods in addition to breast milk or formula. Most commonly, cereals made of rice, oat, or barley are introduced one at a time mixed with breast milk or formula.

Numerous false assumptions are associated with introduction of solid foods. Despite the fact many parents introduce solid foods, especially cereals, during the first month, no nutritional advantage is associated with this practice. The most common reason for early feeding is to help the infant sleep through the night. This naturally occurs between 1 and 3 months of age, with girls typically sleeping through the night earlier than boys. This developmental milestone is not related to what is fed. Foods should be presented to the infant with a spoon, never in a bottle. Disadvantages in starting semisolid foods too early are (1) unnecessary costs, (2) high probability of overfeeding, (3) effects on the immature digestive system, (4) increased risk of food allergies, (5) reduction of milk intake in lieu of a less nutritionally complete food, and (6) decreased iron absorption. After the introduction of foods at 4 to 6 months, formula intake should remain around 32 oz daily.

Fruit juice provides no nutritional benefit for infants younger than 6 months old. To decrease the risk of dental caries, fruit juice should not be given in bottles or sippy cups that allow them to drink easily throughout the day. Too much fruit juice, including apple, pear, and prune, can cause diarrhea, and decreases intake of other foods containing essential nutrients for infants and toddlers. Juices can be diluted with equal amounts of water. Infants receiving breast milk or formula do not need additional water.

As noted in Chapter 12, breastfeeding for at least 4 months helps prevent allergies in infants.[18] Infants are at high risk of developing allergies if they have at least one first-degree relative (parent or sibling) with allergies and are not exclusively breastfed for 4 to 6 months. For these infants, the onset of atopic disease (atopic dermatitis, asthma, food allergy) may be delayed or prevented by using hydrolyzed formulas compared with formula made with intact cow's milk protein.[18] According to the Food Allergy and Anaphylaxis Network, 1 in every 17 children younger than age 3 years has a documented food allergy. Only 2% to 6% of infants have clinically confirmed food hypersensitivity, as opposed to parents reporting a rate of 7% to 14% of infants having adverse reactions to food.[19]

When the infant is 6 months old, 4 to 6 oz of fruit juice diluted with equal portions of water can be introduced in a cup. Solid foods should not be introduced before 4 to 6 months of age. Because of the possibility of a food allergy, only one new food should be introduced at a time. Infant cereal, such as rice cereal, may be introduced at 4 months without an increased likelihood of developing an allergy to wheat.[20] After introducing a new food, a waiting period of 5 to 7 days is recommended before introducing another new food to observe for allergic reactions. Early exposure to some components of foods may increase the risk of allergic disorders in infants. Foods most commonly causing allergies include cow's milk (including ice cream), eggs, peanuts, tree nuts (e.g., walnuts, almonds, cashews, pistachios, pecans), wheat, soy, fish, and shellfish. The recommendation is to wait to introduce these foods until after 12 months of age, eggs at 24 months, and the major allergens (peanuts, tree nuts, and seafood) after the child's third birthday.[21]

The recommended order of introduction for vegetables, meats, and fruits varies among pediatricians. Some advise the introduction of vegetables after cereals, then meats followed by fruits. Meats should be introduced early, especially for breastfed infants to provide essential nutrients, such as iron and zinc.[22,23] Preference for sweet foods is an **innate** (inborn) desire. Because sweet flavors are well accepted, other foods (meats, vegetables) are offered first.

Flavors from the mother's diet are transmitted through amniotic fluid and mother's milk. So a mother's food choices, particularly for fruit and vegetables, influence later preferences and food behaviors.[24] An infant's grimace when offered a new food is innate, not a sign of dislike. When the spoon is offered again, it is very likely to be accepted.[25]

Gradually, junior-type foods with a few lumps are introduced to initiate some chewing. The presence of a few teeth does not mean the infant is ready to masticate foods. Certain vegetables are more difficult to digest and are introduced after 1 year of age—cucumbers, onions, cabbage, and broccoli. Commercial infant food may be used, but foods from the family menu can be pureed for use. The addition of sugar, salt, and other spices to infant foods is not recommended.

When semisolid foods are introduced, the goal should be to include all food groups as soon as possible to ensure a well-balanced diet (Fig. 13-2). Guidelines for feeding infants to provide a balance of nutrients are similar to the *Dietary Guidelines for Americans* except for limiting fat and cholesterol content.

Supplements

Based on the 1997 recommendations of the IOM, breastfed infants need a supplement of 200 IU of vitamin D beginning during the first 2 months to prevent rickets. Several cases of vitamin D deficiency have occurred in the United States in exclusively breastfed infants.[26,27] Vitamin D concentrations do not vary by skin pigmentation or sun sensitivity.[28,29] In 2008, the American Academy of Pediatrics (AAP) recommended increasing intakes, based on more recent research and a history of safe use, of 400 IU per day of vitamin D for exclusively and partially breastfed infants until the infants are weaned and consume ≥1000 mL/day of vitamin D–fortified formula or whole milk. In addition, all non-breastfed infants consuming <1000 m/day of vitamin D–fortified formula or milk should receive a vitamin D supplement of 400 IU daily.[30] Formulas marketed in the United States provide ≥400 IU vitamin D per 1000 mL.[31]

If iron-fortified formula is not used, iron supplementation is recommended for formula-fed infants after 4 months of age, for breastfed infants at 4 to 6 months of age, and for preterm infants after 2 months of age. Iron supplementation (usually ferrous sulfate or ferric ammonium citrate) is ordinarily given as liquid drops. These drops can cause staining on erupting teeth, which can be reduced by putting the drops in water.

Systemically, fluoride supplementation is recommended for infants older than 6 months and children to increase the strength and acid resistance of developing tooth enamel. Before fluoride supplementation is prescribed, however, the AAPD recommends a caries risk assessment along with an evaluation of the dietary sources of fluoride (e.g., fluoridated water).[32] Vitamin supplements containing fluoride may be prescribed by a healthcare provider or dentist (see Table 13-2).

ORAL HEALTH CONCERNS IN EARLY CHILDHOOD

Tooth formation begins before birth and is not completed until about 12 years of age; the structure of the tooth is affected by food intake during this time. A clear relationship

---

🦷 Dental Hygiene Considerations

Assessment
- *Physical*: infant's developmental stage, neuromuscular development, age, lip biting, thumb sucking, tongue thrusting, pacifier use.
- *Dietary*: parent's knowledge of bottle-feeding and feeding solid foods, necessity of providing oral care for the infant, source of iron, fluoride, and use of other supplements.

Interventions
- Avoid recommending sugar-free foods, especially those containing sorbitol. This sugar substitute is a known cause of diarrhea in infants and children. Inform parents that supplements containing fluoride should never be added to milk; fluoride binds with milk and soy proteins, decreasing availability of fluoride significantly.
- Exposure to too much fluoride before enamel maturation may change the structure resulting in fluorosis.
- Nonfluoridated or minimally fluoridated water is recommended for reconstituting powdered formulas to reduce the risk of fluorosis.

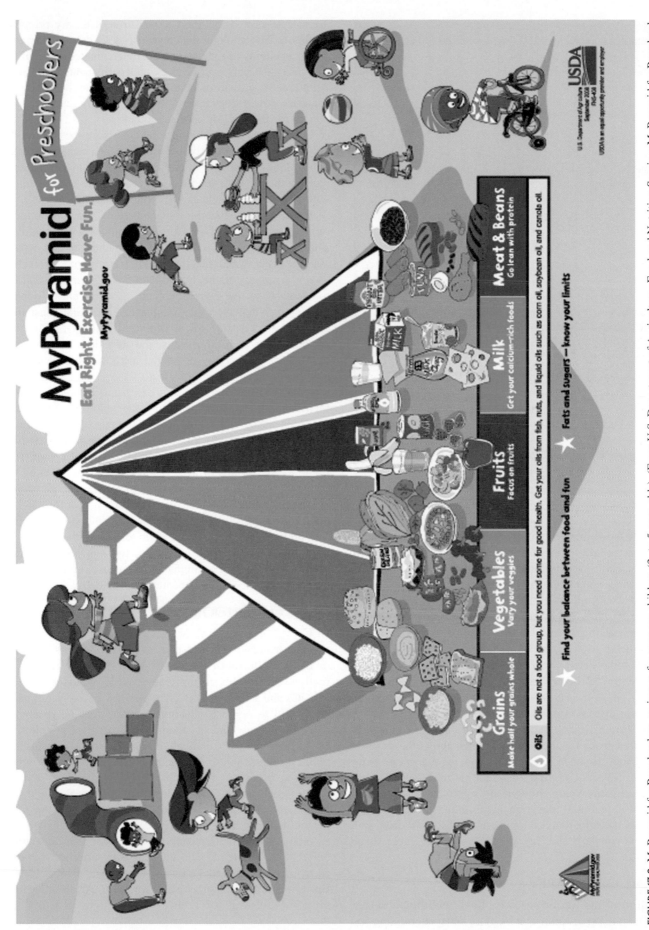

FIGURE 13-2 MyPyramid for Preschoolers, an image for younger children (2- to 5-year-olds). (From U.S. Department of Agriculture, Food and Nutrition Service: MyPyramid for Preschoolers, FNS-408. Washington, D.C.: U.S. Government Printing Office 2008.)

has been shown between nutritional deficiency during tooth development and tooth size, tooth formation, time of tooth eruption, and susceptibility to caries. One occurrence of mild to moderate malnutrition during the first year of life is associated with increased caries in primary and permanent teeth later in life. Calcium and vitamin D must be present for proper calcification of dentin and normal enamel. Vitamin D is crucial to tooth development; later deficiency can promote tooth decay.

Based on *National Health and Nutrition Examination Surveys* (NHANES) (1988-2004) data, 12% of children 6 to 11 years old from families with incomes below the federal poverty line had untreated tooth decay compared with 4% of children from families with incomes above the poverty line.[33] Tooth decay in primary teeth increased among children 2 to 5 years old from 24% in 1994 to 28% in 2004.[33] Dental caries in young children are significantly associated with lower parental education level, living at the poverty level, no breastfeeding, skipping breakfast, low fruit and vegetable intake, and no dental visit for more than 1 year.[34]

INFANT ORAL CARE

Dental problems can begin early. **Early childhood caries (ECC)** is the presence of one or more decayed, missing (as a result of caries), or filled tooth surfaces in any primary tooth in a child younger than 6 years old. Children who have caries as infants or toddlers have a much greater probability of subsequent caries in primary and permanent dentitions. Additionally, growth of infants with ECC may be inhibited because of pain associated with eating. Baby teeth are the pattern for the bite for permanent teeth.

Good dental care starts in infancy, before the first tooth emerges. Decay and early loss can damage permanent teeth before they erupt. The infant's gingiva should be cleaned daily with gauze, or a soft infant toothbrush and water, or with an infant tooth cleaner to remove plaque biofilm.

When teeth begin coming in, parents should continue brushing the teeth with a soft infant toothbrush using a fluoride-free toothpaste. The AAPD recommends the first dental visit to occur when the first tooth has erupted, typically around 6 months of age, but no later than 1 year. The earlier the dental visit, the better the chances of preventing dental problems. When the child is able to expectorate (usually around 2 to 3 years old), a pea-sized amount of fluoride toothpaste can be used. Because the child does not have the dexterity to thoroughly brush the teeth, the parent should continue brushing the child's teeth.

After the first baby teeth begin to erupt, at-will nighttime breastfeeding should be avoided. Older infants and toddlers should never be given a bottle or sippy cup of milk or juice in bed. If the infant is given a bottle in the bed, it should contain only water. Children should be weaned from the bottle by 14 months of age. When children are allowed to take the bottle longer, numerous problems can develop, including speech problems, tooth erosion and deformation, and difficulty in weaning.

Children should be offered a cup as soon as they can hold it in their hands. Between meals, the sippy cup should contain water only. Prolonged use of sugary drinks in sippy cups is a leading cause of pediatric tooth decay.

EARLY CHILDHOOD CARIES

ECC is a leading oral health problem among children younger than age 3; it is also known as nursing bottle caries or **baby bottle tooth decay (BBTD)**. ECC, the term currently used, replaces the terms severe early childhood caries (SECC) and BBTD and is characterized by early rampant decay and associated with inappropriate feeding practices (Fig. 13-3). Any sign of smooth surface caries in children younger than age 3 is indicative of ECC, which is a serious public health problem especially prevalent in lower socioeconomic groups.

Children with ECC weigh less than their ideal weight for height, and their weight for age is frequently below the 10th percentile. Treatment of ECC is costly, requiring extensive extractions or restorations or both, and causing serious future oral health problems and unnecessary suffering. Severe cases are treated under general anesthesia in a hospital. Because it is preventable, healthcare professionals and caregivers need to watch for early warning signs to detect the disease.

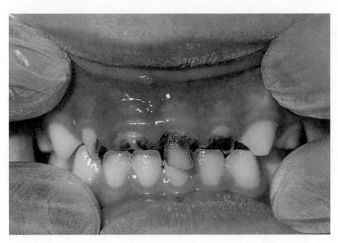

FIGURE 13-3 Early childhood caries. (From Swartz MH: Textbook of Physical Diagnosis, History, and Examination, 5th ed. Philadelphia: Saunders, 2006.)

Box 13-1 Sources of Fermentable Carbohydrates for Infants

Liquids
- Cow's milk, plain and flavored
- Breast milk
- Artificial infant milk
- Unsweetened fruit juice
- Sweetened fruit juice and fruit drinks
- Syrup added to water
- Sweetened soft drinks
- Sodas
- Any sugar-sweetened beverages

Other Sources
- Some infant foods
- Medication
- Use of sweets to comfort or reward infant, or relieve constipation such as a pacifier dipped in honey or corn syrup
- Infant cereals, teething biscuits, crackers
- Dry cereals
- Arrowroot biscuits and other cookies, pretzels
- Fruits

Contributing Factors

The primary contributing factor to ECC is infection with *Streptococcus mutans* (cariogenic bacterium). Colonization of *S. mutans* occurs only after the infant's teeth erupt. Infection with *S. mutans* occurs through transmission of the pathogen from the caregiver to the infant. Kissing and sharing utensils or other objects contaminated with saliva are contributing factors. The infant is more likely to be infected if the caregiver has a high level of *S. mutans*. The addition of frequent or prolonged exposure to a fermentable carbohydrate inoculates *S. mutans*. Destruction of the tooth surface begins and can progress ultimately to rampant caries and abscesses.

Dental caries occur when a sweetened liquid (including milk or juice) pools around the lingual surfaces of the teeth for extended periods (Box 13-1) in the presence of caries-producing bacteria in plaque biofilm. The acid produced by bacteria leads to demineralization of enamel. Allowing the infant to go to bed at night or at naptime with a bottle and frequent daytime bottles or habitual use of a no-spill training cup all are factors related to ECC. Excessive breastfeeding, particularly when the infant sleeps with the mother and nurses as desired throughout the night, also can result in ECC.

As the child sleeps, the cleansing action of saliva is diminished because of reduced salivary flow. The ultimate effect is poor clearance of the liquid. Also, the natural or artificial nipple rests on the palate during sucking, allowing the liquid to pool around the maxillary incisors. The position of the tongue covers and protects the mandibular incisors. Because the disease state follows the eruption pattern, the maxillary incisors are affected, followed by the first molars, and then the canines.

Counseling

Parents must understand their role in preventing dental disease in their children. Begin dietary counseling as soon as the dental team is apprised of the pregnancy. During the initial visit with the child, an assessment can be made to determine the level of fluoride intake and risk of oral problems. Recommendations to parents about controlling oral bacteria and appropriate infant and preschool feeding practices are important. Obtain diet histories of both parents, especially focusing on the primary caregiver to reveal cariogenic eating patterns that may be transferred to the infant. An analysis of the frequency of fermentable carbohydrate intake and oral hygiene habits can be instrumental in creating an awareness of potential problems for the parent (see Chapter 17). Intercepting and modifying damaging health practices before birth can prevent SECC and possibly the development of rampant caries later.

CLEFT PALATE AND CLEFT LIP

One of the most common birth defects in the United States is **cleft lip** or **cleft palate**, or cleft lip/palate, a malformation in which parts of the upper lip or palate fail to grow together. Approximately 1 of 1000 infants is born with cleft lip with or without cleft palate.[35] Scientists believe numerous factors, including drugs, heredity, and nutrient deficiencies (i.e., folic acid), may cause this malformation.

The main priority is to ensure adequate nutrition. Feeding the infant with a cleft palate, with or without a cleft lip, presents unique problems. The length of time needed for feedings to provide adequate nutrients can be exhaustive for the mother and infant. Because of the opening between the roof of the mouth and the floor of the nasal cavity, negative pressure needed for sucking cannot be created (Fig. 13-4). However, breastfeeding sometimes can be successful; the infant adapts by squeezing or chewing the nipple.

Special feeding devices are available if necessary. These are recommended when more than 1 hour is required per

Dental Hygiene Considerations

Assessment

- *Physical*: cursory oral examination to detect decalcification or carious lesions in the teeth; frequency of daily cleaning; destructive habits such as lip biting, thumb sucking, tongue thrusting, or pacifier use.
- *Dietary*: parental knowledge of SECC and what causes it; parental preferences for sweets; sharing of utensils contaminated with saliva; use of bottle propping, especially at night, or continual availability of a sippy cup throughout the day; use of corn syrup in the bottle; dipping the bottle nipple or pacifier in honey or molasses; continued use of the bottle after age 1; and appropriate fluoride consumption.

Interventions

- Recommend routine dental visits, and provide guidance to the parents on feeding practices and nutritional needs.
- Teach parents to clean the infant's gingiva after feedings with a clean cloth. A soft infant toothbrush and water can be used when the infant has several teeth.
- If the water supply is optimally fluoridated, discuss use of a pea-sized amount of toothpaste and avoidance of fluoride-containing dentifrices until the child learns to expectorate.
- If a fluoride supplement is recommended, the tablets should be thoroughly chewed and swished between the teeth before swallowing. The child should not eat or drink for 30 minutes after taking the supplement and should avoid milk products for 1 hour because calcium may interfere with the bioavailability of fluoride.
- Wean the child from the bottle at about 12 months of age or fill the bottle with water.
- Educate all expectant parents and parents of infants about techniques for avoiding ECC: when feeding an infant, hold the infant and bottle; avoid bottle propping or using the bottle or sippy cup as a pacifier at bedtime or throughout the day. Use other methods instead of a bottle at bedtime and naptime to quiet and relax the child, such as rubbing the child's back, rocking in a chair, singing to the child, or providing a stuffed toy.
- Parents should be counseled to avoid saliva sharing practices, such as sharing a spoon when tasting food, to prevent transmission of caries-causing bacteria (*S. mutans*) to the infant.
- Educate parents about ECC when (1) carious lesions are initially noted in a young child, (2) either parent has active caries or dentures, or (3) sweets are used to comfort or reward the infant.
- Explain the importance of primary teeth (appearance, speech, ability to eat). Patients may be under the false impression that because primary teeth fall out anyway, they serve no purpose.

Nutritional Directions

- Do not let the infant suck the bottle unattended.
- Discuss the role of carbohydrates, including those present in milk and fruit juice, in the decay process. Do not put fruit juice or other carbohydrate-containing beverages in a bottle. Offer juice in a cup.
- Describe disadvantages of rampant decay in an infant (discomfort, future dental phobia, infection, cost, tongue-thrust habit).
- Limit the child's access to a sippy cup containing milk or juice.
- Home filtration systems may remove fluoride, so tests should be conducted to measure fluoride content of filtered and treated water. Most state health departments assess the fluoride content of the water for a minimal fee.
- During the first year, foods that require chewing should be added based on the number of erupted teeth.
- Wean the infant from the bottle soon after the first birthday.

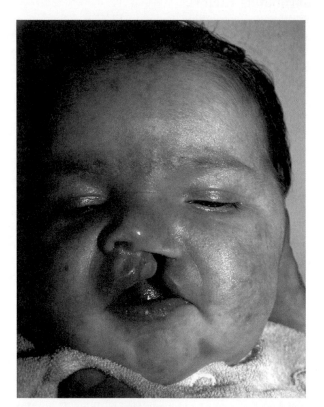

FIGURE 13-4 Cleft lip/palate. (From Kaban L, Troulis M: Pediatric Oral and Maxillofacial Surgery. Philadelphia: Saunders, 2004.)

feeding. The infant is held in a sitting position to prevent formula from entering the nose. Other feeding difficulties include nasal regurgitation, excessive air intake, and frequent burping. As soon as possible, spoon feeding is introduced. In severe cases, a prosthesis is made when the child is older (Fig. 13-5). Patience is required, and extra time for feeding must be allowed to provide needed nutrients.

Infants born with cleft palates are at high risk of developmental delays, including motor skill delays. They also have increased rates of dental abnormalities, including supernumerary, missing, or malformed teeth.

DIETARY RECOMMENDATIONS AND GUIDELINES FOR GROWTH (CHILDREN OLDER THAN 2 YEARS)

MyPyramid has introduced a website for preschoolers (www.mypyramid.gov/preschoolers/index.html) to help

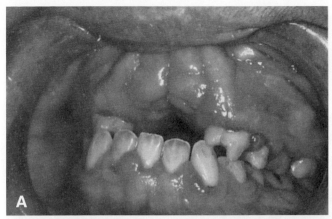

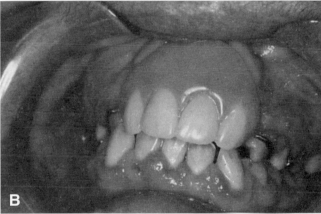

FIGURE 13-5 A, Cleft palate. **B,** Cleft palate with removable prosthesis. (Courtesy of Kathleen B. Muzzin, The Texas A&M University System, Baylor College of Dentistry, Dallas, TX.)

Box 13-2 Suggestions for Feeding an Infant with Cleft Palate

- The infant should consume a specific amount in a feeding that takes no more than 30 minutes.
- Enlarge the hole in the bottle's nipple or use a special feeding device that enables the infant to get milk more easily.
- Boil new nipples before use to soften them.
- Mix pureed foods (fruits, vegetables, meats) with milk or broth for a thinner consistency so that they may be fed from a bottle with an enlarged hole in the nipple.
- Burp frequently to aid in releasing excessive air intake.
- To prevent regurgitation, teach an older child to eat slowly and to take small bites.
- Some children take liquids more easily by using a straw.
- Feeding a child with cleft palate takes longer than feeding a normal child; the mother needs to allow the necessary time. Fatigue on the part of the parent may interfere with the child's receiving adequate nourishment.
- Use saline drops before and after feeding to help clear any food or liquid that is in the nasal passage secondary to the cleft palate.

Nutritional Directions

- Introduce spoon feeding as soon as possible.
- Oral skills develop after surgery to correct the problem.
- Acidic and spicy foods may irritate the delicate tissue in the cleft area.
- Young children with cleft palate are at increased risk for choking on foods that may slip into the trachea.
- Because of the increased incidence of enamel hypoplasia, encourage meticulous oral hygiene practices and limited cariogenic food or liquids to avoid carious lesions at these sites.
- Refer parents to the American Cleft Palate Association for literature and to local support groups.

---

with healthy food choices and an active, healthy lifestyle. MyPyramid Plan creates a customized plan for a child 2 to 5 years of age. It is designed to help mothers help young children (1) grow up healthy, (2) develop healthy eating habits, (3) try new foods, (4) play actively every day, and (5) follow food safety rules. It provides sample meal patterns and snacks, and kitchen and physical activities for preschoolers. Parents can complete a growth chart for the child.

Dental Hygiene Considerations

Assessment
- *Physical*: cleft palate/lip, aspiration.
- *Dietary*: feeding technique and past experiences in feeding infants.

Interventions
- Explain the principal problem is a lack of normal suction, and by modifying feeding techniques, the infant can obtain adequate nutrients.
- Feed the infant slowly at a 60- to 80-degree angle, following the guidelines in Box 13-2 to provide nutrients while minimizing risks.
- After repair, recommend foods requiring the patient to use the tongue and muscles for mastication.

This tool should be very helpful for parents, helping them to instill healthy eating habits when they are the most important influential factor on the child's future food choices.

MyPyramid for Kids (Fig. 13-6) provides age-appropriate information for 6- to 11-year-old children based on the *Dietary Guidelines for Americans 2005*. These pyramids (see Figs. 13-2 and 13-6) promote messages similar to the adult version of MyPyramid. The key message of MyPyramid (variety, moderation, and balance in food choices) applies to childhood nutrition. MyPyramid for Kids (http://www.mypyramid.gov/kids/index.html) represents the recommended proportion of food from each food group and focuses on the importance of making consistent smart food choices. MyPyramid for Kids packs a powerful message with the slogan "Eat Healthy, Exercise, Have Fun."

The website has links to a coloring page, worksheet, and classroom materials for teachers. The Web-based MyPyramid for Kids contains an interactive spaceship-themed game, "MyPyramid Blast Off." Concrete examples are provided on how to choose the right foods from each

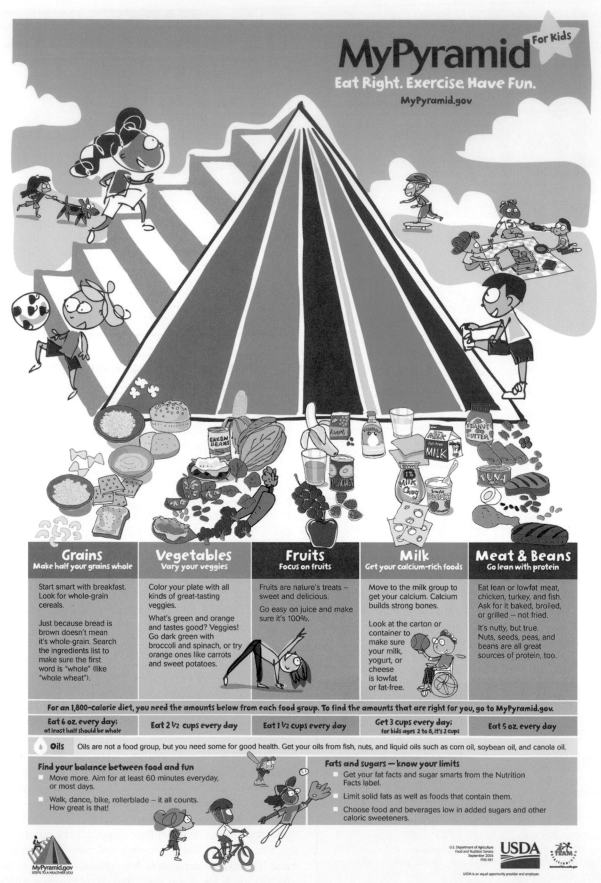

FIGURE 13-6 MyPyramid for Kids, a detailed image for older children (6-to 11-year-olds). (From the US Department of Agriculture, Food an Nutrition Service: MyPyramid for Kids, FNS-381, Washington, DC: US Goverment Printing Office, 2005.)

food group for "lift off." It is a fun way for children to learn about their nutritional needs, and the child must stay engaged in the activity for at least 1 hour to provide the space shuttle that is part of the game with adequate battery power for launching. MyPyramid for Kids was developed to help parents influence their children to make wise food choices.

The main concern with providing dietary recommendations and guidelines for children older than 2 years is to (1) provide adequate kilocalories and nutrients to support growth and development, and (2) reduce the risk of diet-related chronic diseases later in life (Box 13-3). Prepubescent children burn more fat per kilocalorie of energy expended than adults and need fat to fuel growth.[36] Scientific studies have determined that energy and nutrient needs of most children can be met with limited fat intake.

After many studies and much deliberation, the AAP Committee on Nutrition recommends that children older than 2 years gradually adopt a diet consistent with the *Dietary Guidelines for Americans* in regard to fats and cholesterol by age 5. The basic reasoning for implementing the Dietary Guidelines for fat and cholesterol is based on the assumption that childhood obesity and cholesterol levels will continue into adulthood. Fat intake in children should be maintained at a moderate level (25% to 35% of kilocalories) to ensure growth to their genetic potential. Children older than 2 years should consume fat-free or low-fat milk

or equivalent milk products. The average percentage of energy from total fat and saturated fat decreased from 1971 to 2000, but only about 38% of the population 2 years and older met the guideline of 30% or less of energy from total fat, and 41% met the guideline of 10% or less of energy from saturated fat.[37]

A revised policy statement from the AAP recommends screening children 2 to 10 years old who have a genetic predisposition for heart disease, or who have other risk factors for cardiovascular disease (CVD), such as obesity, hypertension, and diabetes mellitus.[38] The statement reinforces that all children older than 2 years should follow the *Dietary Guidelines for Americans* and make lifestyle changes, such as increasing physical activity, and in extremely high-risk cases, taking lipid-lowering medications. Most children with abnormal cholesterol levels should be treated with diet and exercise; a few with very high levels of LDL, the "bad" cholesterol, should consider drug treatment, especially if other risk factors are present. Although there are no studies showing long-term safety or effectiveness of the use of nutritional modifications, lifestyle changes, or use of medications in preventing the development of CVD, the safety and efficacy of these modifications seem similar to effects in adults.

Dietary modifications are similar to those recommended for adults (see Chapter 5). However, these dietary adjustments may require involvement of a dietitian to help families make appropriate changes without compromising good nutrition. When parents have implemented very-low-fat diets without supervision, nutritional insufficiency and failure to thrive have occurred.[39] Children can learn how to read food labels and determine which food choices are wise selections. The entire family usually benefits from implementing these guidelines.

Parents should encourage individual physical activities and model them for the children (Fig. 13-7). The energy needs of children and adolescents are high to support growth and development, and energy expenditure must be in balance with the child's physical activity level (Table 13-3). Childhood obesity in the United States is increasing (see Health Application 13). The energy requirement for children can be affected by physical activity levels or other genetic and environmental factors.

Physical activity is evidenced on MyPyramid for Kids by displaying children participating in various activities. The need for physical activity, which is important for bone mineralization, growth, and cardiovascular health, is promoted. MyPyramid for Kids recommends 1 hour of physical activity over the course of the day. The 2008 Physical Activity Guidelines for Americans recommended by USDHHS advocates 1 hour or more of physical activity for children and adolescents. Most of the 60 or more minutes a day should be either moderate- or vigorous-intensity aerobic physical activity and should include vigorous-intensity physical activity at least 3 days a week. Part of the 60 or more minutes of daily physical activity should include muscle-strengthening physical activity at least 3 days a week. Part

---

Box 13-3	**Acceptable Macronutrient Distribution Ranges**

Acceptable macronutrient distribution ranges (AMDRs) as a percent of energy intake for carbohydrates, fat, and protein are as follows:

Carbohydrates—45% to 65% of total calories

Fat—30% to 40% of energy for 1 to 3 years, and 25% to 35% of energy for 4 to 18 years

Protein—5% to 20% for young children, and 10% to 30% for older children

Added sugars should not exceed 25% of total calories (to ensure sufficient intake of essential micronutrients). This is a maximum suggested intake and not the amount recommended for achieving a healthful diet.

Consumption of saturated fat, *trans* fatty acids, and cholesterol should be as low as possible, while maintaining a nutritionally adequate diet.

Adequate intake for total fiber is as follows:

Children 1 to 3 years: 19 g total fiber per day

Children 4 to 8 years: 25 g per day

Boys 9 to 13 years: 31 g per day

Girls 9 to 13 years: 26 g per day

Data adapted from A Report of the Panel on Macronutrients, Subcommittees on Upper Reference Levels of Nutrients and Interpretation and Uses of Dietary Reference Intakes, and the Standing Committee on the Scientific Evaluation of Dietary Reference Intakes; Food and Nutrition Board; and Institute or Medicine: Dietary Reference Intakes for Energy, Carbohydrate, Fiber, Fat, Fatty Acids, Cholesterol, Protein, and Amino Acids. Washington, DC: The National Academies Press, 2005, p 1357. From Position of the American Dietetic Association: Nutrition guidance for healthy children ages 2 to 11 years. J Am Diet Assoc 2008 Jun; 108(6):1038-1047.

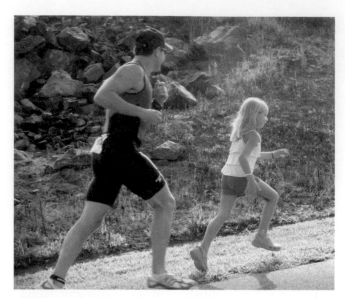

FIGURE 13-7 Parents should encourage individual physical activities and model these behaviors. (Photo courtesy of Sara Birkemeier, Raleigh, NC.)

Table 13-3	Daily Estimated Calories and Recommended Servings* for Children,† by Age and Sex		
	2-3 years old	**4-8 years old**	**9-13 years old**
Calories‡ (kcal)	1000		
Female		1200	1600
Male		1400	1800
Milk/dairy (cup)	2	2	3
Lean meat/beans (oz)	2	5	
Female			3
Male			4
Fruits§ (cup)	1	1.5	1.5
Vegetables§ (cup)	1		
Female		1	2
Male		1.5	2.5
Grains (oz)	3		
Female		4	5
Male		5	6
Oils (g)	14	17-18	20-22
Discretionary	154	163-173	181-190

From Position of the American Dietetic Association: Nutrition guidance for healthy children ages 2 to 11 years. J Am Diet Assoc 2008 Jun; 108(6):1038-1047.
*Nutrient and energy contributions from each group are calculated according to the nutrient-dense forms of food in each group (e.g., lean meats, fat-free milk, low-fat dairy products, and fruits/vegetables with no added fats or sugars).
†Adapted from Tables D1-1 and D1-13, Report of Dietary Guidelines for Americans Committee (2005). Available at www.health.gov/dietaryguidelines/dga2005/report/.
‡Calorie estimates are based on a sedentary lifestyle. Increased physical activity would require additional calories: by 0-200 kcal/d if moderately physically active and by 200-400 kcal/d if very physically active.
§For fruits and vegetables, serving sizes are ⅓ cup for 2-3 years of age, and ½ cup for 4 years of age. A variety of vegetables should be selected from the vegetable subgroups (dark green, deep yellow, legumes, and starchy) during the week.
¶Half of all grains should be whole grains.

of the 60 or more minutes of daily physical activity should include bone-strengthening physical activity at least 3 days a week.[40]

Children should be given the opportunity to participate in a variety of activities, from walking to jumping rope to competitive sports. In reality, children will not be physically active unless they are having fun. Activity is important in helping control weight, and reducing the risk for heart attack, colon cancer, diabetes, and high blood pressure.

MyPyramid for Kids adjusts portion sizes based on children's smaller size and physiological needs, and the number of servings from the bread-cereal group differs (see Table 13-3). Research indicates preschool children do not adjust the amount they eat in response to how much they ate at the previous meal or in the past 24 hours, or the caloric density of their meal.

The most powerful predictor for how much children eat is how much food is put on their plate.[41] One of the keys to the cause and prevention of overweight is knowledge of the caregiver. When parents assume control of food portions or coerce the child to eat rather than allowing him or her to focus on internal cues of hunger, the child's ability to regulate meal size is diminished. Large portion sizes of snack and fast foods parallel dramatic increases in childhood obesity.[42] Family mealtime is essential for children's nutrition, health, and overall well-being. Portion sizes and numbers of servings increase when the child reaches puberty and needs are greater because of accelerated growth rate and increased size, but one of the principal concerns is an inappropriate increase in portion sizes contributing to the prevalence of overweight.

Several organizations have endorsed the recommendation that a reasonable goal for dietary fiber intake during childhood and adolescence is approximately equivalent to the age of the child plus 5 g per day. This formula (age + 5) represents a level that would provide health benefits, such

as normal laxation, without compromising mineral balance or caloric intake in children older than 2 years of age. Based on this formula, minimal dietary fiber intake would be 8 g per day for a 3-year-old, and would gradually increase to 20 g per day for a 15-year-old. The gradual increases are consistent with current guidelines for adult dietary fiber intake (25 to 35 g per day). Average dietary fiber intake among children 3 to 5 years old and 6 to 11 years old is 11.4 g per day and 13.1 g per day.[37]

The *Dietary Guidelines for Americans* and Food Guide Pyramid promote increasing fruit and vegetable consumption to five or more servings daily. Students who eat an adequate amount of fruit, vegetables, protein, fiber, and other components of a healthy diet are more likely to perform better in school.[43] Fresh fruits are preferred over fruit juice—only 4 to 6 oz daily of a vitamin C–rich juice is recommended for children 1 to 5 years old; 8 to 12 oz is recommended for 6- to 12-year-olds. By using whole-grain breads and cereals, as recommended in the Dietary Guidelines, fiber and other nutrient requirements can be met. At least half of the grain servings should be whole grains.

Because of the high calcium requirement to increase bone mineral density in children, milk and dairy products are an essential part of the child's diet. Calcium levels were established to decrease the risk of osteoporosis later in life. Inadequate amounts of calcium and vitamin D during the toddler years, however, could cause rickets as infants are weaned to diets with minimal dairy content. Three servings a day of milk or dairy products are recommended for children, and four servings are recommended for adolescents. In a longitudinal study, children who consumed at least recommended amounts of milk products throughout childhood along with adequate amounts of meats and other protein-containing foods had higher levels of bone mineral content at adolescence.[44] Calcium intake can be favorably increased by using calcium-fortified beverages, such as orange juice with calcium. Between 1977-2001, daily milk consumption decreased from 3.56 servings to 2.75 servings in 2- to 18-year-olds.[37] At the same time, energy intake from sweetened beverages increased.

It is a general consensus most children's diets "need improvement" or are "poor."[37] Nutrients most likely to be consumed in amounts low enough to be of concern include vitamins D and E, calcium, magnesium, potassium, and fiber.[37,45,46] Intake of these and other nutrients may be affected when fats are reduced if milk and meat products are curtailed. However, some studies have reported increased vitamin and nutrient density in the diet with decreased fat intake. By using skim milk instead of reduced-fat or whole milk, lean meats in place of higher fat meats, or lower fat products rather than high-fat products, nutrient requirements can be achieved. Children's diets containing adequate energy and 25% to 35% of total energy from fat have positive effects on health later in life.

TODDLER AND PRESCHOOL CHILDREN

GROWTH

After the child reaches 1 year of age, the growth spurt slows down. The toddler gains approximately 4 to 6 lb until 2 years old, and height doubles by age 4. In a normally growing child, height increases parallel that of weight. Children grow approximately 2 to 3 inches a year and gain around 5 lb a year. One-half of adult height is achieved by 2½ to 3 years of age.

NUTRIENT REQUIREMENTS

Poor nutritional status of children (as measured by growth rate and biochemical indices) is generally more prevalent in lower socioeconomic groups, in which the amounts and variety of foods may be limited. Approximately 10% of all children, regardless of socioeconomic background, may be iron deficient. Iron deficiency during infancy results in lower cognitive abilities and motor skills that continue throughout childhood and adolescence. Zinc, calcium, and vitamin D also are frequently deficient in the diet. During the past 30 years, the nutritional status of children in the United States has improved, with few nutrient deficiencies being observed. As mentioned earlier, research studies note that ensuring vitamin D sufficiency throughout childhood and during the time of maximal bone mineral accrual seems particularly warranted.[47] Therefore the AAP recommends doubling vitamin D intake by children to 400 IU per day.[30,48] Depending on vitamin D intake, a supplement may be needed.

Although most children fail to meet MyPyramid recommendations (especially in the fruit, grain, and dairy groups), average intake of most vitamins and minerals in 2- to 11-year-olds exceeds 100% of the RDA. However, overweight is becoming pandemic. By striving toward healthy eating and physical activity patterns, people may achieve healthful weights, which may prevent lifetime risks of chronic health problems (see Health Application 13).

Because of high activity level, basal metabolic rate, and growth, the caloric requirement is relatively high, roughly 1000 kcal plus 100 kcal per year of life. Younger children need to eat foods with high nutrient and energy density because they are unable to eat large quantities of food at any particular time. Healthy snacks can contribute vital nutrients. The extra nutrient needs for growth and development result in dietary deficiencies occurring more quickly and with more severe consequences than in adults. The dietary reference intakes (DRIs) for major nutrients are listed in Table 13-4.

Table 13-4 Dietary Reference Intakes for Selected Nutrients for Children through Adolescence

Nutrients	Children 1-3 years old	Children 4-8 years old	9-13 years old		14-18 years old	
			Boys	Girls	Boys	Girls
Protein (g)	13	19	34	34	52	46
Vitamin C (mg)	15	25	45	45	75	65
Calcium (mg)	500*	800*	1300*	1300*	1300*	1300*
Iron (mg)	7	10	8	8	11	15
Total fiber (g)	19*	25*	31*	26*	38*	26*

Data from Institute of Medicine, Food and Nutrition Board: Dietary Reference Intakes for: (1) Vitamin C, Vitamin E, Selenium, and Carotenoids (2000); (2) Calcium, Phosphorus, Magnesium, Vitamin D, and Fluoride (1997); (3) Vitamin A, Vitamin K, Arsenic, Boron, Chromium, Copper, Iodine, Iron, Manganese, Molybdenum, Nickel, Silicon, Vanadium, and Zinc (2001); (4) Carbohydrates, Fats, Protein, Fiber, and Physical Activity, Parts 1 and 2 (2002). Washington, DC: National Academies Press.
Note: Recommended dietary allowances (RDAs) are presented in bold type and adequate intakes (AIs) are followed with an asterisk (*).

FOOD-RELATED BEHAVIORS

Lifelong habits and food attitudes are formed during pre-school years that to some extent affect health throughout life. A variety of foods should be available providing the needed nutrients. A basic understanding of the nutrient content of foods, the role of foods in health, and food-related behaviors for these age groups is important for parents to promote food habits conducive to adequate nutrient intake (see Box 13-4). Healthful eating produces benefits in cogni-tive and physical performance, fitness, psychological aspects, physical sensation, and energy level.

Parental attitudes and food preferences, eating habits, and food choices are influential factors in the child's food prefer-ences. Foods disliked by one or both parents are not served often or may not be served at all. Additionally, children model their parents and tend to enjoy foods preferred by their parents. Providing fruits for snacks and serving vege-tables at mealtime affect a preschooler's eating patterns for life.[49]

When planning menus, parents must consider the child's food preferences, but parents can control the options. Without appropriate guidance, young children do not independently make healthy food choices; the parents' role is to offer nutri-tious foods. Children can choose how much or even whether they will eat the food that has been provided. Feeding prob-lems can result when either the parent or the child crosses this line of responsibility. The best predictor of a child's ability to regulate energy intake is parental control of feeding. More food is eaten by the child when the family eats together, rather than just offering food for the child to eat alone.

Toddlers (1 to 3 Years Old)

During the second year of life, development of fine motor skills results in toddlers learning to feed themselves, but skills and capabilities do not occur at exactly the same time for every child. Although this is a messy learning process, this transitional period stabilizes by age 2. Finger feeding may be preferred to spoon feeding; some finger foods should be provided at every meal. A toddler can manipulate a cup by about 18 months of age. Rotary chewing skills develop in the second year. Until then, finely chopped meats are accepted better and minimize the risk of choking.

Toddlers prefer regularity, so eating at the same time is desirable and helps control appetite. Regular meals also help to avoid fatigue, which can lead to an overly emotional situ-ation that interferes with appetite. Tired children eat poorly. If the child has been very active, a short rest period before the meal improves intake.

Small amounts of food should be offered several times a day. Serving sizes should be based on appetite, but initially about 1 Tbsp can be offered for each year of age. Studies show that providing larger than age-appropriate portion sizes may result in children consuming more food and kilo-calories, and they do not compensate for this by decreasing intake of other foods.[50] When children serve themselves from family-size bowls, they choose smaller portions and are less likely to overeat. Brightly colored foods are espe-cially appealing to children. Children older than $1\frac{1}{2}$ years of age who are still taking a bottle containing milk or sweet-ened liquids are more likely than others to be overweight and to have anemia because of low iron intake, in addition to increasing the risk of tooth decay.

Anemia remains a public health concern among young (less than 2 years old) low-income children.[51] The incidence of anemia usually declines with age and is observed consis-tently more often in African-American children than in white, Asian, Native American, or Hispanic children. Iron-rich foods, such as meat, and fresh fruits and vegetables that contain vitamin C, which enhances iron absorption, are expensive compared with calorically dense foods such as chips or candy.

The amount of liquid consumed can affect the child's appetite. Either the child has a poor appetite for foods or consumes more food in addition to the kilocalories provided in the bottles, which can increase the risk of obesity. Milk is a poor source of iron, and large amounts of milk deter absorption of iron.

Food jags—refusing to eat anything except one food for several days—in toddlers and children are common and are a way to assert independence. This typical developmental stage is temporary. The food obsession may cause parental concern, but overreaction may prolong rather than correct such behaviors. Refusing to eat is a way to attract attention. Appetites, which are erratic and unpredictable, are a strong reflection of the current growth rate. Parents should not force children to eat when they are not hungry. When well-bal-anced meals are provided, caloric intake at any given meal varies greatly, but compensation at subsequent meals results in little variability in total energy intake. If sufficient amounts are not eaten at the meal, parents may limit snacking or provide nutrient-dense snacks. Snacks can contribute sig-nificantly to adequate nutrient intake (Box 13-4).

Box 13-4	Healthy Snack Choices

- Cut-up fresh vegetables with low-fat dip or salad dressing
- Air-popped popcorn with a sprinkle of Parmesan cheese
- Fresh fruit*
- Frozen fruit (grapes, bananas)
- Nuts
- Low-fat cheese (sticks, strings, cubes, or slices)
- Low-fat cottage cheese or yogurt
- Peanut butter* on apple slices or celery sticks
- Pretzels*
- Baked chips*
- Hard-boiled eggs
- Animal crackers*
- Graham crackers*
- Sliced turkey or chicken
- Dry, low-sugar cereal*
- Rice cakes*
- Low-fat pudding*
- Sugar-free gelatin with fruit
- Mini bagels*
- Pickles
- Frozen juice bars*

*Cariogenic potential. Encourage tooth-brushing after snacks.

Until age 4, children are at risk for choking on food that gets caught in the airway. Food is not chewed thoroughly until the molars erupt. To prevent choking, children should be closely supervised while eating, and should not be allowed to eat while walking, playing, talking, laughing, crying, or lying down. Additionally, foods most likely to cause choking should be avoided: (1) small nuts and seeds; (2) round, firm, smooth foods such as grapes, hard candy, hot dogs, and round candies; (3) dry or hard foods such as raw carrots, cookies, pieces of pretzels, potato chips, and popcorn; and (4) sticky or tough foods such as peanut butter, raisins, tough meat, and caramel candy.

Preschool Children (4 to 6 Years Old)

Preschoolers are relatively independent at the table and can feed themselves. Certain factors need to be considered to make the mealtime pleasant rather than an ordeal. By allowing children to eat with adults, they imitate adults in manners and food habits. Parental insistence on proper utensil usage, manners, and other demands inappropriate for this age group and may result in less food intake. Parents need to ignore some inappropriate mealtime behaviors and focus on positive nonmealtime activities. Conversation and role modeling can reinforce appropriate eating behavior and promote food intake.

Few children eat the recommended five servings of fruits and vegetables daily. Strong-flavored vegetables (overcooked cabbage and onions) are generally disliked, but are more popular if served raw. Crisp, raw vegetables are well accepted. Tough stringy fibers, such as those in celery or string beans, should be removed. Because preschool children still enjoy eating with their fingers, cutting fruits and vegetables into small pieces increases their acceptance. Preschoolers generally prefer their foods separate; casseroles and stews may not be well accepted. Foods that can be easily chewed are more readily accepted. Snacks are still important for adequate nutrient intake (see Box 13-4). The body uses food more effectively and energy levels are more consistent when children "refuel" every 2 to 4 hours. The number of snacks varies, depending on the family schedule and the child's activity and hunger levels. Parents should lead by example. When parents eat more fruits and vegetables, so do their children.[49]

Preschoolers are likely to be suspicious of any new foods introduced. They may need repeated exposures to the food before they are willing to swallow it. Eight to 15 exposures to a new food are needed to achieve acceptance. Even after they have accepted a food, preschool children may not eat it every time it is served. Rather than bargaining with a child who does not want what is on the menu or become a short-order cook, it is better to give the child the option to eat or not. Children eventually eat more of what we want them to eat if they are not forced to eat it.

ATTENTION-DEFICIT/HYPERACTIVITY DISORDER

Many parents and teachers believe sugar causes hyperactivity, or attention-deficit/hyperactivity disorder (ADHD), in children. ADHD is the fastest growing chronic disorder. Approximately 7.8% of children 4 to 17 years old are diagnosed with ADHD.[52] Hyperactivity is characterized by chronic age-inappropriate behaviors, including inattention, impulsiveness, hyperactivity, or restlessness. For a diagnosis of ADHD, the child must exhibit specific symptoms before age 7. Many theories have been proposed on the causes of hyperactivity, but none has been proven conclusively.

Two theories have been proposed for sugar affecting behavior: (1) an allergic response to sugar and (2) a hypoglycemic response. A meta-analysis of scientific studies (double-blind, placebo-controlled) indicates sugar does not affect behavior or cognitive performance of children.[53] The origin of the idea that sugar is responsible for hyperactivity seems to be purely based on the fact that sugar is a source of energy, as are other carbohydrates. The belief high sugar intake causes ADHD contradicts the findings of many research studies. External cues, such as parties or celebrations, possibly associated with a higher sugar intake, may cause hyperactivity, not the increased sugar intake.

Some studies suggest several food additives (e.g., colorings, flavorings, and preservatives) may increase hyperactivity in children with behavior problems. One study suggests a link between consumption of certain mixtures of artificial food coloring and the preservative sodium benzoate and hyperactivity.[54] Some children with ADHD and a personal or family history of food allergies show some improvement of ADHD by eliminating the allergic foods.[55]

For children showing behavior problems such as hyperactivity, the use of dietary manipulation tends to be a more acceptable approach to treatment than use of drugs. However, evidence of an association between diet and other behaviors is considered weak, and healthcare professionals need to be

---

🦷 Dental Hygiene Considerations

Assessment
- *Physical*: socioeconomic level, child's age, and child's developmental level.
- *Dietary*: eating environment, frequency of meals and snacks, quantity of foods consumed, adequacy of intake, parental beliefs and preferences about food.

Interventions
- Encourage eating meals at regular times. Serve food shortly after being seated to avoid restless behavior.
- If sufficient amounts are not eaten, limit snacking or provide nutrient-dense snacks; offer cheese cubes, fresh fruit, raw vegetable sticks, milk or yogurt, fruit juices, whole-grain cereals, and bread.
- Help parents clarify any misconceptions interfering with a child's ability to consume foods to meet their nutrient needs for growth and development, such as "healthy foods do not taste good" or "healthful eating means eliminating all high-fat foods."
- Refer low-income patients to any government or local social programs (WIC, food stamp program) for which they may be eligible.

Nutritional Directions

- Offer new foods frequently; introduce one- or two-bite portions along with a familiar food for better acceptance. The child is expected to taste each food that is prepared and served, but the taste may be very small.
- Atherosclerosis probably begins in childhood; a reduction of dietary fats (especially saturated) and cholesterol after the second birthday most likely decreases the risk of this disease. However, undue restriction of fat intake could compromise a child's growth and development, and potentially lead to eating disorders or unhealthy attitudes about food.
- Skim milk and other low-fat dairy products may be introduced after the second birthday.
- Until age 6, a good rule of thumb is 1 Tbsp of vegetables, fruit, or meat per year of life.
- Food, especially sweet foods, should not be used as a bribe or reward.
- Children should not be made to clean their plates. Rather, teach children to recognize and honor their hunger and satiety cues.
- Caregivers must understand diet and lifestyle choices during early childhood have an impact on later disease risk. Accelerated weight and fat mass gain seem to predict adult disease conditions.
- Present disliked foods in a matter-of-fact manner, serving small portions (1 to 2 Tbsp); discard without comment if the child does not eat them.
- Successful childhood feeding may be best accomplished by providing a variety of healthful foods and allowing children to eat without coercion. Without some guidance, however, children may fill up on calorie-dense foods that do not provide adequate amounts of necessary nutrients.
- Provide healthy snacks, but prevent the child from grazing throughout the day to ensure a good appetite at meal time.
- Food habits established early in life affect lifelong eating patterns.
- Children who avoid drinking milk are at increased risk for prepubertal fractures.
- Children generally eat better when the family or at least one adult sits at the table and eats with them.
- Offer a wide variety of vegetables and fruits daily, especially dark green, leafy, and deep yellow vegetables and colorful fruits.
- Offer desserts, sweets, sweetened beverages, and salty snacks only occasionally, offering nutrient-dense, age-appropriate foods as alternatives (see Box 13-4).
- Water is the ideal beverage between meals; omitting sugar-sweetened beverages and sodas and their extra kilocalories helps prevent risks of excess weight gain and dental caries.
- If a wide variety of foods is offered to toddlers who are healthy and growing appropriately, parents need not be overly concerned about risk of nutrient deficiency.[57]

critical of scientific claims regarding diet and behavior. The use of dietary treatments alone is unlikely to be sufficient treatment for many children with ADHD.[56] The National Institutes of Health concluded dietary changes other than a well-balanced diet cannot be recommended until clinical significances have been documented. Inappropriate dietary treatment without scientific backing could (1) detract from efforts to identify effective treatment and prevention of delinquent behavior; (2) lead to nutritional deficiencies or excesses; and (3) provide offenders with a dietary excuse for their behavior, rather than assuming responsibility for their own behavior.

CHILDREN WITH SPECIAL NEEDS

Health conditions, such as mental retardation of unknown origin, cerebral palsy, Down syndrome, infantile autism, and muscular dystrophy, have significant oral health and oral hygiene implications. Gum disease is frequently observed in children with Down syndrome. Mastication and swallowing problems occur in all these conditions except Down syndrome. Some children with oral-motor problems can improve; others cannot.

Children with cerebral palsy and Down syndrome may practice bruxism. **Bruxism** is involuntary grinding or clenching of teeth, which results in abnormal wear patterns on the teeth and joint or neuromuscular problems. Loosened teeth interfere with the child eating chewy foods such as meats. Children with cerebral palsy, Down syndrome, and intellectual disabilities are likely to have abnormal sensory input and muscle tone. Difficulties with sucking, swallowing, spoon-feeding skills with semisolid or solid foods, chewing development, and independent feeding are common. Tongue thrust associated with many of these conditions results in significant food waste and may jeopardize nutritional status.

Dental Hygiene Considerations

Assessment

- *Physical*: condition of the oral cavity, presence of dental caries, plaque biofilm, abnormal oral-motor habits, such as tongue thrust, bruxism, oral-motor development, medications.
- *Dietary*: intake of fermentable carbohydrates, frequency of snacking, calcium and vitamin D intake, source of fluoride, pica.

Interventions

- The goal when counseling parents of children is to prevent caries and plaque biofilm formation, and provide appropriate recommendations or referrals.
- Evaluate and assess children's diets at regular intervals.
- Stress the importance of providing adequate amounts of protein; vitamins A, C and D; calcium; phosphorus; and fluoride during the formation and calcification of teeth.
- Consider the parents' attitudes, cultures, beliefs, fears, and educational levels when developing and providing oral health education.
- Recommendations for fluoride usage should be determined by need, based on risk indicators.
- Encourage parents to assume responsibility for the child's oral healthcare and model good oral health behaviors.

Nutritional Directions

- Provide nutritious snacks such as cheese cubes or raw vegetables. Fibrous foods promote salivary flow, increasing the buffering capacity of saliva.
- Vitamin D–fortified milk and cheeses not only provide nutrients needed for healthy teeth, but also are cariostatic.
- Provide an opportunity to brush the teeth after eating; if brushing is impossible, rinse mouth with water.
- Encourage the use of fluoridated toothpastes for children older than 2 to 3 years. Use a pea-sized amount of toothpaste to limit the amount accidentally swallowed.
- Inappropriate dietary habits and unhealthy food preferences developed during childhood have lifetime implications.
- A dental examination is recommended every 6 to 12 months; topical fluoride may be applied if the water supply is not fluoridated. The dental team determines the appropriate fluoride regimen for each child.
- Limit sticky carbohydrate foods, such as candies, cookies, crackers, pastries, and raisins, between meals. If these foods are frequently consumed as snacks, the carbohydrate content and physical properties of these foods may contribute to dental caries risk.
- Encourage children to eat whole fruits rather than drink fruit juices and beverages.
- Good oral health is directly correlated to good dietary habits that promote daily breakfast consumption and fruit and vegetable intake in conjunction with fluoridation.

Dental problems may become exaggerated in these children as a result of difficulty in maintaining good oral hygiene, the child's unique dietary habits and patterns, and the influences of their prescribed medications. Such problems include oral infections, dental caries, and periodontal disease.

The dental hygienist may become involved in team treatment of these children. Treatment is individualized, depending on the potential capabilities and skills of the child. Nutritional intervention for feeding skill difficulties is to assist in planning a diet that is easiest for the patient to eat and still meet the nutritional needs.

SCHOOL-AGE CHILDREN (7 TO 12 YEARS OLD)

The middle childhood years are the result of early growth and development; reserves are laid down for upcoming rapid adolescent growth. New activities and new friends begin to influence choices and broaden the child's horizons. The child is exposed to different foods and food patterns and usually begins to accept more foods. These new ideas may affect food choices at home.

Almost all foods are liked. Vegetables are the least favorite, with only 22% of all children consuming three servings daily. Planning menus around food groups is important to include all the necessary nutrients. Foods containing mostly sugars or fats need not be eliminated, but they should not replace recommended amounts from the food groups. The appetite is usually good; but food habits and intake may suffer because children do not take time for meals (15 to 20 minutes). Enforcement of a specific amount of time to eat may prevent the child from forming the habit of eating too fast. Poor appetite may be caused by stresses, such as schoolwork and emotional difficulties.

Students are ravenous after school. Although bakery products, soft drinks, candy, and chips are favorites, nutritious snacks are preferable. More access to money and the influence of peers and mass media may result in expenditures at fast food restaurants and from vending machines. These foods are usually high in fat, salt, and sugar.

Children may continue to have problems with allergy to milk and eggs. Rather than outgrowing allergies by the time they start to school, as previously thought, only about 20% to 40% of children outgrow their allergy to milk, and about 4% to 26% outgrow their allergy to egg. This condition may persist well into adolescence.[58,59]

DENTAL CARIES IN SCHOOL-AGE CHILDREN

According to the CDC, trends in oral health prevalence of tooth decay in the permanent teeth of children 6 to 11 years old decreased from approximately 25% in 1988-1994 to 21% in 1999-2004, and decreased from 68% to 59% among adolescents 12 to 19 years old during the same periods.[33] Although strides are being made in prevention of tooth decay, this disease remains a problem for some racial and ethnic and lower socioeconomic groups who continue to have more treated and untreated tooth decay compared with other groups. In children from families at less than 200% of the poverty level, one-third have not had a dental visit in the past year.

This age range also generally marks exfoliation of all or most of the primary teeth and the eruption of most of the permanent teeth. This is significant because the application of topical fluoride (professionally applied and self-applied) now becomes as effective as systemic fluoride administration. Systemic fluoride is effective during the mineralization phase of erupting teeth and before eruption. When 1 ppm of fluoride in drinking water is present during tooth formation, caries rate is reduced 60% along with reduction in the prevalence of plaque biofilm and remineralization of teeth. To provide maximum protection, systemic fluoride is recommended through age 16 for children in nonfluoridated or inadequately fluoridated areas.

Topical administration of fluoride to teeth can also result in reduction of tooth decay. Topical fluoride sources include dentifrices, rinses, gels, fluoride supplements, varnishes, and fluoridated water.

Application of **sealants** (a clear or shaded plastic material applied to occlusal surfaces of permanent teeth) acts as a barrier protecting decay-prone areas of the teeth from plaque biofilm and acid. Approximately 30% of children 6 to 11 years old and 38% of teens 12 to 19 years old have had sealants applied.[31] However, use of a toothbrush with dental floss, fluoride toothpaste, and sealants cannot completely control caries formation.

Another factor in caries formation is food selection and patterns of consumption. Cariogenicity of food is influenced by the presence of fermentable carbohydrates, physical properties, and frequency of consumption (see Chapter 17). The use of products (e.g., chewing gum, candy) containing xylitol can be effective in preventing tooth decay by reducing levels of harmful mutans streptococci bacteria in plaque biofilm.[60,61]

Dental Hygiene Considerations

Assessment
- *Physical*: schoolwork or emotional difficulties, activity level, sports interests.
- *Dietary*: nutrient and fluid intake, appetite, food preferences and eating patterns, child's and parent's beliefs about nutrition.

Interventions
- Recommend nutritious snacks be readily available (see Box 13-4). Cutting foods into shapes often creates interest in the snack, such as cheese sandwiches cut into stars.
- Evaluate sources of fluoride to ensure optimal intake to protect erupting and newly erupted teeth, while minimizing excessive intake and risk for fluorosis.
- Antimicrobial agents, such as chlorhexidine, can be used to control existing plaque biofilm and formation of new plaque biofilm by controlling bacteria and limiting acid production.
- Ask low-income patients about the child's participation in governmental child nutrition programs (National School Lunch, School Breakfast, Summer Food Service, and Special Milk).

Nutritional Directions

- Children involved in meal preparation are more likely to eat the food they prepare and to be aware of what is in the food.
- Have nutritious foods available for snacks, such as sliced apples, yogurt, popcorn, low-fat cheese, or dry roasted seeds or nuts.
- As children grow older, they consume larger quantities of food, but food choices deviate more from the *Dietary Guidelines for Americans*.[62]
- Encourage appropriate oral hygiene techniques.

ADOLESCENTS

GROWTH AND NUTRIENT REQUIREMENTS

Major biological, social, psychological, and cognitive changes occur during adolescence. Because of these changes and rapid growth rates, 17% of U.S. teenagers are considered to be at nutritional risk, consuming inadequate amounts of nutrients. Many adolescent eating practices place them at risk for developing chronic diseases later in life. Additionally, fitness levels are declining.

The slow childhood growth rate accelerates with pubescence until the rate is as rapid as that of early infancy. Growth of long bones, secondary sexual maturation, and fat and muscle deposition create an increased nutrient requirement. The end of this adolescent growth spurt is signaled by a deceleration of growth, completion of sexual maturation, and closure of the epiphyses of long bones.

Although the DRIs provide recommended nutrient intakes by chronological age, nutrient needs closely parallel physical development. Adolescent girls need to increase their energy intake sooner and decrease it more quickly than boys because of earlier onset of puberty and lower total body weight after adulthood is reached. Adolescent boys have greater nutritional needs than adolescent girls because of growth rates and body composition changes (see Table 13-4). A very active 18-year-old boy requires approximately 3800 kcal compared with almost 2900 kcal for an 18-year-old girl. Most adolescents need and are able to eat large quantities of food many times a day. However, teens need to be careful of amounts and frequency of eating when the rapid growth rate levels off.

Average protein intake is well above recommendations (see Table 13-4). However, if for any reason, such as weight loss diets or chronic illness, overall intake becomes insufficient, dietary protein may be used to meet energy needs and would not be available for needed growth and repair.

The need for calcium, vitamin D, and iron is of particular importance throughout childhood. Adolescence is a crucial phase in bone development. During adolescence, 45% of adult skeletal mass is formed; calcium needs are greater than at any other time of life. Building good bone mass during adolescence is thought to be the best way to prevent osteoporosis in old age. However, only 9% of girls and 31% of boys 14 to 18 years old get the daily amount of calcium recommended.[63] A daily calcium intake of 1300 mg in addition to exercise during adolescence promotes calcium retention and bone mineral density. Long-term studies also support the importance of vitamin D supplements for bone health in adolescence.[64] Vitamin D deficiency is prevalent in adolescent girls, however, placing them at risk for later osteoporosis. The recommendation to double vitamin D intake by the AAP could necessitate a vitamin D supplement.[30,48]

Increased iron is required because of the expansion of blood volume; increase in red blood cell (RBC) mass and muscle mass, especially in boys; and the need to replace iron losses associated with menstruation in girls. Participation in sports activities leads to RBC destruction. Poor dietary habits result in inadequate intake of folate; riboflavin; vitamins B₆, A, C, and D; iron; and calcium.

Poor food choices result in poor compliance with MyPyramid. The caloric percentage of dietary fat intake for adolescent boys and girls in 2002-2004 was approximately 33%, with about 11% of the kilocalories from saturated fat.[63] Fiber intake is about one-half the recommended amount. These two issues could be corrected by increasing fruit and vegetable consumption and choosing more whole-grain products.

INFLUENTIAL FACTORS ON EATING HABITS

Eating is an important part of socialization and exerting one's independence. Food choices are influenced by complex external factors, such as family, peers, mass media, and economic and sociocultural factors, and internal factors, such as physiological needs, body image, self-concept, food preferences, and personal values and beliefs about health and nutrition. Probably the strongest influential factor among teenagers is peer pressure. Times available to eat may be determined by group activities.

Most adolescents are stressed because of continual changes. Sexuality, body image, scholastic and athletic pressures, relationships with friends and relatives, finances, career plans, and ideological beliefs may cause conflicts as adolescents try to establish and understand their identity. The presence of stress can decrease the use of several nutrients, particularly vitamin C and calcium.

Increasing numbers of children and adolescents are overweight (see Health Application 13). Adolescents, especially girls, are often obsessed about their body image and a desire to be thin. They are eager to try fad diets and other unsafe weight loss methods, which may be inadequate in nutrients. The conclusion of one study was that chronic dieting to control weight by adolescents was not only ineffective, but also seemed to promote weight gain.[65] Dieting is not recommended for adolescents because nutrients during this period are necessary to build and strengthen their bodies to last a lifetime. Obesity, anorexia nervosa, and bulimia are serious health concerns amenable to early treatment. Oral problems associated with eating disorders are discussed in Chapter 16. Prevention may be the only successful treatment in some cases.

Favorite food choices among adolescents are carbonated beverages, sports and energy drinks, flavored milk, steak, hamburgers, tacos, chips, pizza, spaghetti, chicken, French fries, ice cream, oranges, orange and apple juice, apples, bread, candy (sour, hard, or chewy), and snack cakes. Vegetables are unpopular.

Between 1977 and 2001, Americans increased the proportion of total energy obtained from soft drinks and fruit drinks, while decreasing the proportion of total energy obtained from milk. The largest decrease in milk consumption occurred in children and adolescents 2 to 18 years old. In 1977, approximately 13.2% of total energy intake was from milk, but it was only 8.3% in 2001. During this time period, soft drink consumption in this age group increased from 3% to 6.9%, and fruit drink consumption increased from 1.8% to 3.4%. In contrast to consuming 13.1 oz of sweetened beverages in 1977, consumption had increased to 18.9 oz in 1996.[66] In 1977, 12- to 19-year-olds consumed 16 oz of soda; this same group consumed 28 oz a day in 1999.[67] Teens are drinking twice as much soft drinks as milk.[68] This alarming trend has also been linked with lower calcium and vitamin D intake.

Adolescents are particularly vulnerable to an insult to their bones. A lack of calcium or vitamin D can have profound implications for their future skeletal health because a mild deficiency of either can be unrecognized until severe skeletal damage has occurred. The Academy of General Dentistry believes the increase in soda consumption has helped boost the caries rate in teens, which is approaching the levels in teens before fluoridation. The AAP issued a policy statement encouraging restriction of the sale of soft drinks in schools to prevent health problems as a result of overconsumption. The AAP warns of the following potential health problems as a result of high intake of sweetened drinks: (1) overweight attributable to additional caloric intake; (2) displacement of milk consumption, resulting in calcium deficiency with an attendant risk of osteoporosis and fractures; and (3) dental caries and potential enamel erosion.

Adolescents have more access to food outside the home and experiment more with food selections. About 25% of an adolescent's kilocalories come from high-calorie, low-nutrient-dense foods, making overeating easy. This results in such problems as excessive intake of sodium, sugar, and fat; inadequate fiber; frequent snacking and skipping meals, especially breakfast; eating in a hurry; and reliance on convenience and fast foods. Fast food restaurants, vending machines, and convenience stores fit adolescents' busy, active lifestyles.

Older adolescents 15 to 18 years old are notable for skipping breakfast—25% of boys and 35% of girls. Omission of breakfast is more prevalent with children from lower socioeconomic levels, who also have higher rates of overweight and obesity.[69,70] Many studies have shown positive short-term effects of breakfast on cognitive functioning and alertness, and implications of skipping breakfast on mental stability and academic performance are stronger for boys than girls.[71]

Fast foods are acceptable nutritionally when consumed in moderation as a part of a well-balanced diet (see Fig. 13-6). During the transition from middle adolescence to young adulthood, the proportion of boys who reported frequent fast food intake (three or more times weekly) increased from 23.6% to 33%.[72] Lower calorie items and a wider variety of menu selections, such as salads and low-fat milkshakes, can contribute to nutrient requirements without providing excessive kilocalories.

NUTRITION COUNSELING

Despite adolescents being knowledgeable about healthy eating and wise choices, they frequently choose foods they perceive are unhealthy. Promoting change is more important than providing information. Factors negatively affecting food choices are time, availability of healthy foods, and lack of concern about healthy eating. Counseling works well for adolescents who are willing to listen and make changes. Adolescents can frequently be motivated by responsibility, collaboration, fear of failure, and respect for the counselor. Techniques such as negotiation and reflective listening can enhance their critical thinking skills.

Effective tactics for nutrition counseling among adolescents are to appeal to their physical image or their muscular development and competitiveness for sports, and to praise better food choices, ignore choices that are neutral, and discourage harmful choices. By presenting nutrition and health information in terms relevant to adolescent lifestyles and personal interests, health professionals can help teenagers understand how current eating and exercise habits affect their current and future health.

Dental Hygiene Considerations

Assessment
- *Physical*: activity level, growth spurt, use of illicit drugs, use of tobacco products, body image, self-efficacy, influence of peer pressure, stress level.
- *Dietary*: adequacy of nutrient intake based on MyPyramid; amount and frequency of carbonated beverages, and sports and energy drinks; use of fast foods, convenience foods, or vending machine foods; food preferences and personal values and beliefs about health and nutrition; dietary and nutritional supplements; breakfast; and alcohol intake.

Interventions
- Encourage use of calcium-rich and vitamin D–rich foods.
- Praise good eating patterns; collaboratively work with adolescents to modify food choices and suggest substitutions.
- Determine the frequency, quantity, and form of cariogenic foods.
- Encourage a smoking cessation program for adolescents who smoke.
- Provide knowledge to teens regarding risks of using smokeless tobacco and other tobacco products.

Nutritional Directions

- Teenagers should be aware of long-term risks and benefits of good nutrition, but the best approach is to focus on short-term benefits of eating well.
- Restriction of kilocalorie intake during rapid growth period compromises lean body mass accumulation despite a seemingly adequate protein intake.
- Intense physical activity can cause increased urinary loss of calcium and RBC destruction. Referral to a dietitian may be needed to ensure adequate nutritional intake.
- Snacking can have a positive influence on the overall nutritional status of the teenager. Kitchens should be stocked with nutritious snack foods, such as cooked meats, raw vegetables, milk, cheese, fresh and dried fruit, nuts and seeds, peanut butter, pretzels, and popcorn to encourage good eating habits.
- Use of dietary supplements by most adolescents is not needed.
- An inadequate intake of calcium and vitamin D during childhood or adolescence may result in the child not reaching the genetically predetermined peak height and bone mass.
- Children and adolescents who skip breakfast miss the opportunity to consume a nutrient-rich meal; unhealthful dietary behaviors may have an adverse effect on body weight.
- An adolescent with light skin needs to spend about 5 to 10 minutes in the sun with only part of the body exposed (arms or legs) two or three times a week to produce enough vitamin D; an African American needs to spend 15 to 30 minutes. Additionally, calcium intake should be adequate (3 cups of milk or equivalent milk products).

HEALTH APPLICATION 13 Childhood and Adolescent Obesity

"Childhood obesity is the greatest challenge to child health in the 21st century."[73] The prevalence of obesity, body mass index (BMI) ≥95th percentile, increased almost fourfold for 6- to 11-year-old children and threefold for 12- to 19-year-olds between 1963 and 1970 and 1999 and 2000.[74] The most recent statistics from the CDC indicate 11.3% of children and adolescents aged 2 through 19 years are at or above the 97th percentile of the 2000 BMI-for-age growth charts, 16.3% are at or above the 95th percentile, and 31.9% are at or above the 85th percentile.[75] More alarming is the increase in prevalence of overweight and obesity in African American and Hispanic children (21% greater than the 95th percentile for BMI based on age and sex).

BMI is a screening tool, not a diagnostic tool, used to detect weight problems. A BMI for children 2 to 19 years old can be calculated using this CDC website: http://apps.nccd.cdc.gov/dnpabmi/Calculator.aspx. Children with a high BMI do not necessarily have clinical complications or health risks related to increased body fat. A high BMI is a clue necessitating more in-depth assessment of the individual child to ascertain health status. Childhood obesity in the United States is greatest in groups with the highest poverty rates and least education.[76]

Obese children are now more frequently being diagnosed with type 2 diabetes, which was formerly diagnosed only in adults. The CDC predicts American children born in 2000 face a one in three chance of developing diabetes. Other health problems associated with obesity in children include high cholesterol and blood pressure levels, which are risk factors for heart disease; sleep apnea (interrupted breathing while sleeping); orthopedic problems; liver disease; and asthma. Sixty percent of overweight children 5 to 10 years old have at least one risk factor for heart disease. Many diagnosable and treatable conditions arise from childhood obesity. The existence of any of these conditions should be used to motivate change; many patients benefit from lifestyle modification. The cycle of obesity and disease seems to begin before birth: women who are overweight are more likely to give birth to larger infants, who are more likely to become obese.[77] An individual's weight at birth, as a preschooler, and as a teenager seems to have a strong connection to weight problems in adulthood, accompanied by increased health risks and mortality. Weight gain in at-risk children begins in early childhood, before starting school.[78]

Research is supporting the connection between obesity and oral health. It is an important issue for all healthcare professionals to discuss with their patients. Treatment of obesity for any individual requires the expertise of many healthcare disciplines.

Obesity is a difficult subject to discuss even in a clinical setting because of current societal culture and values. Only 31.6% of mothers of overweight children thought that their child was overweight.[79] Parents may become defensive when the issue is mentioned or view comments provided negatively. Individuals from low-income groups may possess different perceptions of weight than the healthcare provider, and may be unconcerned about the child's weight. Children who are modestly overweight often continue to gain during their school years, making weight loss later on even tougher. Perhaps more devastating to an overweight child is social discrimination. Overweight children often experience psychological stress, poor body image, low self-esteem, and depression. Despite these distressing effects on American youth, the consensus seems to be that our environment, especially the sedentary lifestyle, supports a genetic predisposition to gain excessive weight. Children are more concerned about their current appearance and athletic performance than the long-term effects of the weight on their mental and physical capacities and shortened life span.

Although the cause of childhood obesity is multifaceted, factors driving this phenomenon include rapid changes in the modern food and activity environment of children superimposed onto genetic and metabolic predispositions for weight gain. Childhood obesity, similar to adult obesity, is a complex disease caused by an imbalance between kilocalorie intake and output. The problems of American children eating too many high-kilocalorie fast foods and snacks and being inactive are well recognized as contributing factors in this problem.

Weight loss or gain reflects inadequate or excessive intake, which should be balanced with an appropriate amount of exercise. This simple equation is confounded by complex social factors influencing children's eating habits, exercise, and play. Treating obesity in children is not easy. A task force of the Endocrine Society issued new clinical practice guidelines to help clinicians focus on prevention and early intervention of obesity in children. These guidelines stressed that medication or surgical treatment should not be offered to overweight or obese children until more modest measures, including intensive dietary, behavioral, and activity-related lifestyle changes, are attempted.[80]

The goal for obese children has been weight maintenance or reduction in the rate of weight gain while height increases. By "growing into their weight," body fat decreases without compromising lean body mass and growth. Many experts believe overweight children should not be put on a diet because of the importance of providing adequate nutrients to promote optimal linear growth.

The American Dietetic Association advises children 2 to 7 years old with a BMI between the 85th and 94th percentiles or a BMI greater than the 95th percentile with no complications should maintain their weight. If the child's BMI is greater than the 95th percentile with mild complications (e.g., mild hypertension, abnormal lipid levels, and

insulin resistance), gradual weight loss is recommended. The goal for children 7 years or older whose BMI is between the 85th and 94th percentiles with no complications is to maintain their weight. If the BMI is between the 85th and 95th percentiles, and the child has mild complications, or the BMI is equal to or greater than the 95th percentile, gradual weight loss is recommended.

The final goal for all children and adolescents who are overweight or at risk for being overweight is a BMI for age less than the 85th percentile, but this goal should be secondary to healthy eating and activity. Assisting an overweight toddler or school-age child is easier than assisting a teenager because parents have a greater amount of control regarding food choices inside and outside the home. Treating obesity requires a motivated child and parent. Prevention of obesity is important for numerous reasons: (1) it is very expensive to treat; (2) an older child regains most of the weight after an obesity management program; (3) success rates for long-term treatment of morbidly overweight teens is extremely low; and (4) access to any effective weight loss program is limited for high-risk children.

The first intervention is behavior and lifestyle change. The first step in addressing this epidemic is to teach parents of young children how to make healthy choices. Nutritional imprinting starts early, so early childhood is the ideal time to start discussing proper feeding practices. Nutrition education for the child and family is needed to provide a well-balanced diet with some caloric restriction. Many experts believe children should not be required to eat food that is different than the rest of the family; only food portions should be different. Drinks with kilocalories, including fruit juices, should be limited to less than 12 oz daily. Even though juice is natural and healthy, fresh fruits are preferable. When parents change how the whole family eats, and offer children wholesome rewards for not being couch potatoes, obese children begin to shed pounds.

Parents play a vital role in the development of lifestyle habits that contribute to overeating and inactivity in children, and a family approach is needed to manage childhood obesity. In addition to children watching 3 to 5 hours of television daily, they are now spending more hours in front of a computer screen. "Inactive entertainment" has paralleled the disturbing increase in obese and overweight children. Instead of rewarding children with snacks, alternative ways of spending quality time with them is recommended. Environmental change is fostered by restructuring family mealtimes and leisure-time activities, and reinforcing appropriate eating cues (Box 13-5).

Necessary lifestyle changes are challenging to the child and family. Generally, the emphasis is on a healthy lifestyle rather than weight reduction. Physical activity and healthy eating habits are two lifestyle practices that children need to learn to prevent obesity. MyPyramid for Kids (see Figs. 13-2 and 13-6) was developed to help promote activities to offset energy intake. Exercise should be encouraged with consideration of the child's interests and preferences. The whole family should become more active.

Behavioral treatment of obesity may be more effective for children than for adults. A family-based, multifactor intervention can be implemented by a multidisciplinary team after a comprehensive, in-depth assessment when obesity is diagnosed. A behavior modification program should be developed with the support of the whole family. Successful behavioral programs are labor-intensive and require intensive parental involvement. Changes such as taking time to chew food, cutting down on sugar-laden beverages, eating more vegetables, and walking for exercise can be effective in gaining control of the weight problem.

The goal is to establish an environment that supports behavior changes, while minimizing any perceptions of restrictions or limitations on the child. Successful programs focus on encouragement and "small victories" to sustain involvement in improving fitness levels. Parents need help in communicating about eating and exercise habits with their children in positive and encouraging ways and to learn how to help children improve their fitness levels. Because of the lack of success in weight loss and maintenance programs for severely obese children and adolescents, even with intensive behavioral treatment, clinicians have begun investigating medication therapy and are resorting to bariatric surgery to ameliorate pediatric obesity.

Currently, it remains very difficult for overweight children and adolescents to lose weight and even more tedious to sustain that weight loss. The ultimate goal is prevention of the development of overweight in children and adolescents. Experts agree it is much easier to keep weight off a child than to deal with it as an adult. If an answer to this obesity epidemic is not found, for the first time in at least a century, the life span for this generation will be shorter than their parents.

Addressing childhood obesity with parents and children has been a touchy and difficult subject for most professionals. WellPointSM, a leading health insurer, has teamed with the American Dietetic Association to develop helpful information for healthcare professionals to overcome this barrier and communicate with parents and children about obesity. Helpful information is available on the Internet at www.wellpoint.com and www.eatright.com, for professionals and parents to assess and address child and adolescent obesity.

Box 13-5 Help Children Maintain a Healthy Body Weight

- Be supportive. Children know if they are overweight, and do not need to be reminded or singled out. They need acceptance, encouragement, and love.
- Be a positive role model. Note lifestyle habits contributing to overeating and inactivity, and help them avoid the situation.
- Start the day off on the right foot. Breakfast helps spread the kilocalories throughout the day and helps avoid mid-morning unhealthy snacks.
- Set guidelines for the amount of time children spend watching television, playing video games, or playing on the computer.
- Set goals for physical activity; plan family activities involving exercise. Instead of watching TV, go hiking or biking, wash the car, or walk around a mall. Offer choices, and let children decide.
- Be sensitive. Find activities children will enjoy that are not difficult or could cause embarrassment.
- Eat meals together as a family, and eat at the table, not in front of a television. Eat slowly and enjoy the food. Eating at home with family often translates into a healthier diet.
- Avoid using food as a reward or punishment. Spend some quality time together; take a walk or go on a long bike ride.
- Focus on positive goals. Allow children to determine goals they want to achieve, such as being able to swim five laps in a specified time. Focusing on positive goals is better than focusing on weight loss.

- Do not be too restrictive; focus on moderation. Children should not be placed on restrictive diets, unless ordered by a pediatrician (for medical reasons). Encourage kid-sized portions. Sweets and fast foods should be curtailed, but they can be used sparingly. Children need food for growth, development, and energy, but if they are forced to clean their plates, they are doing their bodies a disservice.
- Make eating a family activity. Involve children in meal planning, grocery shopping, and meal preparation. This helps them learn, and gives them a role in the decision making.
- Keep healthy snacks on hand. Good options include fresh, frozen, or canned fruits and vegetables; low-fat cheese, yogurt, or ice cream; frozen fruit juice bars; and cookies such as fig bars, graham crackers, gingersnaps, or vanilla wafers.
- Watch what children drink. High-energy drinks provide a lot of sugar with little health benefit.
- Make small changes as a family. Menu changes should be implemented for all family members. Begin parking the car a little farther away or eating fast food less often.
- Focus on small, gradual changes in eating and activity patterns. This helps form habits that can last a lifetime.
- Get active. Plan activities involving the whole family, such as skating, hiking, or biking. Make an after-dinner walk a regular part of the family's evening.

Adapted from Torgan C: Childhood obesity on the rise. Consumer Health Information Based on Research from the National Institutes of Health. Available at http://www.nih.gov/news/WordonHealth/jun2002/childhoodobesity.htm and Mayo Clinic. Childhood obesity: Parenting advice. Available at: http://www.mayoclinic.com/invoke.cfm?id=FL00058&si=1880 or http://www.eatright.org/cps/rde/xchg/ada/hs.xsl/shop_8119_ENU_HTML.htm.

CASE APPLICATION FOR THE DENTAL HYGIENIST

A mother brings her 3-year-old son in because of the need for a routine oral examination required by the Head Start program he is attending. She knows he has some white spots on his front teeth, but he will not allow her to brush his teeth, and she does not routinely ensure he brushes his teeth. He is still using a sippy cup, but gave up the bottle at age 18 months.

Nutritional Assessment
- Willingness to seek nutritional information
- Desire for increased knowledge of nutritional health habits
- Knowledge of community resources
- Cultural or religious influences
- Knowledge regarding the *Dietary Guidelines for Americans,* food labels, and MyPyramid

Nutritional Diagnosis
Health-seeking behaviors related to lack of knowledge concerning optimal nutrition practices in relation to dental health.

Nutritional Goals
The patient verbalizes correct information concerning the importance of oral hygiene and foods and beverages affecting the oral cavity; is aware of snacks that do not promote dental caries; is able to read food labels; and can name the food groups in MyPyramid, the number of servings needed for the child, and portion sizes from each group.

Nutritional Implementation
Intervention: Ask the parent to write down everything the child ate yesterday from the time he got up until this morning when he got up. Also ask the parent to write down everything she ate.
Rationale: This will help you tailor the information you provide to the needs of the patient. You especially need to know the child's access to the sippy cup during the day, what beverage was in the cup, and whether he went to bed with it. The parent's diet recall reflects the primary caregiver's preferences and habits. Any changes in her diet ultimately help the child.
Intervention: (1) Encourage variety of food intake, using MyPyramid. Review the number of servings needed and what consists of a serving size. (2) Recommend substituting fresh fruit for juices and to limit fruit juice to 4 to 6 oz daily. (3) Instruct her to avoid products that contain fermentable carbohydrates, such as cookies, crackers, or cereal, between meals.
Rationale: It is the total balance of diet that matters, and the best balance incorporates variety to promote optimal nutrition.

Providing the minimal number of servings prevents nutritional deficiencies in healthy individuals. Certain foods, although they may be wholesome and nutritious, may not be advisable for oral health.
Intervention: (1) Explain how to read labels for carbohydrate content. The name of most sugars end in "-ose." (2) Emphasize moderation of sugar intake. (3) Explain that "dietetic" and "sugar-free" do not mean that the product is low in kilocalories or low in cariogenic potential. (4) Explain the relationship between carbohydrate and the caries process; emphasize the importance of proper oral hygiene after its use.
Rationale: Refined sugar contains kilocalories and no other nutrients, but is acceptable when used in items that contain appreciable amounts of other nutrients (e.g., a pudding would provide more nutrients than a gelatin dessert or carbonated beverages).
Intervention: (1) Review an entire label with the mother to help her understand how to use it, (2) determine a serving size, and (3) explain the types of carbohydrates.
Rationale: Knowledge increases compliance and allows one to make informed choices regarding food selections.
Intervention: Discuss the importance of three regular mealtimes and three healthy snacks and avoidance of grazing.
Rationale: Adequate nutrients are important for growth and health of the child; snacking is needed for a 3-year-old to obtain adequate nutrients. Assist the child in tooth brushing after meals and snacks.
Intervention: Refer the patient to governmental programs for which she may be eligible—WIC, food stamps, or expanded nutrition programs.
Rationale: These agencies may help in providing healthy foods and provide practical guidelines via newsletters, workshops, and written materials to improve health.

Evaluation
To determine effectiveness of care, have the patient read labels; have the patient state the number of servings and portion sizes needed for her son. Additionally, the patient should be able to plan a menu using foods recommended, and to state how to obtain or use community information and support. The patient should be able to indicate how changes in food choices will not only improve overall health, but also maintain health of the oral cavity and ensure optimal growth of her son with minimal or no problems in the oral cavity.

STUDENT READINESS

1. Plan meals for 1 day for a family with a 2-year-old toddler, a 10-year-old boy, and a 15-year-old girl.
2. Discuss feeding an infant from birth to age 1.
3. What is considered normal weight for a newborn?
4. Create an outline of a discussion you might have in counseling an expectant parent about ECC.
5. A mother wants to know why snacks are needed and which ones to give her preschooler to lessen the risk of developing dental cavities. What would you tell her? Provide a list of specific suggestions and food choices for the mother.
6. A mother tells you that because her child is hyperactive, she is going to eliminate all sugar. How would you respond?

CASE STUDY

Mrs. C. is at her 6-month recall visit and talks about her 6-month-old daughter, Jennifer. Jennifer weighed 7 lb at birth and now weighs 15 lb. She was bottle-fed from birth. At 3 months, Mrs. C. introduced cereals, but Jennifer has resisted all attempts to increase her solid food intake. She is allowed to go to sleep with a bottle propped in her crib at the daycare center.

1. What additional assessment data do you need?
2. Is Jennifer's weight gain within the expected range?
3. How much should she gain in the next 6 months?
4. What tentative dental hygiene diagnosis could you derive?
5. The dental hygienist encourages Jennifer's mother to discontinue the habit of allowing her to go to sleep with a bottle and to request that the daycare center do the same. Why?
6. The healthcare provider recommends solid foods be introduced gradually to Jennifer. What foods should be introduced first?
7. When will Jennifer be old enough for finger foods?
8. Why should honey be withheld until 1 year of age?
9. Why would the dental hygienist want to assess Mrs. C's dietary intake?

CASE STUDY

R.J. is a large 16-year-old boy (6 feet, 4 inches, 190 lb) who has complained to you about pain from dental caries. He is active in athletics in school and has a part-time job. You determine from his dietary history that his appetite is very good, and his nutrient intake is adequate except for vegetables. Snacking, principally soft drinks, candy, and cookies, constitutes almost 50% of his total caloric intake.

1. How would you counsel R.J.? What motivational factors would you consider for him?
2. What are some dental hygiene nutritional diagnoses and goals and interventions for Raymond?
3. What further data are needed for a complete assessment?
4. When having R.J. choose better snack options, what are some that you would recommend?

CASE STUDY

Norma returns for a 6-month recall visit. Since her last checkup, this 17-year-old girl has developed 12 new dental caries in the mandibular anterior teeth. Norma's parents are in their 50s. Her father has lost numerous teeth as a result of periodontal disease, and her mother is completely edentulous. Norma has no medical problems other than rhinitis (inflammation of the nasal mucous membranes secondary to allergies), which causes her to breathe through her mouth much of the time. The oral examination showed normal color and tone of the oral mucosa, tongue, and gingiva. Her decayed, missing, filled rate was 17. She reports eating a varied well-balanced diet except for fruit and vegetable intake. Because of the dryness in her mouth, she relies heavily on cough drops and chewing gum.

1. What is a possible cause of these new dental caries?
2. What suggestions would you give her to relieve mouth dryness?
3. Based on her dietary habits, what nutrient is apparently inadequate?

References

1. Schack-Nielsen L, Michaelsen KF: Advances in our understanding of the biology of human milk and its effects on the offspring. J Nutr 2007 Feb; 137(2):503S-510S.
2. Glahn RP: Got Milk? How about iron? Agricultural Research, July 2004. Available at http://www.ars.usda.gov/is/AR/archive/jul04/milk0704.htm. Accessed August 1, 2008.
3. Raj S, et al: A prospective study of iron status in exclusively breastfed term infants up to 6 months of age. Int Breastfeed J 2008 Mar; 1(3):3.
4. American Dental Association: Fluoride and fluoridation: infants, formula and fluoride. Available at www.ada.org/public/topics/fluoride/infantsformula.asp. Accessed September 18, 2008.
5. Marshall TA, et al: Associations between intakes of fluoride from beverages during infancy and dental fluorosis of primary teeth. J Am Coll Nutr 2004; 23:108-116.
6. Chouraqui JP, et al: Assessment of the safety, tolerance, and protective effect against diarrhea of infant formulas containing mixtures of probiotics or probiotics and prebiotics in a randomized controlled trial. Am J Clin Nutr 2008 May; 87(5):1265-1273.
7. Skripak JM, et al: The natural history of IgE-mediated cow's milk allergy. J Allergy Clin Immunol 2007 Nov; 120(5):1172-1177.
8. Merritt RJ, Jenks BH: Safety of soy-based infant formulas containing isoflavones: the clinical evidence. J Nutr 2004; 134(5):1220S-1224S.
9. Bhatia J, Greer F; Committee on Nutrition: Use of soy protein-based formulas in infant feeding. Pediatrics 2008 May; 121(5):1062-1068.
10. Von Berg AJ: Preventive effect of hydrolyzed infant formulas persists until age 6 years: long-term results from the German Infant Nutritional Intervention Study (GINI). J Allergy Clin Immunol 2008 Jun; 121(6):1442-1447.
11. Karjalainen S, et al: Association between early weaning, non-nutritive sucking habits, and occlusal anomalies in 3-year-old

Finnish children. Int J Paediatr Dent 1999 Sep; 9(3): 169-173.

12. Labbok MH, Hendershot GE: Does breastfeeding protect against malocclusion? An analysis of the 1981 Child Health Supplement to the National Health Interview Survey. Am J Prev Med 1987 Jul-Aug; 3(4):227-232.

13. Davis D, Bell PA: Infant feeding practices and occlusal outcomes: a longitudinal study. J Can Dent Assoc 1991 Jul; 57(7):593-594.

14. Page DC: Breastfeeding is early functional jaw orthopedics (an introduction). Funct Orthod 2001 Fall; 18(3):24-27.

15. Marshal TA, et al: Associations between intakes of fluoride from beverages during infancy and dental fluorosis of primary teeth. J Am Coll Nutr 2004 Apr; 23(2):108-116.

16. Collins CT, et al: Effect of bottles, cups and dummies on breastfeeding in preterm infants: a randomized controlled trial. BMJ 2004 Jul 24; 329(7459):193-198.

17. Fein SB, et al: Selected complementary feeding practices and their association with maternal education. Pediatrics 2008 Oct; 122(suppl):S91-S97.

18. Greer FR, et al: Effects of early nutritional interventions on the development of atopic disease in infants and children: the role of maternal dietary restriction, breastfeeding, timing of introduction of complementary foods, and hydrolyzed formulas. Pediatrics 2008 Jan; 121(1):183-191.

19. The Food Allergy and Anaphylaxis Network. Available at http://www.foodallergy.org/downloads/AboutFAAN2.pdf. Accessed August 2, 2008.

20. Poole JA, et al: Timing of initial exposure to cereal grains and the risk of wheat allergy. Pediatrics 2006 Jun; 117(6):2175-2182.

21. Adverse Reactions to Foods Committee, American College of Allergy, Asthma and Immunology: Food allergy and the introduction of solid foods to infants: A consensus document. Ann Allergy Asthma Immunol 2006 Oct; 97(4):559-560.

22. Krebs NF, et al: Meat as a first complementary food for breast-fed infants: Feasibility and impact on zinc intake and status. J Pediatr Gastroenterol Nutr 2006 Feb; 42(2):207-214.

23. Krebs NF: Food choices to meet nutritional needs of breast-fed infants and toddlers on mixed diets. J Nutr 2007 Feb; 137(2):511S-517S.

24. Hausner H: Differential transfer of dietary flavour compounds into human breast milk. Physiol Behav 2008 Sep 3; 95(1-2):118-124.

25. Forestell CA, Mennella JA: Early determinants of fruit and vegetable acceptance. Pediatrics 2007 Dec; 120(6):1247-1254.

26. Greer FR: 25-hydroxyvitamin D: functional outcomes in infants and young children. Am J Clin Nutr 2008 Aug; 88(Suppl):529S-533S.

27. Williams AL, Cox J, Gordon CM: Rickets in an otherwise healthy 11-month-old. Clin Pediatr (Phila) 2008 May; 47(4):409-412.

28. Ziegler E, et al: Vitamin D deficiency in breastfed infants in Iowa. Pediatrics 2006 Aug; 118(2):603-610.

29. Gordon CM, et al: Prevalence of vitamin D deficiency among healthy infants and toddlers. Arch Pediatr Adolesc Med 2008 Jun; 162(6):505-512.

30. Wagner CL, Greer FR, American Academy of Pediatrics Section on Breastfeeding: Prevention of rickets and vitamin D deficiency in infants, children, and adolescents. Pediatrics 2008 Nov; 122(5):1142-1152.

31. National Institutes of Health Office of Dietary Supplements. Available: http://ods.od.nih.gov/factsheets/vitamind.asp. Accessed January 30, 2009.

32. American Academy of Pediatric Dentistry: Guideline on fluoride therapy. Available at http://www.aapd.org/media/

Policies_Guidelines/G_FluorideTherapy.pdf. Accessed September 18, 2008.

33. Centers for Disease Control and Prevention (CDC): Oral health improving for most Americans, but tooth decay among preschool children on the rise. Trends in Oral Health Status: United States, 1988-1994 and 1999-2004. Series 11 No 248 (PHS) 2007-1698.

34. Dye BA, et al: The relationship between healthful eating practices and dental caries in children aged 2-5 years in the United States 1988-1994. J Am Dent Assoc 2004 Jan; 135(1):55-66.

35. National Institute of Dental and Craniofacial Research: Prevalence (number of cases) of cleft lip and cleft palate. Available at www.nidcr.nih.gov/DataStatistics/FindDataByTopic/CraniofacialBirthDefects/Prevalence. Accessed August 12, 2008.

36. Kostyak JC, et al: Relative fat oxidation is higher in children than adults. Nutr J 2007, Aug 16; 6:19.

37. Position of the American Dietetic Association: Nutrition guidance for healthy children ages 2 to 11 years. J Am Diet Assoc 2008 Jun; 108(6):1038-1047.

38. Daniels SR, Greer FT; Committee on Nutrition: Lipid screening and cardiovascular health in childhood. Pediatrics 2008 Jul; 122(1):198-208.

39. Lifshitz F, Tarim O: Considerations about dietary fat restrictions for children. J Nutr 1996; 126(4 Suppl):1031S-1041S.

40. USHHS: 2008 Physical Activity Guidelines for Americans. Available online: www.health.gov/paguidelines. Accessed January 10, 2008.

41. Mrdjenovic G, Levitsky DA: Children eat what they are served: the imprecise regulation of energy intake. Appetite 2005 Jun; 44(3):273-282.

42. Colapinto CK, et al: Children's preference for large portions: prevalence, determinants, and consequences. J Am Diet Assoc 2007 Jul; 107(7):1183-1190.

43. Florence MD, Asbridge M, Veugelers PJ: Diet quality and academic performance. J Sch Health 2008 Apr; 78(4):209-215.

44. Moore LL, et al: Effects of average childhood dairy intake on adolescent bone health. J Pediatr 2008 Nov; 153(5):667-673.

45. Gordon CM, et al: Prevalence of vitamin D deficiency among health infants and toddlers. Arch Pediatr Adolesc Med 2008 Jun; 162(6):505-512.

46. Moore CE, Murphy MM, Holick MF: Vitamin D intakes by children and adults in the United States differ among ethnic groups. J Nutr 2005; 135:2478-2485.

47. Svoren BM, et al: Significant vitamin D deficiency in youth with type 1 diabetes mellitus. J Pediatr 2009 Jan; 143(1):132-134.

48. National Institutes of Health Office of Dietary Supplements. Available: http://ods.od.nih.gov/factsheets/vitamind.asp. Accessed January 30, 2009.

49. Haire-Joshu D, et al: High 5 for kids: the impact of a home visiting program on fruit and vegetable intake of parents and their preschool children. Prev Med 2008 Jul; 47(1):77-82.

50. Nielsen SJ, et al: Trends in energy intake in US between 1977 and 1996: similar shifts seen across age groups. Obes Res 2002; 10:370-378.

51. Cusick SE, Mei Z, Cogswell ME: Continuing anemia prevention strategies are needed throughout early childhood in low-income preschool children. J Pediatr 2007 Apr; 150(4):422-428.

52. Centers for Disease Control and Prevention (CDC): Mental health in the United States: prevalence of diagnosis and medication treatment for attention-deficit/hyperactivity disorder—United States, 2003. MMWR Morb Mortal Wkly Rep 2005 Sept 2; 54(34):842-847. http://www.cdc.gov/mmwr/preview/mmwrhtml/mm5434a2.htm. Accessed August 12, 2008.

53. Wolraich ML, et al: The effects of sugar on behavior or cognition in children. JAMA 1995; 274(20):1617-1621.

54. Bateman B, et al: The effects of a double blind, placebo controlled, artificial food colorings and benzoate preservative challenge on hyperactivity in a general population sample of preschool children. Arch Dis Child 2004 Jun; 89(6):506-511.

55. Baumgaertel A: Diet and behavior in children. Nutr MD 2001 Dec; 27(12):1-6.

56. Stevenson J: Dietary influences on cognitive development and behavior in children. Proc Nutr Soc 2006 Nov; 65(4):361-365.

57. Devaney B, et al: Nutrient intake of infants and toddlers. J Am Diet Assoc 2004 Jan; 104(Suppl 1):S14-S21.

58. Skripak JM, et al: The natural history of IGE-mediated cow's milk allergy. J Allergy Clin Immunol 2007 Nov; 120(5):1172-1177.

59. Savage JH, et al: The natural history of egg allergy. J Allergy Clin Immunol 2007 Dec; 120(6):1413-1417.

60. Ly KA, Milgrom P, Rothen M: The potential of dental-protective chewing gum in oral health interventions. J Am Dent Assoc 2008 May; 139(5):553-563.

61. Ly KA, et al: Xylitol gummy bears snacks: a school-based randomized clinical trial. BMC Oral Health 2008 Jul 25; 8(1):20.

62. Knol LL, Haughton B, Fitzhugh EC: Food group adherence scores assess food patterns compared to US Department of Agriculture Food Guide. J Am Diet Assoc 2006 Aug; 106(8):1201-1208.

63. Moshfegh A, Goldman J, Cleveland L: What We Eat in America, NHANES 2001-2002: usual nutrient intakes from food compared to Dietary Reference Intakes. U.S. Department of Agriculture, Agricultural Research Service, 2005.

64. Lamberg-Allardt CJE, Viljakainen HT: 25-hydroxyvitamin D and functional outcomes in adolescents. Am J Clin Nutr 2008 Jul; 88(Suppl):534S-536S.

65. Field AE, et al: Relations between dieting and weight change among preadolescents and adolescents. Pediatrics 2003 Oct; 112(10):900-906.

66. Nielsen SJ, Popkin BM: Changes in beverage intake between 1977 and 2001. Am J Prev Med 2004 Oct; 27(3):205-210.

67. Shenkin J, et al: Soft drink consumption and caries risk in children and adolescents. Gen Dent 2003 Jan/Feb; 51(1):30-36.

68. Bowman SA: Beverage choices of young females: changes and impact on nutrient intakes. J Am Diet Assoc 2002 Sep; 102(9):1234-1239.

69. Affenito SG: Breakfast: a missed opportunity. J Am Diet Assoc 2007 Apr; 107(4):565-567.

70. Parnell W, et al: NZ Food, NZ Children: Key Results of the 2002 National Children's Nutrition Survey. Wellington, New Zealand: Ministry of Health, 2003.

71. Lien L: Is breakfast consumption related to mental distress and academic performance in adolescents? Public Health Nutr 2007 Apr; 10(4):422-428.

72. Larson NI, et al: Fast food intake: longitudinal trends during the transition to young adulthood and correlations of intake. J Adolesc Health 2008; 43(1):79-86.

73. Ponder SW: Childhood obesity: practical considerations for prevention and management. Diabetes Spectrum 2007; 20(3):148-153.

74. NCHS 2005 Prevalence of overweight among children and adolescents: United States, 1999-2002. National Center for Health Statistics. Available at: http://www.cdc.gov/nchs/products/pubs/pubd/hestats/overwght99.htm Accessed January 30, 2009.

75. Ogden CL, et al: High body mass index for age among US children and adolescents, 2003-2006. JAMA 2008 May 28; 299(20):2401-2405.

76. Drewnowski A: Obesity and the food environment: dietary energy density and diet costs. Am J Prev Med 2004 Oct; 27(3 Suppl):154-162.

77. Gillman MW, et al: Developmental origins of childhood overweight: potential public health impact. Obesity (Silver Spring) 2008 Jul; 16(7):1651-1656.

78. Gardner DSH, et al: Contribution of early weight gain to childhood overweight and metabolic health: a longitudinal study (EarlyBird 36). Pediatrics 2008 Dec 29; 123(1):e67-e73.

79. Shibli R, et al: Morbidity of overweight (≥85th percentile) in the first 2 years of life. Pediatrics 2008 Aug; 122(2):267-272.

80. August FP, et al: Guidelines for the Prevention and Treatment of Pediatric Obesity. J Clin Endocrin Metab. First published ahead of print Sept 9, 2008 as doi:10.1210/jc.2007-2458.

Chapter 14

Nutritional Requirements for Older Adults and Eating Habits Affecting Oral Health

LEARNING OBJECTIVES

Upon completion of this chapter, the student will be able to achieve the following objectives:

- Discuss ways to handle typical nutritional problems occurring in older adults.
- Know dental hygiene considerations of nutritional needs that occur in older patients.
- Identify nutrition education needs for older patients.
- Discuss physiological changes altering an older patient's nutritional status.

- Discuss differences in amounts of nutrients needed by older patients compared with younger patients.
- Describe factors influencing food intake of older patients.
- Suggest dietary changes that could be implemented to provide optimum nutrient intake for older patients.

KEY TERMS

Atrophic gastritis
Dysphagia
Functional foods
Homeostatic mechanisms

Hypogeusia
Incontinence
Nocturia
Sarcopenia

Test Your NQ

1. **T/F** Normal physiological changes occurring in older adults do not affect nutritional requirements.
2. **T/F** Nutritional requirements for a 50-year-old patient are different from those for an 81-year-old patient.
3. **T/F** Food selection is highly correlated with dentition.
4. **T/F** Edentulous patients should puree their food.
5. **T/F** Dehydration is seldom observed in older adults.

6. **T/F** Older adults need more vitamins D and B_{12} than individuals younger than 51 years.
7. **T/F** Healthy older women require increased amounts of iron.
8. **T/F** Energy requirements decrease with age.
9. **T/F** Self-medication with vitamins is a healthy practice for older adults.
10. **T/F** Exercise is of no benefit to older adults.

Major shifts in the age of the U.S. population are affecting healthcare needs in the United States. Compared with 2000, when approximately 35 million people were age 65 years and older (12.4% of the population), this population is expected to increase to approximately 80 million people (28.3%) by 2040.[1] The Census Bureau created a classification for older adults: young-old people are 65 to 74 years old, old people are 75 to 84 years old, and oldest-old people are 85 years old and older. The oldest-old group is the fastest growing segment of the older population, increasing the number of four-generation families.

Improved medical care and good nutrition since infancy have helped us increase our life span; it is important to increase the quality of that life by changing lifestyles and food choices. The *Dietary Guidelines for Americans 2005* recognize that people older than 50 years are one of the population groups that need special consideration. Some changes in food habits are needed in later life to adjust to the physical and metabolic changes that occur with aging. Dietary quality and obesity are two modifiable health risks and behaviors that can improve longevity and quality of life.[1] It is never too late to make lifestyle changes to improve one's health.

GENERAL HEALTH STATUS

The most common nutritional disorder in older individuals is obesity. In 2003-2004, about 31% of individuals older than 60 years were obese compared with 24% in 1990.[2,3] Obesity is more common in older women than in older men.[4] Surveys in the U.S. population indicate the prevalence of obesity increases progressively from 20 to 60 years of age and decreases after age 60 years. The rate of obesity in individuals who are older than 80 years is about half that observed in individuals 50 to 59 years old.[5]

Obesity causes serious medical complications and impairs quality of life. Approximately 80% of older Americans have one chronic disease, and 50% have two or more. Obesity contributes to several common chronic conditions in older adults, including cardiovascular diseases (hypertension, congestive heart failure, abnormal blood lipid values, and

stroke), diabetes, cancer, renal disease, and osteoporosis. Most of these conditions increase the risk of poor nutritional status. Routine nutritional care for older adults can help prevent or manage chronic diseases. Obesity can exacerbate the age-related decline in physical function and lead to frailty.[6] Studies reviewing the relationship between obesity-associated mortality risk in patients 75 years and older have yielded conflicting results. Voluntary weight loss seems to have a protective effect, however.

Malnutrition is another nutrition-related problem diagnosed in older adults admitted to hospitals or nursing homes or with serious medical problems. Several major identifiable biological or environmental circumstances or events that increase risk and suggest special care and attention have been identified as key risk factors of poor nutritional status in individuals older than age 65. An example of a nutritional assessment questionnaire is available on the Evolve website. Generally, individuals with less education and income; housebound individuals, especially those living alone; individuals with physical disabilities, depression, and other mental challenges; individuals with recent drastic lifestyle changes, such as death of spouse; and individuals who do not have regularly cooked meals are considered to be at risk of developing malnutrition.

Food choices are also related to oral problems, so a dental assessment should inquire about oral problems affecting intake. Identifying individuals at nutritional risk is critical to cost-effectiveness for the healthcare system and to assist older patients in maintaining their independence and personal well-being.

Dietary restrictions associated with management of chronic diseases, such as diabetes, renal disease, or heart disease, can be confusing, especially if more than one condition exists. Improper food selection or fear of choosing the wrong foods may be a factor for inadequate nutrition. The result of certain treatments, such as with cancer, can affect eating by creating loss of appetite, nausea and vomiting, diarrhea or constipation, xerostomia, or changes in the taste of food.

Many Americans older than 60 years take an average of five prescription medications and may take several over-the-counter medications each day. Some of these drugs can interfere with appetite and nutrient absorption. Although drug-nutrient interactions can compromise anyone's nutritional status, these problems are accentuated in older adults. Physiological and pathophysiological changes, such as decreased hepatic and renal clearance, result in greater variability and less predictability of a drug's effects.

PHYSIOLOGICAL FACTORS INFLUENCING NUTRITIONAL NEEDS AND STATUS

Age has an important impact on body composition. Many organ functions decline with age, some beginning as early as age 30. These physiological changes may significantly influence nutritional requirements of older adults by affecting absorption, transportation, metabolism, and excretion of nutrients. With aging, the body is less able to correct nutrient imbalances, such as increasing absorption when intake is decreased; the precarious physiological balance may be upset by disease, physical and mental challenges, and environmental, economic, and social disabilities. Chronological age and functional capacity do not always correlate, however. Older individuals differ from one another in physiological and health status more than any other age group, meaning that chronological status is not useful in predicting physiological abilities and health status.

Impairment of visual, auditory, and olfactory sensory organs is common. Poor vision makes food preparation difficult and even hazardous in some cases and may be responsible for senior citizens not identifying contaminated foods, which could lead to foodborne illnesses. Poor hearing increases isolation and decreases socialization.

ORAL CAVITY

Oral health problems (chewing, swallowing, and mouth pain) are indicators of nutritional risk and may be primary contributors to malnutrition. Persistent oral health problems are associated with impaired intake of certain foods and nutrients. When the ability to smell declines, cariogenic food choices usually increase. A progressive decline in gustatory and olfactory sensitivity affects food choices and quantity because "nothing tastes good." Olfactory and taste receptors are affected by impaired chewing and swallowing.

Some conditions and certain medications also lead to deterioration of taste sensitivity or perception. **Hypogeusia** (loss of taste) may be associated with certain disorders rather than being a normal component of the aging process. Older adults may confuse taste sensations, describing sour foods as metallic and salty foods as tasteless. Many people gradually begin to lose their sense of smell around age 50, a condition called anosmia. As a consequence of anosmia and hypogeusia, foods may be overly seasoned with salt or sugar. Losses in salt or sugar perception make it difficult to comply with low-sodium or diabetes guidelines. Other seasonings can help replace the taste of salt or sugar.

Xerostomia, which affects half of all older adults, compromises oral processing of foods and use of nutrients. Most individuals taking five medications report problems with xerostomia. Xerostomia causes difficulties with chewing and initiating a swallow. Lack of saliva increases the risk for oral disease because saliva contains antimicrobial components and minerals that can help rebuild tooth enamel after attack by acid-producing, decay-causing bacteria. Although crunchy foods stimulate saliva flow, older patients with xerostomia are more likely to avoid crunchy foods such as vegetables. They also tend to shun dry foods such as bread and sticky foods such as peanut butter. Many patients may choose hard candy or gum to stimulate saliva flow and relieve the dryness; however, this frequent exposure to fermentable carbohydrate promotes root caries and reduces intake of nutrient-dense foods (see Chapter 19 for further discussion of xerostomia).

The prevalence of root caries, discussed in Chapter 19, is much higher in older adults than in younger adults. Only 9.4% of individuals 20 to 29 years old have root caries compared with 31.6% for adults older than 60 years.[7] Recession of gingival tissues exposes root surfaces of teeth to the oral environment. The lack of a protective enamel layer on the root, surface roughness of roots, and demineralization owing to a lower pH make it highly susceptible to dental caries.

Periodontal disease increases the likelihood of weight loss in older adults; the more extensive and severe the disease, the greater the weight loss. Approximately 19% of individuals 55 to 64 years old and 23% of 65- to 74-year-olds have severe periodontal disease that is partially responsible for loss of teeth.[8] The function and position of the remaining teeth seem to indicate chewing ability more accurately than the total number of teeth present.

Edentulism is not inevitable with advancing age. A targeted goal for *Healthy People 2010* to decrease the percentage of older adults who have lost all their natural teeth is close to being met. From a percentage of 46% in 1971-1974, only 24% of adults 65 to 74 years old were edentulous in 2002.[9]

Calcium is readily mobilized from trabecular bone. A negative calcium balance results in loss of calcium from the maxilla and mandible, which are primarily trabecular bone. Normally, alveolar bone is maintained in response to occlusal forces associated with chewing. Age-related bone loss affecting the alveolar bone results in tooth loss and edentulism. Bone resorption accelerates and bone height rapidly diminishes in edentulous patients. The combination of periodontal disease and thinning bones may put postmenopausal women at particular risk of tooth loss. The primary risk factor for tooth loss is the degree of deterioration in the alveolar bones supporting the teeth. Because postmenopausal women lose bone at an increased rate, control of periodontal disease can significantly reduce their tooth loss.[10] Tooth loss and edentulism reflect differences in healthy behaviors, attitudes toward oral health, and dental care.

Most individuals in the United States older than 60 years have 19 teeth, and 25% of 65- to 74-year-olds are edentulous.[7] In the United States, there are significant disparities between socioeconomic groups and edentulism; these disparities have not improved between 1972 and 2001. Approximately 10% to 11% more lower income elderly individuals are edentulous than elderly individuals in higher income brackets.[11] Older people who have no or few teeth at age 70 are more likely to have mobility problems within the next 5 or 10 years, so tooth loss may be an early indicator of accelerated aging.[12]

Food selection is highly correlated with dentition. For partially edentate individuals, nutrient intake decreases as the total number of teeth decreases. Soft foods may replace consumption of some meats. Patients with seriously compromised natural dentition, periodontal conditions, edentulous areas, or ill-fitting appliances tend to alter their food choices to reduce chewing or because of fear of choking. Studies have found individuals with less than 28 teeth had significantly lower intakes of fruits and vegetables, especially raw carrots and tossed salads, and dietary fiber than did individuals with all their teeth, as well as lower serum levels for beta carotene, folate, and vitamin C.[13,14] A Japanese study found total protein, animal protein, sodium, vitamin D, vitamin B_1, vitamin B_6, niacin, and pantothenic acid were significantly associated with the number of teeth present.[15] Other studies indicate individuals who had lost numerous teeth were more likely to be obese than individuals with more teeth.[16] The nutrients beta carotene, vitamin C, and folate are consistently lower among edentulous individuals, but intake is affected more if the patient feels the dentures do not fit well.[17,18] Older women who have difficulty chewing or swallowing with their dentures have a higher risk of malnutrition, frailty, and mortality.[19]

Generally, patients who wear dentures have reduced masticatory efficiency—75% to 85% less than with natural teeth. After edentulous individuals fully adjust to new dentures, caloric intake increases, but magnesium, folic acid, fluoride, zinc, and calcium levels in their diets continue to be low.

Weight changes, often occurring in older adults, can be a reason for an ill-fitting dental appliance. Weight gain (usually secondary to edema) results in a tight-fitting denture, which may cause ulcerations; weight loss resulting in loose-fitting dentures also can increase risk of ulcerations. If severe mandibular resorption occurs, it is very difficult to construct a well-fitting dental prosthesis.

Nutrient intakes of patients with impaired dentition can fall below minimum requirements. Many older individuals or their families do not believe the cost of a new or replaced appliance is warranted because of the patients' perceived life expectancy. Even if they have dentures, some may not wear them, or they may be unable to chew because of a periodontal condition.

GASTROINTESTINAL TRACT

Changes in esophageal motility and deterioration of nerve function may cause **dysphagia** (difficulty with swallowing).

This frequently observed disorder increases risk of aspiration pneumonia and morbidity from inadequate nutrition. Individuals with swallowing problems eat slowly and may be unable to consume adequate amounts.

Atrophic gastritis is a chronic stomach inflammation with atrophy of the mucous membrane and glands and diminished hydrochloric acid production that is frequently observed in older patients. Diminished hydrochloric acid secretion may affect absorption of calcium, iron, and vitamin B_{12}. Additionally, the lack of acid permits overgrowth of bacteria that use much of the available vitamin B_{12}.

Constipation may be a consequence of altered gastrointestinal motility, along with loss of bowel muscle tone, inadequate food and fluid intake, low-fiber diet, and inactivity. Additional causes include chronic laxative use and some medications, especially analgesics, antihypertensives, and narcotics. Constipation may be corrected by increasing fiber-containing foods, fluid intake, and activity level.

HYDRATION STATUS

Decreased thirst sensations are associated with aging. Fluid intake may not increase automatically to offset increased water losses from the compromised kidney; dehydration occurs more frequently in older adults. As a result of poor fluid intake, susceptibility to caries is increased. **Homeostatic mechanisms** indicate the body's ability to correct imbalances, such as decreased nutrient intake accompanied by an increase in the nutrient's absorption or efficiency of use. Certain chronic illnesses (heart and kidney disease) lead to impairment of various homeostatic mechanisms controlling water balance. Fever, which can lead to mild dehydration in healthy individuals, may result in severe dehydration in older adults. Other seemingly mild stresses, such as the presence of infection or diarrhea, or the use of diuretics, can upset the normal homeostasis of an older individual. Dehydration is probably the primary cause of confusion in older hospitalized patients and can occur because of the kidney's inability to concentrate urine, altered thirst sensation, changes in functional status, side effects of medications, and mobility disorders. Dehydration can lead to loose-fitting dentures. Dehydration frequently results in hospitalization as a result of fecal impaction, cognitive impairment, and overall functional decline.

MUSCULOSKELETAL SYSTEM

Bone resorption progresses rapidly in older patients. Trabecular bone loss may be associated with physical inactivity, unavailability of calcium (inadequate dietary intake, imbalance in calcium-to-phosphorus ratio, and decreased calcium absorption), changes in hormones affecting calcium metabolism, lack of vitamin D, or altered vitamin D metabolism associated with impaired renal function. Bone loss increases susceptibility to fractures and possible disability. As discussed in Health Application 8, osteoporosis or shortening and outward bowing of the spine may develop.

Inactivity is responsible for loss of muscle strength and balance, conditions contributing to a fall. Physical activity can also help ameliorate some chronic health problems, yet two-thirds of people older than 65 do not exercise. An active lifestyle is also helpful in improving physiological well-being and relieving symptoms of depression and anxiety. Most older adults can be motivated to make changes that prevent or delay the spiral toward ill health and disability if the information is presented with an understandable rationale. The *2008 Physical Activity Guidelines for Americans* issued by the U.S. Department of Health and Human Services (USDHHS) addressing adults also apply to older adults[20] (see Chapter 6). If the older adult is unable to do 150 minutes of moderate-intensity aerobic activity a week because of health conditions, they should be as physically active as their abilities and conditions allow. Older adults with chronic conditions should understand whether and how their conditions affect their ability to do regular physical activity safely. Exercises that maintain or improve balance are recommended if falling is a risk.

After age 45, lean body mass declines up to 0.4% every year, and adipose tissue increases.[21] The amount of muscle a person has is determined in part simply by how much the muscles are used. Exercising muscles to the limits of their capacity, such as in weightlifting, results in maintaining or even increasing a person's muscle mass and strength.[22] Women have less muscle than men, but lose it more slowly during aging. Older women do not use protein as effectively as men, and it is harder for women to replace muscle that has been lost. Adequate amounts of protein are essential to replace muscle lost during the aging process.

Sarcopenia is the reduction of skeletal muscle mass and replacement by fat that occurs in older adults. This condition affects functional capacity, leading to frailty, reduced mobility, and loss of balance. If enough muscle is lost, it can be debilitating. This condition is not inevitable with aging, however. High-protein foods stimulate muscle protein synthesis, even in older adults.[23] Protein use may be impaired, but this can be overcome by consuming high-quality protein at each meal and doing resistance training. Maintaining muscle is essential in reducing the risk of falls.

Even if an individual's weight has not increased, the percentage of fat is probably increased. With aging, intra-abdominal fat increases more than subcutaneous or total body fat, and there is a greater relative decrease in peripheral than in central muscle mass because of loss of skeletal muscle.[24] As musculature shrinks, fat tissue accumulates. Instead of focusing on losing weight, the goal should be to increase muscle and reduce fat. A slightly higher body mass index (BMI) seems to be protective in maintaining immunity to diseases.

Less lean body mass results in a decreased basal metabolic rate (Fig. 14-1). In older individuals, the basal metabolic rate may be 10% to 12% below the level of 20-year-olds (see Chapter 6). In other words, the body burns fewer kilocalories than during earlier years, so less food is needed to prevent weight gain. Decreases in vital proteins result in an inability to respond to a physiological injury or insult and declining function of many organ systems. Muscle mass can be preserved by increasing physical activity. When older people diet without exercising, they lose more lean muscle

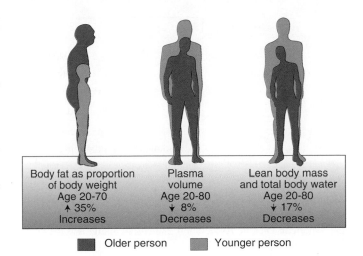

| Body fat as proportion of body weight Age 20-70 ↑ 35% Increases | Plasma volume Age 20-80 ↓ 8% Decreases | Lean body mass and total body water Age 20-80 ↓ 17% Decreases |

■ Older person   ■ Younger person

FIGURE 14-1 Changes in the body with aging. Younger person, age 20. Older person, age 80. (Redrawn from Vestal RE: Drugs and the Elderly. NIH Publication No. 79-1449. Washington, DC: U.S. Department of Health, Education, and Welfare, 1979.)

mass and less fat compared to those who exercise while dieting.[25]

SOCIOECONOMIC AND PSYCHOLOGICAL FACTORS

Many changes occur that may affect food intake of older adults (Fig. 14-2). Most retired people live on fixed incomes significantly lower than when they were employed. Inflation, failing health, and medical bills, especially cost of medications, can have a devastating effect on fixed incomes. The food budget frequently is affected and is a risk factor for inadequate nutrition. Fresh fruit and vegetable choices may be curtailed because of their high cost and limited shelf life. Title III Nutrition Programs for the Elderly (congregate dining and Meals-on-Wheels) are available to improve the nutritional and health status of older patients and possibly prevent or postpone more expensive services of long-term care institutions. Nutritious meals are furnished free to older adults who qualify or at a minimal charge. These programs have been proven to improve dietary intakes of recipients whose diets were previously below the estimated average requirement (EAR).[26]

An inability to drive or lack of access to transportation affects use of health services and availability of food. Approximately one-third of noninstitutionalized individuals older than 65 live alone. Individuals who live with another person and are socially active tend to consume a larger variety of foods. An inactive person who lives alone may lack motivation to prepare well-balanced meals, especially if the appetite is poor.

Apathy and depression can predispose older individuals to decreased appetite and interest in food. Depression is difficult to distinguish from symptoms related to the stresses of later life such as illness and changes in lifestyle. Some older individuals may consider depression as a natural and inevitable component of aging, and treatment may not be obtained. Loneliness is related to dietary inadequacies.

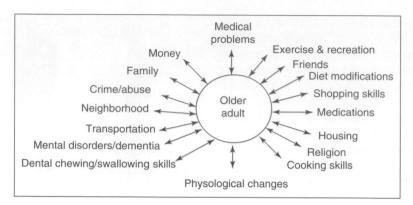

FIGURE 14-2 Multiple interrelated factors affecting nutritional status for older adults. (From American Dietetic Association: Position of the American Dietetic Association: Nutrition, aging, and the continuum of care. J Am Diet Assoc 2000 May; 100[5]:580-594.)

Dental Hygiene Considerations

Assessment

- *Physical*: blood pressure, diagnosis of chronic disease, dentures, swallowing process, xerostomia, condition of oral cavity and gingiva; financial status, socioeconomic status, mental status, educational level, psychological status; types of drugs taken, including over-the-counter drugs and aspirin use.
- *Dietary*: screen for nutritional health (see the assessment available on Evolve); motivation to eat and drink; beliefs and attitudes about foods or products to delay the aging process.

Interventions

- Encourage new denture wearers to swallow liquids with the dentures first, then to chew soft foods, and, last, to bite and masticate regular foods. It is easier to master the complex masticatory movements in this order, and the mouth is protected from becoming sore. New denture wearers need to eat slowly, chew the food longer, and cut raw fibrous foods such as apples and carrots into bite-size pieces.
- Wearing new dentures, especially by edentulous postmenopausal women, may promote positive calcium balance and decrease alveolar resorption. If calcium intake is poor, calcium supplements with vitamin D may help promote positive calcium balance.
- For edentulous patients, inquire about the preferred texture of food. Do not assume edentulous patients require pureed foods; because of lack of visual appeal and flavor, appetite may be affected if only pureed foods are offered.
- Teach older patients about appropriate oral hygiene techniques to minimize recession, followed with a fluoride regimen.
- Assess the fit of a denture or any prosthesis. The dental team may need to make recommendations for adjusting the prosthesis for a better fit or refer the older patient to a healthcare provider for assessment and management of unintentional weight changes.
- Encourage older patients to eat slowly and to chew food well.
- Often healthcare providers recommend lemon glycerin swabs to moisten oral tissues in patients with xerostomia.

This may be detrimental to the mouth for two reasons: (1) Because lemon is an acid, it may cause decalcification of the teeth, and (2) glycerin is a form of alcohol that can dry the oral tissues further. A better alternative would be to moisten a swab with water and apply it to the dry mucosa.
- Avoidance of certain food categories, such as fresh fruit and vegetables and meats, because of masticatory difficulties may aggravate other nutrition-related problems because these foods are major sources of vitamins and minerals.

Nutritional Directions

- Factors that slow the aging process include regular exercise, abstinence from smoking, and reduction of stress. Physical exercise and activity enhance muscle strength and preserve muscle mass.
- Less muscle tissue and a lower activity level result in a reduced caloric requirement.
- If xerostomia is present, use artificial saliva products (oral moisturizers), gum, or hard, sugarless candies (preferably containing xylitol); practice frequent oral hygiene care; and drink adequate noncariogenic fluids.
- For patients with a compromised natural dentition or xerostomia, suggest including fluids, sauces, or gravies with each meal to make chewing easier. However, beverage consumption should not interfere with food intake.
- Because of decreased stomach acid, older adults should take calcium citrate with vitamin D supplements between meals for optimal absorption or use calcium carbonate supplements with meals.
- Moderate exercise, such as walking, is beneficial in reducing cardiovascular risk in older adults.[27]
- By working out 45 minutes a day, older adults can improve muscle strength by 75% to 100% and bone density by 1% to 2%.[28] The promotion of physical activity in older adults should emphasize moderate-intensity aerobic activity, muscle-strengthening activity, reducing sedentary behavior, risk management, and balance exercise for individuals at risk of falling.[28]

Table 14-1 Dietary Reference Intakes for Selected Nutrients for Older Adults

Nutrients	Age 51-70 Years		Age Older than 70 Years	
	Men	Women	Men	Women
Protein (g)	56	46	56	46
Carbohydrate (g)	130	130	130	130
Fiber (g)	30*	21*	30*	21*
Fat-Soluble Vitamins				
Vitamin A (µg)	900	700	900	700
Vitamin E (mg)	15	15	15	15
Vitamin D (µg/IU)†	10/400*	10/400*	15/600*	15/600*
Water-Soluble Vitamins				
Ascorbic acid (mg)	90	75	90	75
Folate (µg)	400	400	400	400
Niacin (mg)	16	14	16	14
Riboflavin (mg)	1.3	1.1	1.3	1.1
Thiamin (mg)	1.2	1.1	1.2	1.1
Vitamin B_6 (mg)	1.7	1.5	1.7	1.5
Vitamin B_{12} (µg)†	2.4	2.4	2.4	2.4
Minerals				
Calcium (mg)	1200*	1200*	1200*	1200*
Phosphorus (mg)	700	700	700	700
Iodine (µg)	150	150	150	150
Iron (mg)	8	8	8	8
Magnesium (mg)	420	320	420	320
Zinc (mg)	11	8	11	8
Selenium (µg)	55	55	55	55

Data from Institute of Medicine, Food and Nutrition Board: Dietary Reference Intakes for: (1) Vitamin C, Vitamin E, Selenium, and Carotenoids (2000); (2) Calcium, Phosphorus, Magnesium, Vitamin D, and Fluoride (1997); (3) Vitamin A, Vitamin K, Arsenic, Boron, Chromium, Copper, Iodine, Iron, Manganese, Molybdenum, Nickel, Silicon, Vanadium, and Zinc (2001); (4) Carbohydrates, Fats, Protein, Fiber, and Physical Activity, Parts 1 and 2. Washington, DC: National Academies Pres.
Note: Recommended dietary allowances (RDAs) are presented in **bold type** and adequate intakes (AIs) are followed with an asterisk (*).
†1 µ cholecalciferol = 40 IU vitamin D.

NUTRIENT REQUIREMENTS

DIETARY REFERENCE INTAKES

Metabolism to maintain body functions requires all the same nutrients, but the requirements for most micronutrients are increased because of the effects of aging on absorption, use, and excretion. Energy needs are lower. The revised dietary reference intakes (DRIs) have separated the recommendations of individuals 51 to 70 years old and older than 70 years. With few exceptions, the recommended amounts for both groups are the same. However, recommendations for several nutrients differ from those for adults 31 to 50 years old, including fiber, calcium, chromium, iron (for women), and vitamins D and B_6 (Table 14-1).

FLUIDS

In normal situations, at least eight glasses of fluids per day are recommended (Fig. 14-3). Fluid intake is of particular concern because older individuals are susceptible to fluid imbalances secondary to the physiological changes. An older patient may intentionally restrict fluids because of **nocturia** (excessive urination at night), **incontinence**

(inability to control urinary excretion), pain associated with movement owing to arthritis, or having to request assistance to go to the toilet.

VITAMINS AND MINERALS

Older patients (especially women) usually have a negative calcium balance and lose bone mass, leading to osteoporosis and spontaneous fractures. Inadequate calcium intake is one possible reason for this, but genetic, hormonal, and environmental factors are also important. Decreased physical activity contributes to calcium loss over the years. The adequate intake (AI) of 1200 mg for calcium is higher than for younger adults to maintain bone mass and reduce risk of osteoporosis.

Some experts believe 90% of adults 51 to 70 years old are deficient in vitamin D.[29] The *Third National Health and Nutrition Examination Survey* (NHANES III) estimated 30% of individuals 60 years old and older who reside in lower latitudes have vitamin D insufficiency in the winter, and 26% residing in higher latitudes have vitamin D insufficiency in the summer.[30] Prevalence of vitamin D deficiency is even higher in homebound or institutionalized older individuals.

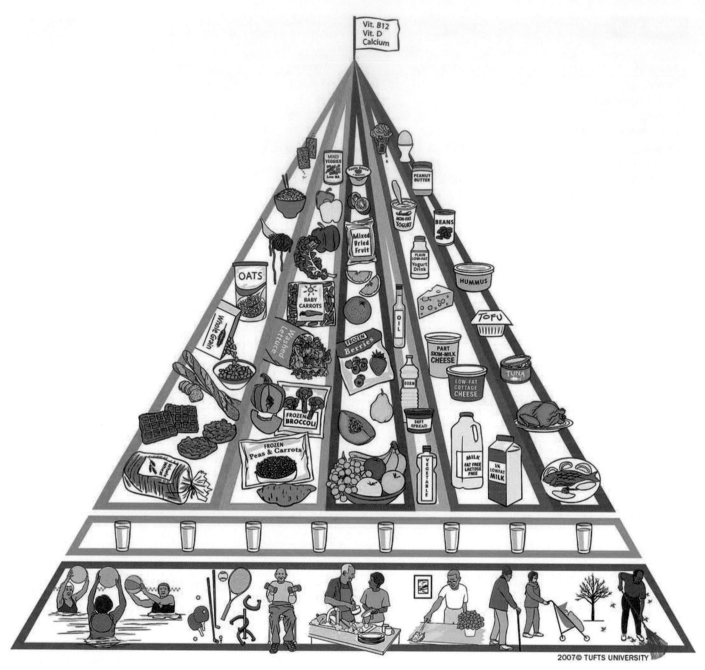

FIGURE 14-3 Modified MyPyramid for Older Adults. The Tufts University MyPyramid for Older Adults is geared to help individuals 50 years or older—and especially individuals 70 and older—eat a healthful diet. As individuals age, less food is needed to maintain weight. Vitamin and mineral requirements may stay the same or even increase, however, and so it is important to choose a variety of nutrient-rich foods every day. Also, older individuals need to include physical activity such as walking, climbing stairs, or yard work as part of their daily routine. (© 2007 Tufts University. Reprinted with permission from Lichtenstein AH, et al: Modified MyPyramid for Older Adults. J Nutr 2008; 138:78-82. Available at http://nutrition.tufts.edu.)

Vitamin D insufficiency leads to reduced active transport of calcium from the intestine. In older individuals with vitamin D insufficiency, supplementation reduces bone loss. Muscle performance also is improved, which reduces the risk of falling and fracture risk.[31,32]

Aging decreases the capacity of the skin to convert vitamin D precursors to the active form in the skin and kidneys. A deficiency may be the result of several causes that reduce production of vitamin D_3 by the skin, such as increased clothing to cover the skin and use of sunscreen. Other causes of vitamin D deficiency include dietary insufficiency, malabsorption, kidney disease, and use of glucocorticoids. To prevent problems with bone mineralization, the recommendation for vitamin D intake is higher than for younger adults: 10 µg daily for individuals 51 to 70 years old and 15 µg for individuals older than 70 years. It is important to ensure that patients receive adequate calcium in addition to vitamin D.

Because 10% to 30% of older adults have decreased absorption of vitamin B_{12}, choosing foods fortified with vitamin B_{12} or taking a vitamin B_{12} supplement is recommended to meet the DRIs. Neurological symptoms similar to dementia may result from deficiencies of vitamins B_6 and B_{12} and folate; intake is reported to be marginal. Economic factors and chewing problems may negatively affect meat consumption, thus negatively affecting vitamins B_6 and B_{12} intake. Physiological requirements for folic acid and vitamins B_6 and B_{12} are increased to prevent a decline in cognitive function associated with aging and to reduce risk for coronary artery disease. Cobalamin (vitamin B_{12}) may be less available in older adults because of atrophic gastritis and bacterial overgrowth. Studies have reported decreased symptoms (confusion, disorientation, and neurological problems) in individuals treated with vitamin B_{12}.[33]

In addition to these neurological symptoms, metabolic abnormalities may occur before vitamin B_{12} levels in the blood decrease; pernicious anemia occurs only in severely vitamin B_{12}–depleted individuals. When serum levels are depressed, low oral doses of vitamin B_{12} can be used rather than the painful and more expensive injections.[34] Oral vitamin B_{12} is effective in benefiting symptoms of depression in some older adults.[35]

Dietary mineral intake, especially sodium, may need to be adjusted based on the patient's physiological status. Excess or even normal dietary levels can have deleterious consequences in certain diseases, particularly chronic illness such as hypertension or congestive heart failure. Rigid and severe restrictions may seriously affect food acceptance. Individualization is crucial.

EATING PATTERNS

DEFICIENCIES

Compared with younger age groups, the diets of Americans older than 65 are rated better because of higher average consumption of fruits and lower consumption of sodium and cholesterol. The only notable deficiency for respondents older than age 65 was a lower proportion (less than one in four) meeting the recommended level of meat consumption. Approximately 21% of individuals 50 to 64 years old, 15% of individuals 65 to 79 years old, and 17% of individuals 80 years old and older consume a poor diet.[36]

Dairy products, fruits, and vegetables are frequently lacking in the diet, especially for individuals living alone. Milk provides needed calcium. However, daily consumption of milk is difficult because of its expense and the frequent trips needed to purchase it. Dry milk, although less palatable than regular milk, can be incorporated into many foods without deleterious effects on taste. Additionally, lactose intolerance may contribute to inadequate calcium intake (see Health Application 2). The choice of soft foods usually results in a decrease in protein and intake of more simple carbohydrates. Inadequate monetary resources to purchase meat products may result in less protein consumption. Elderly individuals at highest risk of consuming minimal amounts of fruits and vegetables are those who are socially isolated, are missing pairs of posterior teeth, have poor self-reported health, and are obese.[37]

SNACKS AND NUTRITIONAL SUPPLEMENTS

For some older adults, energy intakes decline. For those who have experienced weight loss, snacking may ensure older adults consume adequate amounts of kilocalories and protein.[38] Underweight is a recognized risk factor for disease and disability. Between-meal snacks can be used to offset some of the nutrient deficits. Healthy snacks such as cheese, hard-boiled eggs, low-fat milk products, bananas, and canned fruit can be recommended.

Milk-based food supplements, such as an Instant Breakfast mix, are economical and can help prevent nutrient deficiencies. A tasty supplement can augment overall nutrient intake to maintain nutritional status. Commercial liquid nutrition supplements, such as Ensure (Abbott Nutrition) and Sustacal (Mead Johnson Nutritionals), are more convenient and may be preferred. Some of these liquid supplements are lactose-free. Oral nutritional supplements for acutely ill patients can be used to improve nutritional status and avoid hospital admissions.[39] Referral to the healthcare provider or registered dietitian is recommended for these patients.

FOOD SAFETY

Foodborne illness can be very serious for older patients. Many older adults are more susceptible to foodborne illness because of a compromised immune system, decreased hydrochloric acid in the stomach, and reduced senses of smell and taste. Food poisoning (discussed more fully in Chapter 15) is caused by food contaminated with pathogenic bacteria, toxins, viruses, or parasites. The immune system, which helps to fight infection, is compromised in many elderly individuals.

MYPYRAMID FOR OLDER ADULTS

Tufts University developed *MyPyramid for Older Adults* (especially adults older than age 70) to help in selecting foods to ensure adequate amounts of nutrients (see Fig. 14-3). An updated version corresponds with the new MyPyramid. This information is readily accessible for people who may have limited computer skills or not have access to a computer.

MyPyramid for Older Adults emphasizes nutrient-dense food choices and the importance of fluid balance, but has additional guidance about forms of foods that best meet the unique needs of older adults and the importance of regular physical activity. Consistent with MyPyramid, *MyPyramid for Older Adults*, has six food groupings. Icons of foods within the groups include fruits and vegetables in different forms (packaged, frozen or canned, in addition to fresh) more appropriate for older adults. These choices require minimal preparation and have a longer shelf life, minimizing waste. Single-serve portions of canned fruits may be easier to prepare and have a longer shelf life. Fiber-rich foods are included, emphasizing whole-grain products and whole fruits and vegetables rather than juices. Low-fat and nonfat forms of dairy products, including reduced lactose alternatives, are shown in the milk group.

Additionally, *MyPyramid for Older Adults* stresses the importance of consuming fluids with a row of glasses as one of its foundations. Foods with high water content, such as lettuce and soups, can contribute significantly to fluid intake for people who are unaware they are not well-hydrated.

This pyramid also has a foundation depicting physical activities characteristic of older adults, such as walking and swimming. Regular physical activity is linked to reduced risk of chronic disease and lower body weight. It also can improve quality of life for older adults.

VITAMIN-MINERAL SUPPLEMENTS

For older adults, poor appetite, decreased sense of taste and smell, and denture problems all can contribute to a poor diet, as can eating alone and depression. Food is the best source of vitamins and minerals, so if additional food is needed for adequacy, healthy snacks should be encouraged. However, because of the increased need for calcium and vitamins D and B_{12}, along with decreased caloric requirements, *MyPyr-*

amid for Older Adults notes that supplements may be needed.

The flag at the top of *MyPyramid for Older Adults* is a reminder about the increased need for calcium and vitamins D and B_{12}. The older adult should discuss the need for nutritional supplements with the healthcare provider; natural food sources of nutrients are best. The amounts recommended for older adults each day are as follows:

- Calcium—1200 mg. For better absorption, this amount of calcium should be split into two 600-mg doses. Calcium not only keeps bones healthy, but also helps muscles function properly and normalize blood pressure.

Dental Hygiene Considerations

Assessment
- *Physical*: visual appraisal of weight status; dry mucous membranes.
- *Dietary*: adequacy of nutrients and fluid intake based on the Food Guide Pyramid for Older Adults; multivitamin/mineral/herbal use.

Interventions
- To prevent dehydration, encourage older patients to use caffeine in moderation and to take medications with 8 oz of fluid. If the patient refuses to drink water, soups, juices, and milk can be used to increase fluid intake.
- Encourage nutrient-dense foods, especially for older patients whose kilocalorie expenditure is low.
- Older patients who have had an unintentional weight change of 10% (loss or gain) in 6 months should be referred to a healthcare provider.
- Absorption of vitamin B_{12} from vitamin supplements or fortified foods is not affected by atrophic gastritis. Suggest enriched or fortified cereals to increase intake of iron and vitamin B_{12}.
- Encourage consumption of milk and milk products or addition of dry milk powder into foods.
- Encourage consumption of a vitamin C–rich food daily.
- Review economical sources of folate and cooking practices to retain folate.
- Encourage wise selections of convenience foods. Explain how to read food labels to make selections that are appropriate for restricted diets or to provide a well-balanced diet.

Nutritional Directions

- A well-balanced diet following the *MyPyramid for Older Adults* may delay symptoms of aging.
- A lack of vitamin B_{12} can cause poor memory and impaired balance.
- Nutrition counseling by a registered dietitian can provide information on consuming adequate amounts of high-quality protein to help patients living on a limited budget and offer alternatives to eating problems.
- Nonfat or low-fat milk provides an excellent source of calcium and vitamin D. Nonfat dairy products offer the best sources of calcium.
- Dietary intake should strive to optimize immune function and reduce disease risk of older adults.
- Calcium supplements should also contain vitamin D to enhance calcium absorption and increase bone density.
- Discuss economical fruit, vegetable, and meat selections (see Chapter 15).
- Adequate fluid intake is beneficial in preventing and treating constipation.
- Soups, juices, milk products, decaffeinated soft drinks, and decaffeinated tea and coffee can enhance fluid intake.
- Because many older adults cannot efficiently use vitamin B_{12} found in animal foods, vitamin B_{12} foods, such as breakfast cereals or supplements, are better absorbed.
- Older adults should check with their healthcare provider or registered dietitian to find out whether supplements are needed.
- Older patients should contact their healthcare provider when their food choices are limited over a period of time because of illness, chewing problems, lack of appetite, or inability to shop for or prepare food.
- Vitamin supplements more than 100% of the RDIs should be taken only in cases of specific need or recommendations of a healthcare provider. Use of vitamin-mineral supplements does not eliminate the need to consume a nutritionally balanced diet, and supplements do not protect against development of chronic diseases associated with inappropriate food intake.
- Excess supplementation of vitamins and minerals may cause more problems with hypervitaminosis and detrimental effects on other nutrients. Zinc supplements can result in copper imbalance and reduce high-density lipoprotein cholesterol levels. Refer the patient to a healthcare provider or registered dietitian.
- Heed food safety guidelines to ensure foods do not cause illness.

- Vitamin D—400 IU for adults 51 to 70 and 600 IU for adults older than 70 years. This should be taken in conjunction with calcium to increase calcium absorption. This recommendation should not be increased without a recommendation from the healthcare provider.
- Vitamin B_{12}—2.4 μg. Because of poor absorption of vitamin B_{12}, increased amounts are needed, which may help improve cognitive function and symptoms of depression and prevent pernicious anemia.[33,35]

The *Dietary Guidelines for Americans 2005* recommends eating fish twice a week. People who do not eat much fish could benefit from a fish oil supplement (300 mg of omega-3 fatty acid), which can help reduce triglyceride levels.

Sometimes food choices of older adults are not as well balanced as they should be, or less food is consumed to try to control weight. Because of impaired absorption of nutrients and reduced food intake, most individuals would profit from a multiple vitamin-mineral supplement. Daily multivitamin-mineral supplementation at 100% of the RDI levels is helpful in protecting older adults against a decline in immune response and preventing anemia.

The National Institutes of Health (NIH) panel advises elderly patients with early-stage macular degeneration to take antioxidants (vitamins C and E, beta carotene, and zinc). The amount of dietary antioxidants vitamin C, beta carotene, and zinc may be critical in some older adults. With age-related decreases in the activities of antioxidant enzymes, a sufficient supply of dietary antioxidants is important. Oxidative damage is thought to contribute to some deteriorating processes associated with aging and to promote cardiovascular disease, cognitive disorders, cancer, and diabetes mellitus, which occur more frequently in older individuals. Antioxidants are available in special formulations of multivitamin-mineral supplements. Referral to the healthcare provider or a registered dietitian is necessary to assess the need of supplements.

HEALTH APPLICATION Functional Foods

The term **functional foods** is a relatively new concept. "Functional" implies that the food has been identified as having value in providing some type of health benefits. Foods have always been known to provide therapeutic benefits, so all foods, because they provide nutritive value, are functional to some extent. After determining the role for essential elements (e.g., protein, carbohydrates, vitamins) of foods in deficiency diseases, scientists began to recognize physiologically active components from plant and animal products can reduce risk for various chronic diseases or otherwise provide desirable physiological effects. The U.S. Food and Drug Administration (FDA) defines functional foods as "foods and food components that provide a health benefit beyond basic nutrition (for the intended population). These substances provide essential nutrients often beyond quantities necessary for normal maintenance, growth, and development, and/or other biologically active imparting health benefits or desirable physiological effects."[40] Functional foods can include conventional foods; and fortified, enriched or enhanced foods. The American Dietetic Association warns against the implication some foods are "good" and others are "bad."[41] Various terms are used interchangeably—nutraceuticals, phytochemicals, and phoods, to name a few. Dietary supplements are not functional foods. Functional foods are found virtually in all food categories. Foods can be regarded as functional if proven to beneficially affect one or more target functions in the body, beyond adequate nutritional effects, in a way relevant to improved state of health and well-being, reduction of risk of diseases, or both.

Examples of functional foods include natural components of fruits and vegetables, milk, fortified or enhanced foods, and even some foods previously thought of as unhealthy, such as chocolate and wine. More than a dozen classes of biologically active plant chemicals are now known as phytochemicals and antioxidants (Table 14-2).

These natural components found in vegetables such as cabbage, carrots, broccoli, and tomatoes may reduce the risk of cancer. Foods that have been fortified to enhance the level of a specific food component include products such as calcium-fortified orange juice, fiber-supplemented snack bars, or folate enriched cereals. Oat products reduce serum cholesterol, reducing risk of coronary heart disease.

New food products are rapidly being developed with beneficial components, such as cholesterol-lowering margarine and products with soy protein. Red wine and chocolate, long thought of as being unhealthy, are now classified as functional foods. Red wine is associated with a reduced risk of cardiovascular disease, and chocolate has a high antioxidant count that has been shown to boost the immune system, decrease the risk of blood clots, and arrest DNA damage. Tea is associated with an increase in antioxidant activity and is linked to a reduction in cardiovascular disease risk.

Sometimes the press reports the results of a perfectly legitimate scientific study, or firms begin marketing a functional food on the basis of "emerging evidence." (For more information, see Chapter 15.) The scientifically sound approach to labeling and marketing a functional food is through the use of FDA-approved health claims as outlined by the Nutrition Labeling and Education Act (NLEA) discussed in Chapter 1. Under the NLEA, a health claim can be authorized by FDA with the consensus of qualified experts that scientific studies support the validity of the relationship described in that claim. Scientific agreement would require consistent findings from well-designed clinical, epidemiological studies and expert opinions from a body of independent scientists. There is strong evidence for some of the claims, but only weak evidence for others. As research confirms links between food components and health, the FDA will permit more health claims on these foods.

HEALTH APPLICATION 14   Functional Foods—cont'd

In some cases, consumers worry about new technology that may influence the acceptance of these products. They may tend to prefer natural as opposed to synthetic additives. Lack of nutritional knowledge may limit the acceptance of functional foods. Use of health claims may help ensure consumers are aware of the health benefits of a food. However, people should not automatically assume that consuming functional foods will allow them to improve their health. Adding a food containing a particular nutrient does not mean the nutrient will have the desired effect. Whether these foods are beneficial depends on several factors.

Research regarding how foods or food components and dietary supplements may promote health and reduce chronic disease is providing a fast stream of information. Dietary recommendations from established scientific authorities are slow to react to this growing body of information because of the need for a strong, consensus-based body of evidence before changing dietary advice for the public. Increasing the intake of selected foods may not be wise without considering potential negative consequences, and whether or not these specific elements are needed. Factors such as the overall nutritional value and calorie intake of an individual's diet, and whether sound scientific evidence backs the claims on the package labels should be considered before routinely choosing these foods. When evaluating functional foods, safe levels of intake must be considered. In many cases, optimal levels of nutrients and other physiologically active components in functional foods have yet to be determined.

A person who does not have cardiovascular heart disease or an elevated cholesterol level would not benefit from using sterol-enhanced products. The vitamins in vitamin-enhanced drinks are probably well absorbed, but the vitamins may not be the ones lacking in the diet, and most of the products on the market have more sugar than a regular soda. Many products are available indicating improvement of athletic performance, conditioning, recovery from fatigue after exercise, and avoidance of injury. Some of these claims may be valid. However, these foods should be used only when scientific evidence clearly supports the claim, and with understanding of the physiological changes caused by the functional ingredient. The best way a consumer can evaluate the effectiveness of a food product is by trying it for several weeks and seeing if any benefits result.

Functional foods are an important part of wellness offering great potential for consumers to optimize their health through diet, but they are not "magic bullets" or a universal panacea for poor health habits. Functional foods are not a substitute for a well-balanced diet and regular physical activity within the framework of a healthy lifestyle. Consumers will probably continue to choose functional foods they enjoy eating, are familiar and readily available to them. This helps explain why many Americans are unlikely to incorporate foods like soy into their diet. When referring to functional foods, the important thing is that what you do eat may be more important to your health than what you do not eat. The best advice is to counsel consumers about appropriate intake of functional foods and strategies for achieving dietary intake goals in the context of a healthful diet, based on MyPyramid to optimize health and potentially to decrease the risk of chronic diseases.

Table 14-2   Examples of Functional Components*

Class/Component	Source	Potential Benefit
Carotenoids		
Beta carotene	Carrots, pumpkin, sweet potato, cantaloupe	Neutralizes free radicals that may damage cells; bolsters cellular antioxidant defenses; can be made into vitamin A in the body
Lutein, zeaxanthin	Kale, collard, spinach, corn, eggs, citrus	May contribute to maintenance of health vision
Lycopene	Tomatoes and processed tomato products (more effective after heating), watermelon, red/pink grapefruit	May contribute to maintenance of prostate health
Dietary (Functional and Total) Fiber		
Insoluble fiber	Wheat bran, corn bran, fruit skins	May contribute to maintenance of a healthy digestive tract; may reduce risk of some types of cancer
Beta glucan†	Oat bran, oatmeal, oat flour, barley, rye	May reduce risk of CHD
Soluble fiber†	Psyllium seed husk, peas, beans, apples, citrus fruit	May reduce risk of CHD and some types of cancer
Whole grains†	Cereal grains, whole-wheat bread, oatmeal, brown rice	May reduce risk of CHD and some types of cancer; may contribute to maintenance of healthy blood glucose levels

CHD, coronary heart disease.
*Examples are not an all-inclusive list.
†FDA-approved health claim established for component.
Data from Functional Foods. International Food Information Council, July 2006. Available at http://ific.org/nutrition/functional/indext. cfm?renderforprint=1. Accessed August 18, 2008.

Table 14-2	Examples of Functional Components*—cont'd	
Class/Component	**Source**	**Potential Benefit**
Fatty Acids		
Monounsaturated fatty acids (MUFAs)†	Tree nuts, olive oil, canola oil	May reduce risk of CHD
Omega-3 fatty acids—Linoleic acid	Walnuts, flax	May contribute to maintenance of heart health; may contribute to maintenance of mental and visual function
Omega-3 fatty acids—docosahexaenoic acid (DHA) and eicosapentaenoic acid (EPA)	Salmon, tuna, marine, and other fish oils	May reduce risk of CHD; may contribute to maintenance of mental and visual function
Conjugated linoleic acid (CLA)	Beef and lamb; some cheese	May contribute to maintenance of desirable body composition and health immune function
Flavonoids		
Anthocyanins—cyanidin, delphinidin, malvidin	Berries, cherries, red grapes	Bolster cellular antioxidant defenses; may contribute to maintenance of brain function
Flavanols—catechins, epicatechins, epigallocatechin, procyanidins	Tea, cocoa, chocolate, apples, grapes	May contribute to maintenance of heart health
Flavonols—quercetin, kaempferol, isorhamnetin, myricetin	Onions, apples, tea, broccoli	Neutralize free radicals that may damage cells; bolster cellular antioxidant defenses
Proanthocyanidins	Cranberries, cocoa, apples, strawberries, grapes, wine, peanuts, cinnamon	May contribute to maintenance of urinary tract health and heart health
Isothiocyanates		
Sulfoaphane	Cauliflower, broccoli, broccoli sprouts, cabbage, kale, horseradish	May enhance detoxification of undesirable compounds; bolsters cellular antioxidant defenses
Plant Stanols/Sterols		
Free stanols/sterols†	Corn, soy, wheat, wood oils, fortified foods and beverages	May reduce risk of CHD
Stanol/sterol esters†	Fortified margarine, stanol ester dietary supplements	May reduce risk of CHD
Polyols		
Sugar alcohols†—xylitol, sorbitol, mannitol, lactitol	Some chewing gums and other food	Applications may reduce risk of dental caries
Prebiotics		
Inulin, fructo oligosaccharides (FOS), polydextrose	Whole grains, onions, some fruits, garlic, honey, leeks, fortified foods and beverages	May improve gastrointestinal health; may improve calcium absorption
Probiotics		
Yeast, lactobacilli, bifidobacteria, other specific strains of beneficial bacteria	Certain yogurts and other cultured dairy and nondairy products	May improve gastrointestinal health and systemic immunity; benefits are strain specific
Phytoestrogens		
Isoflavones—daidzein, genistein	Soybeans and soy-based foods	May contribute to maintenance of bone health, and healthy brain and immune function; for women, may contribute to maintenance of menopausal health
Lignans	Flax, rye, some vegetables	May contribute to maintenance of heart health and healthy immune function
Soy Protein		
Soy protein	Soybeans and soy-based products	May reduce risk of CHD
Sulfides/Thiols		
Diallyl sulfide, allyl methyl trisulfide	Garlic, onions, leeks, scallions	May enhance detoxification of undesirable compounds; may contribute to maintenance of heart health and healthy immune function
Dithiolthiones	Cruciferous vegetables	May enhance detoxification of undesirable compounds; may contribute to maintenance of healthy immune function

CASE APPLICATION FOR THE DENTAL HYGIENIST

A 75-year-old edentulous patient is not eating because he states he has difficulty chewing, and food does not taste good. He reports he dislikes a lot of red meat and milk. He has lost 14 lb since his last recall appointment (usual weight 170 lb).

Nutritional Assessment
- Height; weight; appropriateness of BMI; significant weight changes, especially loss
- Nutrient and fluid intake in relation to DRIs
- Medications
- Alterations in taste, smell, or vision
- Support group, significant others, living arrangements, social support
- Psychological status

Nutritional Diagnosis
Altered nutrition: less than body requirements related to taste changes and chewing difficulty.

Nutritional Goals
The patient will consume a well-balanced diet (based on the *MyPyramid for Older Adults*) and verbalize ways to increase protein and calcium intake and exercise.

Nutritional Implementation
Intervention: Encourage small, frequent meals.
Rationale: This helps the older patient consume adequate amounts of nutrients by decreasing fatigue and feelings of fullness that may occur with larger meals.
Intervention: Suggest use of spices such as pepper, thyme, and basil.
Rationale: These spices may improve the taste of foods because the older patient's ability to detect tastes is altered.
Intervention: Encourage fluids with meals.
Rationale: Drinking fluids with meals makes chewing and swallowing easier.
Intervention: Examine and question about the fit of the prosthesis. Clinically, conduct an intraoral and extraoral examination, especially noting any deviations from normal of the underlying tissue.
Rationale: The weight change may have created a loose-fitting denture and ultimately difficulty in chewing. An ill-fitting denture may also result in weight loss.

Intervention: Teach the patient to perform an oral self-examination.
Rationale: The patient also can identify oral problems earlier for more effective treatment.
Intervention: Emphasize use of eggs, turkey, chicken, fish, tenderized meat in marinates (e.g., wine or vinegar), and soy products such as tofu and bacon bits.
Rationale: Because he does not like red meats, the patient may obtain needed protein in a more acceptable manner.
Intervention: Emphasize the use of low-fat or nonfat dairy products, such as yogurt, cream cheese, cheese, or frozen yogurt.
Rationale: His dislike of milk lessens the likelihood of his choosing milk; these foods are alternatives to supply the needed calcium.
Intervention: Encourage adding powdered milk to soups, sauces, cereals, and casseroles.
Rationale: These are methods to increase protein and calcium consumption.
Intervention: Encourage the patient to walk outdoors for 10 to 20 minutes daily and to eat foods that require more chewing, such as lettuce salads, raw carrots, and cabbage.
Rationale: Exercise is important to maintain bone density in the mandible and throughout the body. Available dietary calcium is better absorbed because it is dependent on vitamin D, which can be obtained through sunshine.
Intervention: Suggest mixing meat with vegetables.
Rationale: Because he enjoys vegetables, this form may be more palatable for him and would enhance protein intake.
Intervention: Refer the patient to Meals-on-Wheels or another federally funded program (food stamps), community meals centers, or church-sponsored centers.
Rationale: Anorexia may be due to a lack of socialization during mealtimes.

Evaluation
The patient should be eating at least 75% of the number of food servings from MyPyramid and steadily gain weight until desired body weight is achieved. Other behaviors, such as consuming yogurt, eggs, fish, and dry milk in foods, will increase calcium and protein intake.

STUDENT READINESS

1. Plan a day's menus for an older edentulous patient.
2. What are some vitamin and mineral deficiencies that might influence mental attitudes of older patients?
3. Discuss reasons older patients might not eat adequately.
4. Visit a group meal program. Review the menu with the registered dietitian, and discuss beneficial effects of the program's various activities.
5. List nutritional interventions to help a healthy older patient with full dentures to eat a well-balanced diet.
6. Observe the staff at an extended-care facility, and note positive activities related to maintaining good oral health and activities that can be improved.
7. Why are older individuals prone to dehydration? How can dehydration affect oral status?
8. Describe the procedure for introducing food intake for new denture wearers.
9. What are some suggestions you could make for a patient experiencing xerostomia?
10. Name three differences in *MyPyramid for Older Adults* and MyPyramid for Americans.

CASE STUDY

A 75-year-old man widowed for 2 years is seen in the health-care clinic for decreased intake. He states nothing tastes good. He is on a limited, fixed income from Social Security.

He has lost 6 lb within the last year. His current weight is 130 lb, and his height is 5 feet, 7 inches. He is edentulous and refuses to get dentures because he feels he is "too old."

He fixes a bologna sandwich occasionally, but mostly eats frozen food dinners. He thinks meats and fruits are too expensive to buy, and states, "They spoil before I can eat them." He eats overcooked vegetables in the summer because a neighbor shares fresh produce from his garden. He does not want to use any community resources because he objects to "a handout."

1. Explain why "food does not taste good."
2. What psychological and social factors may influence his dietary patterns?
3. What are some practical ways to increase protein and calcium in his diet?
4. How could you address his attitude of not wanting to accept "a handout"?
5. What medical and dental information should you assess on this man to determine nutritional status?
6. What are the strengths and weaknesses of his diet?
7. What behaviors would indicate this patient is meeting his nutritional needs?

References

1. Federal Interagency Forum on Aging-Related Statistics: Older Americans Update 2006: Key Indicators of Well-Being. Washington, DC: U.S. Government Printing Office, May 2006. Available at http://www.agingstats.gov/. Accessed August 16, 2008.
2. Ogden CL, et al: Prevalence of overweight and obesity in the United States, 1999-2004. JAMA 2006 Apr 5; 295(13):1549-1555.
3. Arterburn DE, et al: The coming epidemic of obesity in elderly Americans. J Am Geriatr Soc 2004 Nov; 52:1907-1912.
4. Flegal KM, et al: Prevalence and trends in obesity among US adults, 1999-2000. JAMA 2002 Oct 9; 288(4):1723-1727.
5. Villareal DT, et al: Obesity in older adults: technical review and position statement of the American Society for Nutrition and NAASO, The Obesity Society. Am J Clin Nutr 2005 Nov; 82(5):923-924.
6. Lang IA, et al: Obesity, physical function, and mortality in older adults. J Am Geriatr Soc 2008 Aug; 56(8): 1474-1478.
7. Beltrán-Aguilar ED, et al: Surveillance for dental caries, dental sealants, tooth retention, edentulism, and enamel fluorosis— United States, 1988-1994 and 1999-2002. Centers for Disease Control and Prevention (CDC), 2005 Aug 26; 4(3):1-44.
8. U.S. Department of Health and Human Services: Oral Health in America: A Report of the Surgeon General. Rockville, MD: U.S. Department of Health and Human Services, National Institute of Dental and Craniofacial Research, National Institutes of Health, 2000.
9. Centers for Disease Control and Prevention (CDC): The state of aging and health in America report. Available at //apps.nccd. cdc.gov/saha/HPTargets.aspx. Accessed August 16, 2008.
10. Tezal M, et al: Periodontal disease and the incidence of tooth loss in postmenopausal women. J Periodontol 2005 Jul; 76(7):1123-1128.
11. Cunha-Cruz J, Hujoel PP, Nadanovsky P: Secular trends in socio-economic disparities in edentulism: USA, 1972-2001. J Dent Res 2007 Feb; 86(2):131-136.
12. Holm-Pedersen P, et al: Tooth loss and subsequent disability and mortality in old age. J Am Geriatr Soc 2008 Mar; 56(3):429-435.
13. Nowjack-Raymer RE, Sheiham A: Numbers of natural teeth, diet, and nutritional status in US adults. J Dent Res 2007 Dec; 86(12):1171-1175.
14. Sheiham A, et al: The impact of oral health on stated ability of eating certain food: findings from the National Diet and Nutrition Survey of Older People in Great Britain. Gerontology 1999; 16:11-20.
15. Yoshihara A, et al: The relationship between dietary intake and the number of teeth in elderly Japanese subjects. Gerodontology 2005 Dec; 22(4):211-218.
16. Sheiham A, et al: The relationship between oral health status and body mass index among older people: a national survey of older people in Great Britain. Br Dent J 2002; 192:703-706.
17. Nowjack-Raymer RE, Sheiham A: Association of edentulism and diet and nutrition in U.S. adults. J Dent Res 2003 Feb; 82(2):123-126.
18. Sahyoun NF, Krall E: Low dietary quality among older adults with self-perceived ill-fitting dentures. J Am Diet Assoc 2003 Nov; 103(11):1494-1499.
19. Semba RD, et al: Denture use, malnutrition frailty, and mortality among older women living in the community. J Nutr Health Aging 2006 Mar-Apr; 10(2):161-167.
20. USHHS: 2008 Physical Activity Guidelines for Americans. Available online: www.health.gov/paguidelines. Accessed January 10, 2009.
21. Smith GI, et al: Differences in muscle protein synthesis and anabolic signaling in the postabsorptive state and in response to food in 65-80 year old men and women. PLoS ONE 2008 Mar 26; 3(3):e1875.
22. Tufts University: 10 determinants of aging you can control. Tufts University Health & Nutrition Letter 2006 May; 24(5): 2-3.
23. Symons TB, et al: Aging does not impair the anabolic response to a protein-rich meal. Am J Clin Nutr 2007 Aug; 86(2):451-456.
24. Beaufrere B, Morio B: Fat and protein redistribution with aging: metabolic considerations. Eur J Clin Nutr 2000, 54(Suppl):S48-S53.
25. Amati F, et al: Separate and combined effects of exercise training and weight loss on exercise efficiency and substrate oxidation. J Appl Physiol 2008 Sept; 105(3:)825-831.
26. Roy MA, Payette H: Meals-on-Wheels improves energy and nutrient intake in a frail free-living elderly population. J Nutr Health Aging 2006 Nov-Dec; 10(6):554-560.
27. Tufts University: New exercise rules add goals for seniors. Tufts University Health & Nutrition Letter 2007 Nov 25(9):1-2.
28. Nelson ME, et al: Physical activity and public health in older adults: recommendation from the American College of Sports Medicine and the American Heart Association. Med Sci Sports Exerc 2007 Aug; 39(8):1435-1445.
29. Dawson-Hughes B: Serum 25-hydroxyvitamin D and functional outcomes in the elderly. Am J Clin Nutr 2008 Aug; 88(Suppl):537S-540S.
30. Looker AC, et al: Serum 25-hydroxyvitamin D status of adolescents and adults in two seasonal subpopulations from NHANES III. Bone 2002 May; 30(5):771-777.
31. Wicherts IS, et al: Vitamin D status predicts physical performance and its decline in older persons. J Clin Endocrinol Metab 2007 Jun; 92(6):2058-2065.

32. Dawson-Hughes B: Serum 25-hydroxyvitamin D and functional outcomes in the elderly. Am J Clin Nutr 2008 Aug; 88(Suppl):537S-540S.

33. Clarke R, et al: Low vitamin B_{12} status and risk of cognitive decline in older adults. Am J Clin Nutr 2007 Nov; 86(11):1384-1391.

34. Blacher J, et al: Very low oral doses of vitamin B_{12} increase serum concentrations in elderly subjects with food-bound vitamin B_{12} malabsorption. J Nutr 2007 Feb; 137(2): 373-378.

35. Garibalia S, Forster S: Effects of dietary supplements on depressive symptoms in older patients: a randomized double-blind placebo-controlled trial. Clin Nutr 2007 Oct; 26(5):545-551.

36. Finke MS, Huston SJ: Healthy eating index scores and the elderly. Fam Economic Nutr Rev 2003; 15(1):67-73.

37. Sahyoun NR, Zhang XL, Serdula MK: Barriers to the consumption of fruits and vegetables among older adults. J Nutr Elder 2005; 24(4):5-21.

38. Zizza CA, Tayie FA, Lina M: Benefits of snacking in older Americans. J Am Diet Assoc 2007 May; 107(5):800-806.

39. Gariballa S, et al: A randomized, double-blind, placebo-controlled trial of nutritional supplementation during acute illness. Am J Med 2006 Aug; 119(8):693-699.

40. U.S. Department of Health and Human Services, Food and Drug Administration: Conventional foods being marketed as 'functional' foods. Fed Reg 21 CFT Parts 101 and 170, October 25, 2006. Accessed August 18, 2008.

41. American Dietetic Association: Position of the American Dietetic Association: Functional foods. J Am Diet Assoc 2004 May; 104(5):814-826.

Chapter 15

Other Considerations Affecting Nutrient Intake

LEARNING OBJECTIVES

Upon completion of this chapter, the student will be able to achieve the following objectives:

- Explain how a patient can obtain adequate nutrients from different cultural food patterns.
- Identify reasons for food patterns.
- Respect cultural and religious food patterns while providing nutritional counseling for patients.
- Describe food preparation and storage techniques to retain nutrient value.

- Provide referral sources for nutritional resources.
- Identify patient education necessary for economical food purchases.
- Explain the effects of food processing, convenience foods, and fast foods on a patient's overall intake.
- Discuss reasons why food additives are used.
- List reasons why health quackery can be dangerous.
- Identify common themes of health quackery and why they are contrary to evidence-based research.

KEY TERMS

Dietary acculturation
Food fad
Food insecurity
Food patterns
Food quackery
Irradiated foods

Nanotechnology
Nutrient density
Nutritionist
Organic
Stable nutrients

Test Your NQ

1. **T/F** Religion can affect food patterns.
2. **T/F** Adults usually avoid the foods they ate during childhood.
3. **T/F** The nutritional content of food is the most important determinant for food choices.
4. **T/F** Consumers spend less than 10% of their income on food.
5. **T/F** Fad diets are usually well balanced and nutritious.

6. **T/F** Organic foods are more nutritious.
7. **T/F** All processing of foods is detrimental to the nutritional quality of foods.
8. **T/F** Fast foods are usually a good source of protein.
9. **T/F** Food additives can be used to improve the nutritional value of foods.
10. **T/F** Individual food preferences do not ordinarily influence nutritional adequacy of the diet.

FOOD PATTERNS

In terms of food choices, people are creatures of habit. Patterns throughout societies are quite evident; however, the term *habit* connotes inflexibility. People change their food habits for numerous reasons; hence, the term *food pattern* is more descriptive of food choices. Many factors are associated with formation of **food patterns** and preferences. Food patterns are generally developed during childhood and reflect the family's lifestyle and its ethnic or cultural, social, religious, geographical, economic, and psychological components. All of these influence one's attitudes, feelings, and beliefs about food. However, the factors that seem to predominate in food choices are cultural and economic.

No culture has ever been known to make food choices solely on the basis of nutritional and health values of food. Nutritional value is secondary, especially if a food has established social, religious, or economic status. For example, broccoli is one of the most nutritious vegetables (based on nutrient density) available in the United States, but is a less popular vegetable, whereas the tomato, the most commonly eaten vegetable, rates 16th as a source of vitamins and minerals. **Nutrient density** is the amount of nutrients in a food relative to the number of kilocalories it provides. A raw carrot is more nutrient dense than a candy bar because the carrot contains more nutrients per kilocalorie.

Dental hygienists who recognize good nutrition can be achieved by using many different types of food respect patients' needs to stretch their food dollar and choose culturally acceptable foods. Advice that takes into consideration a patient's needs and food preferences is more likely to be followed.

CULTURAL INFLUENCES

The United States is more culturally diverse today than at any time in its history. The immigrant population has changed dramatically. Dietary needs unique to foreign-born immigrants have a direct impact on the national health of the United States. The ethnic and cultural diversity of the U.S. population presents new challenges to health professionals in offering culturally sensitive interventions to improve the health of these people. One of the most interesting and visible ways cultural identity is expressed is through an individual's food choices. Although milk is the only food used worldwide, many cultures consider it appropriate only for infants and children.

Children of different cultures accept as the norm what adults in their family eat. Cultural food patterns establish the foundation for a child's lifelong eating patterns regarding time and number of meals per day, foods acceptable for specific meals, preparation methods, likes and dislikes, foods suitable for specific members of a group, table manners, the social role of foods and eating, and attitudes toward eating and health. Patterns and attitudes internalized during childhood promote a sense of stability and security for the adult (Fig. 15-1).

Many ethnic groups have brought a rich heritage of various food patterns to the United States that has resulted in distinct and discrete patterns of food consumption. Although American diets are diversified, they have become more homogeneous because of transportation, advertising, mobility, new methods of production, changes in income

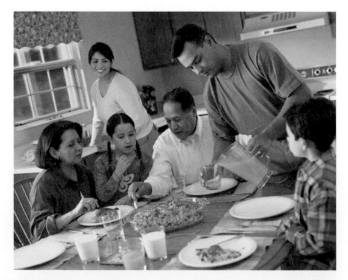

FIGURE 15-1 Eating habits are established at a very young age. (From Food and Nutrition Service, U.S. Department of Agriculture and Food and Nutrition Information Center, National Agricultural Library: Food stamp nutrition collection: photo gallery. Beltsville, MD, 2005. Retrieved December 9, 2005, from http://grande.nel.usda.gov/foodstamp_album.php?mode=mealtime.)

distribution, and appreciation of one another's heritage. Food preferences have remained quite consistent over the past decade in the United States, however—few people in the northern states would routinely choose grits, and many Southerners would not recognize lentils. Individual food preferences do not influence nutritional adequacy of the diet. Insufficient quantities of food groups (milk, fruits, vegetables, cereals, and meats) have the greatest effect on nutritional adequacy rather than specific aversions, such as a dislike of turnips or rye bread.

STATUS AND SYMBOLIC INFLUENCES

Various cultures may regard a food differently. For example, beef is regarded as a high-status food among some people in the United States, but some Hindus from India consider cows sacred and do not eat beef. The choice of different foods is influenced by religious beliefs, availability, cost, cultural values, and traditions, or even the endorsement or condemnation of a highly respected person.

Because of symbolic meanings of food, eating becomes associated with sentiments and assumptions about oneself and the world. Foods sometimes become symbolic because of religious connotations and use as rewards. After a child has fallen, a mother may give the child ice cream or candy to help forget the pain and stop the crying. Food is also withheld for bad behavior.

WORKING WITH PATIENTS WITH DIFFERENT FOOD PATTERNS

RESPECT FOR OTHER EATING PATTERNS

Dental hygienists must be prepared for the unexpected. Eating habits and patterns vary among patients, and characteristic cultural patterns are usually observed among different nationalities and religious groups. People are partial to their own food pattern; however, too many people, including dental hygienists, are convinced their own beliefs, attitudes, and practices are best and assume everyone should follow them. It is important when working with patients who have strong cultural ties to be sensitive to their preferences, avoid being judgmental, and treat each patient with respect. Multicultural competence is the ability to discover each patient's cultural and ethnic preferences, and effectively adapt interventions.

An open-minded dental hygienist who avoids cultural biases is more likely to have patients disclose crucial information that allows the dental hygienist to help them. A heavy accent or lack of English proficiency is not indicative of educational level or intelligence. In addition to being tactful, it may be necessary to allow longer response times for patients from different cultures.

Even when the facts are known, an analysis of the situation may be clouded because of unique individual habits. Information should be obtained regarding food habits using open-ended questions, rather than questions that put words into a patient's mouth. For example, "Tell me everything you had to eat this morning" might elicit a different response than the open-ended question, "What did you have for breakfast this morning?"

Patients sometimes refuse to eat a particular food or to comply with recommended changes because of cultural or religious beliefs. Generally, if these preferences and beliefs are known, an adequate diet can be planned around them, and the patient would be more receptive to minor changes in the diet pattern.

EFFECTING CHANGE

Knowledge of food preferences and attitudes is important for effecting change. The key is to ease patients into change. An empathetic, observant dental hygienist understands and is aware of the customs, behaviors, attitudes, and beliefs of different cultures in the area and treats each patient with respect. Several basic facts help in approaching patients from various ethnic groups to promote sound nutritional practices.

One can find advantages and faults in each cultural food pattern. These patterns have contributed to the survival of the group in a particular environment. People have a remarkable ability to obtain a nutritious diet out of available foodstuffs. Some eating patterns that seem strange may actually be adaptive by enhancing or preserving nutritional value.

Food patterns of other countries are in some instances nutritionally superior or at least comparable to "ordinary" American traditions. When people relocate, they retain their traditional food patterns only if their native foods are available in the new location at an affordable price. They may be challenged to find the native foods their families based their diet on for centuries.

Problems arising within various cultural groups are economic, rather than the fault of traditional food patterns. Foods from the country of origin, which were cheapest at "home," may be very expensive or possibly unavailable in the new location. Immigrants may be able to find their culturally preferred foods easily in urban areas because American people are more interested in exotic and ethnic cuisines, increasing the availability of ethnic foods in supermarkets along with more ethnic restaurants. However, finding native foods may be difficult, especially if the location is a rural, less populated area. In many cases, American food practices adopted by immigrants have been deleterious to their health by contributing to the same chronic diseases typical of the United States.

Each food, food-related behavior, and tradition can be categorized as beneficial, neutral, or potentially harmful. A food that is beneficial promotes health by contributing necessary nutrients. Neutral foods are not especially beneficial, but are not harmful to health. Foods are not usually harmful, but customs affecting nutritional content of the food may be potentially harmful. Efforts should be made to alter only the patterns affecting the nutritional value undesirably. For example, because many water-soluble vitamins are destroyed by heat, the practice of cooking foods (especially vegetables) for long periods is discouraged unless the liquids are consumed or iron cookware is used. The dental hygienist can use an understanding of ethnic food habits to encourage or incorporate beneficial practices into the patient's diet.

Food patterns are generally deeply ingrained, contribute to psychological stability, and are hard to change. If dietary changes are indicated for health or dental reasons, suggest minimal alterations in the patient's normal patterns and, if possible, present the information with options. Rather than indicating a patient should stop eating a food that is a part of his or her cultural heritage, talk about portion control of the food. A main concern is that healthcare workers are not accounting for individual needs by not giving patients information they are comfortable with and will use.[1] Additionally, compliance is improved when the patient has input into changes in food choices, understands the reason changes are indicated, and feels responsible for following the suggestions.

Cultural patterns tend to be used more consistently by older family members. First-generation immigrants are still rooted in their homeland and usually have at least one native meal a day. Dental hygienists should know about the ethnic foods for immigrants in the area so they can assist in offering alternatives or similar types of foods. Gradually, the diet conforms to food resources of the new location, a process called **dietary acculturation**. Second-generation Americans are raised without that direct native connection, and their parents, often struggling with the new foods themselves, may not have the knowledge to educate their children on what to eat. These individuals need to learn which American foods are healthful.

It is impossible to cover the dietary practices of all cultures and religions in this text. A food guide for Mexico is provided in Figure 15-2. The Canadian Food Guide was presented in Chapter 1 (see Fig. 1-5). Additional food guides can be found in the back of the book and on Evolve. Individuals from any culture have unique tastes and preferences; stereotyping members of cultural groups should be strictly avoided. Dental hygienists should become familiar with patterns common in the local area. Table 15-1 categorizes foods of different cultures and regions, and includes brief descriptions that help introduce some unique and interesting foods.

RELIGIOUS FOOD RESTRICTIONS

Religious beliefs affect eating patterns, attaching symbolic meanings to food and drink. Some examples are the bread and wine served during the Christian communion service, and the Hindu reverence for the cow. Many Seventh Day Adventists are vegetarians; some are vegans. These patterns do not usually result in any nutritional problems, but could affect one's food patterns and require consideration before making dietary recommendations.

FOOD BUDGETS

Foods available in the home are primarily the result of food shopping behaviors. If nutrient-dense healthful foods are not purchased, they cannot be consumed; likewise, if more

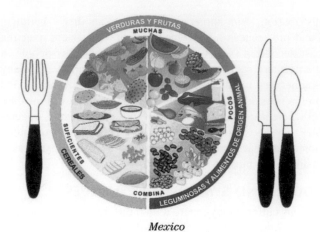

Mexico

FIGURE 15-2 Mexican Food Guide. (From Painter J, et al: Comparison of international food guide pictorial representations. J Am Dietetic Assoc 2002; 102[4]:483, with permission from the American Dietetic Association.)

energy-dense foods are purchased, they compete with more healthful choices even if the healthful foods are available. Despite increasing interest in optimal nutrition, many Americans are anxious about food prices and are attempting to conserve their food dollars. Inflation of food prices began to increase in 2007, with price increases not seen since 1990. Although the precise annual levels of food inflation are difficult to predict, increased commodity prices suggest food prices will continue to increase.[2,3] Evidence of poor or fair health status and malnutrition increases as income level decreases, as discussed in Health Application 15.

Purchasing the most nutritious products using available money is a common concern. The average American family spends less than 10% of their income on food; families at the poverty level may spend 30%. A general awareness of food costs can be used to assist patients in stretching their food dollar (Box 15-1). The amount of money a household spends on food provides insight into how adequately it could be meeting its food needs. In 2007, the typical U.S. household spent $42.50 per person each week for food.[4] Higher priced foods may not be the most nutritious; palatable, nutritious foods can be provided economically. Eating healthier can save money by reduced portion sizes and buying fewer energy-dense foods. Energy-dense foods are the least expensive and are most resistant to inflation.[5]

Research by the U.S. Department of Agriculture (USDA) indicates that low-income households score below higher income households on healthy eating indices (based on the *Dietary Guidelines for Americans*). Compliance with the recommendations for fruits and vegetables is the biggest concern. Households earning below 130% of the poverty line spent less money than other households on groceries, including beef, dairy products, fruit, vegetables, bread and other baked goods, and frozen prepared foods.

An analysis of the *2003 Consumer Expenditure Survey* questioned the effect of small adjustments to lower income households' buying power on food budgets. The analysis found additional income would result in increased

Table 15-1 Cultural and Regional Foods

Name of Food	Culture/Region	Type of Food	Description
Adobo	Filipino	Meat	Meat with soy sauce
Ajinomoto	Japanese	Grain	Wheat germ
Anadama	New England	Grain	Cornmeal-molasses yeast bread
Arroz blanco	Puerto Rican	Grain	Enriched white rice
Bacalao	Puerto Rican	Meat	Salted codfish
Bagels	Jewish	Grain	Bread dough, doughnut-shaped, boiled in water and baked
Baklava	Greek	Dessert	Layered pastry made with honey
Bok choy	Asian	Vegetable	Green leafy, stalklike vegetable
Brioche	French	Grain	Egg-rich cake bread, used as sweet roll or shell for entrees
Bulgur	Middle Eastern	Grain	Granular wheat product with nutlike flavor
Burrito	Mexican	Combination	Tortilla filled with beef-bean mixture and fried or baked
Café con leche	Latin American	Beverage	Coffee with milk
Cape Cod turkey	New England	Meat	Codfish balls
Challah	Jewish	Grain	Sabbath or holiday twisted egg-bread
Chappati	Indian	Grain	Unleavened bread
Chayote	Mexican	Vegetable	Squashlike vegetable
Chitterlings	Southern U.S.	Meat	Intestine of young pigs, soaked, boiled, and fried
Chorizo	Mexican	Meat	Sausage
Cilantro	Mexican	Seasoning	Coriander, similar to parsley
Crackling	Southern U.S.	Snack	Crispy pieces of fried pork fat
Croissants	French	Grain	Buttery, flaky, crescent-shaped rolls
Crumpets	English	Grain	Muffin-like product cooked on griddle then toasted
Cush	Montana	Grain	Cornbread mixed with butter and water and fried
Dandelion greens	Southern U.S.	Vegetable	Leaves from dandelion plant
Dhal	Indian	Meat	Stew with lentils or beans
Dolmathes	Greek	Combination	Grape leaves stuffed with beef
Dosai	Indian	Combination	Pancakes with lentils
Edamame	Oriental	Vegetable	Baby soybean in the pod
Enchiladas	Mexican	Combination	Tortilla filled with meat and cheese
Escargots	French	Meat	Snails
Falafel	Middle Eastern	"Meat"	Vegetarian-type meatball
Fatback	Southern U.S.	Fat	Fat from loin of pig
Feijoada	Brazilian	Meat	Black beans with meat
Feta	Greek	Milk	Soft, salty white cheese from sheep or goat milk
Finnan haddie	Scottish	Milk	Salted, smoked haddock
Frijoles fritos	Mexican	"Meat"	Refried pinto beans
Gazpacho	Spanish	Soup	Cold soup with chopped tomatoes, green peppers, and cucumbers
Gefilte fish	Jewish	Meat	Seasoned fish ground and shaped into balls
Goulash	Hungarian	Meat	Stew seasoned with paprika
Grits	Southern U.S.	Grain	Hulled and coarsely ground corn
Guava	Cuban	Fruit	Small, yellow or red sweet tropical fruit
Gumbo	Creole	Combination	Well-seasoned okra stew with meat or seafood
Hangtown fry	California	Meat	Fried oysters and eggs
Hoe cake	Southeast U.S.	Grain	Thin corn cake
Hog maw	Southern U.S.	Meat	Stomach of pig
Hoppin' John	Southern U.S.	Combination	Black-eyed peas and rice
Hushpuppies	Southern U.S.	Grain	Fried cornbread
Idli	Indian	Combination	Steamed dumplings with lentils
Jalapeños	Latin American	Vegetable	Hot peppers
Jambalaya	Creole	Combination	Well-seasoned combination of seafoods, tomatoes, and rice
Kale	Southern U.S.	Vegetable	Dark green leafy vegetable, similar to spinach
Kasha	Jewish	Grain	Coarsely ground buckwheat, toasted before cooking in liquid
Kelp	Asian	Vegetable	Seaweed
Kibbeh	Middle Eastern	Meat	Fresh raw lamb, ground and seasoned, similar to meat loaf
Kielbasa	Polish	Meat	Sausage
Kimchi	Korean	Vegetable	Peppery fermented combination of pickled cabbage, turnips, radishes, and other vegetables

Table 15-1	Cultural and Regional Foods—cont'd		
Name of Food	**Culture/Region**	**Type of Food**	**Description**
Kuchen	German	Dessert	Yeast cake
Lard	—	Fat	Shortening-like product from pork
Latkas	Jewish	Grain	Pancakes, sometimes from potatoes
Limpa	Swedish	Grain	Rye bread
Lox	Jewish	Meat	Smoked salmon
Matzo	Jewish	Grain	Unleavened bread
Menudo	Mexican	Meat	Stew made with tripe (cow's stomach)
Minestrone	Italian	Soup	Vegetable soup
Miso	Asian	"Meat"	Fermented soybean paste
Moussaka	Greek	Combination	Meat and eggplant casserole
Mush	Southwest U.S.	Grain	Cooked cereal, usually cornmeal
Pan Dowdy	New England	Dessert	Dumplings and fruit
Pasta	Italian	Grain	Macaroni, spaghetti, and noodles in various shapes made from wheat
Pepperoni	Italian	Meat	Hot sausage
Phyllo	Greek	Grain	Paper-thin pastry for making meat, vegetables, cheese, and egg dishes and sweet pastries
Pilaf	Middle Eastern	Grain	Rice enriched with fat and sometimes vegetables, bits of meat, and spices
Poi	Polynesian	Vegetable	Root vegetable, especially taro, cooked and pounded, mixed with water, and sometimes fermented
Polenta	Italian	Grain	Cornmeal or cornmeal mush
Polk	Southern U.S.	Vegetable	Dark green leafy vegetable
Poori	Indian	Grain	Deep-fried whole-wheat bread
Potato latkes	Jewish	Vegetable	Potato pancakes
Pot liquor (likker)	Southern U.S.	Vegetable	Liquid from cooking green vegetables or bones
Prickly pear	Native American	Fruit	Fruit of cactus
Proscuitto	Italian	Meat	Ready-to-eat, cured, smoked ham
Pumpernickel	—	Grain	Yeast bread with wheat, corn, rye, and potatoes
Ratatouille	French	Vegetable	Well-seasoned casserole of eggplant, zucchini, tomato, and green pepper
Red-eye gravy	Southern U.S.	Gravy	Fried ham gravy
Sake	Asian	Beverage	Rice wine
Salt pork	Southern U.S.	Fat	Salted pork fat from the belly
Sancocho	Puerto Rican	Combination	Soup with meat and viandas
Sashimi	Japanese	Meat	Raw fish
Sauerbrauten	German	Meat	Pot roast in spicy, aromatic, sweet-and-sour marinade
Scones	English	Grain	Round, flat, unleavened sweetened bread
Scrapple	Pennsylvania Dutch	Combination	Solid mush from cornmeal and by-products of hog butchering
Shoofly pie	Pennsylvania Dutch	Dessert	Molasses pie
Shoyu	Japanese	Seasoning	Soy sauce
Sofrito	Puerto Rican	Seasoning	Specially seasoned tomato sauce
Sopapillos	Mexican	Grain	Rich fried bread
Spatzle	German	Grain	Small dumplings
Spoonbread	Virginia	Grain	Baked dish with cornmeal
Spumoni	Italian	Dessert	Fruited ice cream
Stollen	German	Dessert	Christmas fruitcake
Strickle sheets	Pennsylvania Dutch	Dessert	Coffee cake
Strudel	German	Dessert	Light pastry, filled with fruit or cheese
Tacos	Mexican	Combination	Fried tortillas, filled with meat, vegetables, and hot sauce
Tamales	Mexican	Grain	Pancake-like leathery bread
Tempura	Japanese	Combination	Deep-fried seafood or vegetables
Teriyaki sauce	Hawaiian	Seasoning	Sweetened soy sauce
Tofu	Asian	"Meat"	Soybean curd
Trotters	Southern U.S.	Meat	Pig's feet
Viandas	Puerto Rican	Vegetable	Starchy tropical vegetables, including plantain, green bananas, and sweet potatoes

From Davis JR, Sherer K: Applied Nutrition and Diet Therapy for Nurses, 2nd ed. Philadelphia: Saunders, 1994.

Box 15-1	**Basic Principles for Economical Food Purchases**

- Take inventory before going to the supermarket.
- Never shop when hungry.
- Purchase the least expensive items in each food group, but pay attention to the amounts. Bonus packages may be super-sizing your waistline.
- Rely on minimal servings of meats. On the average, purchase 1 lb ground beef or turkey for four people. When purchasing steaks, check the weight; most would serve at least two people.
- Use meat substitutes (e.g., legumes, nuts, peanut butter, and cheese) several times each week.
- Serve adequate quantities of grains, cereals, and pasta products (6 to 11 servings per day), but be aware of portion sizes. For instance, one serving of pasta is $\frac{1}{2}$ cup cooked, but pasta labels may identify one serving as 1 cup cooked.
- Purchase smaller quantities of whole-grain products in place of a larger quantity of refined grains. The first ingredient in the bread should be 100% whole grain.
- Prepare most foods from scratch rather than buying convenience items, such as frozen pizza.
- Limit highly processed foods that are expensive or have low nutrient density (e.g., carbonated beverages and chips). Replace these foods with fresh fruits and vegetables.
- Plan weekly menus, using MyPyramid as a guideline.
- Plan menus around seasonal foods or weekly specials.
- Prepare a shopping list and stick to it. Avoid impulse buying, but be prepared to make substitutions if a similar item is a better buy.
- Purchase store brands, which are usually a good buy for the money. Store brands, often found on the lowest shelves, are equal in quality and taste to more popular national brands.

- Read labels to determine nutritive value, and compare with similar products.
- Compare unit prices. Generally, the price per unit (e.g., ounce) stated on the shelf below the grocery item facilitates comparing various sizes.
- Buy larger sizes (which are usually cheaper per serving) if the food will be eaten before it spoils, but purchase individual serving sizes of products such as low-fat yogurt, pudding, and raisins if portion control is important.
- Shop at large supermarkets rather than small stores or convenience stores for more economical purchases.
- Avoid purchasing high-energy snack foods and breakfast cereals with a high sugar content.
- Do most of your shopping around the perimeter of the store, where seasonal items and basic essentials such as fresh meat, milk, and eggs are located. Highly processed foods line the inner supermarket shelves.
- Frozen meats are cheaper and as healthful as fresh meat.
- Eat highly perishable items such as fresh fish or strawberries as soon as possible after purchasing.
- Use convenience foods wisely. In general, the more someone else does in preparing food, the more the product will cost.
- Use dating information on products to select the freshest foods. Do not let food in the pantry or refrigerator go to waste.
- Pay attention at the checkout counter to be sure you are charged the advertised price or the price indicated on the shelf.

purchases of beef and frozen prepared foods. These foods may be priorities over fruit and vegetables because of taste and convenience. With additional income, fruit and vegetable expenditures increased only slightly.[6]

If the amount of kilocalories is not of concern, foods supplying the most nutrients relative to their cost include beef, fresh potatoes, brown rice, wheat germ, milk, eggs, and peanut butter. Foods can be categorized based on their nutrient density. On the basis of nutrient density, spinach, liver, tomatoes, canned tuna, nonfat and low-fat milk, tofu, dry-roasted peanuts, eggs, and fresh carrots are usually the most economical. Some less expensive fruits per serving size are watermelon, apples, grapefruit, grapes, oranges, bananas, and papaya; least expensive vegetables include potatoes, carrots, cucumbers, green beans, onions, celery, mustard greens, kale, romaine and iceberg lettuce, bell peppers, tomatoes, and cauliflower.[7] Buying fruits and vegetables that are homegrown and in season is more economical. Generally, more of the food dollar should be spent for fruits, vegetables, grain products, milk, and dry beans; less is needed for meats and high-sugar, high-fat food items (e.g., candy, carbonated beverages, and chips).

People with limited financial resources are hampered by other constraints. Without transportation, low-income consumers are often limited to shopping in small independent

stores common in inner city areas, or must spend money for travel or delivery services. Prices tend to be higher in small, independent stores. The lack of availability in small grocery stores located in low-income neighborhoods and the higher cost of the healthier market basket may be a deterrent to eating healthier among very-low-income consumers. Availability in small, low income–area grocery stores is less consistent for whole grains, low-fat cheeses, lean ground beef, and larger package sizes.[8]

Families on food stamps or on a very low food budget need to learn skills in buying and storing food. Low-income shoppers spend less on food purchases despite the fact that food prices are higher. Low-income shoppers can buy more food with less money by shopping in discount grocery stores, purchasing and consuming less food, especially kilocalorie-dense foods, than higher income shoppers, and purchasing lower priced (and sometimes lower quality) foods by selecting less expensive meats and fresh fruits and vegetables. Table 15-2 shows the relative cost of 20 g of protein from various sources.

Although the USDA maintains that well-balanced healthy foods can be obtained using their Thrifty Food Plan (TFP), a study investigated the cost and availability of a standard market basket of foods compared with a healthier basket that included low-fat meat and dairy and whole-grain products.

Table 15-2	Cost of 20 Grams of Protein from Various Meats and Meat Alternatives*			
Food	Cost ($)/ Market Unit	AP† to Provide 20 G Protein	EP‡ Amount to Provide 20 G Protein	Cost ($)/20 G Protein
Ready-to-cook turkey	1.29/lb	3½ oz	2⅓ oz	0.19
Dry pinto beans	0.99/lb	¾ cup	1½ cup	0.22
Pork and beans, canned	0.79/15 oz	1⅔ cup	1⅔ cup	0.23
Beef liver	1.59/lb	3½ oz	3 oz	0.30
Cured picnic ham, bone-in	1.99/lb	5½ oz	3½ oz	0.44
Split chicken breasts with bone and skin	2.99/lb	4 oz	2½ oz	0.47
Tuna, canned in water	1.19/6 oz	3 oz	3 oz	0.48
Peanut butter	2.99/16 oz	5 Tbsp	5 Tbsp	0.53
Ground turkey	2.49/lb	3½ oz	2¾ oz	0.55
Bread, white enriched (sandwich slices)	1.99/24 oz	8 slice	8 slice	0.61
Whole fryer	3.99/lb	4 oz	2½ oz	0.62
Skim milk	3.99/gallon	2½ cup	2½ cup	0.62
Loin pork chops (rib with bone)	3.99/lb	4½ oz	2½ oz	0.62
Eggs (large)	2.69/dozen	3	3	0.67
Regular ground beef	4.99/lb	4 oz	2⅔ oz	0.73
Processed American cheese	6.99/2 lb	3½ oz	3½ oz	0.77
Ham, boneless	4.29/lb	3 oz	3 oz	0.80
Beef, chuck roast, bone-in	4.69/lb	4¼ oz	3 oz	0.88
Cod or catfish fillet, fresh	5.99/lb	3½ oz	3 oz	1.12
Beef, round steak, boneless	5.99/lb	3½ oz	3 oz	1.12
Bread, whole-grain (sandwich sliced)	2.79/16 oz	6⅔ slice	6⅔ slice	1.16
Chicken wings	2.29/lb	2 wings	2 wings	1.30
Salmon, fresh fillets	7.99/lb	3⅓ oz	3 oz	1.49
Frankfurters	4.79/lb	5 count	5 count	1.92
Sliced bologna, beef	4.69/lb	6⅔ oz	6⅔ oz	1.95
Sliced bacon	5.79/lb	8 slice	8 slice	2.31
Breaded fish fillets, frozen	7.99/19 oz	4 fillets	4 fillets	3.26

*Prices in Austin, TX, July 2003.
†AP, as purchased, including weight of bone, skin, and fat.
‡EP, edible portion, cooked.

For the 2-week shopping list for a family of four, the average TFP market-basket cost was $194, and the healthier market basket cost was $230.[8] Another study determined that a low-income family would have to spend 43% to 70% of their food budget on fruits and vegetables to consume the amounts recommended by the *Dietary Guidelines for Americans 2005*.[9]

REFERRALS FOR NUTRITIONAL RESOURCES

Frequently, patients need special assistance for nutritional problems. A variety of nutrition resources are available to help financially, assist with food budgeting, or teach basic nutrition and meal planning.

Dental hygienists can identify patients or families with nutritional needs, provide appropriate referrals, and help them participate in applicable programs (Table 15-3). Registered dietitians and nutritionists are trained to assist with dietary problems. A **nutritionist** has at least a 4-year degree in foods and nutrition, and usually works in a public health setting assisting people in the community.

One of the best sources is the city or county health department. State and local health departments usually have

various programs to provide nutrition services, such as well-baby clinics and family health centers. Health departments and county hospitals are excellent resources for information about various programs available. The federal government administers several nutrition programs through the USDA and the U.S. Department of Health and Human Services (USDHHS).

Federal assistance to individuals below the poverty level has declined and failed to keep up with inflation. Historically, changes in U.S. economic conditions significantly affect participation in government nutrition programs.

The Area Information Center (2-1-1) maintains comprehensive databases of resources, including federal, state, and local government agencies, and community-based and private nonprofit organizations. Information and referral (I & R) services is a national dialing code to link people in need of assistance with appropriate providers of services in their community.

The Supplemental Nutrition Assistance Program (SNAP) (formerly the Food Stamp Program) is the cornerstone of the nutrition safety net in the United States. The program was renamed because benefits are provided through an Elec-

Table 15-3	Referral Chart for Community Nutrition Resources		
Population Group	**Risk Factor**	**Referral Source***	**Contact†**
Pregnant and lactating women	Low income	Food stamps	State food stamp hotline number available at www.fns.usda.gov/fsp/contact_info/hotlines.htm
	Anemia, inadequate weight gain, age-related risk factor, inadequate health care, or lack of food and nutrition information	WIC Program	City, county, or state health department
		Maternity and Infant Care Project	State health department
		Expanded Food and Nutrition Education Program (EFNEP)	Land-grant universities
			Prenatal clinic or private healthcare team
Infants	Low-birth-weight, failure to thrive, or poor growth patterns	Prenatal education	City, county, or state health department
	Inadequate health care	WIC Program	State health department
Children	Poor growth patterns or overweight, inadequate diet, or anemia	WIC Program (up to 5 years old)	City, county, or state health department
	Low income	Children and Youth Project (up to 18 years old)	State health department
		Head Start (preschool)	Local community action project
		School lunch	Board of education
		School breakfast	Local school district
Older adult	Low income	Supplemental Nutrition Assistance Program (Food stamps)	State food stamp hotline number available at www.fns.usda.gov/fsp/contact_info/hotlines.htm
		Congregate meal sites	State and local agencies on aging
	Homebound	Meals on Wheels	Locations available at www.mealcall.org/meals-on-wheels/senior-center.htm
General adult	Obesity	Weight Watchers International, Thin Within, Dieters workshop, TOPS, and other weight reduction groups	Local chapters
	Hyperlipidemia, cardiovascular disease, or hypertension	American Heart Association	Local chapter
	Diabetes	American Diabetes Association	Local chapter
	Low income	Food stamps	State food stamp hotline number available at www.fns.usda.gov/fsp/contact_info/hotlines.htm
	Reliable food and nutrition information	EFNEP	Land-grant universities
	General consumer information for all populations	Community nutrition groups and community cooperatives	Local groups
		American Dietetic Association	Available at www.eatright.org/Public/
		Center for Science in the Public Interest	Available at actionnetwork.org/CSPI/home.html
		U.S. Department of Health and Human Services	Available at dhhs.gov/
		Healthfinder	Available at healthfinder.gov

tronic Benefit Card (EBT) to low-income households that meet certain requirements, rather than food stamp coupons. Food stamps are free to individuals who qualify. The program, designed to help low-income households purchase nutritious food, is based on family income and household size. Local offices that administer the program are widely distributed throughout the United States. Recipients can use the EBT card to buy any foods sold in participating grocery stores, with the exception of prepared hot foods. The program was initially designed to boost food consumption and energy intake.

Food stamp usage has hit a new high; the number of people on food stamps has been growing steadily from 21.2 million in 2003 to 26.5 million in 2007. Food price inflation has caused rapid erosion in the purchasing power of food stamp benefits.

The federal government adjusts for inflation annually, and the Food, Conservation and Energy Act of 2008 increased the minimum benefit, indexed to inflation, but with the steep climb in food prices, the monthly food allowance may run out mid-month. The amount of benefits is inadequate to purchase minimal foods for adequate nutrition. Because poor diets exert heavy costs in medical expenditures and lost productivity, measures for promoting healthful food choices could yield considerable benefits. State governments and health advocates are considering additional modifications to reinforce nutrition education, restrict foods allowed with food stamp benefits, and expand benefits to encourage purchases of more healthful foods, such as fruit and vegetables.[10]

The Special Supplemental Food Program for Women, Infants, and Children (WIC) is designed to prevent nutritional problems in this high-risk, low-income group. The WIC program is available to pregnant and lactating women, infants, and children up to 5 years old who are considered to be at nutritional risk. Some of the criteria for nutritional risk are evidence of iron deficiency, inadequate weight gain during pregnancy, teenage pregnancy, failure to thrive, poor growth patterns, and inadequate dietary patterns. Breastfeeding is supported and encouraged. The WIC program is usually available through county and city health departments. In addition to supplemental foods, nutrition education and referrals to healthcare sources are provided. Studies of the WIC program have shown positive effects on iron status and growth and development of infants and children. The program also saves millions of dollars by decreasing the rate of low-birth-weight infants, so funding has remained relatively stable.

After 25 years of providing the same foods to WIC participants, the USDA implemented a new food package that more closely aligns allowable WIC foods with the *Dietary Guidelines for Americans* and the nutrition policies of the American Association of Pediatrics. These new guidelines, which are being implemented by fall 2009, reinforce the importance of breastfeeding, increase variety of the food packages, and accommodate cultural food preferences. The addition of whole-grain cereals and breads or other whole-grain products, use of low-fat milk for all participants older than age 2, and the choice of fruits and vegetables will empower mothers to choose healthy food using WIC vouchers. Additionally, it will improve the availability of healthy foods in low-income community grocery stores. Many items in the current food package are provided in smaller amounts to allow for cost neutrality and to concur with nutritional concerns.

School breakfast and lunch programs provide nutritious meals for children at school. Nutritional standards for school lunch require lunch and breakfast furnish at least one-third and one-fourth of the recommended dietary allowances (RDAs) for children. Free and reduced-price meals are provided based on household income and size. Meals must meet the applicable recommendations of the *Dietary Guidelines for Americans,* which recommend no more than 30% of kilocalories from fat and less than 10% of kilocalories from saturated fat averaged over a 1-week period. A reduction in sodium and cholesterol and increase in fiber are encouraged. Lunches must provide one-third of the RDA for protein, vitamins A and C, iron, calcium, and kilocalories. The Child Nutrition and WIC Reauthorization Act of 2004 included a nutrition component regarding wellness policies restricting foods sold on school campuses during the school day, providing free fruits and vegetables to designated schools, and funding for nutrition education programs that focus on nutrition and physical activity of students.

The Nutrition Program for the Elderly (Title III) provides group and home-delivered meals. The purpose of this program is to improve nutritional and health status of older adults through improved access to food. Most individuals applying for Meals on Wheels are at risk of malnutrition. In addition to providing a hot meal to older adults (containing one-third of the RDAs), various social services are available.

The Expanded Food and Nutrition Education Program (EFNEP) is designed to help lower socioeconomic groups with all aspects of nutrition. EFNEP is available through county extension services of land-grant universities and assists with meal planning, budgeting, cooking, and other food-related and nutrition-related problems. Nutrition aides are low-income homemakers who are trained to visit homes of low-income families to assist in providing well-balanced meals.

Head Start is a preschool educational program for low-income families. Meals are furnished for the children, and nutrition education is available for parents.

Local chapters of many health-related organizations, listed in the telephone directory, furnish free or inexpensive literature, audiovisual material, and health-oriented programs on various topics. Locally funded food agencies providing assistance through food banks and food pantries have increased substantially. Food pantries, which usually do not base eligibility for benefits on income status, currently serve millions of Americans. A survey of food banks in the United States found that all are seeing more participants, with a 15% to 20% increase over 2007. They are having to make difficult choices; 83% of the food banks responded that they are unable to meet the needs of their community adequately.[11] Foods available at food pantries provide inadequate amounts of calcium and vitamins A and C, but many of these facilities are trying to improving the quality of foods they stock. Emergency food providers serve a diverse population with different reasons for needing the assistance. These providers are especially helpful for people during a short-term setback, such as an unexpected emergency medical bill; others need emergency kitchens to receive a hot meal or to supplement food stamps. Referrals can also come from in-hospital sources such as the social worker, dietitian, or nutrition support team. Other referrals are listed in Appendix C.

Dental Hygiene Considerations

- Identify patients needing food assistance, and refer them to appropriate sources.
- If kilocalories, sodium, and fat should be restricted, discourage patronage of fast food establishments or provide suggestions for appropriate fast food selections (e.g., salads or baked chicken).
- Low-income households must allocate a high share of both their income and time budgets to food if they wish to consume palatable, nutritious meals.
- When recommending foods to patients, consider the income level. Suggesting steak or lobster as a protein source for low-income patients would be inappropriate.

Nutritional Directions

- Protein sources are generally the most expensive budget items; however, it is unnecessary to buy choice quality grades of meat for good nutrition. ("Select" and "standard" are more economical grades of meat.)
- Discuss guidelines for economic food purchases (see Box 15-1) to help patients modify food purchases.

MAINTAINING OPTIMAL NUTRITION DURING FOOD PREPARATION

From the time any produce is taken from the plant or a grain product is harvested, nutrient content begins to degrade. Harvesting, processing, and cooking food means nutrient losses are occurring, but good handling processes, such as chilling, minimize losses and bacterial growth.

METHODS OF PREPARATION

In many instances, cooking enhances palatability, increases digestibility of food, and destroys pathogenic organisms. Cooking affects acceptability and nutritional value of food. Following a few guidelines can help preserve nutrients during cooking (Box 15-2).

Adding large amounts of fats during the cooking process, as in frying, is discouraged. Specific methods of preparing meats such as broiling or cooking on a charcoal grill are recommended to lessen natural fat content. Meats cooked to the well-done stage contain less fat. To remove fats during cooking, meats can be boiled, microwaved in a colander or on paper towels, or roasted or broiled on a rack. Cooking increases digestibility of protein in meats.

Cooking generally softens cellulose in fresh produce. Total volume and bulk of the food are decreased, so a greater quantity of these low-calorie foods can be eaten.

A relatively new method of cooking to most Americans is stir-frying, which is an old Asian technique. This method is highly recommended and has the added benefit of being fast. Bite-sized pieces of food are cooked very briefly over high heat with or without a small amount of vegetable oil. Vegetables retain their nutrient value, color, and crispness.

A microwave oven is another time-saver because of the shorter cooking time. The vitamin content of foods cooked

Box 15-2   Guidelines to Preserve Nutrients During Preparation

- Prepare fresh produce as near to serving time as possible to prevent deterioration of many nutrients when they are exposed to air.
- Do not soak fruits and vegetables that have been cut to prevent loss of water-soluble vitamins and some minerals (especially potassium) into the water. If cut-up fruits and vegetables are soaked in water, use the water in food preparation.
- Scrub fruits and vegetables rather than pare them to increase fiber intake. When necessary, pare as thinly as possible to maintain nutrients.
- Boil nonconsumable parings and portions of vegetables in water and incorporate in soup stock or gravies. This is a very rich source of potassium and water-soluble vitamins.
- Leave produce whole or in large pieces so that less surface area is available for oxidation of nutrients.
- Store any fruits or vegetables that have been cut or otherwise processed, such as fruit juice, in airtight opaque containers. Container size should be appropriate for the amount to be stored to prevent excessive oxidation from air inside the container.
- Cook foods for the shortest time possible. A covered pan minimizes cooking time by increasing the temperature inside.
- Use the least amount of liquid possible in cooking. Use left-over liquid, which contains water-soluble vitamins, in gravies and soups.
- Serve vegetables as soon as they are cooked.
- Do not use baking soda when cooking vegetables.

in a home microwave oven is about the same as foods prepared conventionally, especially if a minimal amount of water is added.

FOOD SANITATION AND SAFETY

Food carefully chosen for its nutritional value may be adversely affected by how it is handled and prepared before its consumption. Approximately 76 million illnesses, 325,000 hospitalizations, and 5000 deaths are attributed to known pathogens in food each year.[12] Three pathogens, *Salmonella, Escherichia coli,* and *Listeria,* account for most of these outbreaks. Symptoms include diarrhea, fever, headache, and vomiting. Reported cases of foodborne diseases caused by *Salmonella* and *E. coli* did not decline between 2006 and 2007, whereas cases caused by *Cryptosporidium* increased.[13] For most people, the illness resolves on its own, but for young and older individuals and those with weakened immune systems, these illnesses can be fatal. Illness caused by *Listeria* can result in miscarriage, fetal death, or severe illness or death of a newborn (see Chapter 12).

The Centers for Disease Control and Prevention (CDC) estimates that at least one-third of foodborne disease cases reported could be prevented by thorough hand washing before food preparation and eating. Because of the prevalence of foodborne illness, the *Dietary Guidelines for Americans* address food safety. The five major control factors for pathogens are personal hygiene, adequate cooking, avoiding cross-contamination, keeping food at safe temperatures, and avoiding foods from unsafe sources. Edibles must be handled with care to prevent contamination with foodborne organisms, and sometimes must be properly cooked to kill any organisms naturally present. Many foods, especially meat, poultry, and eggs, require sufficiently high temperatures to destroy microorganisms. Because of large portions provided in restaurants, many people leave with a "doggie bag." This increases risk for foodborne illness. Bacteria and other organisms grow at an astonishing rate between 40° F and 140° F. All leftover foods should be refrigerated as soon as possible and reheated to an internal temperature of at least 165° F. Foods left unrefrigerated for more than 2 hours should be discarded. Leftovers should be eaten within 2 days. Safe practices from the *Dietary Guidelines for Americans* for handling food are listed in Box 15-3.

In recent years, nationwide recalls of tainted food products included meats, peanut butter, vegetables, salad, snacks, fast food, and dessert items because of thousands of people becoming ill and even a few deaths. New foods have been implicated—organically grown spinach and peanut butter were perplexing problems. One reason problems have increased is because more people are consuming increased amounts of fresh produce, which is good nutritionally, but in some instances, harmful microbes on the produce have created problems. Contrary to popular opinion, pathogens that cause illness are odorless, colorless, and invisible, so smelling, tasting, or looking at the food would not reveal whether the food is harmful. Spoilage bacteria evidenced by slimy films on lunch meat, soggy edges on vegetables, or sticky chicken are not as toxic as are pathogens.

Additionally, the government and U.S. citizens are concerned about the possibility of contaminated food caused by terrorist acts. The FDA is authorized in the Public Health Security and Bioterrorism Preparedness and Response Act of 2002 (Bioterrorism Act) to detain suspect food.

PROCESSED FOODS

Active, mobile lifestyles and an increasing number of women working full-time or part-time outside the home have led to a continued increase in consumption of processed foods. Although growing one's own food and making foods from "scratch" can give consumers control over how food is

handled and what is added, this is not feasible for most Americans.

Effect of Processing on Nutrients

Nutrient content of foods can be affected by the way food is handled—that is, the type of processing to which the food is subjected (e.g., milling, cooking, freezing)—and how it is stored. In general, most minerals, carbohydrates, lipids, proteins, and vitamin K and niacin are **stable nutrients**. Nutrients are considered stable if at least 85% of the original level is retained during processing and storage. Thiamin, riboflavin, folate, and ascorbic acid are most likely to be seriously depleted by processing and storage and the method of food preparation. The nutritional value of home-cooked foods is frequently about the same as processed foods. Highly processed foods are usually less nutritious than the fresh form (e.g., potato chips are less nutritious than a baked potato).

Food processing attempts to maintain optimal qualities of color, flavor, texture, and nutritive value. Not everything done to foods by food processors has been good; however, not all processing is detrimental. The milling process removes the bran coat of grains. Removal of the high lipid-containing bran produces a more stable grain, increasing its shelf life. Nutritionally, however, this results in a reduction of fiber and loss of 70% to 80% of thiamin, riboflavin, vitamin B_6, and other nutrients. Enrichment replaces some nutrients (thiamin, riboflavin, niacin, folic acid, and iron) lost in processing, but not all of the ones lost in processing (see Table 1-3).

Fresh fruits and vegetables have a higher nutritive value and better taste immediately after harvest, but rapidly deteriorate if transported long distances or improperly stored. Frozen foods packed immediately after harvesting may be higher in nutritive value than their fresh counterparts available in the supermarket. Because canned vegetables have prolonged exposure to water, they usually lose more nutrients than frozen ones, but even canned vegetables are better than no vegetables at all.

Irradiated Foods

Foods treated with controlled amounts of ionized radiation for a prescribed period to kill the spoilage-causing and disease-causing bacteria and molds in food are known as **irradiated foods**. This process has stimulated a lot of controversy, with opponents criticizing the process as being a stopgap measure that ignores the bigger problem of how food is grown, processed, and sold. The irradiation process breaks down DNA molecules of the harmful organisms. The process, which kills microorganisms that cause food spoilage without significantly increasing the temperature of the food, is often called "cold pasteurization." It can be used on meats and produce. Exposure of food to the irradiation process can lengthen the period of ripeness of fruits and vegetables, prolong the freshness of many foods, and prevent certain foodborne illnesses. Washing fresh fruits and vegetables can reduce the risk of food poisoning, but irradiation

---

Box 15-3 **Keep Food Safe to Eat**

- Wash hands and surfaces often.
- Separate raw, cooked, and ready-to-eat foods while shopping, preparing, or storing.
- Cook foods to a safe temperature.
- Refrigerate perishable foods promptly.
- Check and follow the label.
- When in doubt, throw it out.

From U.S. Department of Agriculture, U.S. Department of Health and Human Services: Nutrition and Your Health: Dietary Guidelines for Americans, 5th ed. Home and Garden Bulletin No. 232. Washington, DC, Government Printing Office, 2000.

can kill bacteria that are beyond the reach of conventional chemical sanitizers, such as inside the leaves of spinach and lettuce.[14]

Foods have been safely irradiated in the United States for more than 30 years, and more than 40 other countries use the process. The process is carefully controlled and monitored by numerous government organizations.

Organic Foods

The organic food industry has grown dramatically over the past 2 decades. Organic foods constitute more than 2% of all food in the United States.[15] This rapid growth may be because consumers perceive that organic foods are healthier, more nutritious, and fresher, and do not contain pesticides. Nearly every supermarket chain now has an organic line of foods.

In 2002, the USDA passed legislation defining organic food and permits use of a seal (Fig. 15-3) for foods meeting the organic standards. Organic certification regulates the way these foods are grown, handled, and processed. Foods labeled **organic** are grown without synthetic pesticides, growth hormones, antibiotics, or genetic engineering. Organic farmers use animal and crop wastes; botanical, biological, or nonsynthetic pest controls; or allowed synthetic materials that can be broken down quickly by oxygen and sunlight. Products labeled "Made with Organic Ingredients" must contain at least 70% organic ingredients. Manufacturers can state the exact percentage of organic ingredients on the display panel. A product containing more than 5% of the Environmental Protection Agency (EPA) pesticide tolerance cannot be labeled organic.

The food manufacturer voluntarily provides information to the USDA about substances and practices used in food production, including how nonorganic and organic foods are kept separate. The USDA is responsible for inspecting the site annually and certifying a producer.

The USDA does not support that organic food is safer or more nutritious than conventionally produced foods. Based on available evidence-based data, most comprehensive reviews comparing nutrient levels in organic and conventional foods are inconclusive, yielding mixed results. Several studies have shown organic foods contain more polyphenols or antioxidants having potential human health benefits. As far as nutritional scientists have been able to determine, conventionally grown produce is a healthy choice, and the benefits of eating a lot of fruits and vegetables outweigh any possible risk of ingesting trace amounts of pesticides. Organic foods are generally fresher, but because stabilizers and chemicals that delay ripening are not permitted in organic processing, these foods may have a shorter shelf life. Any additional nutrients in organic food do not seem to be present in quantities enough to alter a person's health to any significant extent. Although these foods have been on the market for many years, it is premature to say that either organic or conventional foods are superior with respect to safety or nutritional composition.

Animals raised by organic producers cannot be given antibiotics to stimulate growth, so organic meats, poultry, milk, or eggs do not contain residues of these drugs. If an antibiotic is given to treat an infection, the meat, milk, or eggs from the animal cannot be marketed as organic. Nonorganic animals do not contain antibiotic residues either because FDA regulations prohibit farmers from giving feed with antibiotics to conventionally raised animals for a period of time before slaughter. This "withdrawal time" is specific to the antibiotic used to ensure the drug is at a safe level in the animal's system before the meat or milk enters the food supply. Tests rarely detect traces of antibiotics or other drugs in conventionally produced meat, poultry, milk, or eggs.[16]

Organic foods may be less risky than conventional foods with respect to pesticides because lower amounts of pesticide residues are present in organic foods. When given to animals in high doses, pesticides can cause cancer, nervous system damage, and birth defects. The health risks of pesticides in humans are unclear. However, food surveys of conventional foods indicate estimated exposures from 34 pesticides were less than 1% of the United Nations Food and Agriculture Organization/World Health Organization's acceptable daily intake (ADI), and four other pesticides contributed 1% to 4.8% of the ADI. A typical human exposure at 1% of the ADI represents an exposure 10,000 times lower than levels that do not cause toxicity in animals.[17]

Currently, almost all the pesticides used in farming are "nonpersistent." That means they are metabolized quickly and are not stored in the body. A few days after ingesting a pesticide, it is completely gone from the body. Studies have found that pesticide levels in children's bodies dropped to zero a few days after changing from conventional foods to organic foods.[18,19] About 75% of conventionally grown fruits and vegetables contain very small amounts of pesticides,

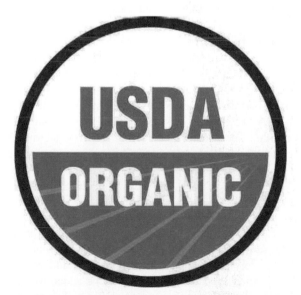

FIGURE 15-3 Official USDA organic seal, available at www.ams. usda.gov/nop/Consumers/Seal.htm. (From the National Organic Program, Agricultural Marketing Service, U.S. Department of Agriculture, Washington, D.C.)

whereas only about 25% of organic fruits and vegetables contained a pesticide in smaller amounts than the amount found on conventional foods.[20]

The use of animal manures as fertilizers presents potential microbiological risks if the manure is composted improperly. Standards for organic and conventional foods require specific procedures regarding the use of manures, or the manure must be applied more than 90 days before harvest. One study indicated certified organic produce poses no higher microbiological risk than conventional produce.[21]

Organic food generally comes at a premium cost for many reasons, including higher production and labor costs, lower yields, and high demand. Also, profit margins are higher than those of conventional foods. Organic products cost about 10% to 50% more than conventional products. When deciding whether the additional cost to purchase organic food is worth it, remember: you are better off eating fruits and vegetables with pesticides than not eating fruits and vegetables.

Several things can be done to ensure minimal intake of questionable chemicals other than purchasing only organic products. Even after washing fruits and vegetables, some foods still contain higher levels of pesticide residue than others. These foods include apples, berries, grapes, spinach, and potatoes, so if possible, choose organic for these foods. Also, buying locally produced fresh vegetables and fruits in season is helpful because fewer pesticides are used when long storage periods and long-distance shipping are not required. Trim tops and the outer portions of celery, lettuce, cabbages, and other leafy vegetables that may contain the bulk of pesticide residues. Eat a wide variety of fruits and vegetables to limit exposure to any one type of pesticide residue. Purchase only fruits and vegetables that are subject to USDA regulations. Imported produce is not grown under the same regulations as enforced by the USDA. Wash produce in cold water; special soaps or washes are not needed and could be harmful.

The term "natural" is popular on food packaging. Consumers assume a product labeled "natural" is probably healthier. "Natural" does not mean organic. The FDA has not established a standardized legal definition for this term, and no organization regulates this claim on food products. The FDA generally interprets "natural" as a product that does not contain synthetic or artificial ingredients that would not normally be expected in the food, including artificial flavors or color additives. "Natural" labels are meaningless and misleading for consumers.

Convenience Foods

Convenience foods are usually popular because they save time in meal preparation, planning, purchasing, and cleanup. The variety of foods available is also expanded. Convenience foods prepared by food manufacturers may cost more because of extra handling and packaging. Convenience foods also require more preservatives and may contain more sodium and fat than home-cooked products.

Fast Foods

Fast food sales have increased dramatically; fast foods have become an integral part of our fast-paced lifestyle. Spending for meals and snacks away from home has increased substantially since 1965 and accounts for more than double the amount spent on food eaten at home.

Although some people believe fast food is junk food, this is not always true. Nutritional analyses by fast food chains and independent studies reveal their menu items contain rich sources of protein (30% to 50% of the RDAs). Additionally, items are available that (if selected) provide 20% to 30% of the RDAs for thiamin, riboflavin, ascorbic acid, and calcium. When a hamburger or roast beef sandwich is selected, substantial amounts of iron are supplied. Most fast food menus lack a rich source of vitamin A. In many cases, salads and other healthier items have been added to menus because of consumer demand. This provides a source of vitamins A and C and dietary fiber; however, the cost may be two to seven times higher than the same foods purchased at supermarkets. Shortages of other nutrients—specifically biotin, folate, pantothenic acid, and copper—are also reported.

Several other problems with fast foods have been of concern: (1) The kilocalorie count of a regular meal is generally 900 to 1800 kcal (33% to 66% of the RDA for young men or 45% to 90% for young women), (2) sodium content is very high (1000 to 2515 mg), (3) fat content of some fast food meals is 51% of kcal consumed, and (4) mega-size portions contain a day's worth of kilocalories in one meal. The impact of fast foods on nutritional status depends on how frequently they are consumed, composition of each item selected, and what other foods are eaten during the day. Wise choices are possible when an individual's nutritional needs and nutrient content of menu items are known. New menu items and reduced portion sizes by several fast food chains make it easier to choose wisely. Nutritional analysis of menu items is available from most fast food chains.

Food Additives

During the 1950s, the Delaney committee investigated food additives. The Delaney clause prohibits use of any food additive if it is found to be carcinogenic in humans or animals. Additives deemed to be harmless were labeled "generally recognized as safe" (GRAS). These substances met certain specifications of safety under what might be called a "grandfather clause"—in other words, they are generally recognized by experts as safe, based on their use in foods for years without any known occurrence of health problems.

In 1960, similar legislation was passed for color additives. Colors currently in use were required to undergo further testing to continue being marketed. Since then, approximately 90 of the original 200 color additives have been classified as safe and continue to be added to foods.

The use of additives is regulated by law. Before a newly proposed additive can be marketed, it must undergo strict testing to establish its safety for the intended purpose. Safety levels of additives have been established by the FDA and limit the quantity and use of the additive. Currently, additives are specific, well-known substances meeting specifications for purity and have been shown as convincingly as possible to be free from harmful effects in the amounts commonly used.

Almost all food additives (99%) are derived from natural sources or are synthetically produced to be identical to the natural chemical substance. In many instances, effects of chemicals naturally present in a food are observed, and this chemical is added to other foods to achieve a similar effect. For instance, after calcium propionate in Swiss cheese was observed to retard mold, it was added to bread to inhibit mold growth.

Currently, additives are as safe as science can make them. "Absolute safety" cannot be guaranteed for anything in life. They are designed not to be toxic, and most of them would have to be ingested in very large amounts to produce acute symptoms. Some people experience allergic reactions to food additives, just as allergies to specific foods can occur. **Nanotechnology,** or the ability to measure and detect molecular structures nonometes or smaller, is allowing the ability to determine minute amounts of substances in the food supply. While some experts are urging foods or food additives containing nanoscale materials be subject to new safety testing to ensure their use does not pose unintended risks, current scientific evidence demonstrating the safety of a nanoscale food additive is not sufficient to meet the GRAS standard.[22]

The use of food additives makes many foods more readily available by preventing spoilage and keeping food wholesome and appealing. Complicated chemical names found on labels can be intimidating. Even names of vitamins on labels (e.g., thiamin mononitrate or cyanocobalamin) can cause apprehension for consumers unfamiliar with the terms. Food additives have the following benefits (Table 15-4):

1. They improve nutritional value. Enrichment and fortification have helped reduce malnutrition in the United States. Nutrients added help ensure adequate intake of vitamins or minerals. All added nutrients must be listed on product labels.
2. They maintain wholesomeness and palatability of foods. Bacterial contamination can cause foodborne illnesses. Preservatives retard spoilage caused by mold, air, bacteria, fungi, or yeast, and preserve natural color and flavor. Antioxidants prevent oxidation of fats and oils, fruits, and vegetables.
3. They maintain product consistency. Emulsifiers enable particles to mix and prevent separation. Stabilizers and thickeners contribute to a smooth, uniform texture.
4. They provide leavening or control pH. Leavening agents, such as yeast and baking powder, are used to make foods light in texture and baked goods rise.
5. They enhance flavor and appearance. These substances are the most widely used and controversial additives. Included in this category are coloring agents, natural and synthetic flavors, spices, flavor enhancers, and sweeten-

ers. Sugar, corn syrup, and salt are used in the largest amounts. Without these products, foods are less appealing, a factor that influences selection and nutrient intake.

Dental Hygiene Considerations

- Stress following the recommendations on how to preserve nutrients during preparation listed in Box 15-2.
- Clarify any misinformation about use of organic foods, but respect patients' beliefs and assist them in obtaining economical products that are acceptable to them.

Nutritional Directions

- Products that can be stored at room temperature should be kept in cool, dry areas in airtight containers.
- Regular ground beef is more economical than ground round, and total fat content can be significantly reduced by using a low-fat cooking method and by rinsing crumbled ground beef after cooking.
- Organic foods cost more but are not more nutritious or significantly different in taste. Fresh, locally grown produce is ideal.
- Organic produce does not look as attractive and unblemished as traditionally grown produce; organically processed foods have a shorter shelf life than products containing preservatives.
- The terms "natural" and "organic" were used interchangeably in the past to describe food that was minimally processed and free of artificial additives or preservatives; however, consumers should be aware that only products with the organic label have met USDA standards. Legally, use of terms such as "natural" or "all-natural" can mean anything the manufacturer wants them to mean.
- Food additives are tested before use. They are considered safe, but should be consumed in moderation. Choosing fresh foods is usually the ideal situation; these foods may have fewer additives.

FOOD FADS AND MISINFORMATION

Nutrition is a very popular subject, but even with all the current knowledge, it is no easier to understand today than it was in 1938:

More food notions flourish in the United States than in any other civilized country on earth, and most of them are wrong. They thrive in the minds of the same people who talk about their operations; and like all mythology, they are a blend of fear, coincidence, and advertising.[23]

As consumers' interest in nutrition increases, myths surrounding nutrition continue to confuse. Purveyors of nutritional misinformation capitalize on fears and hopes by exaggerating and oversimplifying health virtues or curative properties of foods. Too few consumers understand the effects of various nutrients on the body and how the body uses these nutrients, opening the door to food faddism or nutrition quackery.

Table 15-4 Guide to Food Additives

Type or Function	Commonly Used Additives	Food Usage
Vitamins and minerals improve nutritive value of foods	Vitamin D	Milk and margarine
	Potassium iodide (iodine)	Iodized salt
	Thiamin mononitrate (vitamin B₁), riboflavin (vitamin B₂), niacin (vitamin B₃), folate and ferrous sulfate (iron)	Enriched or fortified breakfast cereals, macaroni, pastas, breads and flour
	Ascorbic acid/sodium ascorbate (vitamin C)	Fruit juices and fruit drinks, cured meats, cereals
Preservatives maintain wholesomeness and palatability of foods	Butylated hydroxyanisole (BHA)	Cereals, chewing gum, potato chips, vegetable oil
	Tocopherols (vitamin E)	Vegetable oils
Antioxidants prevent unsaturated fats and oils, flavorings, and colorings from oxidation, which would result in rancidity, flavor changes, and loss of color	Citric acid	Instant potatoes, fruit drinks, sherbet
	Ascorbic acid (vitamin C)	Cured meats, fruit drinks
	Propyl gallate	Vegetable oils, meat products, potato sticks
	Erythorbic acid	Cured meats
Other preservatives control growth of mold, bacteria, and yeast	Sodium benzoate	Pickles, preserves, fruit juice
	Calcium (or sodium) propionate and potassium sorbate	Breads, rolls, pies, and cakes
	Sulfites	Dried fruit, frozen potatoes, and wines
	Sodium nitrite/nitrate	Bacon, ham, frankfurters, luncheon meats, smoked fish
	Sorbic acid, potassium sorbate	Cheese, syrup, jelly, cake, wine, dry fruits
Processing aids product consistency and texture. Emulsifiers keep oil and water mixed together with uniform dispersement of tiny particles	Monoglycerides and diglycerides	Baked goods, margarine, candy, peanut butter
	Lecithin	Baked goods, chocolate ice cream
	Polysorbate 60	Frozen desserts, imitation dairy products
Stabilizers, other processing aids, help maintain smooth texture and uniform color and flavor	Alginate and propylene glycol alginate	Ice cream, cheese, yogurt
	Carrageenan	Ice cream, jelly, chocolate milk, artificial breast milk
Thickeners, still other processing aids, provide desired thickness or gel	Various gums (Arabic, guar, xanthan)	Beverages, salad dressing, cottage cheese, frozen pudding
	Casein/sodium caseinate	Ice cream, sherbet, coffee creamers
	Pectin	Jelly
	Gelatin	Powdered dessert mixes, yogurt, ice cream, cheese spreads
	Starch/modified starch	Soup, gravy, baby food
Acids and bases control the pH of many foods and may act as buffers or neutralizing agents, or as leavening agents	Citric acid and sodium citrate	Frozen desserts, fruit drink, candy, instant potatoes
	Fumaric acid	Powdered drinks, pudding, pie fillings, gelatin desserts
	Lactic acid	Olives, cheese, powdered foods, cured meats, carbonated beverages
	Phosphoric acid	Breads, pastries, and baked goods
	Sodium bicarbonate	
Colorings, cosmetic additives in natural and synthetic forms, enhance the appearance of foods	Beta carotene	Margarine, shortening, nondairy whiteners
	Caramel color	Carbonated beverages, candy
	Artificial colors	Beverages, candy, baked goods, cherries in fruit cocktail, sausage, gelatin desserts
	Ferrous gluconate	Black olives
Flavoring agents, cosmetic additives available in natural and synthetic forms, enhance flavors	Artificial and natural flavoring	Carbonated beverages, candy, breakfast cereals, gelatin desserts
	Hydrolyzed vegetable protein (HVP)	Instant soups, frankfurters, sauce mixes, beef stew
	Vanillin (substitute for vanilla)	Ice cream, baked goods, beverages, chocolate, candy, gelatin desserts
	Monosodium glutamate (MSG)	Tonic water, bitter lemon
	Quinine	Soup, potato chips, crackers
	Salt (sodium chloride)	

Table 15-4	Guide to Food Additives—cont'd	
Type or Function	**Commonly Used Additives**	**Food Usage**
Sweeteners are cosmetic additives used to increase sweetness	Dextrose (corn syrup, glucose)	Candy, toppings, syrups, snack foods, imitation dairy foods
	High-fructose corn syrup	Soft drinks and other processed foods
	Invert sugar	Candy, soft drinks
	Sugar (sucrose)	Table sugar, sweetened foods
	Lactose	Whipped topping mix, breakfast pastry
Alternative sweeteners are cosmetic additives replacing sugar in products to reduce kilocalories or to reduce risk of dental decay	Acesulfame-K	Baked goods, chewing gum, gelatin desserts, soft drinks
	Aspartame	Soft drinks, drink mixes, frozen desserts, gelatin desserts
	Mannitol	Chewing gum, low-kilocalorie foods
	Saccharin	"Diet" products, soft drinks
	Sorbitol	Dietetic drinks and foods, candy, shredded coconut, chewing gum
	Sucralose	Diet foods
Other additives needed for processed foods to be prepared, stored, and shipped include anticaking agents; humectants; curing agents; sequestrants; and firming, bleaching, and maturing agents	Calcium (or sodium) stearyl lactylate	Bread dough, cake fillings, processed egg whites
	Ethylenediamine tetraacetic acid (EDTA)	Salad dressing, margarine, processed fruits and vegetables, canned shellfish
	Glycerin	Marshmallows, candy, fudge, baked goods

Food fad is a catchall term covering all aspects of nutritional nonsense, characterized by exaggerated beliefs about the value of nutrition in health and disease. A food fad may be based on a food fact or fallacy. People often begin a diet or believe claims for specific foods or supplements on the basis of something they read or hear without investigating its validity or effectiveness. Although some fads are physically harmless, they may create an economic hardship for individuals with limited income because the foods or supplements may be expensive. Others are nutritionally inadequate and could lead to serious deficiencies. A fad is sometimes harmful because this therapy is substituted for the advice of a healthcare provider, and the consumer delays medical treatment.

Fad diets are prevalent in the United States as Americans continue to search for a magic formula to lose weight and defy the aging process. According to promoters of weight loss diets, specific foods or food combinations facilitate weight loss, implying that a specific food or combination of foods oxidizes body fat, increases the metabolic rate, or inhibits voluntary food intake. These diets are frequently deficient in essential nutrients. Results of fad diets can be devastating and have even led to death. Other benefits, such as rapid weight loss, may not be long-lasting (see Evolve website).

Fad diets may promise to melt away fat without exercise while eating without limitation and with an immediate result of losing several pounds. Miraculous promises are a good reason to run the other way. Diets that provide adequate nutrients and changes in lifestyle behaviors are desirable and more effective. Fads, whether for weight loss or other purposes, can be recognized instantly when they promise secret formulas to "cure all."

Food quackery is the promotion of nutrition-related products or services having questionable safety or effectiveness or both for claims made. These claims or promises may be due to ignorance, delusion, misconception, or intent to deceive. Americans spend more than $10 billion annually for cures scientists deem as quackery.

The unknowns of medicine and disagreement among reputable scientists regarding interpretation of research findings foster nutritional misinformation. Given the right circumstances, such as confronting a chronic or incurable disease, everyone is potentially capable of exchanging sound judgment and common sense for the promise of a miraculous cure.

Numerous unproven theories abound regarding food allergies and intolerances, ranging from illegitimate diagnostic testing to treatment with diets and supplements not proven effective in scientific studies. Unconventional procedures for nutritional assessment are numerous. Hair analysis is used to recommend vitamin and mineral supplements. Hair analysis can indicate exposure to toxic heavy metals, but vitamins are not present in hair except in the roots below the skin. Hair grows very slowly and does not reflect current body status. Hair mineral content can be affected by shampoos, bleach, dye, and many other factors, including environmental and geographical factors. Frequently, a computer-scored questionnaire is used to diagnose nutrient deficiencies. These computers are programmed to recommend supplements for almost everyone, regardless of health problems or the presence or absence of symptoms.

Many theories have been proposed regarding the aging process. Nutritional manipulations are used based on these theories to extend a person's life. To date, no proven methods exist to extend the life span. Chelation therapy has been proposed to rejuvenate the cardiovascular system, treat cancer and immune disorders, and retard aging. This treatment has caused kidney damage and may result in people not seeking competent medical treatment.

Numerous concerns are associated with use of herbs as supplements. Herbal medicine should not be regarded as quackery, but should be approached with caution. Herbs, including herbal teas, and other plant-based formulations, are marketed as being the only natural method to prevent and cure numerous conditions. Deaths and severe health problems, including cardiovascular disease, cirrhosis, and renal failure, have occurred from use of herbal preparations in the United States.

No governmental organizations monitor the production and marketing of herbal supplements. The supplements may or may not perform as advertised. Many dietary and herbal supplements on the market have an inconsistent quality, and claims about their benefit are misleading and unsubstantiated by reliable studies. Any product can be marketed as a supplement if the label does not claim to affect a disease; it can state that the product affects a "structure or function" of the body, as long as the FDA is notified. A supplement is presumed safe until the FDA becomes aware of adverse reactions. The FDA can warn the public, request the manufacturer to change the product to make it safer, or recall the product. A supplement can be seized only if the FDA proves the product is unsafe.

Another problem is whether the product contains as much of the active ingredient as purported and in an effective form. Only about 50% to 70% of herbal products tested by ConsumerLab.com, an independent company that acts as a watchdog over the supplement industry, contain the active ingredient in the amount listed on the label. In some cases, the product contains harmful ingredients. Research has shown that some herbal supplements can interact with life-saving medications, making them either ineffective or occasionally even toxic. People can reduce the risks of these problems by (1) avoiding herbs if pregnant or nursing (herbs should not be given to infants), (2) not taking large amounts of any single herbal preparation on a daily basis, (3) buying only preparations that list all ingredients on the label (still no guarantee of safety), and (4) alerting the healthcare provider about use of herbs (see Health Application 10).

IDENTIFYING SOURCES OF NUTRITION MISINFORMATION

How do unscrupulous health promoters get away with their lies and fake products? Strict laws protect against false advertising and mislabeling, but health food deception and "food terrorism" thrive. The government actively pursues health swindlers, but enforcement agencies lack adequate staff and resources needed to handle all the problems reported.

The First Amendment to the U.S. Constitution protects free speech and a free press; it also protects a person's right to dispense false, misleading, or deceptive health claims. If a food product makes false or misleading claims on its label,

the FDA can take action because of mislabeling. For many years, health-related claims on a food product were prohibited by the FDA. Health claims are now permitted on food labels if (1) it is well documented that a particular nutrient can reduce risk, and (2) the benefits of this nutrient are not offset by another ingredient present. (For instance, a high-fiber cereal high in fat could not be touted as being beneficial to health because of its fat content.)

The Federal Trade Commission can take action if false claims are made in advertising, so claims made on labels or in promotions are not usually false. However, products can be legally promoted in books and magazine articles and on radio and television talk shows because of protection under the First Amendment.

Consumer interest in health and nutrition information is high as consumers are taking more responsibility for their own health care. Our culture is bombarded with nutrition information—television, radio, magazines, newspapers, books, Internet, infomercials, family and friends, and healthcare providers. People are frequently influenced by testimonials. Celebrities, sports figures, fitness experts, and others without nutrition expertise frequently are featured in advertisements purporting a nutritional product. The Internet is an unregulated source of nutrition information, reaching millions of people with sales of fraudulent and illegal nutritional and medical products. Probably the best way to begin a search on the Internet is to go to credible websites of trusted health organizations with names you recognize, universities, and state and national government agencies and offices, and click on links provided on these websites. Reliable nutrition websites are given throughout this text and on the Evolve website. Information provided in Box 15-4 is helpful in the evaluation of oral or written claims.

The news media often have a poor understanding of research methods and statistics, and seldom report the extent and limitations of the information or the important nuances of a research study. They generally report medical findings as "facts." Consumers are confused by listening to journalists presenting research studies that provide conflicting information. Two physicians developed four valuable guidelines for an editorial in the *New England Journal of Medicine* to help prevent misinterpretation of scientific studies:[24] (1) an association between two events is not the same as a cause and effect, (2) demonstrating one link in a postulated chain of events does not mean that the whole chain has been proven, (3) probabilities are not the same as certainties, and (4) the way a scientific result is framed can greatly affect its impact.

Evaluating nutritional information for its legitimacy and validity can be tedious. Healthcare professionals, regardless of where the nutrition information is presented—on the Internet, on television, or in print—should evaluate the findings in light of well-established nutrition principles. Dental hygienists and consumers should begin by checking the credentials of the person making a questionable claim. Most articles appearing in established medical and scientific journals were submitted to a board of other scientists for evalu-

Box 15-4	**Scrutinizing for Fraudulent Information**

1. Under the Food, Drug, and Cosmetic Act, a product is a drug if medical claims are made, or if it affects body functions. All medical manufacturers marketing products interstate must register and list the products with FDA. FDA prohibits introduction of any food, drug, device, or cosmetic not labeled correctly. (a) Even though the FDA must approve products before they are marketed, the term FDA is not permitted in any claim suggesting approval. (b) Ask to see the firm's FDA registration letter, product's listing letter, or FDA marketing approval letter.
2. Look for use of superlative terms, such as "amazing," "exclusive," "miracle," or "breakthrough," or extravagant terms, such as "cure" or "long life," or emotionally appealing terms, such as promises of "youth," "beauty," or "glamour." Scientific literature does not use these terms. Serious medical problems cannot be cured with remedies marketed mail order, door to door, or on the Internet.
3. Study the label on the product. (a) The instructions on the label should clarify the benefits for the user. (b) The information in the advertisement or promotional material should agree with the product label. Most false claims do not appear on the label because of FDA regulations. Unsubstantiated false claims are usually found in books, television, brochures, infomercials, and promotional materials. Because of the First Amendment that allows free speech and press, these types of materials are not regulated.
4. Insist on full identification of the institution or researcher promoting the product. Determine whether this information is from a credible source, or if the credentials of the promoter are from an accredited college or university. Medical clinics or medical personnel willingly provide full names, addresses, and phone numbers.
5. Beware of cures for serious diseases, or products that claim to cure multiple health problems.
6. Be careful of self-diagnosis based on a person's symptoms. Symptoms of many illnesses are similar, and a misdiagnosis can be hazardous if the condition is not being treated appropriately. A proper diagnosis requires an assessment, including a physical examination, by a health professional. Delaying treatment may allow progression of the disease beyond help.
7. Investigate information based on testimonials or case histories or promoted by movie stars, sports figures, or any "big name" person. This is not scientific evidence. The FDA cannot regulate a testimonial about a product.
8. Be cautious of recommendations for vitamin or mineral doses more than the RDAs or over the tolerable upper intake levels (ULs) for the nutrient. Reliable sources recommend only vitamin and mineral doses in line with the RDAs. Nutrients in amounts over the RDA or UL may be used as medications, as is done when niacin is used to reduce blood cholesterol levels. Only certain conditions use doses beyond the RDAs, and a legitimate medical source should monitor the effects.
9. If it sounds too good to be true, it probably is.

ation before publication. If the peer reviewers consider conclusions to be well supported by the research, it is published for others to read. A single study is never perfect, providing conclusive information, but provokes more questions for further studies. A single study is not meaningful by itself, but it serves as another piece of the puzzle if it can be replicated. Many types of studies—epidemiological, case-control, placebo-controlled, randomized, crossover-design, double-blind, clinical trials or interventions, meta-analysis—together help provide conclusive information. Research studies can be evaluated using the questions in Box 15-5.

ROLE OF DENTAL HYGIENISTS

What role can the dental hygienist play in combating nutrition fads and misinformation? Natalie Van Cleve stated in 1938, when times were different but widespread misinformation on diet was just as prevalent as today:[25]

It is the duty of all professions active in the field of food and nutrition to cooperate in clarifying any misconceptions of the laity. If the [healthcare providers] do not know their vitamins, the patients will find a radio announcer who does.

Healthcare providers, dental hygienists, and even dietitians have sometimes promoted nutritional misinformation by failing to apply their knowledge, misunderstanding how nutrients are used, or searching for fame and fortune. The dental hygienist is in a unique position to understand the causes of food fads and to recognize their dangers. First,

Box 15-5	**Questions to Ask About a Research Report**

- Was the research done by a credible institution? Was the research done by a qualified researcher?
- Is this a preliminary study? Have other studies reached the same conclusions?
- Was the study done with animals or humans?
- Was the research population large enough? Was the study long enough?
- Who paid for the study? Might that affect the findings? Is the science valid despite the funding source?
- Was the report reviewed by peers?
- Does the report avoid absolutes, such as "proves" or "causes"?
- Does the report reflect appropriate context, such as how the research fits into a broader picture of scientific evidence and consumer lifestyles?
- Do the results apply to a certain group of people? Do they apply to someone your age, gender, and health condition?
- What do follow-up reports from qualified nutrition experts say?

From Position of the American Dietetic Association: Food and nutrition misinformation. J Am Diet Assoc 2002 Feb; 102(2):260-266.

understanding patients and their love of "miracle" answers should help in recognizing the appeal of such misinformation. Second, a scientific background permits assessment of potential effects or uselessness of food fads. Dental hygienists can help patients understand the true essence of nutritional science—the process of nourishing or being nourished—rather than the polypharmacy of supernutrition. Many legitimate resources include governmental and professional organizations; these are referenced in Appendix C to help evaluate the legitimacy of nutritional claims. Many legitimate medical journals are also available on the Internet, as listed in Appendix D.

Nutritional Directions

- Populations consuming large amounts of fruits and vegetables, even with the use of fertilizers and pesticides, have a lower rate of cancer.
- Wash produce thoroughly. Some fruits and vegetables should be scrubbed with a brush under running water.
- In addition to government health agencies already mentioned, numerous health and professional organizations listed in Appendix C provide health information. Other organizations, such as the Better Business Bureau, may also be helpful.

Dental Hygiene Considerations

- Assess patients' use of food fads, economic level, and educational level, and the nutrient adequacy of any fad diet undertaken.
- If a patient restricts food choices because of a food fad or belief, ensuring nutrient adequacy is more difficult. A thorough assessment and evaluation by the dental hygienist may indicate the risk for a nutritional insufficiency or deficiency. Referral to a registered dietitian may be needed.
- Help patients choose a variety of foods to ensure a balanced intake and decrease the amount consumed of any one food to decrease risk of excessive contaminants from any one source. For instance, consumption of fish is encouraged because of beneficial substances to prevent coronary heart disease. However, too much fish, especially large fish such as sword-

fish, shark, mackerel, tilefish, and tuna, contain methylmercury that can potentially cause neurological problems.
- Provide patients with positive advice based on a broad knowledge base and understanding of nutritional concepts and current research findings.
- Answer any questions about therapies, products, or treatments a patient may be contemplating, or refer the patient to a reliable source.
- Speak out to protect the public from misinformation.
- Do not offer remedies unless they have been shown to be safe and effective.
- If a patient is using or contemplating using a food fad or diet you are unfamiliar with, do not hesitate to consult a registered dietitian, home economist, or nutrition professor.

HEALTH APPLICATION Food Insecurity in the United States

Food security, or access to enough food for an active, healthy life by all people at all times, is a universal dimension of household and personal well-being and considered a fundamental requirement for a healthy and well-nourished population. However, food insecurity and hunger continue to exist in the United States. **Food insecurity** refers to the lack of access to enough food to meet basic needs fully at sometime during the year because of lack of money or resources for food. Food insecurity is often episodic and may involve a low-quality diet that is monotonous and lacking in nutrients. Hunger, or an uneasy or painful sensation caused by lack of food, typically precedes food insecurity.

Food-secure households typically spend more on food than food-insecure households.[26] Hunger rates decrease as income increases, but food insecurity is not exclusive to very-low-income families. In 2007, census surveys indicated food insecurity rates were 10.1, essentially unchanged from 2005 and 2006.[27] The prevalence was about 30% for households with poverty-level incomes.[26] About one in three food-insecure households (4.7 million or 4.1%) of all U.S. households, had very low food security at some time in 2007. Rates of food insecurity were substantially higher than the national average for households with children headed by a single woman (30.8%) and in households with children (15.6%). Black and Hispanic households had rates of food insecurity more than twice those of white non-

Hispanic households.[28] A work-limiting disability substantially increases the risk of food insecurity for low-income families. In addition to the disabled individual being unable to work and incurring burdensome medical costs and other expenses, having a household member with a work-limiting disability can reduce the work opportunities and hours of other adult caretakers.[27] Several factors may account for the increase in food insecurity—the state of the U.S. economy; welfare reform legislation (e.g., Supplemental Nutrition Assistance Program); and the changing composition of the U.S. population, particularly households headed by single women.

Households attempt to avoid hunger by using various strategies, such as eating less varied diets, skipping meals, participating in federal food assistance programs, or getting emergency food from community food pantries. When individuals skip meals or postpone mealtimes, they are more likely to consume more kilocalories at each occasion.[29] A 5-hour interval between meals instead of 4 hours resulted in an additional intake of 52 kcal; extending that interval from 4 to 6 hours would add about 91 kcal to the meal.

The mental and physical changes accompanying inadequate food intakes can have harmful effects on learning, development, productivity, physical and psychological health, and family life. In the United States, food insecurity may be hidden because individuals may be malnourished in the sense of being overweight or obese. The homeless make up a large percentage of the hungry. Millions of people in the United States maintain a home and may even work full-time but live below the poverty level. (Poverty was defined as an annual income less than $20,000 for a family of four in the 48 contiguous states in 2006.) Low income, coupled with high housing and healthcare costs, can result in hunger and food insecurity. Approximately one-third of the monthly income for poverty-level families is spent on food.

Most studies have focused on food-insecure households with children. In 2000, 18% of children in the United States lived in food-insecure households. In most households, older family members protect children, especially younger ones, from substantial reductions in food intake and ensuing hunger. However, in 0.6% of households with children, food insecurity was sufficiently severe that at least one child was hungry on 1 or more days during the year because of insufficient funds.[30]

Acute and chronic effects on health and behavior have been observed. Insufficient food intake affects mental and physical health. Food-insecure children younger than 3 years old were nearly twice as likely to be in "fair or poor" health, and a larger percentage of children were more likely to have been hospitalized since birth than were food-secure children.[31] Ensuring food security may reduce health problems and hospitalizations. Growth stunting without muscle wasting is characteristic of homeless children who experience moderate chronic nutritional stress. Hungry children are more likely to experience undesired weight loss, fatigue, irritability, concentration problems, and dizziness, and frequent headaches, ear infections, and colds.

Cognitive and academic performance are also detrimentally affected. Missing a meal such as breakfast can reduce a child's ability to respond to the environment, negatively affecting learning. Apathy, disinterest, irritability, and a low tolerance for frustration are common behaviors in hungry children. These hungry children are unable to concentrate in school and are less likely to reach their potential to become fully productive adults. Additionally, psychosocial problems are observed more often: difficulty getting along with peers, suspension from school, and adolescent suicide.

The existence of hunger and food insecurity in the low-income adult population has been questioned because of the high prevalence of overweight and obesity in this group, especially in women. Information from the *Third National Health and Nutrition Examination Survey* (NHANES III) from 1988-1994 showed that adults, especially women, who participated in the Supplemental Nutrition Assistance Program had a greater body mass index (BMI) than adults who did not participate.[32] A consensus of research indicates participation in the program does not increase the likelihood of being overweight or obese for men or children. For nonelderly women, who account for 28% of all participants, multiple studies show a potential link between food stamp use and an increase in obesity and BMI, although this effect seems to be only about 3 lb.[33] Currently, food stamps participants can choose how to spend their benefits. Women who experienced food insecurity with hunger had greater BMIs than women who

were food secure. However, food insecurity without hunger was not significantly related to maternal obesity.[34] When adequate food supplies are not always available, people may find themselves in a cycle of overeating and then hunger when money or food stamps run out. Similar to people who frequently engage in a restrictive diet but return to their normal eating pattern, the "feast or famine" cycle can lead to weight gain.

Nutritionally, adults and children from food-insufficient households are more likely to consume substantially less than recommended amounts for certain food groups and nutrients. The first food group eliminated from an impoverished person's diet is produce.[35] Over the long-term, these deficits increase the risk of developing chronic diseases, including cancer and heart disease, more frequent and severe disease complications, and increased demands and costs for healthcare services.

Food-insecure elderly individuals have poorer dietary intake, nutritional status, and health status than do food-secure elderly individuals. The U.S. Census Bureau indicates that 9.4% of older adults had incomes below the poverty level in 2006.[36] The prevalence of food insecurity was lower (6.4%) than the national average in households with elderly members older than 65. Low intakes and concentrations of certain nutrients may compromise immune function and increase the risk of developing major chronic diseases, including osteoporosis, macular degeneration, and cataracts.

Food insecurity represents a major public health and public policy challenge by causing health problems, increasing education costs, and less than optimal productivity. Yet this serious health problem is treatable with a simple inexpensive cure: providing food. Proper nutrition can decrease money spent on health problems. Education may be the key to helping these families understand that cost of a food is important, but from a nutritional point of view, certain purchases are poor choices. Adults in food-insufficient families need nutrition education to help them know how to choose healthy foods within their limited financial means. Use of dietary supplements containing the recommended amounts of vitamins and minerals has been proposed because the average cost of one tablet is less than a dime. However, dietary supplements do not provide energy, which is especially important for children and older adults.

The goal of *Healthy People 2010* is to increase quality and years of healthy life and to eliminate health disparities; this requires improved food and nutrition security. By increasing food security among U.S. households to 95% (from the baseline of 89%), hunger would also be reduced. Federal assistance programs discussed earlier in this chapter are available to address hunger in the United States. Full use of these programs, with increased availability and benefits, and increased awareness of programs are good starts. Millions of eligible families are unaware of options for obtaining assistance or are declared ineligible for food stamps by onerous regulations.

The dental hygienist can help by referring patients to appropriate resources and agencies or to a social worker for assistance in filling out forms. These embarrassing issues should be discussed in a matter-of-fact manner.

HEALTH APPLICATION   Food Insecurity in the United States—cont'd

Patients may benefit by ventilating feelings and beliefs about food "handouts." Information should be presented in a positive manner, stating how it would benefit the patient and family. Most parents desire the best for their children; it is important to stress benefits children would receive (e.g., increased growth, learning, productivity) by participating. Help patients recognize that having inadequate funds for food is not a sign of failure, and that asking for help shows strength, courage, and wisdom. In due time, they may be able to help someone else. Dental hygienists can also help by offering to serve at community food resource centers or food donation drives. Some centers offer dental care using volunteer dental hygienists and dentists.

CASE APPLICATION FOR THE DENTAL HYGIENIST

A patient reports he has found a miracle cure for his advanced periodontal disease. He plans to follow a diet and take recommended supplements "to strengthen my gums." This diet eliminates all foods from two food groups in MyPyramid.

Nutritional Assessment
- Dietary intake, especially which of the food groups are omitted; nutrients most likely to be lacking
- Nutrition knowledge
- Supplements used and dosage
- Economic status
- Where most meals taken; food preparation

Nutritional Diagnosis
Knowledge deficit related to nutritional requirements.

Nutritional Goals
The patient will receive adequate nutrients to maintain oral health status by consuming a well-balanced diet.

Nutritional Implementation
Intervention: Discuss MyPyramid—different groups, numbers of servings needed from each group, portion sizes, and nutrients provided from each group.
Rationale: Healthy oral structures depend on a variety of nutrients that can be obtained by following this guideline.

Intervention: Discuss the nutrients that are deficient in his proposed diet and why those nutrients are important.
Rationale: When essential nutrients are omitted, the body cannot function effectively, and its immune response is compromised.
Intervention: Discuss the importance of obtaining nutrients from foods rather than supplements.
Rationale: Foods are the natural way of obtaining nutrients; when supplements are used, many times they are in proportions that cannot be absorbed, or they may interfere with the absorption of other nutrients. Other components of the food may affect the use of the nutrient. In general, most supplements are not as effective as the food itself (see Health Application 10).
Intervention: Discuss specific foods and oral care that would be helpful in preventing further deterioration.
Rationale: Adequate nutrition and oral self-care promote healing and repair of disease tissue. Maintaining a well-balanced diet provides the nutrients needed to support a healthy periodontium and resist disease activity.

Evaluation
The patient will practice effective oral care and consume a well-balanced diet; as a consequence, his periodontal health will improve.

STUDENT READINESS

1. What ethnic groups are most prevalent in your area?
   - Identify at least one thing good about this ethnic group's food pattern.
   - List at least one potential dietary problem of this ethnic group, and provide some suggestions for altering the diet.
   - Plan a 2-day menu that would fulfill the RDAs and use many of their favorite foods or habits.
   - Would a patient have any problem being able to follow that menu, such as economic hardship or the local availability of special foods?
   - Does that ethnic group have any predominant dental problems?
2. Other than good foods to eat, what other lifelong eating customs are learned as a child?
3. State some reasons why people in the United States do not have the same eating patterns.
4. Plan an inexpensive menu for 1 day, using low-cost foods.
5. A patient wants to know about convenience and fast foods. What would you tell him or her?
6. Study the meats at a grocery store. Categorize the types of meats that contain nitrate preservatives. Look at your own daily intake for 3 days, and evaluate how frequently you are consuming nitrate-containing foods.
7. Americans are dependent on commercially prepared frozen foods or purchased foods outside the home. Look at the caloric density of the foods consumed in commercial restaurants and the nature of the diseases that relate to obesity and cardiovascular health. What has consumer demand done to change selections offered in commercial food service establishments?
8. Prepare a rough budget showing how your personal funds are expended on a month-to-month basis. Evaluate the percentage of your own personal income that is earmarked for food prepared at home versus food prepared commercially in a restaurant or convenience items

purchased in a grocery store. How well do you spend your own food dollar? Make some conclusions about how you could better use your dollar to provide nutrient-dense foods for you and your family.

9. Compare the cost of three foods from a health food store or the health food section of a supermarket with the cost of similar items in a supermarket. Can you think of any reasons to justify the more expensive product?

10. Locate an advertisement in a popular magazine or newspaper for a health food product, and list merits of the product stated in the ad. List information about the product that might have been omitted or should be questioned.

11. Compare the cost of three organic foods with the same foods that are not labeled organic. Which would you choose to purchase and why?

12. Why are food faddism and quackery a problem for the medical profession?

13. Discuss current food fads and how they may have adverse effects.

14. How can one spot a food quack?

15. Discuss the pros and cons of allowing nutritional claims on products.

16. A patient states, "I want to follow the _____ diet because my favorite actor follows it." How would you respond?

17. Read a nutrition research article from a reputable journal. Using the information provided in this chapter, point out some problems with the validity and applicability of the research. Does the article identify these as problem areas? Summarize the article in one page or less as if presenting to a patient.

CASE STUDY

A young couple with three children, ages 3, 5, and 7, has been living on unemployment insurance payments for 9 months. The mother expresses concerns because of inadequate funds to feed the children. She is worried about their dental health.

1. Prepare a list of social services or federal service agencies in the community that should be contacted to determine potential sources of assistance to support the recovery of this couple.

2. What are some nutritional concerns the dental hygienist could address with the patient?

3. What are some foods that are nutrient-dense and economical purchases?

4. List some snack foods for the children that are nutritious, economical, and noncariogenic.

5. What methods of food preparation could be suggested to the mother that would preserve the nutritional quality of the food?

References

1. Sequist TD, et al: Physician performance and racial disparities in diabetes mellitus care. Arch Intern Med 2008 Jun 9; 168(11): 1145-1151.
2. Jones T, Fergus MA: Prices take bite out of aid. Chicago Tribute, April 8, 2008. Available at www.chicagotribut.com/news/chi-food-stampsapr08,0,4965983,print.story. Accessed April 19, 2008.
3. Doering C: USDA: Food prices to post biggest rise this year since 1990. USA Today, August 22, 2008. Available at //usatoday.printthis.clickability.com/. Accessed August 22, 2008.
4. Nord M, Andrews M, Carlson S: Household food security in the United States, 2007. ERR-66, U.S. Department of Agriculture, Econ Res Serv, November 2008.
5. Monisivais P, Drewnowski A: The rising cost of low-energy-density foods. J Am Diet Assoc 2007 Dec; 107(12): 2071-2076.
6. Stewart H: Lower income households spend additional income on foods other than fruit and vegetables. Amber Waves 2008 June. Available at www.ers.usda.gov/AmberWaves/June08/Findings/Lower_Income.htm. Accessed July 4, 2008.
7. Reed J, Frazão E, Itskowitz R: How much do Americans pay for fruits and vegetables? Economic Research Service/USDA, AIB-790. Available at http://www.ers.usda.gov/Publications/AIB790/. Accessed August 20, 2008.
8. Jetter KM, Cassady DL: The availability and cost of healthier food alternatives. Am J Prev Med 2006 Jan; 30(1):38-44.
9. Cassady D, Jetter KM, Culp J: Is price a barrier to eating more fruits and vegetables for low-income families? J Am Diet Assoc 2007 Nov; 107(11):1909-1915.
10. Guthrie JF, et al: Improving food choices—can food stamps do more? Amber Waves, May 2007. Available at www.ers.usda.gov/AmberWaves/May07SpecialIssue/Features/Improving.htm. Accessed January 12, 2008.
11. Braley G: George Braley testimony to the Joint Economic Committee. America's second harvest: The Nation's Food Bank Network. May 1, 2008. Available at www.secondharvest.org/learn_about_hunger/public_policy/braley_testimony.html. Accessed Aug 20, 2008.
12. Government Food Safety Network. J Am Diet Assoc 2008 May; 108(5):897. Available at www.foodsafety.gov. Accessed July 4, 2008.
13. Centers for Disease Control and Prevention (CDC) Statistics: Preliminary FoodNet Data on the incidence of infection with pathogens transmitted commonly through food—10 states, 2007. MMWR Wkly 2008 Apr 11; 57(14):366-370. Available at www.cdc.gov/mmwr/preview/mmwrhtml/mm5714a2.htm. Accessed April 18, 2008.
14. Niemira BA: Relative efficacy of sodium hypochlorite wash versus irradiation to inactivate *Escherichia coli* O157:H7 internalized in leaves of Romaine lettuce and baby spinach. J Food Prot 2007 Nov; 70(11):2526-2532.
15. Organic Trade Association: U.S. organic industry overview. OTA's 2006 manufacturer survey. Greenfield, MA, 2006.
16. 2005 National Residue Program Data, Red book. Available at www.fsis.usda.gov/Science/2005_Red_Book/index.asp. Accessed Aug 20, 2008.
17. Winter, CK, Davis S: Scientific status summary: organic foods. J Food Science 2006 Nov-Dec; 71(9):R117-R124.
18. Lu C, et al: Organic diets significantly lower children's dietary exposure to organophosphorus pesticides. Environ Health Perspect 2006 Feb; 114(2):260-263.
19. Lu C, et al: Dietary intake and its contribution to longitudinal organophosphorus pesticide exposure in urban/suburban children. Environ Health Perspect 2008 Apr; 116(4):537-542.

20. Organic food: Worth the price? Nutrition Action Health Letter 2007 Jul/Aug; 34(6):1, 3-7.

21. Mukherjee A, et al: Preharvest evaluation of coliforms, *Escherichia coli, Salmonella,* and *Escherichia coli* O157:H7 in organic and conventional produce grown by Minnesota farmers. J Food Protect 2004 May; 67(5):894-900.

22. Finan C: Nan food-additives require new oversight say experts. Medical News TODAY. www.medicalnewstoday.com/printerfriendlynews.php?newsid=133727. Accessed December 29, 2008.

23. Anonymous, cited by Wilder RM: Fads, fancies, and fallacies in adult diets. Sigma Xi O 1938; 26:73.

24. Angel M, Kassuer JP: Clinical research—what should the public believe? (editorial) N Engl J Med 1994 Jul 21; 331(3):189-190.

25. Van Cleve N: Food: Facts, fad, and fancy. Am J Nurs 1988; 38(3):285.

26. Nord M, Prell M: Struggling to feed the family: What does it mean to be food insecure? AmberWaves Jun 2007. Available at www.ers.usda.gov/AmberWaves/June07/Findings/Disability.htm. Accessed June 30, 2007.

27. Nord M, Andrews M, Carlson S: Household Food Security in the United States, 2007. ERR-66, U.S. Dept of Agriculture, Econ. Res. Serv. November 2008.

28. Nord M: More households had difficulty meeting their food needs. AmberWaves Feb 2006. Available at www.ers.usda.gov/AmberWaves/February06/findings/Findings_DH2.htm. Accessed August 20, 2008.

29. Mancino L, Kinsey J: Is dietary knowledge enough? Hunger, stress, and other roadblocks to healthy eating. ERS Report Summary, ERR-62, USDA, Aug 2008. Available at www.ers.usda.gov. Accessed Aug 20, 2008.

30. Nord M, Andrews M, Carlson S: Household food security in the United States, 2002. October 2003. Washington, DC: USDA/ERS FANRR No 21. Available at http://www.ers.usda.gov/publications/fanrr35/fanrr35researchbrief.pdf. Accessed Aug 20, 2008.

31. Cook JT, et al: Food insecurity is associated with adverse health outcomes among human infants and toddlers. J Nutr 2004 Jun; 134(6):1432-1438.

32. Ploeg MV, Mancino L, Lin BH: Food stamps and obesity: ironic twist or complex puzzle? AmberWaves February 2006. Available at www.ers.usda.gov/AmberWaves/February06/Features/feature4.htm. Accessed January 12, 2008.

33. Ploeg MV, Ralston K: Food stamps and obesity: what we know and what it means. Amber Waves 2008 June. Available at http://www.ers.usda.gov/AmberWaves/June08/Features/FoodStampsObesity.htm. Accessed June 21, 2008.

34. Dinour LM, Bergen D, Yeh MC: The food insecurity-obesity paradox: a review of the literature and the role food stamps may play. J Am Diet Assoc 2007 Nov; 107(11):1952-1961.

35. Hampton T: Food insecurity harms health, well-being of millions in the United States. JAMA 2007 Oct 24/31; 298(16):1851-1853.

36. Center for American Progress: Elderly poverty: The challenge before us. July 30, 2008. Available at http://www.americanprogress.org/issues/2008/07/elderly_poverty.html. Accessed August 20, 2008.

Chapter 16

Effects of Systemic Disease on Nutritional Status and Oral Health

OUTLINE

LEARNING OBJECTIVES

Upon completion of this chapter, the student will be able to achieve the following objectives:

- Recognize various diseases, conditions, and treatments that commonly have oral signs and symptoms.
- Recognize diseases, conditions, and treatments likely to affect nutritional intake.

- Critically assess the implications of the patient's systemic diseases or conditions for optimal oral health.
- Plan appropriate dental hygiene interventions for patients with systemic diseases or conditions with oral manifestations based on dietary guidelines.

KEY TERMS

Aneurysm
Atherosclerosis
Binges
Bradykinesia
Chemotherapy
Epilepsy
Esophagitis
Gastroesophageal reflux disease (GERD)
Gastrostomy
Genome
Genomics
Glossodynia
Gluten
Herpetic ulcerations
Hiatal hernia
Ischemia
Kaposi's sarcoma
Leukemia

Leukoplakia
Lipodystrophy
Mucositis
Neutropenia
Nutrigenomics
Nutritional genomics
Odynophagia
Osteonecrosis
Osteosclerosis
Parkinson's disease
Pocketed foods
Purging
Renal osteodystrophy
Stomatitis
Syrup of ipecac
Thrombus
Uremic
Variants

Test Your NQ

1. **T/F** Anorexia, associated with a chronic disease, can result in an increased susceptibility to infection.
2. **T/F** Antihypertensive, anticholinergic, and antidepressant drugs often cause a decrease in salivary flow.
3. **T/F** Iron supplements should be recommended to a patient who has anemia.
4. **T/F** It is within the scope of practice for a dental hygienist to provide nutritional counseling to a patient recently diagnosed with diabetes.
5. **T/F** A patient with a hiatal hernia should be cautioned against eating before a dental appointment to prevent regurgitation while lying in a supine position.

6. **T/F** The healthcare provider should monitor protein intake closely in a patient with chronic renal failure.
7. **T/F** Kaposi's sarcoma is a tumor that occurs frequently in patient's with epilepsy.
8. **T/F** Phenytoin (Dilantin) can cause gingival hyperplasia and vitamin deficiencies.
9. **T/F** A dental hygienist should not confront a patient suspected to have an eating disorder, but should casually refer the patient to a healthcare provider.
10. **T/F** Patients with bulimia generally have low body weight.

As you have already learned, nutritional deficiencies frequently are manifested in the oral and head and neck areas. Oral lesions can be a reflection of or a marker for disease elsewhere. The oral cavity cannot be isolated from and is not immune to what is occurring in the body because oral tissues are nourished by the same blood supply providing oxygen and nutrients to cells throughout the entire body. Oral tissues may reflect changes in the nutrient supply or other metabolic alterations. Oral manifestations are only a single part of the total systemic state.

Oral problems may develop due to disease processes or therapies, or by nutritional deficiencies. The subsequent oral issues can cause inadequate intake. Systemic diseases or medications usually prescribed for these conditions may cause alterations in the oral cavity, such as oral lesions, xerostomia, or muscular weakness (Table 16-1). These oral

alterations may lead to changes in eating patterns, which frequently have a general debilitating effect on the entire body. For example, food preferences are affected by one's ability to chew. Patients with reduced masticatory efficiency usually choose soft foods, which may not provide adequate amounts of essential nutrients. Patients with tooth loss, malocclusion, or ill-fitting dentures or partials may be at increased risk of inadequate intake of nutrients such as protein, some B vitamins, vitamin D, calcium, iron, magnesium, and phosphorus.[1] The body depends on nutrients from foods eaten to regenerate and repair diseased tissues; provisions must be made to provide these nutrients in adequate amounts on a regular basis.

All disease processes result from a combination of factors: the presence of an etiologic agent (e.g., plaque biofilm), the susceptibility or resistance of the host (or activation of

Table 16-1 Oral Problems Associated with Systemic Diseases

Condition	Xerostomia	Taste Alterations	Oral Lesions	Immune Response	Masticatory Efficiency	Delayed Wound Healing	Dysphagia	Sore Tongue	Risk of Bleeding	Dental Caries
Anemias										
Iron-deficiency	X	X	X	X		X		X		
Plummer-Vinson	X	X	X	X		X	X	X		
Megaloblastic		X	X	X				X		
Thalassemia					X					
Aplastic			X						X	
Other Hematological Diseases										
Polycythemia									X	
Neutropenia			X	X						
Gastrointestinal Problems										
Medications for reflux	X	X						X		
Malabsorptive conditions		X	X			X				
Cardiovascular Conditions										
Cardiovascular accidents	X						X			
Antihypertensive medications		X								
Lipid-lowering medications									X	
Skeletal Anomalies										
Systemic bone disturbances					X					
Metabolic Problems										
Diabetes mellitus	X	X		X		X				X
Acromegaly					X					
Hypopituitarism					X					
Cushing's syndrome					X			X		
Hypothyroidism					X					X
Hyperparathyroidism					X					
Renal Disease										
Diminished kidney function			X		X	X			X	
Neuromuscular Problems										
Parkinson's disease	X				X		X			
Developmental disabilities					X		X			
Epilepsy	X									
Neoplasia										
Cancer		X								
Kaposi's sarcoma			X							
Leukemia				X						
Acquired Immunodeficiency Syndrome										
AIDS	X		X	X						
Mental Health Problems										
Anorexia nervosa/bulimia				X						X
Medications for mental illness	X									

immune response), and environmental factors. One of the most important factors in one's ability to combat hostile agents is the availability of nutrients acquired from food. Infections can spread rapidly when the immune response is depressed.

The ramifications of a patient's systemic health are important to the dental hygienist because they provide cues to possible oral problems; may change treatment goals, priorities, or scheduling; or may influence dietary recommendations provided to the patient. The dental hygienist's dietary recommendations should take into consideration the systemic health of a patient and should not contradict dietary instructions provided by the patient's other healthcare providers. In other words, dietary counseling for oral health problems must be done in the context of the entire patient. Many conditions require referral to a healthcare provider or registered dietitian.

This chapter presents oral problems frequently caused by systemic health conditions or their treatment because these problems typically affect eating patterns. No attempt is made to cover pathophysiology, and the information given should not be used to diagnose conditions. If the cause of oral signs and symptoms is unknown, refer the patient to a healthcare provider, who can perform a thorough assessment, including diagnostic laboratory evaluation, for accurate diagnosis and treatment.

EFFECTS OF CHRONIC DISEASE ON INTAKE

ANOREXIA AND APPETITE

The term *anorexia nervosa* refers to a disease associated with a distorted body image, but *anorexia* may also refer to a condition in which a patient has a poor appetite for a variety of reasons (e.g., cancer treatment). Appetite is associated with enjoyment of food. Most healthy individuals have a good appetite with no problems eating adequate amounts of food. However, during illness, appetite may decrease because of pain, apathy, anorexia, drugs, inactivity, or many other reasons. Individuals may become depressed after the diagnosis of a chronic illness, causing mental stress about problems related to living with, or dying because of, the condition. A modified diet may be prescribed for a patient with a chronic illness, which may adversely affect intake. Because poor food intake may lessen the desire to eat further, in some situations it may be unknown whether anorexia is a cause of the illness or an effect of the illness. Malnutrition and other stresses such as infection, surgery, and injuries resulting in anorexia deplete body stores of kilocalories, macronutrients (e.g., protein), and micronutrients (e.g., vitamin C) needed to regenerate and repair cells; the body is more susceptible to bacterial or viral invasion.[2]

TASTE AND SMELL DISORDERS

Taste and smell can dramatically affect appetite and food intake. Various conditions (e.g., respiratory diseases, cancer) and medications and treatment for the conditions may result in chemosensory disorders (i.e., disorders of taste and smell). Reactions to loss of taste and smell vary. Recent research found patients with loss of smell reported they eat less (29%), use more spices (39%), and eat and drink fewer sweets (37% and 48%). Patients experiencing taste changes tend to have inadequate food intake and weight loss resulting in malnutrition.[3,4] Individuals taking three or more medications are likely to have less taste sensitivity and require greater amounts of sodium (11.6 times higher) and sugar (2.7 times higher) to perceive these tastes.[4] The loss of saliva in disease and drug-induced xerostomia reduce the solubility of flavors and the ability to taste.

XEROSTOMIA

Saliva protects hard and soft oral tissues from mechanical, thermal, and chemical irritants in addition to its roles in buffering acids, antimicrobial activity, and remineralization.[5] It is estimated xerostomia is experienced by about 30% of individuals 65 years and older, primarily as a result of prescription and over-the-counter medications used to treat disease.[6] Medications (e.g., antidepressants, antihypertensives, and diuretics), diseases or conditions (e.g., Sjögren's disease), and therapies (e.g., radiation) may cause xerostomia.

Xerostomia can affect nutritional status in several ways, as follows: (1) chewing is difficult because a bolus cannot be formed without additional moisture, (2) chewing is painful because the mouth is sore, (3) swallowing is difficult because of loss of lubrication from saliva, and (4) food intake may decrease because of changes in taste perception. Individuals with xerostomia tend to avoid dry, crunchy foods and sticky foods, which may result in inadequate intake of fiber, potassium, vitamin B_6, iron, calcium, and zinc.[7]

ANEMIAS

Typical symptoms of all the anemias are pallor of the skin, oral mucosa, and conjunctival tissues, along with overall weakness as a result of inadequate oxygen-carrying power of the blood. The occurrence and severity of clinical symptoms depend on the degree of anemia and speed of onset. The type of anemia can be determined only after evaluation of blood tests.

IRON-DEFICIENCY ANEMIA

Iron-deficiency anemia can be caused by a deficiency of dietary iron or by excessive bleeding, and may occur during periods in which iron requirements are high, such as during infancy or pregnancy. Gradual depletion of iron stores may progress to iron-deficiency anemia and levels of iron inadequate to maintain hemoglobin levels to provide oxygen to cells. Lethargy and fatigue in addition to glossitis, aphthous ulcers, and xerostomia associated with iron-deficiency anemia can lead to changes in appetite and food intake.[8] Clinical symptoms in the oral cavity include gingival and mucosal pallor (Fig. 16-1), angular cheilosis, and atrophic glossitis. Atrophic glossitis is described as atrophy of the filiform and fungiform papillae beginning at the tip and

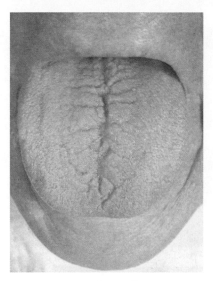

FIGURE 16-1   Clinical symptoms of iron-deficiency anemia include pallor of the gingiva, mucosa, and tongue. (Courtesy DW Beaven and SE Brooks. From McLaren DS: A Colour Atlas and Text of Diet-Related Disorders, 2nd ed. London: Mosby-Yearbook Europe Ltd, 1992.)

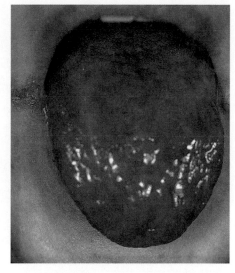

FIGURE 16-2   Iron-deficiency anemia. (From Cawson RA, Odell EW: Cawson's Essentials of Oral Pathology and Oral Medicine, 8th ed. Edinburgh: Churchill Livingstone, 2008.)

lateral borders of the tongue and gradually spreads to the entire dorsum of the tongue. As the papillae gradually shrink in size, bald spots appear on the tongue, and it becomes smooth, shiny, and red (Fig. 16-2).[9]

Iron-deficiency anemia affects the immune response and places a patient at increased risk for fungal infections, such as candidiasis. After iron supplementation is initiated, oral symptoms begin to resolve in 48 hours, and filiform papillae regenerate in 3 to 4 weeks.[10] Depending on the severity of iron-deficiency anemia, wound healing may be impaired in response to more invasive dental treatments, such as tooth extraction, nonsurgical periodontal therapy, and periodontal surgery.

Nutritional Directions

- If the iron supplement is liquid, dilute with water or juice, and drink with a straw to minimize tooth staining.
- Iron stores are replenished very slowly; therapy should be continued for at least 1 year.

MEGALOBLASTIC ANEMIA

Vitamin B_{12} deficiency can result in a megaloblastic anemia (a small number of large red blood cells [RBCs]) also called *pernicious anemia*. This condition occurs when vitamin B_{12} is deficient in the diet, absorption is inadequate, or requirements are increased. With vitamin B_{12} malabsorption or no dietary source (as occurs in vegans), normal body stores are usually sufficient for 3 to 4 years. Vitamin B_{12} deficiency is most common among vegans who consume no animal products.

Oral changes of vitamin B_{12} deficiency may be the only clinical evidence of the disease preceding significant anemia.[10] Patients with pernicious anemia (Fig. 16-3) may initially present with angular cheilosis, recurrent aphthous ulcers (and erythematous **mucositis** [flat lesions with inflamed, red borders]), and pale or yellowish oral mucosa (Fig. 16-4).[10] Patients may also complain of a painful, sore, burning tongue with signs of atrophic glossitis associated with a beefy red color. Replacement therapy with vitamin B_{12} injections relieves symptoms within 36 to 48 hours with evidence of regeneration of tongue papillae within 4 to 7 days, and the tongue may be normal in 3 to 4 weeks.[10]

Dental Hygiene Considerations

Assessment
- *Physical*: burning sensation of the tongue, xerostomia, gingival and mucosal pallor, atrophy of the filiform and fungiform papillae, atrophic glossitis, angular cheilosis, dysphagia, candidiasis.
- *Dietary*: adequacy of dietary intake, especially red meats, dark green vegetables, enriched cereals and bread; use of vitamin-mineral supplements.

Interventions
- Encourage iron-rich foods (see Table 11-9); if principally nonheme sources are consumed at a meal, a source of vitamin C enhances absorption of nonheme iron.
- If the iron supplement causes nausea, suggest the patient take the supplement with food, or discuss the problem with the healthcare provider, rather than discontinue the supplement.

Evaluation
Successful outcomes include the patient's consuming iron-rich foods and taking the ordered supplement.

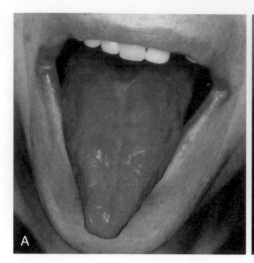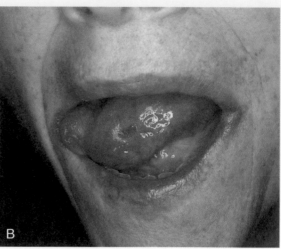

FIGURE 16-3 **A** and **B,** Pernicious anemia. (From Ibsen OAC, Phelan JA: Oral Pathology for the Dental Hygienist, 5th ed. St Louis: Saunders, 2009.)

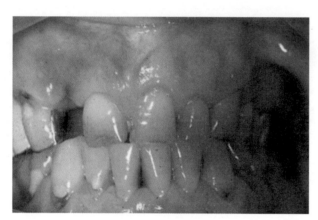

FIGURE 16-4 Gingival pallor owing to anemia. (Courtesy Dr. Edward V. Zegarelli. From Ibsen OAC, Phelan JA: Oral Pathology for the Dental Hygienist, 2nd ed. Philadelphia: Saunders, 1996.)

Another type of megaloblastic anemia, caused by folic acid deficiency, is frequently associated with poor diets or medications that interfere with folate absorption or metabolism, such as phenytoin (Dilantin) or methotrexate. Oral manifestations are similar to the manifestations present in pernicious anemia: glossitis, atrophy of the papillae, ulcerations, and pain in the tongue or **glossodynia**. Angular cheilitis and fungal infections in the perioral area may also be seen.

Folate replacement is necessary because diet alone is inadequate to replace lost stores. Iron supplements also may be ordered because when folate is deficient, iron is usually low as well. Folate supplementation in a patient deficient in vitamin B_{12} may produce hematological improvement, whereas neurological damage from vitamin B_{12} deficiency continues to progress.

Dental Hygiene Considerations

Assessment
- *Physical*: sex; age; glazed, red, sore or painful tongue; pale skin and oral mucous membranes; shortness of breath; malabsorption, previous gastrointestinal surgeries.
- *Dietary*: dietary intake, especially of dark green leafy vegetables, animal products, whole-grain breads, and fortified foods; alcohol intake.

Interventions
- If the patient has megaloblastic anemia caused by folate deficiency, encourage rich food sources of folate along with a supplement meeting the recommended dietary allowance (RDA) for folate (400 µg) (see Table 10-10).
- If the patient is not a vegan, encourage intake of foods from animal sources high in vitamin B_{12} for pernicious anemia (see Table 10-12). If the patient is a vegan, encourage intake of fortified foods or supplementation. Dietary intake helps re-establish depleted stores.
- Refer the patient to a registered dietitian; patients with megaloblastic anemia especially need nutritional counseling because of undesirable eating habits.

Evaluation
Desired outcomes include the patient's consuming a well-balanced diet and foods high in folate or vitamin B_{12} (as appropriate) and taking supplements to enhance the formation of RBCs or erythropoiesis.

OTHER HEMATOLOGICAL DISORDERS

NEUTROPENIA

Neutropenia is a diminished number of white blood cells (WBCs) (neutrophils) in the blood and may predispose an immunocompromised patient to life-threatening infection. The risk of infection is directly proportional to the duration

Nutritional Directions

- Raw vegetables are a better source of folate than cooked vegetables; heat destroys folate.
- Daily intake of dietary folate is necessary.
- Patients with permanent gastric or ileal damage need monthly intramuscular or oral vitamin B_{12} supplementation for life.
- Vitamin B_{12} shots are not always indicated for "tired blood."
- When oral vitamin B_{12} or iron supplements are ordered, take with vitamin C–rich foods to enhance absorption.
- Large doses of folate can negate therapeutic effects of anticonvulsants, so consultation with the healthcare provider is recommended.

and severity of neutropenia. Neutropenia results from drugs (e.g., chemotherapeutic agents or antibiotics), autoimmune disease (e.g., rheumatoid arthritis, systemic lupus erythematosus), hematological disease (e.g., leukemia), nutritional deficiencies (e.g., severe vitamin B_{12} or folate deficiency), or bacterial or viral infection.[11]

Oral mucous membrane surfaces are common sites for infection as a result of neutropenia. The most common oral manifestations are mucositis, and viral and fungal infections (e.g., candidiasis). Mucositis may result in large ulcerative and necrotic lesions with extensive tissue destruction. Periodontal disease can be a source of bacterial infection leading to systemic infection. In a small group of patients with leukemia, 28% of systemic infections were reported to be of periodontal origin. Ideally, this condition is treated and managed before initiation of treatment that may result in neutropenia.[12] Patients with neutropenia must perform meticulous oral hygiene to prevent the progression of periodontal disease. When neutropenia is present, invasive

Dental Hygiene Considerations

Assessment
- *Physical*: painful oral mucosal ulcerations (mucositis), candidiasis.
- *Dietary*: folate and vitamin B_{12} intake.

Interventions
- For neutropenia, encourage foods high in folate (see Table 10-10) and vitamin B_{12} (see Table 10-12) if the patient's intake is questionable.
- Stress the importance of frequent oral prophylaxis and meticulous oral self-care.
- Refer the patient to a registered dietitian for nutritional counseling if eating habits are poor.

Evaluation
Successful outcomes include patient adherence to a diet encompassing a variety of foods, concentrating on iron, vitamin B_{12}, or folate; use of supplementation as recommended by a healthcare provider or registered dietitian; and frequent dental hygiene recalls and maintenance of good periodontal health.

Nutritional Directions

- To ensure adequate iron intake, choose meat, fish, or poultry regularly.
- To enhance iron absorption, choose a vitamin C–rich food with a meal or eat a small amount of meat with each meal.

dental treatment is usually contraindicated until WBC counts increase. If treatment is indicated, a consultation with the healthcare provider is necessary to determine if antibiotic prophylaxis is needed.[12]

GASTROINTESTINAL PROBLEMS

GASTROESOPHAGEAL REFLUX, HIATAL HERNIA, AND ESOPHAGITIS

Heartburn 30 minutes to 1 hour after eating is the most common symptom of **gastroesophageal reflux disease (GERD)**, a return of gastric contents into the esophagus. This condition is commonly associated with **hiatal hernia** (partial protrusion of the stomach through the esophageal opening into the chest cavity), pregnancy, and obesity. Normally, the lower esophageal sphincter prevents caustic gastric acid from refluxing into the esophagus. Acidity from the stomach, alkalinity, pepsin, or bile may damage the esophageal mucosa, and esophagitis may result if left untreated. **Esophagitis** is an inflammation of the lower esophagus and may cause discomfort swallowing.

Patients are normally advised to decrease their intake of foods that precipitate reflux, such as fatty foods (e.g., gravy, pastries, chocolate, fatty meats, cheese, nuts, chips, salad

Dental Hygiene Considerations

Assessment
- *Physical*: type of medications used; heartburn; bitter taste; visual appraisal of weight; enamel erosion; sensitivity of the dentin.
- *Diet*: adequacy of intake; frequency of intake; caffeine, fat, alcohol intake; knowledge of foods that increase reflux or irritate the esophagus.

Interventions
- If weight loss is needed, refer to a registered dietitian or weight loss program, such as Weight Watchers or TOPS (Take Off Pounds Sensibly), for counseling and a nutritionally sound reduction program.
- To reduce risk of regurgitation during dental treatment, the patient's head and neck should be positioned above the stomach in the operatory chair; encourage the patient not to eat for 2 hours before the appointment; omit the use of nitrous oxide because it may relax the lower esophageal sphincter.

Evaluation
The patient plans frequent well-balanced meals, avoiding foods that cause reflux and irritate the esophagus.

Nutritional Directions

- The effectiveness of avoiding or limiting foods that increase the likelihood of reflux to avoid irritation of esophageal tissue varies among patients and is based on individual tolerances. General recommendations include limiting caffeine, chocolate, alcohol, mint, and carbonated beverages. However, evidence-based research does not support the modifications.
- Because citrus fruits and tomato products should be avoided, other sources of vitamin C should be selected, including cantaloupe, potatoes, and strawberries.
- Heartburn is not caused by inadequate digestion; digestive enzyme tablets are inappropriate.
- Eat small meals, evenly distributed throughout the day.
- Reduce or eliminate cigarette smoking, which stimulates gastric acid secretion.

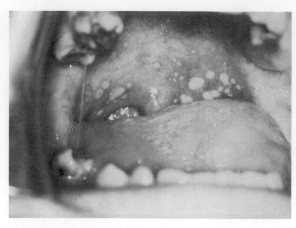

FIGURE 16-5 Oral ulcers (ulcerative colitis). (From Ibsen OAC, Phelan JA: Oral Pathology for the Dental Hygienist, 5th ed. St. Louis: Saunders, 2009.)

dressing, mayonnaise), peppermint and wintergreen, caffeinated foods (e.g., coffee, tea, chocolate, and some carbonated beverages), alcohol, and onions. Other foods to avoid are those directly irritating to the esophagus, such as citrus juices, tomato products, and red peppers. If appropriate, weight loss is recommended. Other suggestions to help reduce pain include eating small, frequent meals; using antacids to buffer gastric juices; wearing loose-fitting clothing; and sleeping with the head and shoulders elevated.

Anticholinergic medications prescribed for GERD may interfere with absorption of vitamin B_{12} and folic acid. Observation for oral signs of vitamin deficiency is appropriate for patients taking these medications. Anticholinergic medications may also cause xerostomia.

MALABSORPTIVE CONDITIONS

Many chronic diseases are associated with poor nutrient absorption, including Crohn's disease, ulcerative colitis, cystic fibrosis, gluten-sensitive enteropathy (sprue or celiac disease), and AIDS. **Gluten** is a protein found mainly in wheat and to a lesser degree in rye, oat, and barley. Different parts of the gastrointestinal tract are affected in these disorders, and manifestations differ from one individual to another with the same condition. Malabsorption may occur with many macronutrients (e.g., gluten [protein], fat, carbohydrates) and micronutrients (e.g., vitamin B_{12}).

Oral problems associated with Crohn's disease and ulcerative colitis include swollen, bleeding, erythematous gingiva; diffuse pustular eruptions on the buccal gingiva; oral ulcerations (Fig. 16-5); swelling of the lips, and cobblestone-like, raised hypertrophic lesions. Additionally, taste alterations (metallic dysgeusia) and reduction in taste acuity for acidic foods may occur in Crohn's disease.[13] Enamel defects and deep aphthous ulcerations may be a marker of Crohn's disease, ulcerative colitis, or celiac disease, and precede gastrointestinal symptoms. These clinical signs appear when the disease is in the acute stage and disappear when it is inactive.

Diarrhea and malabsorption associated with these disease states create deficiencies of nutrients and trace elements. Nutritional requirements of these patients are usually increased; however, cramping abdominal pain precipitated by food intake, and anorexia and intolerance to many different food components (gluten, fat, lactose, fiber) inhibit intake. As a result, patients are finicky and apprehensive about eating; they may present with anemia, protein and energy malnutrition, poor wound healing, and suppressed immune response.

Different nutritional modalities are used with these conditions. A diet high in kilocalories and protein with limited fat and fiber, and possible lactose restriction may be recommended for patients by their healthcare provider or registered dietitian. Small, frequent feedings are better tolerated and increase adequacy of intake. Irritating foods are excluded. Extremely hot and cold foods and high-fiber foods are avoided because they increase peristalsis.

Dental Hygiene Considerations

Assessment
- *Physical*: edema, anemia, weight loss, abdominal pain, diarrhea, fatigue, swollen bleeding gingiva, enamel defects, aphthous ulcers (canker sores), and emotional stress.
- *Dietary*: iron, folate, vitamin B_{12}, and adequate protein and kilocalories.

Interventions
- Encourage the patient to eat a nutrient-rich, well-balanced diet. Reassess the diet frequently to monitor nutrient adequacy.
- The use of stress management techniques during the appointment can prevent aggravating symptoms associated with the disease.
- Consult with the healthcare provider about the need for supplemental steroids and prophylactic antibiotics before the dental appointment. The healthcare provider or registered dietitian may also recommend vitamin and mineral supplementation.

CARDIOVASCULAR CONDITIONS

Cardiovascular disease encompasses numerous prevalent chronic heart problems, including hypertension, congestive heart failure, myocardial infarction, cerebrovascular accident, and arteriosclerosis. A meta-analysis suggests the relative risk of cardiovascular disease resulting from systemic exposure to periodontal pathogens (as measured by antibodies to *Actinobacillus actinomycetemcomitans* and *Porphyromonas gingivalis*) may be 75%.[14] Evidence is mounting that periodontal infections may be a contributing risk factor for cardiovascular disease. In contrast to its many ill effects in other sites of the body, cardiovascular disease produces few oral effects and usually does not have any oral manifestations that affect food intake. However, medications prescribed for cardiovascular conditions may have oral effects. Dietary adjustments recommended for these patients affect the information the dental hygienist provides.

CEREBROVASCULAR ACCIDENT

A cerebrovascular accident or stroke results if occlusion or ischemia occurs in an artery supplying the brain, or if hemorrhaging in the brain occurs. **Ischemia** (inadequate blood flow and lack of oxygen because of constriction or obstruction of arteries) occurs as a result of blockage of one of the arteries serving the brain. Approximately 80% of strokes fall into this category. An artery may become blocked from atherosclerosis or a **thrombus** (blood clot).

Atherosclerosis is caused by an accumulation of fatty materials, such as cholesterol, on smooth inner walls of arteries. As this plaque thickens, arteries become progressively narrow and rough, and blood flow—which carries oxygen and nutrients—may be disrupted.

Hemorrhagic strokes may occur as a result of a bleeding **aneurysm** (weak or thin spot in an arterial wall). Meta-analyses and evidence-based research have inconsistent results in regard to the association between periodontal disease and stroke.[14]

Occasionally, patients who have ministrokes do not seek medical care even though dysphagia can occur as a result of a cerebrovascular accident. The patient may realize that things are not normal, but may attribute these deficits to the aging process. A dental hygienist may suspect dysphagia in a patient who has facial muscle weakness (drooping mouth) or slurred speech; in a patient with weak oral, neck, or tongue muscles; or in a patient who coughs or chokes frequently when taking foods or fluids and on secretions (e.g.,

saliva and mucus). Neurologically impaired patients may deny having swallowing problems. Patients suspected to have dysphagia should be referred to a healthcare provider. Normally, a speech-language pathologist and registered dietitian work closely with these patients to ensure adequate fluid and nutrient intake. Patients may receive their nutrition through a tube that provides the feeding directly into the stomach until the swallowing reflex improves.

Liquids are very difficult to control in the mouth, especially in the oral stage of the swallow. Because of this issue, the use of water for rinsing or ultrasonic instrumentation may be contraindicated during dental care. The patient may be unable to lie in a supine position for fear of choking on saliva. Water should be used sparingly, and use of high-speed evacuation may be necessary to prevent aspiration.[15]

Neurological deficits may cause some patients to be unaware of the presence of food in the mouth. After meals, the mouth should be checked for any **pocketed foods** (foods retained in the mouth, especially in the vestibule) that should be removed to decrease risk of aspirating the food and developing dental caries.

HYPERTENSION

According to the Joint National Committee on Prevention, Detection, Evaluation, and Treatment of High Blood Pressure, blood pressure consistently 140/90 mm Hg or higher is known as stage 1 hypertension. Patients with diagnosed hypertension or congestive heart failure may have been told to increase fruits and vegetables, use more low-fat or nonfat dairy products, limit sodium, limit intake of alcohol and caffeine, quit smoking, exercise, lose weight, and reduce stress. When many older adults are told to limit salt in their diet because of high blood pressure, they may consume less food because it does not taste good to them (see Health Application 11) or not adhere to the recommendations because of limited food choices and lack of palatability.

Diuretics are frequently prescribed for patients with congestive heart failure or hypertension to help eliminate excess fluid. These medications also have side effects on salivary flow causing xerostomia.

HYPERLIPIDEMIA

Patients with other types of heart disease involve elevated cholesterol levels or increased risk of atherosclerosis normally have a total fat, saturated fat, and cholesterol restriction (discussed in Health Application 5). Low-fat diets normally result in weight loss, which is beneficial to many. However, for patients who are trying to maintain their weight, snacks may be needed. Dental hygienists need to recommend noncariogenic snacks relatively low in fat, such as low-fat or nonfat cheese or skim milk.

Long-term use of bile acid sequestrants (e.g., cholestyramine and colestipol), prescribed to reduce serum lipids, may cause malabsorption of fat-soluble vitamins and folic acid. Several bile acid sequestrants may cause gastrointestinal disturbances and affect overall food intake. Patients with heart disease may also be taking anticoagulants, such as warfarin (Coumadin), which may increase risk of bleeding and affect dietary intake because foods with vitamin K are limited.

Dental Hygiene Considerations

Assessment
- *Physical*: medications prescribed, xerostomia, blood pressure.
- *Dietary*: dietary recommendations, adequacy of food intake.

Interventions
- Because stress is a negative risk factor for most patients with hypertension or heart conditions, the dental hygienist needs to minimize stress and consider the effects of the disease on the proposed dental treatment. A shortened appointment and the use of nitrous oxide may need to be considered.[15]
- Generally, hypertension has no typical physiological symptoms; monitoring blood pressure at each appointment is necessary.
- Refer the patient to the registered dietitian for medical nutrition therapy.

Evaluation
The patient's blood pressure is within a normal range; the patient takes prescribed medications and follows recommended dietary guidelines.

Nutritional Directions

- Most salt substitutes contain potassium and chloride. Remind patients to check with the healthcare provider or registered dietitian for advice on the use of salt substitutes to minimize the intake of excessive dietary potassium.
- Help the patient determine low-sodium, low-fat, and low-cholesterol foods feasible for the their lifestyle.
- Antihypertensive drugs may be responsible for a reduced salivary flow. Fluoride therapy may be necessary. Xylitol gum or mints also may be used to promote salivation and remineralization of early carious lesions.
- Calcium channel blockers can cause gingival hyperplasia. Encourage optimal oral hygiene.

SKELETAL SYSTEM

Systemic bone disturbances initially may be detected by the following changes in the maxilla or mandible during an oral examination: (1) significant increase in size or alteration in contour of the maxilla or mandible, (2) alteration in radiographic pattern, (3) mobility of individual teeth without significant periodontal disease, (4) pain or discomfort in the jaw without obvious dental pathology, (5) increased sensitivity of the teeth without obvious dental or periodontal disease, (6) changes in occlusion of the teeth, or (7) abnormal sequence of deciduous tooth loss or eruption of permanent molars in young patients. These changes may be caused by osteoporosis, metabolic disturbances such as hyperparathyroidism, or other conditions such as Paget's disease or fibrous dysplasia. For denture-wearing patients with osteoporosis, rapid resorption of the alveolar ridges may lead to continuous loosening of the dentures with resultant oral lesions or the inability to consume foods that require chewing.

In addition to referring the patient to a healthcare provider for correct diagnosis and treatment, the dental hygienist needs to provide guidance to ensure the patient obtains adequate calcium and vitamin D in the face of missing teeth, sensitivity to hot or cold foods, or pain when hard foods are chosen. A growing concern for patients receiving bisphosphonates to treat osteoporosis and multiple myeloma is the risk for **osteonecrosis** (bone death of the jaw) after dental treatment (Fig. 16-6). Patients at risk for osteonecrosis of the jaw have a history of intravenous bisphosphonates (although patients taking oral bisphosphonates for long periods may also be at risk) with poor oral health requiring invasive dental procedures (e.g., extractions, dental trauma, or surgery).[16,17]

METABOLIC PROBLEMS

DIABETES MELLITUS

Diabetes mellitus and nutrition recommendations are discussed in Health Application 6. Patients with uncontrolled

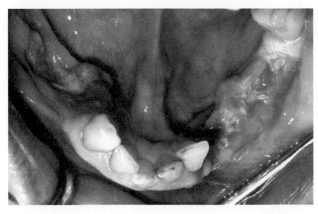

FIGURE 16-6 Bisphosphonate-associated osteonecrosis of mandibular arch. (From Neville BW, et al: Oral and Maxillofacial Pathology, 3rd ed. St. Louis: Saunders, 2009.)

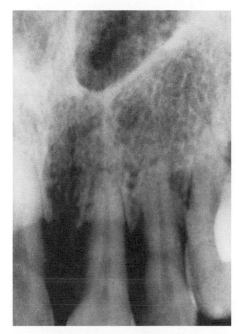

FIGURE 16-7 Alveolar bone loss in diabetes. (From Ibsen OAC, Phelan JA: Oral Pathology for the Dental Hygienist, 5th ed. St. Louis: Saunders, 2009.)

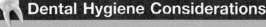

Dental Hygiene Considerations

Assessment
- *Physical*: changes involving bone.
- *Dietary*: variety and a well-balanced meal plan.

Interventions
- Encourage consultation with a healthcare provider to evaluate bone mineral density (BMD), possibly with dual energy x-ray absorptiometry.
- As a part of the healthcare team, the dental professional can explain oral concerns related to bisphosphonate use and risk of osteonecrosis of the jaw.
- Resorption of the edentulous alveolar ridge requires frequent relining of the mandibular denture to avoid oral lesions and ensure the ability to masticate food.
- Provide counseling for tobacco cessation, if necessary.

Evaluation
The patient seeks medical guidance and adheres to prescribed recommendations.

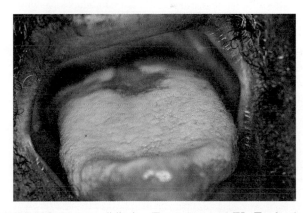

FIGURE 16-8 Oral candidiasis. (From Swartz MH: Textbook of Physical Diagnosis: History and Examination, 5th ed. Philadelphia: Saunders, 2006.)

Nutritional Directions

- A combination of sodium fluoride, calcium, and vitamin D may slow or increase bone mass.
- Avoid excessive alcohol consumption.

or undiagnosed diabetes may have a characteristic fruity-smelling breath (more prevalent in type 1 diabetes), increased thirst, unexplained weight loss, or frequent urination. These symptoms are associated with elevated blood glucose levels. Conversely, patients may be asymptomatic until complications become evident.

Current evidence supports an interrelationship between diabetes and periodontal disease. Studies are inconsistent in regard to the impact of periodontal treatment on improving glycemic control, but because periodontal disease is an infection, it may affect glycemic control. Poorly controlled diabetes results in more severe periodontal disease and alveolar bone loss even in children and adolescents (Fig. 16-7).[18,19] Resistance to infections is lowered, and the normal healing process is slow. In poorly controlled diabetes, minor trauma to the gingiva may result in extensive tissue necrosis with eventual denudation of the underlying bone and the possibility of osteonecrosis.[19] Treatment of oral problems should be reserved until the diabetes is under good control.

Xerostomia is also prevalent and is partially responsible for altered taste, general tenderness or burning of the mucosa, and carious lesions, all of which may affect nutrient intake. Individuals with uncontrolled diabetes have a higher percentage of candidal infections (Fig. 16-8), which may be due in part to increased glucose levels present in the saliva, which provides a substrate for fungal growth.[20]

Dental Hygiene Considerations

Assessment
- *Physical*: polyuria, polydipsia, xerostomia, weight loss, weakness, ketosis, or asymptomatic.
- *Dietary*: polyphagia (increased hunger); adherence to prescribed lifestyle modifications.

Interventions
- To prevent hypoglycemia during dental treatment, the patient must eat at the usual time and take prescribed medications.
- Patients taking insulin or an oral diabetes medication in which hypoglycemia can occur may require at least 15 g of a carbohydrate source to bring blood glucose levels to a normal range.
- Some oral diabetes medications (e.g., α-glucosidase inhibitor) do not cause hypoglycemia by themselves; however, they are often combined with an oral agent that does. In this scenario, the patient requires a glucose source. Have three to four glucose tablets available for such events.
- Periodontal infections may need to be managed with systemic antibiotic therapy and topical antimicrobials.
- Request that the patient bring the blood glucose monitor to each appointment to check the blood glucose level before treatment. Long and stressful appointments may require testing during the appointment. Testing at the end of the appointment is also suggested. Individuals with blood glucose values of less than 70 mg/dL should be treated.
- Before a dental procedure begins, the patient's blood glucose level should be between 70 mg/dL and 200 mg/dL.

Evaluation
The patient's fasting blood glucose levels are normal, and the glycated hemoglobin A_{1c} is less than 7%, indicating the diabetes is well controlled.

Nutritional Directions

- Read labels carefully for sources of carbohydrates, and choose predominately complex carbohydrates. Foods labeled "sugar-free" may contain carbohydrates other than sucrose.
- Because of the risk of periodontal disease, meticulous daily oral self-care is imperative in conjunction with regular supportive periodontal therapy.

HYPOPITUITARISM

The pituitary gland releases seven different hormones, including antidiuretic hormone, growth hormone, thyroid-stimulating hormone, and the sex hormones. Hypopituitarism may occur congenitally. In childhood hypopituitarism, decreased skeletal growth results in disproportionate retardation of mandibular growth. Prepubertal hypopituitarism, or decreased production of growth hormone, is usually caused by pressure from a cyst or tumor. Because of normal size teeth erupting into the small mandible and maxilla, proper alignment is impossible. In addition to delayed eruption, malocclusion is the principal oral problem.

Hypopituitarism may also occur secondarily to a tumor, head trauma, stroke, radiation, or infections of the brain. In adulthood, symptoms of hypopituitarism include loss of appetite, weight loss, low blood pressure, fatigue, headache, and visual disturbances.

CUSHING'S SYNDROME

Pharmacological use of corticosteroids and endogenous secretion of excess cortisol, as seen in Cushing's syndrome, result in a state of hypercortisolism. Physical signs of Cushing's syndrome include high blood pressure, glucose intolerance or diabetes, obesity, muscle weakness, tendency to bruise, acne, hirsutism, osteoporosis, and depression.[21] The muscle weakness resulting from excess amounts of cortisol may affect muscle of mastication and the tongue. The presence of diabetes and osteoporosis may also affect management of periodontal disease and associated bone loss.

HYPOTHYROIDISM

Hypothyroidism may be related to (1) inadequate consumption of iodine, (2) an inborn error of metabolism, (3) high intake of goitrogens, (4) treatment of hyperthyroidism (surgical excision, irradiation, antithyroid drugs), (5) thyroid gland disorder, or (6) deficient secretion of thyrotropin (thyroid-stimulating hormone) by the pituitary gland. Goitrogens are chemicals present in broccoli, kale, kohlrabi, cabbage, rutabagas, turnips, cauliflower, Brussels sprouts, horseradish, and soybeans that inhibit thyroid uptake of iodine. When hypothyroidism occurs at birth or in young children, the child is short in stature and has intellectual disabilities. Poor muscle tone results in a large, protruding tongue (macroglossia), showing indentations on the lateral borders caused by pressure from the teeth (Fig. 16-9), and a tendency to choke. Eruption of the teeth is delayed, causing severe malocclusion, which makes proper oral hygiene dif-

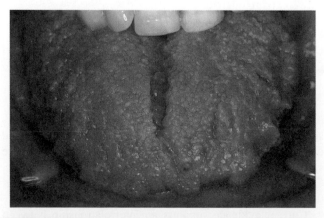

FIGURE 16-9 In hypothyroidism, the large tongue often protrudes from the mouth, showing indentation on the lateral borders caused by pressure from the teeth. (From Neville BW, et al: Oral and Maxillofacial Pathology, 3rd ed. St. Louis: Saunders, 2009.)

ficult. Additionally, it places the patient at increased risk of dental caries and periodontal disease.

When hypothyroidism occurs in an adult, the tongue becomes enlarged and has decreased flexibility. Gingivitis and chronic periodontal disease may be a result of the patient's lack of interest in maintaining normal oral hygiene.

HYPERPARATHYROIDISM

Hyperparathyroidism results from hypersecretion of the parathyroid hormone, leading to alterations in calcium, phosphorus, and bone metabolism. Primary hyperthyroidism is seen more often in women older than 50 years of age. As a result of improved screening of serum calcium levels with routine laboratory tests, most cases of hyperparathyroidism are identified and treated before severe skeletal disease occurs. Clinical manifestations result from increased osteoclastic bone resorption,[22] decreasing bone integrity. This extensive bone disease is known as brown tumors that occur in the head and neck, particularly in the mandible. Systemic bone disturbances are reflected in the mouth by jaw enlargement and reduced bone density. These brown tumors may cause discomfort and may affect the patient's ability to consume an adequate diet.

RENAL DISEASE

The kidney is the primary organ that eliminates significant amounts of waste products; it also has metabolic and endocrine functions are affected when disease is present. Progressive loss of nephrons in the kidney leads to chronic failure. As kidney function diminishes, complications arise as byproducts accumulate from protein metabolism, and alterations occur in electrolyte levels and acid-base balance. Patients with renal disease may be on dialysis while awaiting a kidney transplant.

Nutritional care for these individuals is extremely complex. Anorexia is often present because of the dietary restrictions, uremia, and bad taste that many patients with chronic renal disease experience. High-quality protein intake is recommended to reduce nitrogen waste products (urea) and to minimize accumulation in the blood between dialysis treatments. In addition to protein, intake of minerals and electrolytes (e.g., sodium, potassium, and phosphorus) must be adjusted; adequate energy intake must be maintained; and potentially harmful intake of phosphorus, magnesium, aluminum, and some vitamins must be avoided. Fluid intake must be carefully monitored to prevent excess fluid buildup, which has a negative impact on blood pressure. For this reason, nutritional counseling should be left to a registered dietitian.

The oral cavity reflects many signs of systemic involvement. Platelet abnormalities may result in gingival bleeding and bruising. Anemia is common, so gingival tissues may be pale in color. Other oral manifestations of chronic renal failure include complaints of a bad taste; malodor from urea buildup; xerostomia from fluid restriction; a variety of oral mucosal lesions (e.g., **uremic** [accumulation of urea and waste products in the blood owing to kidney failure] **stomatitis** [inflammation of the mouth], lichen planus, oral hairy **leukoplakia** [an asymptomatic white, yellow, or gray patch or plaque on the oral mucosa that cannot be removed by scraping or rubbing; Fig. 16-10], black hairy tongue, pyogenic granuloma, and nonspecific ulcerations); and oral infection (e.g., candidiasis and viral infections).[23] Wound healing is slow because of general loss of tissue resistance and an inability to withstand normal traumatic insults. Evidence does not suggest an increased caries risk.

Because of calcium-phosphorus imbalances, various changes in bones are observed—a syndrome called **renal osteodystrophy**. This term describes various changes in bones associated with renal failure, such as classic hyperparathyroidism, osteomalacia, osteoporosis, and sometimes **osteosclerosis** (the hardening or abnormal density of bone). Patients with chronically high urea levels may exhibit facial changes. The changes in facial dimensions increase in terms of width (skull base, mandible, and nose), length (mandible and nose), and depth of the mandible. The facial changes may result in a larger maxilla with a tendency toward more prominent lips.[24] Manifestations that may be seen in the teeth and periodontium include delayed eruption, enamel hypoplasia, loss of the lamina dura, widening of the periodontal ligament, severe periodontal destruction, tooth mobility, drifting, and pulp calcifications. Numerous manifestations are seen in the bone, such as bone radiolucent

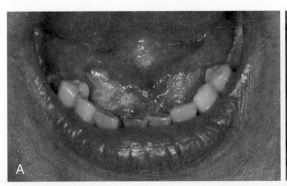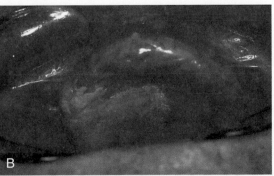

FIGURE 16-10 A, Leukoplakia on the floor of the mouth. **B,** Leukoplakia on the maxillary alveolar mucosa and palate. (From Ibsen OAC, Phelan JA: Oral Pathology for the Dental Hygienist, 5th ed. St. Louis: Saunders, 2009.)

fibrocystic lesions, metastatic soft tissue calcifications, decreased trabeculation and thickness of cortical bone, jaw fracture after trauma or surgery, and abnormal bone healing after extraction.[23]

Dental Hygiene Considerations

Assessment
- *Physical*: oral manifestations and deteriorating physical status.
- *Dietary*: appetite, prescribed diet, adequacy of oral intake.

Interventions
- Consult the healthcare provider before treatment because of the bleeding tendency as a result of platelet dysfunction and anticoagulant medication and to determine the need for antibiotic prophylaxis to prevent infective endocarditis or infection of the vascular access site for dialysis or both.
- Because of the increased occurrence of oral complications, perform a careful and thorough oral examination to detect problems early.
- Because of fluid restrictions for patients on dialysis, minimize the water used during treatment. If the patient does not tolerate the water generated when using ultrasonic units, this may be contraindicated.
- Consult with and refer to a registered dietitian as needed.
- Schedule the dental appointment for a patient who is receiving dialysis the day after dialysis treatment.

Evaluation
The patient is able to describe the relationship between the condition and the effects of dietary intake on oral health.

Nutritional Directions

- Meticulous oral hygiene and frequent recall appointments prevent or reduce oral infections commonly associated with metabolic problems that can lead to difficulties in eating certain foods.
- Antimicrobial mouth rinses are helpful to minimize possible bacterial and fungal infections.

NEUROMUSCULAR PROBLEMS

PARKINSON'S DISEASE

Parkinson's disease is a progressive neurological condition characterized by involuntary muscle tremors, **bradykinesia** (slowness of movement), muscular weakness, rigidity, stooped posture, decreased fine motor coordination, mask-like expression with absence of blinking, orthostatic hypotension, and a peculiar gait. It affects the oral cavity by causing an abnormal swallow pattern, with frequent drooling and tremor of the mandible, lips, and tongue. Decreased voluntary muscle movement affects muscles used to masticate food. Patients with Parkinson's disease may have many problems associated with feeding and receiving adequate

nourishment: (1) mechanical difficulties may interfere with the transfer of food from the plate to the mouth, and (2) oral disturbances may alter normal chewing and swallowing mechanisms. These problems may necessitate a change in the form or consistency of food, or special eating utensils, or both.

Dysphagia may affect the oral phase of swallow or the pharyngeal stage of swallow. This can lead to problems such as pneumonia, dehydration, and malnutrition. The results include drooling of saliva, holding food in the mouth for extended periods, inability to tear food apart and mix it with saliva, food or liquid leaking from the nose, regurgitation, a gurgly voice, and food coating the tongue and palate after the swallow. Because of poor tongue control, a flowing, noncohesive bolus could spill over the base of the tongue before a swallow reflex is initiated, increasing risk for aspiration.

Other dental implications of Parkinson's disease include burning mouth, mucositis, increased plaque accumulation because of challenges with oral self-care, bruxism, orthostatic hypotension, and less caries and more teeth than age-matched controls.[25] In the past, the use of medication was delayed until functional disability occurred, with the goal being to suppress or reduce the symptoms with the fewest adverse effects. A major focus of current research is to find neuroprotective therapies to prevent the progression of disease. Vitamins C and E were tested as a neuroprotective therapy in some studies, but they were not effective, and guidelines do not recommended their use for neuroprotection.[26]

The Parkinson's Disease Foundation recommends eating a balanced diet to maintain a healthy weight, maintaining bone health, bowel regularity, and balancing medications and food. Medications used for Parkinson's disease include levodopa, which has drug-nutrient interactions with protein reducing the effectiveness of the drug. Despite these interactions, adequate protein intake is crucial. Nausea and poor appetite resulting from medications can also negatively affect dietary intake.[27] Because of the challenges in maintaining body weight and health, a registered dietitian should be consulted to tailor diet to meet the patient's needs.

Parkinson's disease cannot be prevented. However, epidemiologic data suggest dietary patterns with high intake of fruits, vegetables, legumes, whole grains, nuts, fish, and poultry; low intake of saturated fat; and moderate intake of alcohol may protect against Parkinson's disease.[27] This is one more reason why dental hygienists need to encourage healthy eating.

DEVELOPMENTAL DISABILITIES

Many disabilities may impair development of normal feeding reflexes (discussed in Chapter 13) and coordination of these reflexes with respiration. These feeding reflexes may be absent or weak and difficult to elicit. Abnormal oral-motor patterns and difficulties associated with feeding may result when structural malformations such as cleft palate, macroglossia, and micrognathia are present. Neuromuscular dis-

Table 16-2	Feeding Problems
Condition	**Description**
Tonic bite reflex	Strong jaw closure when teeth or gingiva are stimulated
Tongue thrust	Forceful and often repetitive protrusion of an often bunched or thick tongue in response to oral stimulation
Jaw thrust	Forceful opening of the jaw to its maximal extent during eating, drinking, attempts to speak, or general excitement
Tongue retraction	Pulling back the tongue within the oral cavity at presentation of food, spoon, or cup
Lip retraction	Pulling back the lips in a very tight, smilelike pattern at the approach of food, spoon, or cup toward the face
Sensory defensiveness	A strong adverse reaction to sensory input (touch, sound, light)

From Lane SJ, Cloud HH: Feeding problems and intervention: An interdisciplinary approach. Top Clin Nutr 1988; 3(3):23-32.

eases such as cerebral palsy, muscular dystrophy, and Down syndrome may be associated with abnormal oral-motor development. The feeding experience, which is normally pleasurable, becomes a frustrating, time-consuming situation for everyone involved in the patient's care.

Oral-motor impairment may become evident during the spoon-feeding phase of feeding development. Tongue retraction, tonic bite reflex, tongue thrusting, and persistence of a suckling pattern interfere with placing the spoon in the mouth and result in loss of food from the mouth (Table 16-2). A patient with tonic bite reflex may clamp down on a spoon inserted in the mouth and be unable to release the bite. Attempting to free the spoon by pulling is ineffective and may cause continued biting.

With tongue thrusting and tongue retraction, the tongue is unable to form a bolus and move it to the back of the mouth. Placing food in the mouth can be difficult with a severe tongue thrust, which also may affect the individual's ability to suck, chew, and swallow.

With lip retraction, lips may be unable to remove food from the spoon, and drinking or sucking may be impossible. Sensory defensiveness is associated with a strong emotional reaction to the unwanted tactile stimuli and can result in a severe food intake problem.

Inadequate chewing skills are associated with jaw thrusting, hyperactive or hypoactive gag reflex, abnormal intraoral sensation, poor tongue lateralization, and tongue thrusting. Oral-motor impairments make providing optimal nutritional care very difficult. Whenever intake of food is limited, because of an oral-motor problem or an inability to self-feed, these patients are at nutritional risk.

With extremely severe oral-motor impairment, adequate nutrition cannot be provided with oral feedings, and nutrition is provided via **gastrostomy** (feeding tube) feedings. Treatment is facilitated using an interdisciplinary team to determine the best treatment promoting development of feeding skills and providing foods in a form that can be safely handled.

EPILEPSY

Epilepsy, or psychomotor seizures, in itself does not usually result in any specific oral or feeding problems. However, the type of treatment, or the use of phenytoin or phenobarbital,

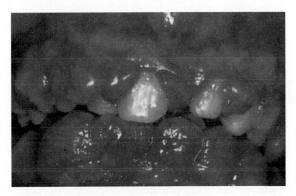

FIGURE 16-11 Hyperplasia associated with phenytoin use. (Courtesy of Barbara D. Altshuler, BSDH, MS, Clinical Assistant Professor, Caruth School of Dental Hygiene, The Texas A&M University System, Baylor College of Dentistry, Dallas, TX.)

Dental Hygiene Considerations

Assessment
- *Physical:* oral complications related to neuromuscular disorders; medications prescribed; nutrient supplements; orthostatic hypotension.
- *Dietary:* adequacy of intake, signs of malnutrition.

Interventions
- Carefully assess oral status of patients taking anticonvulsants.
- To reduce stress and anxiety, keep appointments brief and relaxing.
- Assess saliva flow, and provide tips for preventing xerostomia associated oral problems (see Chapter 19).
- After supine positioning, have the patient sit upright for at least 2 minutes before standing to avoid orthostatic hypotension.
- Refer the patient to the healthcare provider or registered dietitian if nutrient supplementation is reported. Some nutrients may interfere with absorption of the prescribed medication.
- Educate the patient or caregiver on the use of an electric toothbrush if there is difficulty holding a conventional toothbrush.

Evaluation
The patient's dental health is maintained, and prescribed medications are taken.

Nutritional Directions

- Check the fit of a dental prosthesis. An improper fit may impact nutritional status.
- Encourage small, frequent nutrient-dense meals and snacks for patients experiencing anorexia. Refer to a registered dietitian.
- Salivary substitutions and topical fluoride treatments may be recommended for patients experiencing xerostomia.
- Antimicrobial rinses are helpful to decrease the chance of bacterial and fungal infections.
- Patients with Parkinson's disease are often at risk for osteoporosis. Foods high in or fortified with calcium, magnesium, and vitamins D and K may be suggested.
- Patients taking levodopa or carbidopa should avoid eating foods high in vitamin B_6 (e.g., dry skim milk, peas, beans, sweet potatoes, avocados, fortified cereal, oatmeal, wheat germ, yeast, pork and beef organs, tuna, and fresh salmon) when they take the medication.
- Calcium supplements are not recommended for patients taking phenytoin and phenobarbital unless closely monitored by the healthcare provider because large amounts of calcium decrease bioavailability of the drug and the mineral.
- Pyridoxine and folate supplements may alter response of phenytoin and result in increased seizure activity.
- Carbamazepine (Tegretol), another popular anticonvulsant, causes xerostomia, altered taste, and oral sensitivity.

may affect the gingiva. Gingival hyperplasia is noted with long-term phenytoin use (Fig. 16-11). When good oral self-care techniques are routinely practiced, inflammation and gingival overgrowth are reduced.

Phenytoin increases the metabolism of vitamins D and K and folate, which may increase the risk for loss of BMD. Research suggests that 1 year of treatment with phenytoin resulted in significant bone loss even though the participants consumed 1000 mg of calcium and were physically active.[28] This research raises concerns about long-term bone health for these patients. Phenobarbital, which is also used to manage convulsions in epilepsy, may also affect bone health by increasing the turnover of vitamins D and K. Despite the increased need for these nutrients, supplementation of folate or vitamin B_6 may decrease bioavailability of phenytoin and must be carefully monitored by a healthcare provider.

NEOPLASIA

Tumors cause problems not only in the primary site, but also in regional and remote areas. The manifestations at secondary sites away from the primary lesion may be the presenting feature in some cases. The mouth and jaw may be involved in generalized malignant disease.

Nutritional requirements for patients with neoplasms are generally increased to maintain lean body mass and immune responses. Anorexia is an important symptom of an underlying neoplasm. Oral symptoms or signs may be secondary to malnutrition or nutrient deficiencies. Abnormalities in taste perception have been noted in some patients with cancer, such as an elevated threshold for sweets and a reduced threshold for bitter flavors. Altered taste sensations may be secondary to a deficiency of zinc. Hormonal factors affect the hypothalamic feeding center to reduce oral intake. Early satiety may be related to decreased digestive secretions or impaired gastric emptying.

The location of the tumor itself also may be a factor in reduced food intake, especially when the alimentary tract is affected. Intake is reduced in patients with cancer of the oral cavity, pharynx, or esophagus because of **odynophagia** (pain on swallowing) or dysphagia. Gastric cancer may lead to reduced gastric capacity or partial gastric outlet obstruction, resulting in early satiety, nausea, and vomiting.

Psychological factors undoubtedly affect appetite. Depression, grief, or anxiety resulting from the disease or its treatment may lead to poor appetite and abnormal eating behaviors.

KAPOSI'S SARCOMA

Kaposi's sarcoma is a highly malignant tumor of blood vessel origin that occurs on the skin and oral mucosa (Fig. 16-12). It is characterized by bluish red cutaneous nodules, usually on the lower extremities, and occurs frequently in immunocompromised individuals. These lesions appear in many HIV-positive patients. Red-purple macular lesions in the mouth may progress to raised, indurated lesions with central areas of necrosis and ulceration. The lesions can cause obstruction of the esophagus, compromising food intake.

LEUKEMIA

Several types of **leukemia** are classified according to how quickly they progress (acute or chronic). Leukemia is a generalized malignant disease characterized by distorted proliferation and development of WBCs. It is another neoplastic process with many oral manifestations that detrimentally affect food intake. Gingival tissues are especially susceptible to gingivitis because of an exaggerated inflammatory response to local etiologic factors (e.g., calculus,

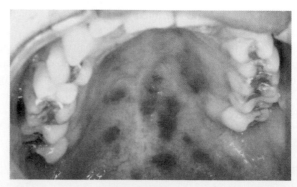

FIGURE 16-12 Kaposi's sarcoma lesions on the hard palate. (From Silverman S Jr: Color Atlas of Oral Manifestations of AIDS, 5th ed. St. Louis: Mosby, 1996.)

plaque biofilm, and materia alba). Rather than the normal response of chronic marginal gingivitis, the gingiva may become severely inflamed with tissue hyperplasia, areas of ulcerations, necrosis, and spontaneous bleeding. This is believed to be caused by the body's depressed immune response. Susceptibility to infection is increased, and healing responses are delayed.

CANCER TREATMENTS

Cancer treatment may include surgery, radiation therapy, **chemotherapy**, biological therapy, or combinations of these modalities. When tumors involve the gastrointestinal tract, the ability to ingest foods orally or digest and absorb nutrients adequately may be affected. Radical surgery in the oropharyngeal area may present problems in chewing and swallowing, and alterations in taste sensations.

Radiation therapy significantly affects the alimentary tract. Early transient effects include general loss of appetite, nausea and vomiting, and diarrhea caused by malabsorption secondary to mucosal damage in the gastrointestinal tract. Food intake is affected because of a loss of taste sensation, xerostomia, difficulty in swallowing, and a burning sensation in the mouth when the larynx or pharynx area is irradiated. When a patient is exposed to a food or beverage before radiation treatment or chemotherapy, the item may become associated with the therapy, causing the patient to develop an aversion to that particular food. Rampant caries and loss of teeth may complicate adequate dietary intake further.

Chemotherapeutic drugs are used to destroy malignant cells without loss of an excessive number of normal cells. Chemotherapy has more widespread effects on the body than either radiation or surgical treatment. Rapid cell turnover rate in the alimentary tract leads to stomatitis or mucositis, oral ulcerations, and decreased absorptive capacity. As a result, changes in taste sensation and learned food aversions occur.

🦷 Dental Hygiene Considerations

Assessment
- *Physical*: fatigue, caries, adequate weight, weight loss, oral ulcerations, medications.
- *Dietary*: maintaining caloric intake, adequate fluids, food aversions (especially food groups), alterations in taste.

Interventions
- Use of an antimicrobial mouth rinse (i.e., nonalcohol chlorhexidine) may be indicated to reduce inflammation associated with cancer treatment.
- A soft or bland diet (refer to diet in Chapter 18) may be recommended as deemed necessary by oral conditions.
- Discuss the relationship between fermentable carbohydrate intake, effects of xerostomia, plaque biofilm formation, and caries. Caution against eating hard candy containing fermentable carbohydrates to relieve the xerostomia.

Evaluation
A dietary recall reveals adequate nutrients and kilocalories with a minimum of fermentable carbohydrates.

Nutritional Directions

- Small, frequent meals are appropriate to provide additional kilocalories and to counteract nausea and vomiting.
- Meticulous oral hygiene, frequent recalls, and fluoride therapy are essential.
- Adequate food and fluid intake not only improve the physical response to cancer treatment, but also create a more positive psychological outlook.
- Avoid foods that are hot, spicy, or acidic (e.g., citrus fruit and juices).
- Avoid alcohol-containing beverages and mouth rinses.
- Commonly used chemotherapeutic agents (bleomycin, cyclophosphamide, and methotrexate) generally cause complications such as stomatitis, nausea, vomiting, diarrhea, and anorexia.

ACQUIRED IMMUNODEFICIENCY DISEASE

Human immunodeficiency virus (HIV) debilitates the body's immune system. Following identification of HIV antibodies in the blood, a positive diagnosis of HIV is made. This retrovirus causes a dysfunction in the genetic core of T lymphocytes or WBCs that normally function to resist infection. Retroviruses are characterized by the presence of reverse transcriptase, which interferes with the production of DNA from RNA. Susceptibility to various opportunistic infections (especially *Pneumocystis carinii, Cryptosporidium, Candida, Mycobacterium,* and herpes simplex) and certain neoplasms (Kaposi's sarcoma, non-Hodgkin's lymphoma, and oral warts) is increased. These infections can appear in virtually every organ system. Because of the body's inability to fight infections, acquired immunodeficiency syndrome (AIDS) develops.

With the advent of highly active antiretroviral therapy (HAART), HIV positive individuals no longer exhibit the classic gaunt appearance typical of wasting. Patients receiving HAART may still lose lean body mass, but because of a fat redistribution syndrome called **lipodystrophy,** it may be harder to diagnose. Research suggests that wasting or anorexia is still prevalent in patients receiving HAART.[29] The course of HIV/AIDS is often complicated by weight loss, wasting of lean body mass, cachexia, opportunistic infections, malignancies, diarrhea, multiple nutrient deficiencies, and, particularly, protein-energy malnutrition. The cause of malnutrition is multifactorial and may involve inadequate intake, malabsorption, or hypermetabolism.

Anorexia may be attributed to respiratory and other infections, fever, dysgeusia, gastrointestinal complications, adverse effects of drugs, and depression. Specific nutritional deficiencies may depress appetite and exacerbate anorectic behavior. Oral and esophageal pain during eating also may decrease intake. Oral candidiasis, which produces pain and inhibits production of saliva, is present in many patients with AIDS. Many oral problems in HIV-positive patients have predictive value for development of AIDS. Pharyngeal or esophageal lesions of Kaposi's sarcoma may cause obstruction, whereas herpetic ulcerations or other ulcerations on the tongue or esophagus or both can cause difficulty in swallowing. **Herpetic ulcerations** are painful ulcerations of the oral mucosa with a red center and yellow border. The development of thrush may be attributed to herpesvirus, candidiasis, chemotherapy, or drugs such as interferon.

Oral hairy leukoplakia (Fig. 16-13) is found predominantly on the lateral borders of the tongue or occasionally on the buccal or labial mucosa in patients who are HIV-positive. These white lesions or filamentous growth do not rub off. HIV-infected patients frequently have ulcerations that resemble aphthous ulcers. These appear as well-circumscribed ulcers with an erythematous margin. These painful ulcers may become extremely large and necrotic; they may persist for several weeks.

The level of HIV control by HAART determines how the patient responds to periodontal therapy. Patients who are not well controlled may not respond normally to standard periodontal therapy; a mild case of gingivitis can progress to severe periodontitis in a few months, resulting in the need for extraction of the affected teeth. HIV-positive patients may have parotid gland swelling accompanied by xerostomia. Spontaneous oral bleeding may be associated with small purpuric lesions or ecchymoses or gingivitis.

At present, nutritional status is not known to affect the length of time for HIV infections to progress to AIDS. Good nutrition does not cure AIDS, but malnutrition may hasten the progression of the disease and affect outcome. Adequate dietary intake can help maintain strength, comfort, and level of functioning. Providing optimal nutrition improves resistance to opportunistic infections.

MENTAL HEALTH PROBLEMS

ANOREXIA NERVOSA AND BULIMIA

Although anorexia nervosa and bulimia are two different conditions, they are symptomatically related (Fig. 16-14).[30] Anorexia nervosa is a disease primarily affecting adolescent

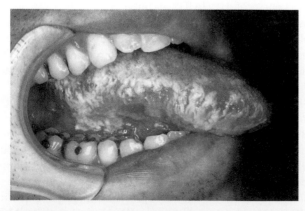

FIGURE 16-13 Hairy leukoplakia. (From Silverman S Jr: Color Atlas of Oral Manifestations of AIDS, 5th ed. St. Louis: Mosby, 1996.)

Dental Hygiene Considerations

Assessment
- *Physical*: weight change, oral infections and malignancies, candidiasis, periodontitis, viral load.
- *Dietary*: oral sensitivity, adequate levels of all nutrients.

Interventions
- Perform a careful oral examination to identify signs of HIV-infected patients so that they can be treated appropriately.
- Individualize the care plan and treatment for each AIDS patient related to special needs.
- Systemic antibiotic therapy may be indicated for infections.
- A consultation with the healthcare provider is necessary to gather information about laboratory values (e.g., platelet and WBC counts, viral load), medications, and history of opportunistic infections, and to determine if antibiotic prophylaxis is needed.
- The patient should use a nonalcohol antimicrobial rinse and antifungal and antiviral agents as prescribed by the dentist or healthcare provider.
- Encourage the patient to maintain the highest possible level of oral self-care and regular preventive dental care.
- Refer the patient to a registered dietitian for medical nutrition therapy.
- Side effects of HAART include diarrhea, nausea, and vomiting. Frequent vomiting can cause enamel erosion. Preventive dental care and use of topical fluoride therapy at home is essential.

Evaluation
The patient exhibits increased attention to oral hygiene care and is maintaining current weight.

Nutritional Directions

- To promote healing and maintenance of oral tissues, encourage attention to nutrient intake. The *Dietary Guidelines for Americans* recommendation to decrease fat intake may be inappropriate for patients with HIV/AIDS.
- To add kilocalories and protein, add nuts and dried fruits to hot and cold cereals; use cream instead of milk; add ground meat or poultry or grated cheese to soups, sauces, casseroles, and vegetable dishes; use peanut butter on fruit or crackers; dip vegetables in sour cream mixes; use nutritional supplements or instant breakfast drinks as snacks.
- Limit caffeine-containing and alcohol-containing beverages if xerostomia is present.

---

girls and young women who have an exaggerated, intense fear of becoming fat. Zealous self-imposed restriction leads to extreme weight loss.

Individuals with anorexia nervosa may be described as achievement-oriented perfectionists who seek to rule their lives by controlling their body by refusing to eat. These young individuals are generally surrounded with all the evidences of success. Individuals with anorexia nervosa may become excellent gourmet cooks, spending hours planning

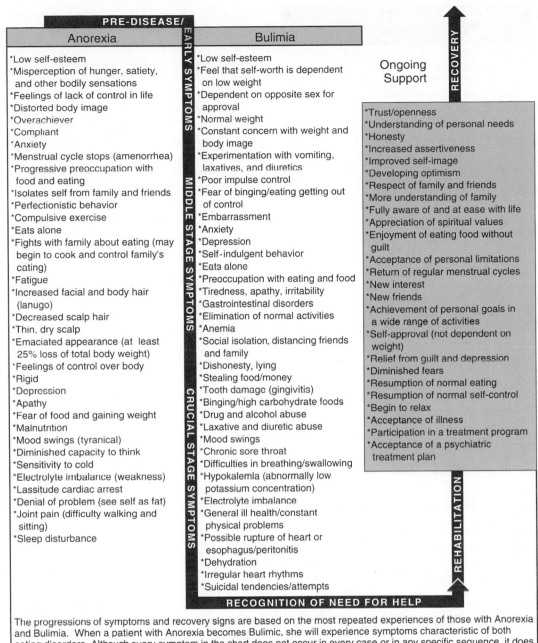

The progressions of symptoms and recovery signs are based on the most repeated experiences of those with Anorexia and Bulimia. When a patient with Anorexia becomes Bulimic, she will experience symptoms characteristic of both eating disorders. Although every symptom in the chart does not occur in every case or in any specific sequence, it does portray an average progression pattern. The goals and resultant behavior changes in the recovery process are similar for both eating disorders.

FIGURE 16-14 Anorexia nervosa and bulimia: a multidimensional profile.

menus, finding special recipes, and shopping for exotic ingredients. In-depth knowledge of nutritional and caloric value of foods is commonly exhibited by individuals with anorexia.

Criteria for diagnosis of anorexia nervosa include a weight loss equal to or exceeding 15% below expected or original body weight, amenorrhea (for women), and an excessive desire for slimness with a distorted body image (Box 16-1). Dental complications in advanced stages of malnutrition are generally observed in patients with anorexia nervosa.

Bulimia occurs more frequently than anorexia nervosa. Bulimia is an eating disorder that is not associated with significant weight loss (Box 16-2). An individual with bulimia might even be normal weight or slightly overweight and appear healthy. Bulimia is characterized by intentional, although not necessarily controllable, secret **binges** (periods of overeating) usually followed by **purging** (a means of counteracting the effects of overindulgence).

Typically, bulimia and anorexia nervosa occur for the same reason: fear of becoming fat. However, individuals with bulimia try to control this fear by repeatedly restraining

Box 16-1 Diagnostic Criteria for Anorexia Nervosa

- Refusal to maintain body weight at or above a minimally normal weight for age and height (e.g., weight loss leading to maintenance of body weight less than 85% of that expected, or failure to make expected weight gain during period of growth, leading to body weight less than 85% of that expected).
- Intense fear of gaining weight or becoming fat, even though underweight.
- Disturbance in the way in which one's body weight or shape is experienced, undue influence of body weight or shape on self-evaluation, or denial of the seriousness of the current low body weight.
- Amenorrhea in postmenarcheal women, that is, the absence of at least three consecutive menstrual cycles. A woman is considered to have amenorrhea if her menstrual periods occur only after hormone (i.e., estrogen) administration.

Specific Types

- *Restricting type*: During the episode of anorexia nervosa, the individual does not regularly engage in binge eating or purging behavior (i.e., self-induced vomiting or the misuse of laxatives, diuretics, or enemas).
- *Binge eating/purging type*: During the current episode of anorexia nervosa, the individual has regularly engaged in binge eating or purging behavior (e.g., self-induced vomiting or the misuse of laxatives, diuretics, or enemas).

Modified with permission from American Psychiatric Association: Diagnostic and Statistical Manual, 4th ed. Washington, DC: American Psychiatric Association, 2000.

Box 16-2 Diagnostic Criteria for Bulimia Nervosa

- Recurrent episodes of binge eating. An episode of binge eating is characterized by both of the following:
  - Eating, in a discrete period (e.g., within any 2-hour period), an amount of food that is definitely larger than most people would eat during a similar period and under similar circumstances
  - A sense of lack of control over eating during the episode (e.g., a feeling that one cannot stop eating or control what or how much one is eating)
- Recurrent inappropriate compensatory behavior to prevent weight gain, such as self-induced vomiting; misuse of laxatives, diuretics, enemas, or other medications; fasting; or excessive exercise.
- Binge eating and inappropriate compensatory behaviors occur, on average, at least twice a week for 3 months.
- Self-evaluation is unduly influenced by body shape and weight.
- The disturbance does not occur exclusively during episodes of anorexia nervosa.

Specific Types

- *Purging type*: The individual regularly engages in self-induced vomiting or the misuse of laxatives, diuretics, or enemas.
- *Nonpurging type*: The individual uses other inappropriate compensatory behaviors, such as fasting or excessive exercise, but does not regularly engage in self-induced vomiting or the misuse of laxatives, diuretics, or enemas.

Modified with permission from American Psychiatric Association: Diagnostic and Statistical Manual, 4th ed. Washington, DC: American Psychiatric Association, 2000.

eating, but this backfires and leads to binging and purging. Individuals with bulimia exhibit many of the same characteristics as individuals with anorexia, but those with bulimia are more sociable, while underneath they feel profoundly separated from other people. Usually they appear very mature, but this is a defense mechanism to hide insecurities. Appearance is extremely important.

Individuals with bulimia acknowledge their eating behaviors are not normal. They have strong appetites and may binge several times a day, with intakes of 1200 or more kcal per episode.[3] Binges may last minutes to several hours and may be planned or spontaneous, but ordinarily are related to stress. Compulsive stealing of food and money to buy food is another common characteristic. Individuals binge on mainly high-carbohydrate, easily digested food.

These binges occur most often in the late afternoon or evening and end with purging. Self-induced vomiting is the main method of purging. Vomiting may be induced by sticking a finger or other object down the throat, applying external pressure to the neck, or drinking **syrup of ipecac** (emetic drug). Eventually, some individuals with bulimia can vomit by merely contracting their abdominal muscles.

In addition to poor overall health status, nutritional effects of bulimia stem from purging and the method employed for purging. Frequent episodes of self-induced vomiting can cause oral cavity trauma; bruises and irritations in the oral cavity may be observed. Frequent vomiting causes erosion of tooth enamel (predominantly on the lingual surfaces of the maxillary teeth) (Fig. 16-15), dentin hypersensitivity, and enlargement of the parotid glands. Erosion usually occurs in 6 months after continued regurgitation (Fig. 16-16). Signs of malnutrition may also be present and observed during the oral examination.

There are two additional categories of eating disorders: binge-eating disorder and eating disorders not otherwise specified (Boxes 16-3 and 16-4). Dental hygienists should not falsely assume oral problems result from poor dental hygiene practices; rather, these oral problems develop secondary to frequent vomiting. Another classic sign of bulimia associated with self-induced vomiting is the presence of abrasions and calluses on dorsal surfaces of fingers and hands secondary to friction of the teeth.

Successful outcomes require comprehensive treatment by a multidisciplinary team that addresses individual psychosocial, nutritional, and medical problems. The team usually comprises a psychoth erapist or psychiatrist, registered dietitian, nurse, social worker, and healthcare provider. This pooling of specialties provides effective treatment for the patient and a support system for team members when difficult decisions are necessary or progress seems slow.

MENTAL ILLNESS

A few of the many different mental illnesses that occur include schizophrenia, depression, and bipolar disorder or mania. These disorders do not usually display any oral manifestations; however, drugs frequently prescribed to treat the conditions may have side effects that affect oral status. Antipsychotics (e.g., haloperidol, thioridazine, fluoxetine, and

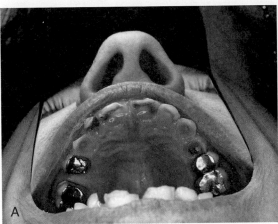 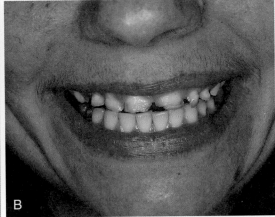

FIGURE 16-15 A and **B,** Enamel erosion caused by bulimia nervosa. (From Ibsen OAC, Phelan JA: Oral Pathology for the Dental Hygienist, 5th ed. St. Louis: Saunders, 2009.)

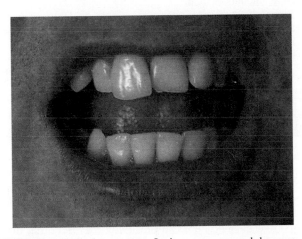

FIGURE 16-16 Bulimia nervosa. Incisor was capped because of dental caries. Continued vomiting has diminished the size of the surrounding teeth, while prosthesis remains unchanged. (Courtesy Dr. J. Treasure. From McLaren DS: A Colour Atlas and Text of Diet-related Disorders, 2nd ed. London: Mosby-Yearbook Europe Ltd, 1992.)

Dental Hygiene Considerations

Assessment

- *Physical*: signs of malnutrition (e.g., thinning hair, always cold, facial hair), fatigue, dehydration, trauma to the soft palate from fingernails or objects used to induce vomiting, location of enamel erosion, parotid enlargement, weight changes.
- *Dietary*: high-carbohydrate diet, very low caloric intake or other unusual dietary habits, obsession with diet or weight.

Interventions

- An increased caries rate can be indicative of high-carbohydrate binging, low pH of saliva from vomiting, and xerostomia. Office and home fluoride therapy should be recommended.
- Treatment of an eating disorder involves a multidisciplinary team of healthcare professionals, including the dental hygienist. It is the responsibility of the dental hygienist to be able to recognize the signs and symptoms of a suspected eating disorder and refer patients to a healthcare provider or

Box 16-3   Diagnostic Criteria for Binge-Eating Disorder

- Recurrent episodes of binge eating. An episode of binge eating is characterized by the following:
  - Eating, in a discrete period (i.e., within any 2-hour period), an amount of food that is definitely larger than most people would eat in a similar period under similar circumstances
  - A sense of lack of control over eating during the episode (i.e., a feeling that one cannot stop eating or control what or how much one is eating)
- Binge-eating episodes are associated with three or more of the following:
  - Eating much more rapidly than normal
  - Eating until feeling uncomfortably full
  - Eating large amounts of food when not feeling physically hungry
  - Eating alone because of being embarrassed by how much one is eating
  - Feeling disgusted with oneself, depressed, or very guilty after overeating
  - Marked distress regarding binge eating is present
  - Binge eating occurs at least 2 days a week for 6 months
- Binge eating is not associated with the regular use of inappropriate compensatory behaviors (e.g., purging, fasting, excessive exercise), and does not occur exclusively during the course of anorexia nervosa or bulimia nervosa.

Modified with permission from American Psychiatric Association: Diagnostic and Statistical Manual, 4th ed. Washington, DC: American Psychiatric Association, 2000.

a local hospital or eating disorder facility for assessment and treatment. Document the findings.
- Chronic use of syrup of ipecac can affect skeletal muscle and cardiac action, which can result in congestive heart failure, arrhythmia, and sudden death.
- Discuss the specific characteristics observed in the dental assessment with the patient.
- Encourage meticulous oral hygiene.

Evaluation

The patient is making realistic changes by protecting the hard and soft tissues, being plaque-free, and being treated by a multidisciplinary healthcare team.

thiothixene) used to treat schizophrenia frequently cause xerostomia. Anticholinergic properties of tricyclic antidepressants, monoamine oxidase inhibitors, and trazodone used to treat depression also cause xerostomia, dental caries, ulcerations, and periodontal disease. Trazodone can also cause an unpleasant taste in the mouth.

Nutritional Directions

- To prevent further damage to the teeth, caution the patient against brushing immediately after vomiting; avoid the use of hard toothbrushes, abrasive toothpaste, and a "scrubbing" toothbrush method; avoid rinsing with tap water because it reduces the protective effects of saliva; encourage use of a mouth guard during vomiting episodes; rinse with sodium bicarbonate to neutralize the oral environment; and encourage use of daily fluoride and dentinal hypersensitivity products.
- Inform the patient about various ways to relieve xerostomia and the effect of lack of saliva on hard and soft tissues.

Box 16-4 | Diagnostic Criteria for Eating Disorders Not Otherwise Specified

Eating disorders that do not meet the criteria for any specific eating disorder, including the following:

- For women, all of the criteria for anorexia nervosa are met except that the individual has regular menses.
- All of the criteria for anorexia nervosa are met except that despite significant weight loss, the individual's current weight is in the normal range.
- All of the criteria for bulimia nervosa are met except that the binge eating and inappropriate compensatory mechanisms occur at a frequency of less than twice a week or for a duration of less than 3 months.
- The regular use of inappropriate compensatory behavior by an individual of normal body weight after eating small amounts of food (i.e., self-induced vomiting after the consumption of two cookies).
- Repeatedly chewing and spitting out, but not swallowing, large amounts of food.
- Binge-eating disorder: recurrent episodes of binge eating in the absence of regular use of inappropriate compensatory behaviors characteristic of bulimia nervosa.

Modified with permission from American Psychiatric Association: Diagnostic and Statistical Manual, 4th ed. Washington, DC: American Psychiatric Association, 2000.

HEALTH APPLICATION 16 Genomics

The word **genome** refers to the entire DNA sequence of an organism. In April 2003, scientists associated with the Human Genome Project announced completion of the mapping for the reference sequence of the human genome.[31] The sequence is a "representative" or generic sequence that is a composite of multiple people. Another project called the International HapMap Project used the information from the Human Genome Project to publish a comprehensive map of human genetic variation in October 2005. This information is being used to identify specific genes associated with common conditions and diseases such as cancer and heart disease.

Genomics is the scientific discipline of mapping, sequencing, and analyzing the genome.[32] Differences in gene makeup account for variability in the risk for developing diseases such as diabetes, heart disease, and cancers. Research has taken this information and used it to develop more effective diagnostic tools with a future vision of using it to understand health needs and design individualized approaches to prevention and treatment.

Genomics and related areas of research have advanced knowledge of the cellular mechanisms underlying diet-disease relationships. This knowledge has led to development of "-omics" disciplines (e.g., genomics, proteomics, and metabolomics) that help us to understand what is going on inside cells in response to nutrients, and to see how those responses differ from person to person.[32] The scientific study of the way foods or their components interact with genes, and how individual genetic differences affect response to nutrients (and other naturally occurring compounds) in food is referred to as **nutrigenomics** or **nutritional genomics**.[32] Integration of genomics and nutrition in research is needed to develop programs aimed at prevention and control of chronic disease through nutritional interventions.

Because of increasing obesity and chronic disease, interest in functional foods and in the idea that foods can have health-promoting or disease-preventing properties beyond the basic nutritional value has increased. Functional foods contain non-nutrient compounds (bioactive food components) that have a beneficial physiological effect that may delay or prevent the onset of chronic disease.[32] This increased interest in the medicinal uses of foods or their components is not a new idea. Hippocrates is often quoted as suggesting almost 2500 years ago "to let food be thy medicine and medicine be thy food."

Folate is an example of a nutrient extensively studied because of its impact on DNA synthesis in the human genome. **Variants** (different forms) of genes that are responsible for folate-dependent enzymes can alter the efficiency of DNA synthesis and provide protection from and risk for developmental conditions such as neural tube defects (NTDs). Folate fortification in the food supply was targeted at a distinct group—women of childbearing age who were at genetic risk for having an infant with an NTD, to prevent this developmental disorder.[33] This public health measure has been successful, and the rate of NTDs has declined.[33] This is just one example of how a nutritional intervention might be individualized based on knowledge of nutrigenomics.

As noted in a 2003 World Health Organization report on chronic diseases, genes help "define opportunities for health and susceptibility to disease, while environmental factors, including diet, determine which susceptible individuals are most likely to develop illness."[34] For the first time, researchers have the tools to understand how genes and nutrients interact on the molecular level. In the coming years nutrigenomics promises to become an area in which some of the most exciting and cutting-edge research in biology will take place, resulting in a wealth of benefits to human health.

CASE APPLICATION FOR THE DENTAL HYGIENIST

Janie, a 17-year-old cheerleader in high school, came in for her 6-month recare appointment. She complained that "my teeth seem to be wearing down," and "I'm getting holes in my front teeth." Further questioning indicated frequent vomiting to control her weight because "everyone does it."

Nutritional Assessment
- Weight changes
- Oral assessment
- Food, nutrient, and kilocalorie intake
- Awareness of the relationship between health and nutritional intake
- Dietary habits

Nutritional Diagnosis
Consumption of large amounts of high-carbohydrate, low-nutrient foods in a short time, several times a week, followed by regurgitation.

Nutritional Goals
Patient will limit fermentable carbohydrates to reduce the incidence of decay.

Nutritional Implementation
Intervention: Conduct an oral examination to note if any of the following complications are present: trauma to the soft palate, erythematous pharyngeal area, enamel erosion, angular cheilosis, salivary gland enlargement, and xerostomia.
Rationale: These self-inflicted oral complications can indicate to the dental professional the need to investigate further the possibility of an eating disorder in a patient who denies the problem.
Intervention: Discuss effects of frequent vomiting on the oral cavity and appropriate methods to prevent further damage.
Rationale: Not brushing immediately after purging, use of mouth guards during purging, and use of daily fluoride and desensitizing agents are practices Janie is encouraged to adopt to decrease further problems in the oral cavity. Providing such information to the patient may be a factor in her reduction of vomiting episodes.
Intervention: Become the dental liaison in the medical/psychological healthcare team for this patient.
Rationale: Because of the complicated issues involved with an eating disorder, several health disciplines are required to treat patients. The dental hygienist plays a crucial role in the overall care of these patients.
Intervention: Discuss specific foods that help to prevent further deterioration of the teeth.
Rationale: Adequate nutrition is essential to support a healthy periodontium and prevents destructive dental activities. Frequent intake of simple carbohydrate foods is a factor in the high caries rate.

Evaluation
The patient is actively seeking treatment for her eating disorder. She plans to achieve small goals as she works toward improving intake of all nutrients and decreasing episodes of binging and purging to improve her oral hygiene status.

STUDENT READINESS

1. List ways to make a low-fat diet more appealing. Using favorite foods, create a low-fat diet for yourself for 1 day.
2. Describe several oral manifestations seen in various systemic diseases that create a painful mouth, making eating difficult and less enjoyable.
3. Identify strategies for a patient who is experiencing (a) nausea and vomiting, (b) bitter or metallic taste in the mouth, (c) chewing and swallowing difficulties, (d) stomatitis, and (e) xerostomia.
4. What factors contribute to anorexia in a patient with HIV/AIDS?
5. What are some of the treatments for cancer, and what oral problems can result from these therapies?

CASE STUDY

A new patient is seen in the office with complaints of recurrent aphthous ulcers. These ulcers have made it very difficult for him to eat, and he has been losing weight. During an oral examination, candidiasis, hairy leukoplakia, and a flat, bluish, nonsymptomatic lesion on the palate, indicative of Kaposi's sarcoma, are noted. HIV/AIDS may be a possible diagnosis.

1. What additional information would you like to obtain from this patient?
2. Would this patient benefit from nutrition counseling by the dental hygienist? If so, on what areas should the dental hygienist concentrate?
3. What dietary modifications and dental care instructions would you make to this patient?
4. Create a list of helpful additional resources or agencies to refer this patient.

References

1. Marshall TA, et al: Oral health, nutrient intake and dietary quality in the very old. J Am Dent Assoc 2002; 133(10):1369-1379.
2. Field CJ, Johnson IR, Schley PD: Nutrients and their role in host resistance to infection. J Leukocyte Biol 2002; 71(1):16-32.
3. Aschenbrenner K, et al: The influence of olfactory loss on dietary behaviors. Laryngoscope 2008; 118(1):135-144.
4. Schiffman SS, Graham BG: Taste and smell perception affect appetite and immunity in the elderly. Eur J Clin Nutr 2000; 54(6):S54-S63.
5. DePaola DP: Saliva: The precious body fluid. J Am Dent Assoc 2008; 139(S2):5S-10S.
6. Turner MD, Ship JA: Dry mouth and its effects on the oral health of elderly people. J Am Dent Assoc 2007; 138:15S-20S.

7. Bäckström I, et al: Dietary intake in head and neck irradiated patients with permanent dry mouth symptoms. Eur J Cancer B Oral Oncol 1995; 31(4):253-257.

8. Osaki T, et al: Clinical and physiological investigations in patients with taste abnormality. J Oral Pathol Med 1996; 25:38-43.

9. Long RG, Hlousek L, Doyle JL: Oral manifestations of systemic diseases. Mt Sinai J Med 1998; 65(5-6):309-315.

10. Lu A, Wu H: Initial diagnosis from sore mouth and improved classification of anemias by MCV and RDW in 30 patients. Oral Surg Oral Med Oral Pathol Oral Radiol Endod 2004; 98:679-685.

11. Schwartzberg LS: Neutropenia: etiology and pathogenesis. Clin Cornerstone 2006; 8(Suppl 5):S5-S11.

12. Raber-Durlacher JE, et al: Periodontal infection in cancer patients treated with high-dose chemotherapy. Support Care Cancer 2002; 10(6):466-473.

13. Ojha J, et al: Gingival involvement in Crohn disease. J Am Dent Assoc 2007; 138(12):1574-1581.

14. Mustapha IZ, et al: Markers of systemic bacterial exposure in periodontal disease and cardiovascular disease risk: a systematic review and meta-analysis. J Periodontol 2007; 78(12):2289-2302.

15. Fatahzadeh M, Glick M: Stroke: epidemiology, classification, risk factors, complications, diagnosis, prevention, and medical and dental management. Oral Surg Oral Med Oral Pathol Oral Radiol Endod 2006; 102(2):180-191.

16. Hoff AO, et al: Frequency and risk factors associated with osteonecrosis of the jaw in cancer patients treated with intravenous bisphosphonates. J Bone Miner Res 2008; 23(6):826-836.

17. Pazianas M, et al: A review of the literature on osteonecrosis of the jaw in patients with osteoporosis treated with oral bisphosphonates: prevalence, risk factors, and clinical characteristics. Clin Ther 2007; 29(8):1548-1558.

18. Sandberg GE, et al: Type 2 diabetes and oral health: a comparison between diabetic and non-diabetic subjects. Diabetes Res Clin Pract 2000; 50(1):27-34.

19. Mealey BL, Oates TW; American Academy of Periodontology: Diabetes mellitus and periodontal diseases. J Periodontol 2006; 77(8):1289-1303.

20. Guggenheimer J, et al: Insulin-dependent diabetes mellitus and oral soft tissue pathologies, II: prevalence and characteristics of Candida and candidal lesions. Oral Surg Oral Med Oral Pathol Oral Radiol Endod 2000; 89(5):570-576.

21. Arnaldi G, et al: Diagnosis and complications of Cushing's syndrome: a consensus statement. J Clin Endocrinol Metab 2003; 88:5593-5602.

22. Daniels JS: Primary hyperparathyroidism presenting as a palatal brown tumor. Oral Surg Oral Med Oral Pathol Oral Radiol Endod 2004; 98(4):409-413.

23. Proctor R, et al: Oral and dental aspects of chronic renal failure. J Dent Res 2005; 84(3):199-208.

24. Ferrario VF, et al: Facial changes in adult uremic patients on chronic dialysis: possible role of hyperparathyroidism. Int J Artif Organs 2005; 28(8):797-802.

25. Suchowersky O, et al: Quality Standards Subcommittee of the American Academy of Neurology. Practice parameter: neuroprotective strategies and alternative therapies for Parkinson disease: Report of the Quality Standards Subcommittee of the American Academy of Neurology. Neurology 2006; 66(7):976-982.

26. Traviss K: Nutrition and Parkinson's disease: What matters most? Parkinson's Disease Foundation News & Review, Winter 2006/07: 1-2.

27. Gao X, et al: Prospective study of dietary pattern and risk of Parkinson disease. Am J Clin Nutr 2007; 86(5):1486-1494.

28. Pack AM, et al: Bone health in young women with epilepsy after one year of antiepileptic drug monotherapy. Neurology 2008; 70(18):1586-1593.

29. Polsky B, Kotler D, Steinhart C: AIDS. Patient Care STDs 2001; 15(8):411-423.

30. Position of the American Dietetic Association: Nutrition intervention in the treatment of anorexia nervosa, bulimia nervosa, and eating disorders not otherwise specified. J Am Diet Assoc 2006; 106(12):2073-2082.

31. National Human Genomic Research Institute: A Brief Guide to Genomics. National Institutes of Health. Available at http://www.genome.gov/18016863. Accessed July 4, 2008.

32. Yaktine AL, Pool R: Nutrigenomics and Beyond: Informing the Future—Workshop Summary. Washington, D.C.: National Academy Press, 2007.

33. Stover PJ, Caudill MA: Genetic and epigenetic contributions to human nutrition and health: managing genome-diet interactions. J Am Diet Assoc 2008; 108(9):1480-1487.

34. WHO: Genomics and Policy. Available at http://www.who.int/genomics/policy/Genomicsandpolicy/en/index.html. Accessed September 6, 2008.

PART III

Nutritional Aspects of Oral Health

Chapter 17

Nutritional Aspects of Dental Caries: Causes, Prevention, and Treatment

LEARNING OBJECTIVES

Upon completion of this chapter, the student will be able to achieve the following objectives:

- Explain the role each of the following play in the caries process: tooth, saliva, food, and plaque biofilm.
- Identify foods that stimulate salivary flow.
- Suggest food choices and their timing to reduce the cariogenicity of a patient's diet.

- Describe characteristics of foods having noncariogenic or cariostatic properties.
- Provide dietary counseling to a patient at risk for dental caries.

KEY TERMS

Casein
Macrodontia

Test Your NQ

1. **T/F** Cariogenic carbohydrates are the only reason for the development of carious lesions.
2. **T/F** Nutrients have a role in the composition and structure of teeth during development.
3. **T/F** The bicarbonates, phosphates, and proteins in saliva dilute and neutralize plaque acids in the mouth.
4. **T/F** Sucrose, fructose, glucose, and maltose have equal potential to cause dental caries.
5. **T/F** Most sugar alcohols, including sorbitol, mannitol, and xylitol, are cariogenic.
6. **T/F** For a tooth to demineralize, the plaque pH needs to be 6 or higher as a result of consuming cariogenic foods.

7. **T/F** The total quantity of sugar is of greatest importance when assessing the patient's diet.
8. **T/F** A fermentable carbohydrate consumed with a meal is less cariogenic than the same food consumed as a snack.
9. **T/F** The revised RDAs provide helpful nutrition information for patients trying to reduce dental caries.
10. **T/F** Providing patients with information about the process of caries leads to desirable dietary and oral behavior changes.

In the United States, approximately 51 million school hours are missed annually by school-age children and 164 million work hours are lost by employed individuals because of a dental problem or visit.[1] The lost income and missed school have a significant economic impact and negative effect on school performance and mental and social well-being.[2]

Nutritional status and oral health have a strong interrelationship. Countless research studies have shown the importance of diet in the development, maintenance, and repair of oral tissues. Dental caries is an oral infectious disease that is multifactorial, transmissible, and of bacterial origin (Fig. 17-1).

Diet and nutrients play a role in dental caries. Some foods exert a cariogenic effect, whereas others are cariostatic or anticariogenic and offer protection to reduce caries. Nutrients also have topical and systemic effects, which can be primary or secondary factors in the development of dental caries. However, many factors must be considered if the situation is to be defined as cariogenic. A list of cariogenic foods would be misleading because no food is cariogenic in all situations.

PREVALENCE

The primary oral health goal of *Healthy People 2010* is to "Prevent and control oral and craniofacial diseases, conditions, and injuries and improve access to related services." In 2003, the U.S. Surgeon General released the "National Call to Action to Promote Oral Health," reflecting initiatives formulated by government and interested organizations, including the American Dental Hygienists' Association (ADHA). The Surgeon General's Call to Action emphasizes prevention, a goal in which dental hygienists have an active role. Box 17-1 identifies the five action areas in this initiative.

Even with advancements in the quality of digital radiography, emerging technology for early detection of caries (e.g., laser fluorescence, light fluorescence, fiberoptic transillumination, and ultrasound), improved restorative materials, multiple fluoride options, application of sealants, frequent dental care appointments, dental health education, and increased access to care, dental caries remain the most common chronic childhood disease. Although a remarkable reduction in caries has been observed in school-age children

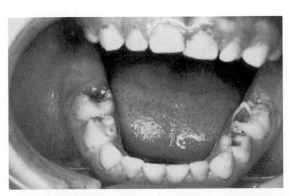

FIGURE 17-1 Dental caries. (Courtesy of Alton McWhorter, DDS, MS, Associate Professor of Pediatric Dentistry, The Texas A&M University System, Baylor College of Dentistry, Dallas, TX.)

Box 17-1	National Call to Action to Promote Oral Health

1. Change perceptions of oral health care
2. Overcome barriers to care by duplicating effective programs and proven efforts
3. Build the science base and accelerate science transfer
4. Increase oral health workforce diversity, capacity, and flexibility
5. Increase collaboration

From U.S. Department of Health and Human Services: A National Call to Action to Promote Oral Health. Rockville, MD: U.S. Department of Health and Human Services, Public Health Service, Centers for Disease Control and Prevention, National Institutes of Health, National Institute of Dental and Craniofacial Research. NIH Publication No. 03-5303, May 2003.

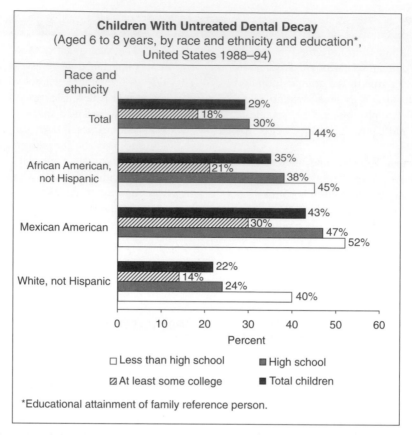

FIGURE 17-2 Children with untreated dental decay. (From National Center for Health Statistics [NCHS]: National Health and Nutrition Examination Survey, 1988-1994. Hyattsville, MD: Centers for Disease Control and Prevention [CDC], unpublished data. In U.S. Department of Health and Human Services [USDHHS]: Healthy People 2010: Objectives for Improving Health. Rockville, MD: USDHHS, 1999. Available at http://www.healthypeople.gov/document/HTML/Volume2/21Oral.htm.)

since the 1970s, certain racial, ethnic, and lower income population groups continue to be problematic (Fig. 17-2).[3] Barriers to dental care include cost; lack of dental insurance, public programs, or providers for underserved groups; fear of dentistry; difficulties in accessing services; or poor awareness of the importance of oral health maintenance.

The caries rate increases as children get older. *National Health and Nutrition Examination Survey* (NHANES) data from 1999-2002 found that among children 2 to 5 years old, 28% had dental caries in their primary teeth. Among older age groups, 49% of children 6 to 11 years old, 68% of adolescents 12 to 19 years old, and approximately 90% of adults had dental caries in their permanent teeth. Dentate non-Hispanic white adults older than 20 years had higher coronal caries experience (93.3%) than did non-Hispanic black (84.6%) and Mexican-American (83.5%) adults. Dentate adults with family income greater than 200% of the federal poverty level had a higher caries experience (93.2%) than did dentate adults with lower incomes.

Overall, caries experience among dentate adults older than 20 years was reduced 3.3%, from 94.6% in 1988-1994 to 91.3% in 1999-2002.[4] Caries on the root surfaces of teeth where gingival recession has occurred is common in older adults. Prevalence of root caries increases with age: 9.4%

among adults 20 to 39 years old, 17.8% among adults 40 to 59 years old, and 31.6% among adults older than 60. Approximately 8% of adults older than 20 years had lost all their natural teeth (edentulism). Prevalence of edentulism increases with age: less than 1% among adults 20 to 39 years old, 4.9% among adults 40 to 59 years old, and 24.9% among adults older than 60.[4] Simple carbohydrate consumption, such as added sugar, "hidden" sugar, and snack foods, has not declined in the United States, and in 2007 was approximately 13 tsp daily per person. Therefore providing dietary advice to reduce caries risk related to sugar consumption is an essential role for the dental hygienist.

MAJOR FACTORS IN THE DENTAL CARIES PROCESS

No single parameter is responsible for formation of a carious lesion (Fig. 17-3). A combination of factors is involved, including a susceptible host or tooth surface, a sufficient quantity of cariogenic microorganisms in the mouth, the presence of fermentable carbohydrates, and a particular composition or flow of saliva. All of these must be present simultaneously for an adequate time to allow decay to occur.

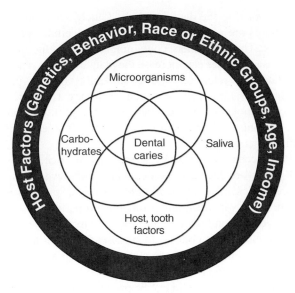

FIGURE 17-3 Major factors that interact in the dental caries process.

TOOTH STRUCTURE

Increasing resistance of the tooth against demineralization begins in the pre-eruptive phase. It is essential to maintain an adequate intake of nutrients during growth and development of enamel and dentin. The most influential nutrients include calcium; phosphorus; vitamins A, C, and D; fluoride; and protein. Indirectly, some fermentable carbohydrates play a role in the formation of caries before tooth eruption. Consider a child who snacks on cookies, candy, or ice cream throughout the day and is not hungry for meat, vegetables, fruit, and milk offered at mealtime. A child's diet high in low-nutrient (or calorie dense) carbohydrates may be deficient in required nutrients for optimal growth and development of the dentition. Other factors, such as genetic or metabolic disturbances, can be responsible for poor tooth formation. Dental anomalies include **macrodontia** (abnormally large teeth) and enamel hypoplasia.

After the tooth erupts, the depth of the natural anatomical pits and fissures and the position of the teeth are relevant factors in the development of dental caries. Deep pits and fissures increase susceptibility for dental caries because of the potential for plaque biofilm and food to be trapped in these areas. Overlapping and crowding of teeth also offer areas for these materials to collect and ferment, compounded by the difficulty of keeping these areas clean.

HOST FACTORS

Food selection, dietary patterns, oral hygiene habits, genetics, race or ethnic groups, age, and income are factors that determine susceptibility to caries.

SALIVA

Availability of essential nutrients during the development of salivary glands, which begins during the fourth week in utero, has a significant impact on the amount of saliva and its composition. Of particular importance are vitamin A, iron, and protein, which have a role in normal growth, development, and secretion of saliva from the salivary glands.

The protection provided by an adequate salivary flow and saliva's buffering capacity ultimately reduce the destructive capabilities of fermentable carbohydrates on teeth. This fact is recognized in patients with xerostomia, who are at high risk for development of caries because of decreased salivary production.

Saliva provides protection against caries in several ways. First, saliva acts as a buffer by neutralizing much of the acids produced by plaque biofilm as a result of carbohydrate metabolism. Second, normal saliva contains bicarbonate, phosphate, and protein, which dilute and neutralize acids to maintain the pH in the mouth. A neutral pH is around 7. After an acidic drink is consumed, the pH of the oral cavity is rapidly normalized by the components of saliva. However, if the frequency or duration of the acidic drink is extended, it becomes more difficult for saliva to buffer the continuous supply of acid, and it no longer offers caries protection.

Particularly important to the prevention of dental caries is the flow of saliva. An adequate salivary flow enables rapid transport of foods from the mouth, decreasing the length of time harmful bacteria and food particles are able to attach to the tooth and cause caries to develop. Consumption of citrus fruits promotes saliva formation by means of their citric acid content, but intake needs to be monitored because of the potential to cause enamel erosion.

Because saliva is saturated with calcium, phosphate, and fluoride ions, the potential for remineralization (restoration of damaged enamel) and resistance to enamel dissolution exists. Finally, antimicrobial elements in saliva, such as IgA, either interfere with adherence of bacteria or compete with bacteria to attach to the tooth surface. An alkaline saliva offers protection, whereas an acidic saliva increases susceptibility to caries.

PLAQUE BIOFILM AND ITS BACTERIAL COMPONENTS

Plaque biofilm is a complex environment of bacteria, polysaccharides, proteins, and lipids. Plaque biofilm forms a local barrier on enamel and may interfere with demineralization. However, acids produced in plaque biofilm have harmful properties offsetting the benefit of its barrier effect.

The composition of plaque biofilm is altered as it matures and is strongly influenced by the diet. As a by-product of the metabolism of sucrose and glucose, bacteria produce acids that lower the pH, resulting in a more favorable environment for the development of certain bacteria, such as *Streptococcus mutans*.[5] *S. mutans*, a gram-positive, anaerobic, spherical bacterium, is widely implicated in the initiation of dental caries. Other microorganisms, such as bacteria from other mutans streptococci and the *Lactobacillus* species, are capable of fermenting carbohydrates. They also thrive in an acidic environment.

When a carbohydrate has been ingested, its metabolism by salivary amylase begins within 2 to 3 minutes and can persist for hours. The metabolic products are acetic, butyric, formic, lactic, and propionic acids. The concentration of the acids escalates as carbohydrate intake continues, whereas the pH of the plaque decreases. Demineralization of enamel occurs when the "critical pH" of 5.5 is reached. The pH can increase to 6.7 for incipient demineralization of cementum and dentin to occur; this is a real concern for areas of gingival recession. In addition, demineralization is approximately twice as fast on root surfaces as in enamel because the dentin contains less mineral content.[6] In interproximal areas or in deep pits and fissures, the pH can decrease to 4 and remain at that pH for an hour. The pH of acids produced by the bacteria in the plaque biofilm is eventually neutralized after elimination of cariogenic foods as saliva exerts its protective action.

🦷 Dental Hygiene Considerations

- Evaluate patient for deep pits and fissures, amount of plaque biofilm in the oral cavity, and composition and flow of saliva. Promote the use of sealants in deep pits and fissures to prevent plaque biofilm accumulation.
- Encourage meticulous oral hygiene habits, including regular recall visits.
- For patients with a high caries rate, recommend use of chlorhexidine or other antimicrobial agents. Educate the patient that this practice can suppress harmful plaque and organisms. Counsel the patient regarding the potential of chlorhexidine staining teeth.
- Caution parents to avoid sharing utensils with children, a practice allowing transfer of the cariogenic microorganism S. mutans.
- Recommend a combination of fluoride sources for patients at high risk for caries. Fluoride in plaque biofilm and saliva inhibit demineralization and enhance remineralization of tooth surfaces.

Nutritional Directions

- Eating a variety of foods in moderation ensures adequate nutrient intake, and the development of healthy eating habits is a factor in growth, development, and maintenance of the teeth; prevention of dental caries; and general good health.
- Firm, fibrous foods, such as raw fruits and vegetables; chewing gum; sour foods; and citrus fruits stimulate salivary flow. An increase in the flow rate has a positive impact on resistance of teeth to caries.

CARIOGENIC FOODS

As previously discussed, fermentable carbohydrates are a factor in the development of caries. The small size of sugar molecules allows salivary amylase to split the molecules into components that can be easily metabolized by plaque bacteria. Sucrose is not the only culprit; other monosaccharides and disaccharides, such as fructose, glucose, and maltose, all produce similar amounts of substrate for metabolism by plaque bacteria to produce acid. Sucrose is used to produce glucans facilitating the adherence of bacteria, such

as *S. mutans,* to the dental pellicle. Glucose and other carbohydrates are also used to produce extracellular polysaccharides. Therefore diets containing sucrose, glucose, and other disaccharides can increase the plaque biofilm mass and facilitate the retention and colonization of the plaque biofilm.[5] "Natural sugars," such as honey (fructose and glucose), molasses (sucrose and invert sugar), and brown sugar (sugar and molasses), have cariogenic capabilities similar to sucrose.

Polysaccharides—starchy foods such as rice, potatoes, and corn—are less cariogenic than monosaccharides and disaccharides. The physical and chemical properties of starches are very different from the properties of simple carbohydrates, and render complex carbohydrates less damaging to enamel. In contrast to sucrose, the large number of glucose units needed to form a starch make it almost insoluble. Because starch must be hydrolyzed (split into smaller glucose units) before acid can be produced, the time a starch is in the mouth is usually not long enough for it to be completely metabolized if oral self-care is completed. Normal saliva flow readily neutralizes any acids produced.

These unique properties prevent starch from providing a readily available energy source for cariogenic microflora, and it is less likely to produce caries than other carbohydrates. When starches and simple carbohydrates are combined (as in pastries or sugar-coated cereals), their potential to produce caries is equal to or greater than that of sucrose. Also, processed starches, as found in instant oatmeal, are often more fermentable than their nonprocessed counterparts because of partial hydrolysis or diminution of particle size. The cariogenic activity is also related to the form of the starch (discussed in Chapter 3).

Fresh fruit is another food group of low cariogenicity because of its low percentage of carbohydrate and high percentage of water. Firm fruits such as apples play a protective role by stimulating saliva flow. The high concentration of fructose found in juices is potentially a source of substrate for plaque bacteria that may influence caries risk; this is shown in early childhood caries (also known as baby bottle tooth decay), which occurs in children given unlimited amounts of fruit juice and other fermentable carbohydrate drinks. The sticky nature of dried fruit (e.g., raisins) also increases risk of decay. Each of these foods is important in its nutritional value, however, and should not be eliminated from the diet.

Box 17-2 lists examples of fermentable carbohydrates potentially increasing risk to dental health. The role of the dental hygienist is to know which foods and situations have the potential to be cariogenic, create awareness of the potential harm, and offer suggestions for appropriate consumption of sweetened foods or alternative choices for sugar-containing foods.

ANTICARIOGENIC PROPERTIES OF FOOD
Sugar Alcohols

Some food components can provide a protection to teeth by decreasing demineralization, enhancing the remineralization process, or increasing salivary flow, even in the presence of a fermentable carbohydrate. Sugar alcohols, such as mannitol and sorbitol, are often used as substitute sweeteners. They are viable alternatives to sugar because of their sweet taste, but have the added benefit of being noncariogenic (see Table 3-1). Sugar alcohols are fermented more slowly in the mouth than monosaccharides and disaccharides; buffering effects of saliva competently neutralize destructive acids produced by plaque bacteria.

Another sugar alcohol, xylitol, is found naturally in plants and is equal to or sweeter than sucrose. Xylitol is classified as anticariogenic because oral flora do not contain enzymes to ferment xylitol, and metabolizing microorganisms, such as *S. mutans*, are inhibited. Chewing gums, mints, and

Box 17-2	Foods That Can Cause the pH of Human Interproximal Plaque to Fall to Less than 5.5

- Alcohol
- Bananas
- Beans, baked
- Bread
- Candy
- Cereals, non-presweetened, ready-to-eat
- Cereals, presweetened, ready-to-eat
- Chips
- Cookies
- Crackers
- Doughnuts, plain
- Fruit, dried
- Fruit drinks
- Gelatin, flavored
- Honey
- Ice cream
- Jams and jellies
- Marshmallows
- Oatmeal, instant cooked
- Pasta
- Peanut butter
- Pretzels
- Rice, cooked
- Snack cakes
- Soft drinks
- Sports drinks

candies containing xylitol inhibit enamel demineralization. This inhibitory effect is enhanced by increased salivary flow, increased oral clearance, and greater buffering capabilities. Compounded by increased mastication, the outcome can be remineralization of incipient decay.

Non-nutritive Sweeteners

Aspartame, saccharin, sucralose, neotame, and acesulfame are a few examples of non-nutritive sweeteners. These sweeteners are not metabolized by microorganisms and do not promote dental caries. Foods made from these sweeteners are generally higher in cost, however, and may not be feasible for low-income patients. Other components of foods using these substitutes, such as raisins, may offset the benefits of using non-nutritive sweeteners to prevent dental caries.

Protein and Fat

Protein and fat are two nutrient classes considered cariostatic because they do not lower the plaque pH. Generally, protein may contribute to buffering effects of saliva. Consuming foods with fat and protein following a fermentable carbohydrate may increase plaque pH. Meat, seafood, poultry, eggs, nuts, seeds, margarine, and oils are examples of cariostatic foods.

Phosphorus and Calcium

Phosphorus and calcium also provide qualities protecting against caries. Dispersion of these minerals throughout plaque biofilm may provide a buffering effect, reducing plaque pH. Ultimately, this action curtails demineralization of enamel.

Cheese and Milk. Protein, **casein** (principal protein in milk), phosphorus, and calcium all are ingredients of other anticariogenic or even cariostatic foods, such as cheese and milk. Despite the fact lactose is cariogenic (although the least cariogenic of all saccharides), these other elements in milk and milk products decrease risk of dental caries (Fig. 17-4). Cheese, produced from milk, contains several anticariogenic properties and has the potential to reduce demineralization (or enhance remineralization) of tooth enamel.

An increase of salivary flow occurs when hard cheeses are chewed. This increased salivary flow provides a neutral

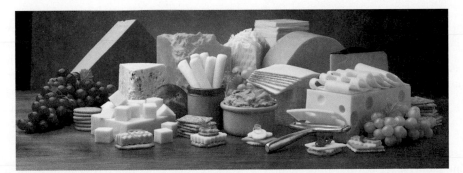

FIGURE 17-4 Milk and milk products contain anticariogenic properties. (Courtesy of National Dairy Council.)

Dental Hygiene Considerations

- Educate the patient about the caries process and how to prevent demineralization of enamel, including the role diet plays in initiation and progression of decay. Use terms that are appropriate and understandable for the patient.
- Use of topical and systemic fluoride, use of products containing xylitol, and application of sealants increase tooth resistance.
- Consider using an antimicrobial agent to control existing plaque biofilm, reduce the number of *S. mutans,* and prevent the formation of new plaque biofilm.[8]

Nutritional Directions

- Using the *Dietary Guidelines for Americans* and MyPyramid, evaluate the patient's diet for adequate nutritional intake and frequency of fermentable carbohydrate consumption.
- Substitute non-nutritive sweeteners for sucrose, if practical. Use aspartame to sweeten coffee or tea instead of table sugar, especially if the coffee or tea is consumed between meals.
- "Natural sugars," such as honey and molasses, are as cariogenic as refined carbohydrates.
- Caution against frequent use of medications, including antacids and cough drops, containing fermentable carbohydrates.
- Increased use of products containing sugar alcohols (e.g., chewing gum, hard candy, dentifrices, and some medications) can cause gastrointestinal distress.
- Although sorbitol and mannitol ferment slowly in the mouth, which allows saliva to neutralize the acids produced, frequent use has the potential to cause caries. This occurs especially in a patient with xerostomia using these products to relieve xerostomia.
- Xylitol-containing chewing gums inhibit growth of microorganisms, reducing caries rate. Use of these gums after eating when patients cannot brush is recommended.
- High-sugar foods are generally high in fat as well. MyPyramid recommends intake of high-sugar and high-fat foods should be limited.
- Compare some low-fat or nonfat foods that compensate for flavor by increasing sugar or sodium content (e.g., frozen dairy products).
- Exercise caution in recommending high-fat foods for their anticariogenic properties to patients with chronic diseases such as heart disease or diabetes mellitus because of their deleterious effects on these conditions.
- Because physical properties of milk are comparable to saliva, increasing low-fat milk intake as a saliva substitute may also offer protection against caries for an older adult with xerostomia.
- Encourage proper oral hygiene techniques to avoid complications associated with exposure to the lactose in the milk, as seen in early childhood caries.

environment and increases clearance of carbohydrates from the oral cavity. Following the MyPyramid recommendation from the low-fat milk, cheese, and yogurt group would be prudent advice for a dental hygiene patient. Eating these foods as snacks or at the end of a meal could provide anti-cariogenic effects.

Other Foods with Protective Factors

A constituent in chocolate, known as the cocoa factor, has shown anticariogenic properties. The Vipeholm study compared the caries rate of individuals consuming chocolate with the rate for individuals consuming other types of "non-chocolate" candies under similar circumstances. The results indicated a slightly lower caries incidence in individuals consuming chocolate.[7] Glycyrrhiza, the active ingredient in licorice, can also be considered anticariogenic. However, glycyrrhiza is contraindicated with some antihypertensive medications, has a staining capability, and can cause sodium retention and increased blood pressure. Grapefruit and other fruits containing citric acid can stimulate saliva production. However, they are generally not considered noncariogenic because of their ability to lower salivary pH and increase caries risk.

OTHER FACTORS INFLUENCING CARIOGENICITY

The amount and type of carbohydrates are not the only determinants of diet related to caries prevalence and severity. Other considerations include retentiveness of the carbohydrate, how often or how long teeth are exposed, sequence in which a carbohydrate is consumed, and whether food is eaten with a meal or as a snack. Some foods thought to have low cariogenic potential (e.g., cornflakes, crackers, or potato chips) may be more acidogenic than simple-carbohydrate foods because of their retentiveness in embrasures, pits, and fissures. Preventive practices, such as regular recall appointments, appropriate oral hygiene practices, sealants, xylitol, and fluoride use, should also be considered when discussing cariogenicity.

Physical Form

How quickly a cariogenic food is cleared from the mouth is a factor related to caries development. Ingestion of hard candy results in prolonged exposure. A sticky and retentive carbohydrate (e.g., raisins) remains in contact with the enamel surface for a longer period than sweetened fluids. Slow oral clearance of fermentable carbohydrate means longer exposure of the tooth to acid attack.

Fermentable carbohydrates that are chewy, such as caramels, adhere to the teeth. However, the additional mastication required to process these foods stimulates saliva flow, making these foods less retentive and damaging than dry, sticky foods, such as pretzels. Caramels are higher in sucrose than pretzels, supporting the concept of quantity of fermentable carbohydrates having a limited impact.

Frequency of Intake

Closely related to the physical form of a food in caries potential is frequency of fermentable carbohydrate intake.

Longer periods of exposure to a fermentable carbohydrate in the oral cavity lead to a greater risk of demineralization and less opportunity for teeth to remineralize. Two individuals can eat equal amounts of fermentable carbohydrates, but the one who eats more frequently throughout the day has the greatest potential for decay. With each exposure, a decrease in pH begins within 2 to 3 minutes; at a pH of 5.5 or less (the critical pH), enamel decalcification occurs. Within 40 minutes, the pH has increased to its initial value. The classic Stephan curve shows the pH changes of dental plaque after rinsing with a sugar solution (Fig. 17-5). Using a similar scenario, if a person eats a candy bar within a 5-minute period, the teeth would be exposed to a critical pH that lasts for approximately 40 minutes before the pH returns to the original level. If another person eats the same candy bar in five bites, but only takes a bite every hour until it is gone, the total acid exposure would be approximately 200 minutes (5 bites × 40 minutes = 200 minutes of acid exposure).

Frequent consumption of soft drinks, sports drinks, energy drinks, and flavored coffees and teas compounded with a decline in dairy products can also influence caries risk and erosion despite the rapid oral clearance of these beverages (Fig. 17-6). The pH of diet and regular soft drinks, bottled iced teas, and sports drinks ranges from 2.5 to 3.5. Although these drinks are popular snacks, low-fat dairy products, 100% fruit juice, and water are preferable beverage alternatives. Fruit juice should be limited to 4 to 6 oz per day for children 1 to 6 years old and 8 to 12 oz per day for children 7 to 18 years old.[9]

Timing and Sequence in a Meal

Another consideration is whether cariogenic food is eaten with meals or snacks. Participants in the Vipeholm study who ate foods high in sugar between meals in addition to mealtime had a significantly higher decay rate than participants who consumed these foods at mealtime only. Despite these results, recommendations to eliminate snacks are not always realistic. Children cannot eat enough food in three meals to get all the nutrients they need, and snacks are warranted. Foods chosen for snacks should produce little or no acid (Box 17-3), and oral self-care should follow a snack.

The location of an acidogenic food within a meal presents another consideration for caries potential. Drinking coffee with sugar after a meal has been determined to lower plaque pH, whereas consuming cheese after a fermentable carbohydrate within a meal prevents the decrease of plaque pH that would occur if this fermentable carbohydrate were eaten alone. Cariogenic foods create less risk of enamel demineralization if followed by a noncariogenic or cariostatic food.

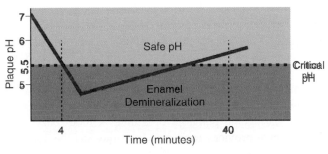

FIGURE 17-5 Stephan curve: time involvement of carbohydrate consumption and enamel demineralization.

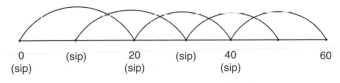

FIGURE 17-6 The increased consumption of soft drinks and sports drinks results in an enhanced caries risk. Although oral clearance is rapid, consuming such drinks over an extended time creates a cariogenic environment. If only soda is consumed, each sip results in at least 20 minutes of acid exposure. In this example, the patient took a sip at approximately 10-minute intervals and finished the drink in 5 sips for a total of 60 minutes of acid exposure.

Box 17-3	Foods That Produce Little or No Plaque Acid

- Cheeses*
  - Blue cheese
  - Brie
  - Cheddar
  - Gouda
  - Monterey jack
  - Mozzarella
  - Swiss
  - Cheese spread
  - Cream cheese
  - American
- Yogurt†
- Nuts
- Licorice
- Chewing gum with xylitol
- Cocoa products
- Protein foods‡
  - Meat
  - Seafood
  - Poultry
  - Eggs
- Fats‡
  - Margarine
  - Butter
  - Oils

*These natural cheeses are high in fat. Reduced-fat or low-fat cheeses can be recommended.
†Encourage use of low-fat or skim versions.
‡Follow the Food Guide Pyramid and Dietary Guidelines for serving sizes and low-fat choices and preparation methods.

Dental Hygiene Considerations

- Review diet history for patterns of fermentable carbohydrate consumption, frequency, form, and time consumed.
- Further questioning can reveal dietary habits the patient failed to recognize as being relevant to oral health.

Nutritional Directions

- When consuming fermentable carbohydrates, do so at mealtimes when possible to allow other foods to neutralize acids in saliva.
- Foods that require chewing (e.g., chewing gum, raw fruits and vegetables) help increase salivary flow. This aids in providing additional buffering effects and accelerated removal of retentive foods.
- Noncariogenic snacks include raw fruits and vegetables, low-fat cheese, skim milk, low-fat yogurt, peanuts, popcorn, whole-grain bagels, seeds, pizza, and tacos.
- Cariogenic snacks before bedtime should be omitted or followed by careful oral hygiene. Salivary flow is reduced when sleeping; clearance of plaque acids is limited. Uninterrupted acid production for 2 hours can be harmful.
- Consume fermentable carbohydrates within a meal, or eat a noncariogenic food last.
- Carbohydrate foods that are retentive (e.g., graham crackers or potato chips) are retained in the mouth longer, creating a greater potential for decay.
- Products made with a non-nutritive sweetener, such as aspartame, should be used in moderation (two to three products per day). Some patients may not tolerate large amounts of aspartame or other non-nutritive sweetener or choose not to use them. Recommend alternative noncariogenic food items and oral self-care.
- Encourage the patient to limit purchasing of soft drinks and sports and energy drinks in large, resealable containers in an effort to decrease the frequency and duration of consumption.
- Athletes require fluid for hydration. In most events lasting less than 4 hours, water is the preferred source of hydration rather than high-carbohydrate sports drinks.

DENTAL HYGIENE PLAN

Dietary counseling is an essential component of the preventive program. Although all patients benefit from nutritional counseling, certain populations (Box 17-4) require special attention by the dental hygienist. As mentioned, the quantity of fermentable carbohydrates consumed is of concern, especially nutritionally. However, the form of the carbohydrate, how often it is consumed, and whether it is eaten with meals or snacks are more important than the amount consumed.

ASSESSMENT

When a dental nutrition care plan is necessary, many factors must be considered. Anthropometric measures (i.e., height and weight), clinical signs, dental and dietary assessment, health and dental history, and laboratory data (if applicable)

Box 17-4   Situations Presenting High Caries Risk

Early Childhood Caries
- Parents before pregnancy
- Parents during pregnancy
- Parents of young children

Root Caries and Xerostomia
- Older adults
- Periodontal patients
- Chronic disease states
- Polypharmacy
- Radiation therapy
- Gingival recession

Habits
- Frequent use of hard candy or chewing gum, cough drops, chew tobacco, medication containing a fermentable carbohydrate source
- Frequent vomiting
- Poor oral hygiene
- Orthodontic patients
- Adolescents
- Challenged dexterity

Dental Issues
- Intake of low-fluoridation or nonfluoridated water
- Unsealed deep pits and fissures
- Family history of high caries risk
- Levels of cariogenic bacteria

Adapted from Barber LR, Wilkins EM: Evidence-based prevention management, and monitoring of dental caries. J Dent Hyg 2002; 76:270-275.

---

are addressed in Chapter 20. In addition, an assessment takes into account a patient's learning style, literacy level, cultural heritage, and socioeconomic status.

Gathering information about the quality of the patient's meal pattern and eating habits is an important step in assessing the cariogenic potential of a diet. A food diary (Fig. 17-7), which provides food data for 1 day, can be obtained through an interview by the dental hygienist, or the patient can be asked to return the completed form at a recall appointment. This practical assessment tool is helpful in determining the adequacy of the overall diet and habits related to carbohydrate intake.

Using MyPyramid as a guide, the dental hygienist can assess adequacy of food intake with the participation of the patient. Actively involving the patient in as many steps as possible is necessary to enhance motivation and adherence. Have the patient highlight all fermentable carbohydrates on the food diary (see Fig. 17-7). Review the food diary, and discuss any oversights with the patient as needed. Classify each of the fermentable carbohydrates as cariogenic or noncariogenic to assess the caries potential (Fig. 17-8). This classification requires identifying the carbohydrate according to its form, frequency of consumption, and when it was eaten. More than 2 hours of acid exposure in 1 day is generally considered high.

Food Diary

Day _____

Time	Place	Food Eaten	Amount Eaten	How Prepared
Example: 6:00 A.M.	Kitchen	Orange juice Whole wheat bread Diet margarine Egg	1/2 c 2 slices 1 tsp 1	Unsweetened Toasted Tub Fried in oil

Instructions:
1. List EVERYTHING you eat or drink on 3 consecutive, typical days.
2. Use 2 weekdays and 1 weekend day.
3. Include extras such as chewing gum, sugar and cream in coffee, or mustard on a sandwich.

FIGURE 17-7 Food diary. Typically used for 1 to 7 days. (A customizable version is available on Evolve.)

Carbohydrate Intake Analysis Worksheet

Fermentable CHO	Cariogenic?	Reason	Period of Exposure to Enamel
Banana and coffee with sugar	Yes	2 carbohydrates eaten at the same time; banana is retentive.	40 minutes
Pizza and regular soda (consumed together)	No	If soda is consumed with meal, carbohydrates in pizza (crust, sauce) and soda will be neutralized by fat and protein of other components of pizza.	0 minutes
Pizza and regular soda (consumed separately)	Yes	If consumption of soda is continued after the meal, there are no components to neutralize the carbohydrates in the soda.	20 minutes

TOTAL EXPOSURE TIME: _____

FIGURE 17-8 Example of a carbohydrate intake analysis. (A customizable version is available on Evolve.)

GOALS

When all the facts are gathered, help the patient develop realistic goals. These goals need to be flexible to meet the patient's needs, preferences, and lifestyle. Achievement of long-term goals is possible only if the patient is able and motivated to make behavioral changes, such as altering choices of cariogenic snacks or limiting frequency of cariogenic foods.

EDUCATION

Providing current information about detrimental dietary habits is instrumental in determining appropriate goals. Education alone does not guarantee behavioral change. For example, a patient may recite the process of decay and list components responsible for caries development, but if several areas of decay are evident at each 6-month recare visit, change has not occurred. Individualize dietary advice based on the patient's lifestyle, rather than requesting a change in lifestyle to accommodate recommendations. The patient's assessment and goals are the basis for any recommendations. The dental hygienist should attempt to dispel myths, redirect inappropriate habits, and provide new thoughts.

CASE APPLICATION FOR THE DENTAL HYGIENIST

At his 6-month recare visit, John S. presented with six new areas of decay: one occlusal area (class I carious lesion), two proximal surfaces of posterior teeth (class II), and three proximal surfaces of anterior teeth (class III). There is bleeding on probing, suggesting active periodontal disease. John admits his busy schedule prevents him from flossing his teeth. He stopped smoking and replaced it with chewing gum and hard candy since his last appointment. When asked about work, John states he takes antacids to settle his stomach because of the added pressures of his job.

Nutritional Assessment
- Food, nutrient, and caloric intake
- Frequency of eating between meals
- Eating habits
- Motivation level
- Knowledge level

Nutritional Diagnosis
Altered nutrition: frequent intake of chewing gum, hard candy, and antacids at various intervals throughout the day compounded by an increased plaque index, a measure of the quantity and location of plaque biofilm.

Nutritional Goals
The patient will improve his overall nutrient intake and make substitutions or modify the habits increasing his caries risk.

Nutritional Implementation
Intervention: Provide a food diary (see Fig. 17-7) with an explanation for its use and instructions emphasizing listing everything put into his mouth.
Rationale: The food record provides additional information about John's intake and reveals habits that he may have neglected to mention, thinking they were not relevant to his dental needs.
Intervention: Review the food record with John to identify health aspects and aspects needing revision. Allow John to make the necessary changes.
Rationale: The probability of a patient adhering to a recommended regimen is enhanced when the patient is actively involved in the decision-making process. The dental hygienist can suggest possible solutions and direct misguided changes. The patient ultimately makes required changes.
Intervention: Explain the caries process, factors involved, and that several of the carious lesions are in places usually unaffected.

Rationale: Understanding the total picture of his particular dental status can be motivating for John and may help him make needed changes.
Intervention: Stress that not only the quantity of fermentable carbohydrates in his diet, but also spacing, duration, frequency, and form of intake leading to caries. Use the example Carbohydrate Intake Analysis (see Fig. 17-8) as an educational tool to enhance the explanation.
Rationale: Each time the patient consumes a fermentable carbohydrate, even if it is a small mint, he is decreasing the plaque pH to an acid level for 40 minutes. By consuming sugar-containing mints six times throughout the day, the acid produced by the plaque bacteria may be present for 4 hours.
Intervention: Educate John about the cariogenic potential of sugar-containing antacids, and discuss options to avoid or reduce use of antacids. Another option may be to use sugar-free antacids, although his condition should be evaluated by his healthcare provider if it persists.
Rationale: Sugar-containing antacids contain simple carbohydrate and have cariogenic potential. Antacids are high in sodium and can interfere with absorption of many nutrients. Suggestions to decrease use of antacids include consuming small, frequent meals; eating slowly; avoiding excessive amounts of caffeine products and alcohol; reducing or eliminating cigarette smoking; and reducing stress. Referral to the healthcare provider is necessary for persistent heartburn to ensure diagnosis and management of gastroesophageal reflux, which may increase the risk for caries and dental erosion and esophageal cancer.
Intervention: Recommend fluoride treatments in the office and at home; sealants, if applicable; an antimicrobial rinse; and optimum oral self-care practices.
Rationale: Omitting the carbohydrate source is not the only factor involved in the caries process. In John's situation, protecting susceptible tooth surfaces and removing plaque biofilm also serve to eliminate the potential for caries.

Evaluation
The patient returns for his 6-month recall appointment caries-free with a reduction in gingival bleeding. He is still not smoking and uses a chewing gum and mints with xylitol. He has begun an exercise program, which is helping to relieve his stress, and he has decreased his use of antacids.

STUDENT READINESS

1. Explain the role of firm, fibrous foods in protecting the tooth against caries.
2. List several noncariogenic substitutions for fermentable carbohydrate snacks.
3. What are the different roles carbohydrates, protein, and fat play in the decay process?
4. Identify at least four nutritional foods contraindicated for a caries-active patient.
5. Complete a 1- to 3-day food diary (see Fig. 17-7). Assess for nutrient adequacy, comparing it with MyPyramid. Highlight the fermentable carbohydrates.
6. Based on the food diary from question 5, complete the example Carbohydrate Intake Analysis worksheet (see Fig. 17-8). Determine your cariogenic behaviors and the number of minutes of acid production. Based on this intake record, create a realistic and appropriate meal pattern. Discuss the rationale for modifications and substitutions.

CASE STUDY

Carol is a 42-year-old married high school graduate with three teenage children. She is a homemaker and does all the cooking and grocery shopping. Each member of Carol's family continues to have new areas of decay at each recall visit. The dental hygienist decides to have Carol write down her food consumption from the previous day while waiting for her appointment. Her food record showed the following:

Breakfast: skipped

Morning snack: glazed doughnut, coffee with cream and sugar

Lunch: grilled cheese sandwich, taco chips, gelatin salad with fruit and whipped cream, coffee with cream and sugar

Afternoon snack: candy bar and two or three homemade cookies throughout the afternoon

Dinner: meat loaf, fried potatoes, buttered carrots, roll with margarine

Evening snack: chocolate chip ice cream

1. What other information needs to be obtained before starting the counseling?
2. What dental information does Carol need to have?
3. What dietary recommendations should a dental hygienist suggest? What are some specific substitutions and modifications that can be made?
4. Approximately how many minutes of acid production occurred on the enamel surfaces this day?

CASE STUDY

As a new mother, Barbara wanted to take precautionary measures to prevent her daughter from having rampant dental decay like the neighborhood children. She breastfed the infant until 9 months of age and refused to allow any sugar-containing foods, including ice cream. The daughter was frequently observed carrying a box of crackers and her sippy cup around the house. By age 3, she has six caries.

1. When should dietary counseling have first been initiated for Barbara? Explain.
2. Describe the procedure a dental hygienist would take to counsel Barbara.
3. What suggestions would you recommend?

References

1. CDC, NIDCR: Oral Health, U.S. 2002 Annual Report: Social and Economic Impact of Oral Disease. Available at http://drc. hhs.gov/report/17_1.htm. Accessed September 7, 2008.
2. Ramage S: The impact of dental disease on school performance: the view of the school nurse. J Southeastern Soc Pediatr Dent 2000; 6(2):26.
3. U.S. Department of Health and Human Services (USDHHS): Oral Health in America: A Report of the Surgeon General. Rockville, MD: USDHHS, National Institutes of Health, National Institute of Dental and Craniofacial Research, 2000.
4. Beltran-Aguilar ED, et al: Surveillance for dental caries, dental sealants, tooth retention, edentulism, and enamel fluorosis— United States, 1988-1994 and 1999-2002. MMWR Surveill Summ 2005; 54(3):1-43.
5. Bowden GH, Li YH: Nutritional influences on biofilm development. Adv Dent Res 1997; 11:81-89.
6. Burgess JO, Gallo JR: Treating root surface caries. Dent Clin North Am 2002; 46(2):385-404.
7. Gustaffson BE, et al: The Vipeholm dental caries study: the effect of different levels of carbohydrate intake on caries activity in 436 individuals observed for 5 years. Acta Odontol Scand 1954; 11:232-364.
8. Emilson CG: Potential efficacy of chlorhexidine against mutans streptococci and human dental caries. J Dent Res 1994; 73:682-691.
9. American Academy of Pediatrics, Committee on Nutrition: The use and misuse of fruit juice in pediatrics. Pediatrics 2001; 107:1210-1213.

Chapter 18

Nutritional Aspects of Gingivitis and Periodontal Disease

OUTLINE

PHYSICAL EFFECTS OF FOOD ON PERIODONTAL HEALTH
Food Composition
Food Consistency

NUTRITIONAL CONSIDERATIONS FOR PERIODONTAL PATIENTS

GINGIVITIS

CHRONIC PERIODONTITIS
Periodontal Surgery

NECROTIZING PERIODONTAL DISEASE
Necrotizing Ulcerative Gingivitis and Necrotizing Ulcerative Periodontitis

LEARNING OBJECTIVES

Upon completion of this chapter, the student will be able to achieve the following objectives:
- Identify the role nutrition plays in periodontal health and disease.
- List the effects of food consistency and composition in periodontal disease.
- Describe nutritional factors associated with gingivitis and periodontitis.
- Discuss components of nutritional counseling for a periodontal patient.
- List major differences between full liquid, mechanical soft, bland, and regular diets.

KEY TERMS

Clinical attachment loss (CAL)
Fibrotic
Full liquid diet

Mechanical soft diet
Purulent exudates
Suppuration

Test Your NQ

1. **T/F** Supplementation beyond recommended levels is ineffective in controlling or preventing periodontal disease.
2. **T/F** Firm, fibrous foods physically remove plaque biofilm from the gingiva and tooth surface.
3. **T/F** A deficiency of vitamin C causes gingivitis.
4. **T/F** A bland, soft diet is commonly prescribed for a patient with necrotizing ulcerative gingivitis (NUG)/necrotizing ulcerative periodontitis (NUP).
5. **T/F** An appropriate instruction to a patient after periodontal surgery is, "Eat whatever foods you can manage."
6. **T/F** An individual with uncontrolled diabetes should be referred to a registered dietitian for nutrition counseling if the diet needs to be modified because of oral discomfort, such as with NUG/NUP or after a periodontal procedure.
7. **T/F** Whole milk and milkshakes mixed with Instant Breakfast powder are acceptable on a full liquid diet.
8. **T/F** A mechanical (dental) soft diet is similar to a regular diet except in consistency and texture.
9. **T/F** It is acceptable for a dental hygienist to recommend an Instant Breakfast drink or liquid supplement to a periodontal patient who is temporarily following a full liquid diet.
10. **T/F** The dental hygienist should complete the nutritional assessment and provide nutritional counseling immediately after periodontal surgery.

The target for *Healthy People 2010* is reduction of gingivitis from the 1988-1994 baseline of 48% to 41% of U.S. adults 35 to 44 years old and a decline from 22% to 14% of advanced periodontal disease.[1] The *Healthy People 2010* midcourse review of progress toward the targets indicates a reduction from 22% to 20% in advanced periodontal disease in adults 35 to 44 years old. Reductions in gingivitis were not measured because of a change in the data collection protocol.

Gingivitis is characterized by inflammation, swelling, changes in contour or consistency, presence of plaque biofilm or calculus or both, no evidence of attachment loss, and bleeding on probing (Fig. 18-1A). There is no loss of connective tissue or bone support. Gingivitis is often reversible with appropriate oral hygiene techniques. If left untreated, gingivitis can progress to periodontal disease.

Periodontal disease is a chronic, inflammatory, and infectious disease (Fig. 18-1B). It is the result of a loss of connective tissue and alveolar bone. Common findings are gingival bleeding, pain, infection, **suppuration** (formation or discharge of pus), tooth mobility, and tooth loss.

The inflammatory process of gingivitis and periodontal disease is affected by the host's immune response or the body's ability to protect itself from the destructive periodontal pathogens and infection that are present. Nutritional deficiencies can modify the body's response to periodontal disease. It can occur from adolescence through adulthood. Periodontal disease is the leading reason for tooth loss for patients older than 35. The bacteria associated with periodontal disease are connected with an increased risk of cardiovascular disease, stroke, premature births, respiratory infections, and high blood glucose levels in individuals with uncontrolled diabetes.

The involvement of nutrition in periodontal disease is not as clear as it is for dental caries. The predisposing, etiological, and contributing factors of periodontal disease are

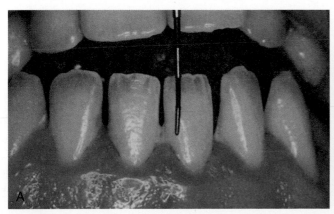
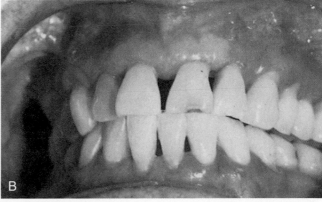

FIGURE 18-1 A, Gingivitis. **B,** Periodontal disease. (**A,** From Perry DA, Beemsterboer P: Periodontology for the Dental Hygienist, 2nd ed. St. Louis: Saunders, 2007. **B,** Courtesy Barbara D. Altshuler, BSDH, MS, Clinical Assistant Professor, Caruth School of Dental Hygiene, The Texas A&M University System, Baylor College of Dentistry, Dallas, TX.)

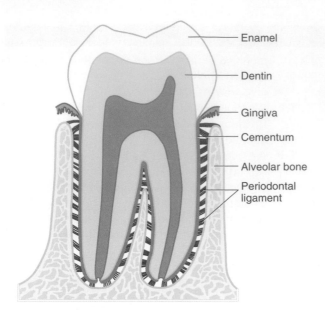

FIGURE 18-2 The periodontium consists of the gingiva, alveolar bone, cementum, and periodontal ligament. (From Bath-Balogh M, Fehrenbach MJ: Illustrated Dental Embryology, Histology, and Anatomy, 2nd ed. St. Louis: Saunders, 2006.)

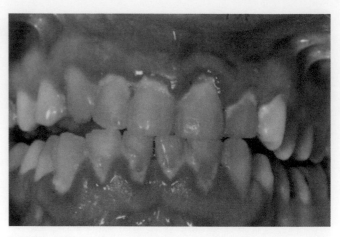

FIGURE 18-3 Gingivitis-related malnutrition. (From Perry DA, Beemsterboer P: Periodontology for the Dental Hygienist, 2nd ed. St. Louis: Saunders, 2007.)

diverse; however, the primary initiating agent is plaque biofilm accumulation around teeth and gingiva. Nutrient deficiencies, excesses, or imbalances do not initiate periodontal disease, and megadoses of supplements do not cure or prevent periodontal disease. Indirectly, nutrition may alter development, resistance, or repair of the periodontium (Fig. 18-2), which ultimately affects the severity and extent of the disease. In addition, a patient's health, medications, and food choices influence the properties of plaque biofilm and saliva. The buffering and antimicrobial effects of saliva make it a significant factor in periodontal disease. A change in composition or amount of saliva can influence the development and maturation of plaque biofilm (see discussion of xerostomia in Chapter 19).

PHYSICAL EFFECTS OF FOOD ON PERIODONTAL HEALTH

FOOD COMPOSITION

The classes of macronutrients and micronutrients having a role in growth, maintenance, and repair in the body include carbohydrates, proteins, fats, vitamins, minerals, and water. At least 50 nutrients are provided by food, most of which are required for a healthy periodontium. An imbalance of one or more nutrients can be a factor in the disruption of tissue integrity and immune response. Consuming adequate amounts of each is the dietary goal. Normal growth and development of periodontal and oral mucosal tissues depend on sufficient intake of vitamin A (salivary glands, epithelial tissue), vitamin C (collagen, connective tissue), and vitamin B complex (epithelial and connective tissue). Calcification of the alveolus and cementum requires amino acids, calcium,

phosphorus, vitamin D, and magnesium. Maintenance of oral tissues and integrity of the host's immune and repair responses requires sufficient amounts of vitamins A, C, and D; proteins; carbohydrates; calcium; iron; zinc; and folic acid. Higher kilocalorie ranges also are indicated for increased metabolic needs. (Refer to Chapters 3 through 11 for more descriptive information on the effects of specific nutrients on the periodontium.) Gingivitis related to malnutrition is depicted in Figure 18-3; note the inflammation, bulbous tissue, edema, and suppuration.

Supragingival plaque biofilm adhesion and formation is influenced by frequent consumption of monosaccharides (e.g., glucose) and disaccharides, particularly sucrose, in the diet. Subgingival plaque biofilm seems to be protected from the local effect of sugars.

Nutritional intervention needs to be a component of the treatment plan for periodontal disease because poor nutrition can affect the entire body and has an adverse effect on the periodontium. In combination with local irritating factors, such as plaque biofilm or tobacco use, systemic factors can increase the risk or severity of periodontal disease of a host, but is not solely responsible for periodontal disease. A nutrition assessment by the dental hygienist can reveal dietary deficiencies that should be corrected for optimal healing. Referral to a registered dietitian may be indicated, particularly for a medically compromised patient, such as patients with diabetes.

FOOD CONSISTENCY

Another factor affecting periodontal health is the texture of food. Chewing firm, coarse, and fibrous foods, such as raw fruits and vegetables, stimulates salivary flow. The increase in saliva enhances oral clearance of food, reducing food retention. By decreasing the amount of food debris remaining in the mouth, less debris accumulates on the teeth. Plaque biofilm is not physically removed by eating firm foods, however. Soft, sticky foods increase accumulation of food, which enhances dental biofilm growth.

NUTRITIONAL CONSIDERATIONS FOR PERIODONTAL PATIENTS

Increased nutrients and energy are required by periodontal patients experiencing stress, tissue catabolism, or infection. A thorough assessment of the periodontal patient, as described in Chapter 20, provides valuable data needed to formulate a nutrition plan.

A medical and social history can indicate whether a patient is at risk of nutrient deficiencies because of alcoholism, anorexia, or other health problems. These patients would benefit from medical nutrition therapy by a registered dietitian to normalize nutrient levels before treatment. Dietary counseling of all periodontal patients by the dental hygienist facilitates tissue repair and wound healing, improves resistance to infection, and reduces the number and severity of complications. Optimally, good nutritional status results in a shorter recovery and a more rapid return to health (Box 18-1).

GINGIVITIS

Gingivitis is a progressive inflammatory process beginning in the interdental papillae and advances to the attached gingiva. The color of the gingiva varies from slight redness to a darker reddish blue. The gingiva bleeds easily and is either edematous and spongy or **fibrotic** (formation of fibrous tissue of the gingiva owing to chronic inflammation). The stippling of the gingiva disappears, and probing depths may increase without loss of attachment. Gingivitis is associated with a large accumulation of plaque biofilm and calculus on the teeth (Fig. 18-4), which is exacerbated by frequent exposure to fermentable carbohydrates and retentive foods.

Gingival disease may be an indication of metabolic disease, such as diabetes mellitus. In combination with local factors, systemic factors, including an immunocompromised system (e.g., AIDS); use of certain medications, hormonal changes (e.g., pregnancy, puberty); and a vitamin C deficiency can be elements in the development of gingivitis. Scurvy, a disease associated with vitamin C deficiency, is rarely seen in the United States because of the availability of fruits, vegetables, and foods fortified with vitamin C. Hemorrhage, bluish red gingiva, a widened periodontal liga-

ment, and tooth mobility are characteristic oral symptoms of scurvy. Correcting the vitamin C deficiency through appropriate food choices or possible supplementation improves gingival health.

A lack of nutrients does not cause gingival inflammation, but may be a predisposing factor in that it disrupts the process of tissue repair. Adequate nutrients can hasten the healing and repair processes. Controlling or modifying the etiological factors can reverse clinical characteristics. Nutritional interventions for the varying severities of gingivitis are the same as those for promoting overall health by encouraging adequate intake of all food groups and analyzing the fermentable carbohydrate intake to determine potentially damaging habits that intensify the gingivitis.

🦷 Dental Hygiene Considerations

Assessment
- *Physical*: gingival tissue is red to reddish blue, or pink if fibrotic; interdental papillae are often bulbous; spontaneous bleeding on probing; the gingival margin is coronal to the cementoenamel junction; periodontal condition may be asymptomatic.
- *Dietary*: adequate nutrient and kilocalorie intake; frequency and amount of alcohol consumption.

Intervention
- Educate the patient that the tissue damage associated with gingivitis is reversible.
- Encourage tailored oral self-care regimens.
- Oral prophylaxis, including débridement and deplaquing.

Evaluation
Satisfactory response to therapy, resulting in health of tissue; patient is able to demonstrate adequately appropriate oral hygiene techniques; adequate dietary intake.

🪥 Nutritional Directions

- Encourage nutrient-dense foods that are not retentive. Soft foods are followed by appropriate oral hygiene.
- Encourage vitamin C–rich foods and a well-balanced diet using MyPyramid as a guide.

Box 18-1	Nutritional Involvement in Periodontal Disease

A patient's dietary intake plays a role in periodontal health, directly and indirectly:
- Growth and development of the periodontium
- Amount and type of supragingival plaque
- Inflammation and immune response
- Integrity of the periodontium
- Amount and type of saliva
- Host resistance
- Repair and healing processes

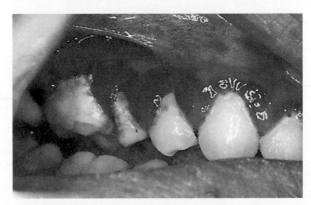

FIGURE 18-4 Gingivitis, with heavy calculus present. (From Darby ML, Walsh MM: Dental Hygiene: Theory and Practice, 2nd ed. St. Louis: Saunders, 2002.)

CHRONIC PERIODONTITIS

Periodontitis involves **clinical attachment loss (CAL)** (Fig. 18-5), the separation of collagen fibers from the cementum, and the apical movement of the junctional epithelium onto the root surface. This destructive process results in bone loss. Inflammation is also present, affecting the gingiva and other components of the periodontium. The severity of the gingival inflammation, recession, bone loss (Fig. 18-6), tooth mobility, and periodontal pocket formation varies according to duration of the disease and the individual's resistance level or immune response. It can be localized or generalized in the mouth with the possibility of **purulent exudates**, or the drainage of fluids from the gingival sulcus.

Initiation and progression of periodontitis do not occur unless plaque biofilm and calculus are present. As with gingivitis, certain types of food (e.g., soft, retentive, or fermentable carbohydrate) can enhance food retention and severity of gingival inflammation. In addition to retentive carbohy-

drates, excess glucose and sucrose have been shown to result in an increased rate of bacterial growth in the early stages of biofilm development. The biofilm development eventually reaches a steady state at this point, and the influence of diet is thought to be less important in the process of maturation of the plaque biofilm.

Systemically, nutritional status determines the immunocompetence of the periodontium. A deficiency of calcium, phosphorus, and vitamin D can contribute to the severity of bone loss (although the deficiency is not the primary cause). Recovery from periodontitis also is enhanced by the positive effect of adequate nutrient reserves and intake on the immune system. Adequate vitamin C reserves can help ensure wound healing. Intake of nutrients beyond the recommended amounts does not improve the healing process or cause it to occur at a faster rate, and can be detrimental because of interference with other nutrients or drugs. With the assistance of the dental hygienist, the patient can make dietary adjustments necessary to meet the stresses and increased nutrient requirements of the disease and to ensure optimal wound healing.

The nutrition recommendations for a patient with gingivitis can be adapted to meet the needs of a patient with periodontitis. Emphasis is placed on maintaining a nutritionally adequate diet; the *Dietary Guidelines for Americans* and MyPyramid are invaluable educational tools. The patient maintains a nutritionally adequate diet, while avoiding retentive foods; the dental hygienist analyzes the food intake for the amount and frequency of fermentable carbohydrate intake (see Fig. 17-8). By working toward improving or eliminating the etiological factors related to periodontitis, the healing process can minimize irreversible damage.

PERIODONTAL SURGERY

Preoperative

If periodontal surgery is indicated, the body's immunological competency is important for optimal healing and to prevent or minimize infections. The dental hygienist can conduct a preliminary assessment of the patient for adequate

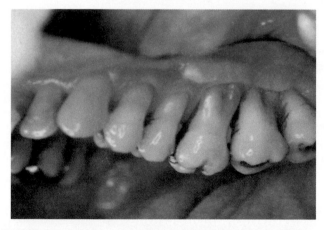

FIGURE 18-5 Clinical attachment loss. (From Perry DA, Beemsterboer P: Periodontology for the Dental Hygienist, 2nd ed. St. Louis: Saunders, 2007.)

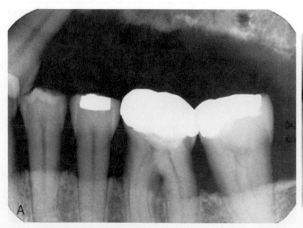
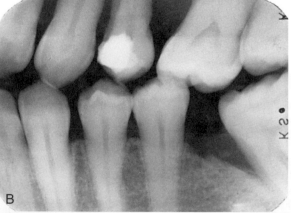

FIGURE 18-6 A and **B,** Horizontal (**A**) and vertical (**B**) bone loss. (From Haring JM, Howerton LJ: Dental Radiography: Principles and Techniques, 3rd ed. St. Louis: Saunders, 2006.)

nutrient reserves before the dental procedure. If the recommendations of the Dietary Guidelines and MyPyramid are met, the patient's dietary intake can be considered adequate. Generally, minor periodontal surgical procedures on a healthy patient with an adequate intake do not require special dietary modification. Surgery on a chronic alcoholic or a patient with anorexia nervosa could require preoperative replenishment of nutrient reserves. An elective surgery may need to be postponed for 1 or 2 weeks to allow nutritional status to be improved. A medically compromised patient is best served by a registered dietitian who can appropriately assess and determine energy and other nutrient requirements. Recommendation of a liquid nutritional supplement (e.g., Ensure) or multivitamin with minerals (MVM) may be warranted. Coordinating efforts with a registered dietitian provides the patient with continuity of care. The dental hygienist can provide the patient with a clear understanding of the relationship of nutrition to periodontal status to enhance compliance.

Before surgery, the patient should be given a tailored meal plan listing nutrient-dense foods and beverages to consume during the recovery period. Milk and 100% fruit juices contain many more nutrients than soft drinks, even if caloric value is similar. The dental hygienist should consider the extent of the surgery, its potential discomfort, and the patient's ability to eat after the periodontal procedure, and instruct the patient to make food choices that avoid tissue trauma. The patient's food preferences and dislikes are other factors to be taken into consideration.

Postoperative

Because of blood loss, increased catabolism, tissue regeneration, and host defense activities after periodontal surgery, adequate nutrient intake by the patient is required. The requirements for kilocalories, proteins, vitamins, minerals, and decaffeinated fluids (8 to 10 glasses a day) enhance recovery.

Dietary intake can be influenced by complications of anorexia, nausea, dysphagia, and oral discomfort. The texture of foods depends on the extent of the surgery and symptoms of the patient. A full liquid diet may be required the first 1 to 3 days (Box 18-2). A **full liquid diet** provides food in a liquid form for patients who are unable to chew. It should consist of high-protein, high-kilocalorie fluids to promote optimal healing. Fluids can be taken by a cup, without the use of spoons and straws. The full liquid diet is used only temporarily because the nutrient and caloric value is usually inadequate. Any special diet modifications (e.g., low sodium, low fat) and patient preferences should be considered.

The full liquid diet can progress to a mechanical soft diet when tolerated. A **mechanical soft diet** (Box 18-3) is a regular diet altered in consistency and texture for ease in mastication when chewing may be compromised. This diet

---

Box 18-2	**Full Liquid Diet: Oral Surgery**

Purpose

To provide a high-protein, high-kilocalorie liquid diet to promote healing in cleft lip and cleft palate repair, dental surgery, or mouth irritations when solid foods are not tolerated.

Adequacy

This diet meets the dietary reference intakes (DRIs) for protein, calcium, and vitamin C for children and adults. It may be inadequate in all other nutrients. Nutritional adequacy can be improved by the addition of a commercial nutritional supplement. For prolonged use, a vitamin-mineral supplement should be considered.

Diet Principles

All foods are of a consistency that can be taken by a cup without the use of spoons or straws (to avoid penetrating the repaired palate tissue).

Sample Menu for Full Liquid Diet for Oral Surgery Patients

Breakfast	Lunch	Dinner
½ cup apple juice	½ cup pineapple juice	½ cup grape juice
6 oz hot chocolate	6 oz blended beef noodle soup made with additional beef	6 oz tomato soup made with milk and additional milk powder
1 cup Instant Breakfast	12 oz milkshake mixed with Instant Breakfast powder	12 oz milkshake mixed with Instant Breakfast powder
1 cup whole milk	8 oz whole milk	1 cup whole milk

Approximate Nutrient Composition for Sample Full Liquid Menu for Oral Surgery

Kilocalories 2183	Sodium 3503 mg
Carbohydrate 304 g	Potassium 4438 mg
Protein 81 g	Calcium 2570 mg
Fat 74 g	Iron 11 mg
Cholesterol 233 mg	Vitamin A 1102 RE
Dietary fiber 5 g	Vitamin C 78 mg

Box 18-3	Mechanical (Dental) Soft Diet

Purpose

To provide a well-balanced diet, soft in texture and consistency, for patients with chewing difficulties.

Adequacy

If a variety of foods are selected, this diet meets the dietary reference intakes (DRIs) for nutrients for all adults.

Diet Principles

1. The diet consists of a regular diet with alterations in consistency and texture.
2. Foods are generally finely chopped, ground, or pureed, although very soft whole foods may be eaten as tolerated.
3. Patient tolerance to food texture and consistency may vary; modifications should be made accordingly.

Mechanical (Dental) Soft Food List

Food	Allowed	Avoid
Soup	Any except those to "Avoid"	Soup with large pieces of food or whole meats or crunchy vegetables
Meat and meat substitutes	Any chopped or ground meat or poultry, very tender whole meat, fish, or poultry; cheese and cottage cheese; eggs; smooth peanut butter; soft dried beans and peas	Whole cuts of meat; fried meat, fish, and poultry; hot dogs and other meat in casings; crunchy peanut butter; chili with beans
Potato and substitutes	Any white or sweet potatoes, mashed, baked, or boiled; macaroni, noodles, rice, pasta	Fried potatoes, potato chips, potato skins; whole grain or brown rice
Vegetables	Vegetable juice; any well-cooked, soft vegetable without seeds or skins; peeled raw tomatoes	Corn and other raw vegetables, unless tolerated
Bread	Any such as plain bread, soft rolls, doughnuts, pancakes, crackers	Hard crusty bread; bread containing nuts, seeds, or dried fruit; bagels; crackers containing seeds or made from whole wheat; taco shells; popcorn
Cereals	Cooked cereals, cereals that soften in milk	Cereals containing nuts, seeds, dried fruit; shredded wheat cereal; granola; cereals that remain crunchy in milk
Fats	Any except those to "Avoid"	Olives, nuts, seeds, bacon
Fruits	Any fruit juice; all canned or cooked fruit without seeds; bananas, orange, or grapefruit segments	All other raw fruits, dried fruits
Milk	Any	
Desserts	Any except those to "Avoid"	Desserts containing coconut, nuts, seeds, dried fruits; fried, tough, or chewy items
Beverages	Any	None
Miscellaneous	Honey, iodized salt, sugar, sugar substitutes, syrup, jelly, ketchup, mustard, pepper, herbs, ground spices	Whole spices, pickles, popcorn, nuts, coconut

Sample Menu for Mechanical Soft Diet

Breakfast	Lunch	Dinner	Snack
½ cup orange juice	2 oz ground turkey	3 oz ground roast beef	1 Tbsp smooth peanut butter
1 cup Cream of Wheat	½ cup mashed potatoes	1 medium baked potato	3 squares graham crackers
1 slice rye toast	¼ cup cottage cheese	½ cup well-cooked broccoli	½ cup apple juice
1 tsp margarine	2 slices peeled tomato	1 slice whole-wheat bread	
1 cup 2% milk	1 ripe banana	1 tsp margarine	
Coffee	1 slice whole-wheat bread	½ cup orange sherbet	
	1 tsp margarine	1 cup 2% milk	
	1 oatmeal cookie		
	1 cup 2% milk		

Approximate Nutrient Composition for Mechanical Soft Diet

Kilocalories 1898	Sodium 1838 mg
Carbohydrate 261 g	Potassium 3502 mg
Protein 89 g	Calcium 927 mg
Fat 61 g	Iron 21 mg
Cholesterol 190 mg	Vitamin A 712 RE
Dietary fiber 22 g	Vitamin C 138 mg

With permission of Greater Cincinnati Dietetic Association: The Cincinnati Diet Manual, 7th ed. Cincinnati: Greater Cincinnati Dietetic Association, 2004.

includes soft, ripened, chopped, ground, mashed, and pureed foods. The foods are generally moist. Most raw fruits and vegetables are avoided, as are any foods containing seeds or nuts. The mechanical soft diet is recommended for 3 to 7 days until the patient is able to eat regular foods. Consuming small, frequent meals (e.g., six small feedings one-half the size of a regular meal) may allow for adequate intake and is easier for the patient. A bland diet may be necessary to avoid irritating the tissue. A liquid nutritional supplement, such as Ensure, or MVM or both may be recommended to ensure adequate nutrients and to shorten duration of recovery.

Periodontal dressing may be used to cover and protect the surgical site; shield the tissue from irritation; help control postoperative bleeding, edema, and infection; and prevent accumulation of food debris and bacteria. Instruct the patient to avoid hard, sticky, and brittle foods, and to follow the guidelines for a mechanical soft diet for 1 to 2 days. Also, encourage cool liquids and foods for the first 24 hours to allow the dressing to harden and to prevent swelling. Discourage smoking and the use of straws because sucking pressure could dislodge a blood clot.

Dental Hygiene Considerations

Assessment
- *Physical*: pale pink to purplish red gingival tissue (firm to spongy); interdental papillae may not fill the interdental spaces; bleeding on probing and suppuration may exist; probing depths of 4 mm or more; tooth mobility, furcation involvement, and pain may be present.
- *Dietary*: adequacy of dietary and fluid intake; avoidance of alcohol; use of vitamin-mineral supplements.

Interventions
- Oral prophylaxis to débride and deplaque the teeth to eliminate or suppress the infectious microorganisms.
- Recommend an antimicrobial therapy for the patient.
- Encourage appropriate techniques for appropriate oral self-care.
- Provide smoking cessation counseling, if needed.
- Control of systemic disease, such as diabetes.

Evaluation
Absence of inflammation and other signs of periodontal issues, such as pain and ulcerations; patient adhering to an adequate diet, avoiding alcohol and smoking; patient maintaining regular recall appointments with a healthy periodontal clinical assessment.

Nutritional Directions

- Postsurgical patients may require a full liquid or mechanical soft diet until the patient is comfortable chewing.
- A patient requiring a therapeutic meal plan, such as for diabetes, may need a referral to a registered dietitian.
- Educate the patient that alcohol abuse may contribute to periodontal issues because of enhanced bleeding tendencies and a propensity toward malnutrition.

NECROTIZING PERIODONTAL DISEASES

NECROTIZING ULCERATIVE GINGIVITIS AND NECROTIZING ULCERATIVE PERIODONTITIS

Necrotizing ulcerative gingivitis (NUG) and necrotizing ulcerative periodontitis (NUP) are classified as acute periodontal diseases and are prevalent in young adults. NUG is characterized by red and shiny marginal labial and lingual gingivae that bleed when probed, cratered interdental papillae, grayish sloughing of the marginal gingiva, foul breath, metallic taste, occasional fever, and pain (Fig. 18-7). Common complaints include a burning mouth and anorexia. The etiology of NUG involves bacteria (e.g., *Borrelia vincentii*); systemic factors (e.g., increased susceptibility to infection, as in patients with diabetes or HIV/AIDS); local factors (e.g., smoking, poor oral hygiene); and psychological factors (e.g., stress, fatigue) predisposing a patient to the disease.

Nutrient deficiencies, such as protein or vitamin C or B complex deficiency, are contributing factors to NUG because of lowered host resistance. These deficiencies commonly occur in young adults with poor eating habits, such as high-kilocalorie and low-nutrient intake, who rely primarily on convenience or fast food meals. Also, patients with NUG may lose the desire to eat because of pain, or they may choose soft foods that are easier to eat. Excessive alcohol intake and food impacted in the interproximal areas of open contacts are other possible factors related to the condition.

Tissue infection and destruction increase physiological requirements for all nutrients. When fever is present, a 12% increase in total nutrient and energy intake is recommended for each degree above normal body temperature. Also, additional nutrients and energy are necessary for optimal repair and healing of tissue. If left untreated, NUG can progress to NUP, in which attachment loss is present.

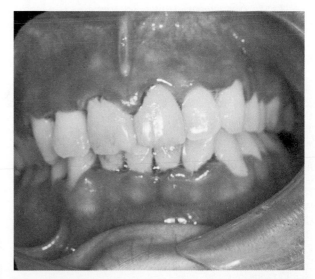

FIGURE 18-7 Necrotizing gingivitis. (Ibsen OAC, Phelan JA: Oral Pathology for the Dental Hygienist, 5th ed. St. Louis: Saunders, 2009.)

Obtaining the patient's health, dental, and social histories is the first step in nutritional management, followed by an extraoral and intraoral examination. In addition, a 24-hour food recall provides important insights into dietary practices and potential nutrient deficiencies. A 3- to 7-day food record may be needed to report a more accurate picture of food intake. Information gathered provides valuable clues regarding causes of the disease needing to be altered or eliminated. Dietary information allows the dental hygienist to make recommendations suited to the patient's eating patterns and take into consideration why the patient selects certain foods (e.g., food preferences, financial resources). Maintaining the patient's regular food intake as closely as possible generally results in greater compliance.

The severity of NUG determines the initial dietary recommendations. The goal is to provide adequate nutrients and kilocalories, avoid alcohol, and consume noncaffeinated fluids to maintain hydration. Based on the information obtained, a liquid nutritional supplement, such as Carnation Instant Breakfast, Ensure (Ross Nutritionals), or Boost (Mead Johnson Nutritionals), or MVM supplement may be suggested to ensure nutrient and caloric adequacy during acute periods of the disease. As soon as a nutritionally adequate diet is being consumed regularly, nutritional supplements can be eliminated.

Lip and tongue ulcers, extremely painful inflamed gingival tissue, and possibly initial removal of calculus may warrant a full liquid diet for 1 to 3 days (see Box 18-2). As tolerated, the patient progresses to a mechanical soft diet (see Box 18-3). A patient's tolerance to consistency varies; the dental hygienist needs to tailor the dietary information to the patient. A patient with ulcerations may need to eliminate nuts and seeds because potentially they may lodge in the ulcer causing further discomfort. Encourage fluids with meals to make chewing foods easier.

Provide examples of acceptable bland and soothing foods (e.g., gelatin), while recommending avoidance of spicy and acidic foods (e.g., citrus fruits and tomatoes), which can irritate the oral mucosa (Box 18-4). Frequent, small meals are beneficial for a patient who is having difficulty eating; choosing a variety of foods from each of the food groups is important. Additional protein intake (in the form of beans, low-fat cottage cheese, or skim milk) is effective in meeting the increased needs owing to fever and infection. Adequate decaffeinated fluid intake is essential. When a regular diet can be reinstated, concentrate efforts on continuing to follow the *Dietary Guidelines for Americans* and MyPyramid. Recurrence of NUG is possible, and preventive guidelines should be emphasized. Each episode of NUG increases the risk of progression to NUP.

Dental Hygiene Considerations

Assessment
- *Physical*: inflamed, hemorrhagic, and red labial and lingual gingivae; cratered interdental papillae; grayish sloughing of the marginal gingivae; metallic taste; foul odor; pain; fever; malaise.
- *Dietary*: adequate nutrient, kilocalorie, and fluid intake; amount and frequency of alcohol consumption.

Interventions
- Explain the extrinsic and intrinsic etiological factors associated with the type and severity of periodontal disease the patient is experiencing.
- Teach appropriate self-care procedures, and recommend use of non–alcohol-containing antimicrobial mouth rinses.
- Explain how fermentable carbohydrates enhance plaque biofilm formation by providing substrates for bacterial growth and biofilm maturation. Also, explain how soft and retentive foods cling to the tooth, allowing adherence of plaque biofilm.
- When nutrient requirements are increased because of a periodontal condition, and therapeutic treatment is needed, a multivitamin supplement may be recommended. Care should be taken to ensure the nutrients in the supplement do not exceed 100% of the recommended dietary allowances (RDAs) unless recommended by a registered dietitian.
- Many foods on a full liquid diet are milk-based. Consider the needs of a patient who is lactose intolerant. A referral to a registered dietitian may be needed.
- A proper balance of calcium and phosphorus is associated with bone mineralization (see Chapter 8). A calcium-to-phosphorus ratio of 1:1 is recommended; however, higher amounts of phosphorus are common. One hypothesis suggests that inadequate dietary intake of calcium combined with excessive amounts of phosphorus creates a nutritional secondary hyperparathyroidism (NSH). Calcium from bone stores (e.g., alveolar bone) may contribute calcium to maintain this ratio. NSH may be associated with abnormal absorption of the alveolar bone.
- Check with the patient for possible allergies to antibiotics.
- The methyl red sugar test can be incorporated into nutritional counseling as a practical motivational and educational tool. Its purpose is to determine a low pH (acid environment) in the oral cavity. Plaque is removed from the oral cavity and placed on a porcelain tile. A few drops of methyl red indicator are added to cover the plaque, and sugar is sprinkled on top. A change of color from red to yellow within 10

Box 18-4 Bland Diet

Purpose
To provide a temporary well-balanced diet for dental patients with ulcerations.

Foods and Fluids to Avoid
Caffeine-containing beverages (coffee, tea, cola, cocoa)
Alcohol
Peppermint
Chocolate
Black and red pepper
Chili pepper
Chili powder
Acidic foods
Citrus fruits

Intolerance to these and other foods varies. Foods that cause discomfort should be avoided.

to 30 minutes indicates a decrease in the pH level. The patient should be taught not only about caries production, but also how carbohydrates increase plaque biofilm adhesion and maturation.

Evaluation

The patient improves the nutritional adequacy of the diet; limits or avoids smoking and alcohol consumption; oral hygiene improves with each visit; and the clinical signs and symptoms of NUP/NUG improve.

Nutritional Directions

- Initially, a liquid diet may be needed; advancement to a mechanical soft diet is followed by a regular diet, depending on the patient's tolerance and comfort.
- Antibiotics (e.g., tetracycline or penicillin) may be prescribed for oral infection to suppress oral microorganisms, such as periodontal pathogens.
- Liquid nutrition supplements may need to be recommended. Most of these products contain cariogenic sweeteners; these should be followed by appropriate oral hygiene care.
- Cooler temperature foods are more soothing when ulcerations are present in the oral cavity.

CASE APPLICATION FOR THE DENTAL HYGIENIST

Jenny is a 20-year-old college student. It has been 9 months since her last recare visit because of her busy school and work schedule. She continues to smoke despite the dental hygienist's encouragement to quit. An oral examination exhibits inflamed gingiva bleeding on touch and a grayish pseudomembrane covering the marginal gingiva. The dental hygienist also notices an unusual odor from the patient's mouth. A 24-hour dietary recall is as follows:

7:30 AM: large coffee with cream and sugar; pastry
10:00 AM: 12 oz cola; potato chips
2:30 PM: 3 slices pizza; 12 oz cola
7:30 PM: 12 oz can of ravioli; 8 oz milk
11:30 PM: hot chocolate; 8 sandwich cookies

Nutritional Assessment

- Food, nutrient, caloric intake
- Eating habits
- Social history
- Motivation level
- Knowledge level

Nutritional Diagnosis

Identify the patient's irregular eating patterns; choices of high-calorie, low nutrient-dense foods; stress from school and work; and smoking.

Nutritional Goals

Jenny will attempt to discontinue smoking or avoid smoking during periods of acute inflammation. With the help of the dental hygienist, she will review her busy schedule and prioritize events to incorporate a variety of foods, including some choices that are quickly prepared, or more nutritious selections from vending machines.

Nutritional Implementation

Intervention: Question Jenny further on the level of oral discomfort she is experiencing. Determine whether a relationship exists between oral health and food choices. Depending on her response, a full liquid diet may initially be suggested, followed by a mechanical soft diet within 1 to 3 days, as tolerated.

Rationale: Oral conditions can interfere with chewing or swallowing. Jenny might be eating too little or omitting foods too painful to eat. Consequently, she may be experiencing a deteriorating nutritional status, which is negatively affecting her oral status. Altering the consistency of her diet can increase the nutrient value by minimizing the task of chewing and swallowing. Every patient's oral situation is unique, and tolerance levels vary greatly. The dental hygienist should listen closely to Jenny's response to individualize recommendations to meet her needs.

Intervention: Encourage Jenny to eat a variety of foods, making choices as similar to her normal eating behaviors as possible.

Rationale: Systemic factors, such as nutrient deficiencies, influence the inflammatory response of the gingiva. The dental hygienist should explain the role of nutrients in maintaining a healthy periodontium, suggesting food choices that vary only slightly from Jenny's regular food intake to enhance compliance. Essential education tools include MyPyramid and *Dietary Guidelines for Americans*. Temporary use of MVM may be recommended.

Intervention: Identify the frequency and form of fermentable carbohydrates in Jenny's diet, along with soft and sticky foods.

Rationale: Foods and drinks, such as coffee with sugar, pastries, potato chips, and cookies, influence the formation of plaque. With Jenny's cooperation, practical and realistic modifications can be established in her diet that fit in with the demands of her busy lifestyle. The dental hygienist should discuss use of milk and milk products (e.g., cheese on pizza and hot chocolate) in her diet.

Intervention: Continue efforts to eliminate smoking. Evaluate Jenny's readiness to quit tobacco use. Refer her to the National Network of Smoking Cessation quitlines at 1-800-QUITNOW or www.smokefree.gov or the state quitline.

Rationale: Smoking may promote plaque biofilm accumulation and inhibit the healing process. The heat, staining, and smoke from cigarettes can lead to unfavorable gingival changes. According to the American Dental Hygienists' Association (ADHA), evidence suggests that quitlines are convenient, effective, and preferred by smokers.

Intervention: During an oral examination, note any areas of ulceration.

Rationale: Depending on the patient's tolerance, a bland diet may be recommended because discomfort may be experienced from highly seasoned or acidic foods. Nuts, popcorn hulls, and seeds can become lodged in an ulcerated area and lead to pain, so they should be avoided. Finally, cooler temperature foods are more soothing.

Evaluation

The patient comes to each of her scheduled appointments, with improvement in oral health noted each time. At a 1-month re-evaluation appointment, Jenny is (1) consuming a regular diet including a variety of foods; (2) eating fermentable carbohydrates only with meals; (3) choosing firm, fibrous foods more frequently; and (4) attending a smoking cessation program. She is also able to verbalize reasons for these lifestyle changes.

STUDENT READINESS

1. List at least four factors detrimentally affecting nutritional status in a periodontally involved patient. Why is it important to concentrate on nutrient intake?
2. Discuss the difference between a mechanical soft and a full liquid diet. What dental situations benefit from use of each of these diets?
3. Describe a periodontal situation in which small, frequent meals should be recommended. Explain the rationale to a patient.
4. What dietary strategies can be offered to a patient experiencing oral discomfort?

CASE STUDY

A 43-year-old man comes to his recare appointment complaining of "sore and bleeding gums, especially after brushing." He is a busy executive and entertains his clients frequently. Consequently, he dines out often and averages two to three alcoholic drinks each day. His medical history is uneventful—no medications or health alerts. An oral examination reveals bleeding on probing with pocket depths generalized at 4 to 6 mm with moderate gingival inflammation.

The dental hygienist asks him to recall everything he has eaten on the previous day. His food consumption is high in fat, kilocalories, and sodium because of heavy reliance on dining out. His diet also lacks variety and is low in nutrient value.

1. List several secondary factors precipitating the periodontal problem. What changes in his lifestyle could be suggested?
2. From the limited information presented, what additional data can the dental hygienist gather to help him modify his diet?
3. What vitamins and minerals might be deficient in this patient's diet and could cause the progression of his periodontal condition?
4. What diet should be suggested? What is the rationale? Provide a realistic menu for 1 day on the recommended diet.

Reference

1. U.S. Department of Health and Human Services: Healthy People 2010, 2nd ed. With Understanding and Improving Health and Objectives for Improving Health, 2 vols. Washington, DC: U.S. Government Printing Office, November 2000.

Chapter 19

Nutritional Aspects of Alterations in the Oral Cavity

OUTLINE

ORTHODONTICS

XEROSTOMIA

ROOT CARIES AND DENTIN HYPERSENSITIVITY

DENTITION STATUS

ORAL AND MAXILLOFACIAL SURGERY

LOSS OF ALVEOLAR BONE

GLOSSITIS

TEMPOROMANDIBULAR DISORDER

LEARNING OBJECTIVES

Upon completion of this chapter, the student will be able to achieve the following objectives:

- Describe the common signs and symptoms of xerostomia and glossitis.
- Synthesize appropriate dietary and oral hygiene recommendations for a patient with orthodontics,

xerostomia, root caries, dentin hypersensitivity, temporomandibular disorder, and removable prosthetic appliances.

- Identify dietary guidelines given to a patient undergoing oral surgery and a patient with a new denture, before and after insertion.

KEY TERMS

Crepitus

Dentin hypersensitivity

Temporomandibular disorder (TMD)

Tinnitus

Following the *Dietary Guidelines for Americans* and MyPyramid is practical nutritional advice for optimum general and oral health. Various oral conditions can interfere with food intake and influence a patient's nutritional status. These situations require modifications of eating patterns based on individual needs. The oral health team is in an ideal position to provide dietary advice to a patient or to be a valuable member of a multidisciplinary team in complicated cases, such as a patient with renal disease.

ORTHODONTICS

Individuals undergoing orthodontic treatment present with unique nutritional implications. Risk of decalcification and gingival inflammation are a concern that may compromise orthodontic outcomes and long-term oral health.

Chaotic meal patterns and snack habits of many adolescents create an additional challenge during orthodontic treatment. Health and science courses at school provide adolescents with knowledge needed to make better choices, but this information is often ignored.[1] Choosing snacks or meals from vending machines, convenience stores, or fast food restaurants is commonplace.

- After initial placement, adjustments or repair in orthodontic care may require a liquid (see Box 18-2) or mechanical soft diet for 1 to 2 days (see Box 18-3).
- Emphasize the importance of oral self-care, daily fluoride use, and possibly an alcohol-free antimicrobial rinse.
- Because fermentable carbohydrates are a factor in demineralization and plaque biofilm formation, counsel the orthodontic patient to use caution, and include recommendations to modify the frequency of consuming fermentable carbohydrates.
- Remind the patient appliances can be damaged with sticky, hard, or firm foods or chewing on ice.
- Soft tissue trauma caused by sharp appliances can lead to discomfort and avoidance of certain foods. Warm saltwater rinses (8 oz water with 1 tsp of salt) and use of utility wax to cover the offending surface of the appliance provide comfort for the patient until the situation can be resolved.

Evaluation
The patient has demonstrated acceptable plaque biofilm control abilities; the soft tissues are free of trauma; the patient is choosing a variety of foods based on MyPyramid.

Dental Hygiene Considerations

Assessment
- *Physical*: gingival inflammation, dental caries, decalcification of teeth, soft tissue lesions from sharp appliances, root resorption, and accumulation of food debris around brackets.
- *Dietary*: frequency and the time fermentable carbohydrates are consumed, form of food intake.

Interventions
- Individualize nutrition counseling for adolescents to motivate them to improve their eating and oral hygiene habits. For any plan to succeed, the adolescent must be willing to change. Remind adolescents this procedure is to help improve their appearance.

Nutritional Directions

- The mechanical soft diet consists of soft, sticky, and retentive foods that can adhere around the brackets, contributing to plaque formation, and consequently result in gingival inflammation and increased caries risk. Encourage and educate the patient regarding an optimal oral self-care regimen.
- Foods such as carrots and apples should not be avoided, but cut into small pieces.
- Soft drinks, energy drinks, and sports drinks with fermentable carbohydrate along with citric acid should be avoided to minimize enamel decalcification.
- An adequate nutritional intake is indispensable for maintenance and repair of hard and soft tissue, and to withstand the stresses of tooth movement.
- Foods with a low nutrient value and fermentable carbohydrates minimize success of orthodontic treatment and increase the risk of oral complications.

XEROSTOMIA

Good oral health depends on adequate salivary flow. Common factors contributing to xerostomia are listed in Box 19-1. Because xerostomia is characterized by diminished or absent salivary flow or a change in the viscosity of saliva, xerostomia has a negative impact on oral tissues and dietary intake (Fig. 19-1). Chapter 2 provides some basic information about the functions of saliva and xerostomia.

The dental hygienist should determine from the medical history whether the patient is at risk for xerostomia. Salivary flow does not significantly decrease as a result of aging. Adults most frequently experience xerostomia in relation to taking multiple medications (see Box 19-1). Xerostomia can also be a result of one or more chronic diseases, such as Sjögren's syndrome (Fig. 19-2). Xerostomia results in various oral complications compromising a patient's nutrient intake (Box 19-2). Overall, the goals for a patient with xerostomia are to protect the oral cavity from the destructive effects of xerostomia and improve the quality of the diet.

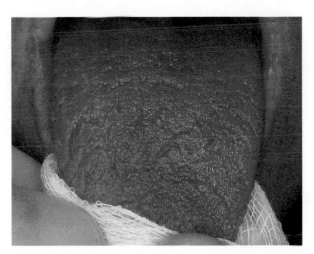

FIGURE 19-1 Xerostomia. (From Ibsen OAC, Phelan JA: Oral Pathology for the Dental Hygienist, 5th ed. St. Louis: Saunders, 2009.)

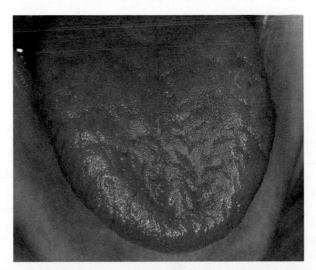

FIGURE 19-2 Sjögren's syndrome. (From Ibsen OAC, Phelan JA: Oral Pathology for the Dental Hygienist, 5th ed. St. Louis: Saunders, 2009.)

Box 19-1	Factors Contributing to Xerostomia

Medications
- Analgesics
- Antianxiety agents
- Anticholinergics
- Anticonvulsants
- Antidepressants
- Antihistamines
- Antihypertensives
- Anti-inflammatories
- Antiobesity agents
- Anti-Parkinson agents
- Antipsychotics
- Bronchodilators
- Decongestants
- Diuretics
- Gastrointestinal agents
- Narcotics

Other Considerations
- Antineoplastic therapy (chemotherapy and radiation)
- Systemic diseases (diabetes, Sjögren's syndrome)
- Stress and depression
- Significant nutrient deficiency (e.g., vitamins A and C, protein)
- Liquid diets, owing to lack of mastication
- Dehydration

Box 19-2	Consequences of Xerostomia That Influence Nutrient Intake

- Increased rate of root caries and oral infections
- Inability to keep mouth moist
- Sticky or tacky saliva
- Absence of salivary pooling
- Difficulty in chewing and swallowing
- Burning or sensitive oral mucosa
- Dry, crusty, smooth, or shiny mucosa
- Low tolerance to spicy and acidic foods
- Ulcerations
- Food sticks to hard palate or tongue
- Painful tongue—atrophied, fissured, inflamed, edematous, burning sensation
- Angular cheilosis—cracking or burning at the corners of the mouth
- Altered or lack of taste—lack of interest in eating, possible unintentional weight loss
- Difficulty with use of dentures
- Dentin hypersensitivity—hot, cold, sweet, touch
- Dry nose—impairs sense of smell
- Dry throat—difficulty with swallowing

Dental Hygiene Considerations

Assessment

- *Physical*: dry mouth; dysgeusia; burning sensation of the tongue or oral mucous membranes; dry and crusty mucosa; difficulty in swallowing and speaking (see Box 19-2); medications (see Box 19-1); antineoplastic therapy (chemotherapy and radiation); systemic diseases (diabetes, Sjögren's syndrome, AIDS); stress and depression; dehydration; and weight loss.
- *Dietary*: inadequate intake of vitamins A and C, fluid, fiber, potassium, vitamin B$_6$, iron, calcium, zinc, and protein; taste changes; lack of interest in eating; and poor appetite.

Interventions

- If the patient complains of oral dryness, the dental hygienist can place a mouth mirror or tongue blade on the oral mucosa and watch for stickiness on removal. Milking the major salivary glands (submandibular, sublingual, and parotid) to observe the amount of saliva produced is another assessment option.
- Because burning mouth syndrome cannot be identified clinically, listen to the patient's symptoms. Patients may compare the burning sensation to consumption of hot peppers, typically complaining of having an intense burning sensation on the anterior two-thirds of the tongue or oral mucous membranes; this is commonly associated with taste changes and xerostomia.[2]
- Discomfort with a removable appliance may be due to the tongue sticking to the prosthesis, an inability to retain the appliance properly, and gingival lesions created by an improperly fitting denture.
- A complete assessment, as described in Chapter 20, allows the dental hygienist to formulate appropriate intervention strategies for xerostomia.
- Each patient's situation is unique, and therapy must be individualized.
- Counsel the patient about techniques and procedures to relieve symptoms of xerostomia, which would be effective in minimizing oral discomfort and related conditions, especially increased dental caries.
- After assessing food intake, note any changes in appetite affecting overall dietary adequacy and resulting in weight changes.
- More than 400 over-the-counter and prescription medications indicate xerostomia is a possible side effect. Because drugs are a common cause of xerostomia, review the patient's medications to identify drug or drugs associated with xerostomia (see Box 19-1). The patient may want to discuss an alternative medication or a reduction in dosage with the healthcare provider. If the medication cannot be changed, or the dosage cannot be reduced, alternative measures for maintaining oral health need to be considered.
- Enhance appetite by presenting foods in interesting, appealing, and appetizing ways. Suggestions to improve the appearance and appeal of food can involve colorful combinations of foods. Imagine the lack of appeal of a plate with cauliflower, mashed potatoes, and baked white fish compared with a colorful plate of baked salmon, steamed broccoli, and a baked yam.

Evaluation

The patient uses oral hygiene and dietary interventions to relieve xerostomia.

Nutritional Directions

- Use products designed to relieve xerostomia (e.g., alcohol-free mouthwash).
- Use lip balm to help keep lips moist.
- Consume fluids with meals and between meals; frequent sips of fluids between bites facilitate chewing and swallowing.
- Use a humidifier to maintain the humidity in the air.
- Choose nutrient-dense, soft, moist foods (e.g., macaroni and cheese, cottage cheese, applesauce).
- Use gravies and sauces to moisten dry foods (e.g., roast beef).
- Choose foods principally made with a non-nutritive sweetener or sugar alcohols (e.g., gum, hard candy, popsicles), especially between meals.
- Avoid dry (e.g., saltines), crumbly (e.g., whole-wheat muffins), sticky (e.g., peanut butter), and spicy (e.g., salsa, chili peppers) foods; alcohol; commercial mouthwashes containing alcohol; tobacco; and caffeine.
- Suck on ice chips between meals.
- Tart, sour, and citrus foods and drinks may help stimulate saliva flow (e.g., sugar-free lemonade, sour candy, and dill pickles).

ROOT CARIES AND DENTIN HYPERSENSITIVITY

Because the population of older adults who have retained their teeth is increasing, root caries are more commonplace. New carious lesions in adults are typically located on the root, below the cementoenamel junction (CEJ), in areas of gingival recession. The area around the CEJ is particularly susceptible because it often has an anatomically thin layer of enamel. The cementum, which is thinner and contains fewer minerals than enamel, is also more susceptible. It is often more difficult to remove plaque biofilm adequately from exposed root surfaces because of root morphology allowing the bacteria and cariogenic material to accumulate. Caries risk increases. Xerostomia frequently compounds the risk for root caries because of limited buffering and dilution capacity of decreased amounts of saliva along with poor oral clearance. Also, prevalence of root caries is increased when carbohydrates are consumed frequently.

In addition to root caries, other problems often associated with gingival recession are abrasion and erosion of enamel and cementum. Erosion is the major cause of hypersensitivity and often occurs as a consequence of exposure to acids such as those found in food and beverages and acid from gastroesophageal reflux. Erosion and abrasion produce dentin exposure, which can lead to dentin hypersensitivity. **Dentin hypersensitivity** is an extremely painful feeling of dentin resulting from a stimulus.

Dental Hygiene Considerations

Assessment
- *Physical*: gingival recession, oral infections, a narrow region of attached gingiva, toothbrush abrasion, use of fluoridated water, oral hygiene status, and xerostomia.
- *Dietary*: diet history, frequency of eating, use of sugar-sweetened medications (cough syrup), or intake of hard candy.

Interventions
- Patients who complain of a sudden, sharp pain in areas where dentin is exposed and recession exists may be experiencing dentin hypersensitivity.
- Onset of dentin hypersensitivity is often related to temperature, primarily cold, or touch.
- Recommend a 3-month recare visit, meticulous oral hygiene, topical fluoride treatments at home, and fluoridated water. Self-applied fluoride gels reduce enamel solubility and oral bacteria.
- For patients with areas of hypersensitivity, recommend the following: (1) brushing before consuming acidic foods to neutralize the pH of saliva, (2) using a straw for acidic drinks, (3) decreasing frequency of intake or following with a chewing gum containing xylitol or a noncariogenic food (e.g., cheese or milk), or (4) avoiding foods causing discomfort (e.g., hot coffee or ice water).[3]
- Brushing immediately after consuming acidic foods can hasten the erosion process. Wait at least 40 minutes to brush.

Evaluation
The patient is free of pain, can eat comfortably, avoided the controllable risk factors, and has incorporated appropriate oral hygiene procedures into a home care regimen.

Nutritional Directions

- Carbonated beverages (regular and diet), sports drinks, energy drinks, pickled products, wine, citrus products (e.g., grapefruit juice), yogurt, and ciders are acidic foods to minimize because they can contribute to erosion.[3]
- Because dairy products, especially cheddar cheese, are cariostatic, their consumption with or without cariogenic foods can decrease the risk of caries. A reduced-fat cheese (5 g of fat per oz or less) or smaller portion size is appropriate for many patients.

DENTITION STATUS

Over the decades, a steady reduction in tooth loss has occurred. However, 26% of individuals 65 to 74 years old still incur loss of all natural teeth.[4] Although many mistakenly believe tooth loss is a normal element of aging, education level of the patient is the strongest determinant of tooth loss.[5] Although a complete dentition is not required for adequate nutrient intake, loss of teeth or supporting periodontium and an improperly fitting prosthesis are frequently

Dental Hygiene Considerations

Assessment
- *Physical*: masticatory efficiency, biting force, number of teeth and location, and fit of dentures.
- *Dietary*: adequacy of nutrients, especially fiber, vitamins A and C, magnesium, folic acid, iron, zinc, and fluids; interest in foods.

Interventions
- Most tooth loss is a result of caries or periodontal disease. Tooth loss can be prevented with education, early diagnosis, and regular care. As a dental health educator, it is important to educate the patient and community continuously regarding prevention and recognition of signs and symptoms of oral disease.
- Nutrient deficiencies frequently interfere with maintenance and repair of oral soft and hard tissues.
- During the appointment preceding placement of a new denture, counsel the patient about the initial days of adaptation so that appropriate foods can be available for the adjustment period.
- Swallowing foods may initially present a challenge to a new denture wearer because a full upper denture interferes with the ability to determine the location of food in the mouth. Days 1 and 2 of placement may necessitate a full liquid diet (see Box 18-2) to allow the patient to master swallowing with the new prosthesis before having to deal with chewing or biting firmer textured foods.
- A liquid nutritional supplement may be needed to meet caloric and nutrient needs to promote healing from extractions or sore spots or both.
- Encourage intake of dairy products fortified with vitamin D to slow the rate of bone loss.
- Discuss the possible decline in taste, owing to the full upper denture covering taste buds located on the palate, and a limited ability to identify texture and temperature of foods.
- As sore spots heal, the patient should add firmer textured foods. This process is essential for masticatory efficiency and stability of the denture, enhancing the patient's nutritional status.
- Examine the denture for fit. An appointment to reline or make new dentures may be needed. Explain the significance of a properly fitting denture to the patient, including its relationship to a poor-quality diet.
- During the next 2 to 3 days, the patient should advance as tolerated to a mechanical soft diet (see Box 18-3), which slowly introduces foods that require limited mastication.
- Patients with a compromised dentition status frequently have inadequate intake of whole grains, fruits, vegetables, and meats.
- Chewy, hard, or fibrous foods are often avoided because of low masticatory performance.
- Ensure adequate nutrient intake.

Evaluation
The patient is choosing a variety of foods from each of the MyPyramid groups, and understands the importance of a complete and functioning dentition to overall general health.

Nutritional Directions

- Fortified foods may improve nutrient intake.
- Cut food into small pieces.
- Peel and chop fruits and vegetables; cooked fruits and vegetables may be better tolerated.
- Chew food well and longer.
- Evenly distribute food on both sides of mouth.
- Chew in a straight up-and-down motion rather than a rotary motion and avoid biting with anterior teeth.
- Avoid foods such as chewing gum, sticky foods (e.g., caramels), berries with seeds, and nuts.

associated with poor food selection and limited chewing ability. Compromised nutritional intake may be a result of tooth loss, tooth mobility, edentulous status, and discomfort from removable appliances. Malnutrition or inability to comply with nutritional recommendations of some chronic diseases may result from declining dentition status.

A patient with dentures may have approximately one-fifth of the chewing ability of a patient with adequate dentition.[6] The patient's masticatory efficiency and biting force increasingly decline with each tooth lost. The number of teeth and presence of advanced mobility determine food choices. Well-fitting dentures can improve the quality of the diet, but with loss of chewing ability, the patient may choose predominantly soft foods.

ORAL AND MAXILLOFACIAL SURGERY

Oral and maxillofacial surgeries include extractions, orthognathic surgery, dental implants, and maxillomandibular fixation. The dental hygienist is a vital part of the dental team providing comprehensive treatment to a patient for optimal outcomes.

The role of the dental hygienist includes obtaining an assessment of the nutritional needs for patients before a surgical procedure to cope better with the postsurgical demands and to minimize complications. The patient must have an adequate nutrient and fluid intake to meet the stress of surgery (e.g., blood loss and catabolism), provide for optimal healing, and increase resistance to infection, which shortens the recovery period. Patients who are malnourished as a result of various chronic diseases and conditions, such as anorexia nervosa, chemotherapy, or alcoholism, are at increased risk because they are likely to be immunosuppressed. A compromised immune response may compound the severity of complications. These patients should be referred to a registered dietitian for medical nutrition therapy before the procedure. The result of a nutritional assessment and consideration of the procedure allow the dental hygienist to provide recommendations to help the patient plan for and purchase appropriate food for the recovery period.

Dental Hygiene Considerations

Assessment
- *Physical*: oral dysfunction that affects speech, mastication, or swallowing; medical history.
- *Dietary*: dietary intake, including noncaffeinated fluids.

Interventions
- When general anesthesia is used for the surgical procedure, the stomach should be empty of food at the time of the operation to avoid aspirating vomitus.
- If the patient loses weight unintentionally, healing seems delayed, history of bisphosphonate use exists, or overall health declines, the patient should be referred to a healthcare provider or dietitian.
- Provide written instructions to reinforce counseling. Tailor the information to meet the patient's needs, attitudes, and behaviors.
- For successful nutritional intervention, it is important to obtain information before the dietary counseling, including food preferences, eating patterns, living conditions, economic status, lifestyle, and physical capabilities.
- Emphasize meeting the recommendations of the MyPyramid. The key factor for optimal healing during the recovery process is adequate intake of kilocalories, carbohydrates, protein, fat, vitamins, minerals, and fluids.
- Depending on severity of the operative procedure, the patient may tolerate solid foods after surgery. If not, the dental hygienist can suggest a full liquid diet (see Box 18-2) for 1 to 2 days with progression to a mechanical soft diet (see Box 18-3) and then to a regular diet when tolerated.
- Suggest nutrient-dense and fortified foods that the patient enjoys.
- Because nutrient requirements increase after surgery, patients may find it difficult to consume adequate amounts of food. A liquid nutritional supplement or multivitamin with minerals may be necessary.

Evaluation
The patient is able to verbalize the problem and discuss ways to continue maintaining a healthy oral cavity and an adequate nutrient intake.

Nutritional Directions

- Cold foods may be soothing to the oral cavity postsurgically.
- Frequent small meals with nutrient-dense foods help meet nutrient needs.

LOSS OF ALVEOLAR BONE

Several factors, including a poor calcium intake over a lifetime, create a physiological negative calcium balance. To maintain a normal serum calcium level, the body obtains calcium from other internal sources. The calcium from spongy trabecular bone, the primary component of the alveolar process, can readily be absorbed. The status of the alveolus, which may undergo resorption before other bones, may be an early indicator of osteoporosis. When osteoporotic change in the alveolus is detected, the dental professional should refer the patient to a healthcare provider for further evaluation. Progressive loss of the alveolar ridge leads to tooth loss.

After tooth extractions, accelerated atrophy of alveolar bone occurs (within months). Resorption is greater in the mandible than the maxilla.[7] A reduction in masticatory efficiency, as occurs in individuals with dentures, also increases resorption, loss of bone mass, or alveolar osteoporosis. As the alveolar ridge reduces in height and volume, it becomes increasingly difficult to fit dentures properly, and relined or new dentures are necessary. Management of osteoporosis is discussed in Health Application 8.

GLOSSITIS

Inflammation of the tongue, or glossitis, is very painful. Food intake deteriorates, and nutritional requirements may not be met. Several systemic disorders affect the tongue.

Glossitis is caused by bacterial, fungal, and viral infection or disease. Drugs cause toxic glossitis. Psychogenic glossitis is related to psychological stress. Also, nutrient deficiency (e.g., B vitamins) or an allergic reaction to food or drugs can result in glossitis.

During an oral examination, the dental hygienist's assessment may note slight to total atrophy of the filiform and fungiform papillae. Depending on the degree of atrophy, the tongue inevitably appears shiny, smooth, and red (see Figs. 10-6 and 10-7). The atrophy can be localized or generalized. The tongue size can shrink because of dehydration or become enlarged (macroglossia) as a result of edema. A thorough assessment of the patient determines the extent and cause of glossitis.

TEMPOROMANDIBULAR DISORDER

When a patient complains of orofacial pain, frequent headaches, impaired mandibular movement, or **tinnitus** (ringing in the ears), and the extraoral examination reveals clicking, **crepitus** (crackling or crunching sound), and popping of the temporomandibular joint, the resultant diagnosis can be **temporomandibular disorder (TMD)**. Clenching, grinding, stress, malocclusion, injury, and bone abnormalities are common conditions that result in TMD. Limited jaw opening and associated discomfort can inhibit nutritional intake. Recommendations may include avoiding gum chewing and foods that require significant chewing, such as caramels, taffy, and bagels. A mechanical soft diet (see Box 18-3) may also be warranted.

CASE APPLICATION FOR THE DENTAL HYGIENIST

Mrs. Owen is a 73-year-old patient with complete dentition in the maxillary arch and a removable mandibular partial denture. The mandibular canines and incisors are present, all of which have periodontal involvement with 3 to 5 mm of gingival recession. Root caries are present on the mandibular right and left canine. Examination reveals dry, cracked lips; a lack of salivary pool; and an ill-fitting mandibular prosthesis. The medical history reveals high blood pressure and a 10-year history of antihypertensive drug use. Mrs. Owen complains of difficulty in swallowing dry food, xerostomia, and taste alterations.

While obtaining a 24-hour food recall, the dental hygienist realizes that Mrs. Owen has lost interest in food. She states: "I just don't feel like eating. Food doesn't taste good, and I don't feel like cooking for myself." If she eats breakfast, she typically has orange juice and a doughnut; for lunch, she has canned soup; and before bedtime, part of a frozen dinner. A jar of hard candy sits in her living room from which she periodically takes a piece throughout the day, and she is constantly drinking soda for relief of the xerostomia.

Nutritional Assessment
- Food intake for nutrient deficiencies
- Oral factors affecting motivation to eat
- Social and medical factors affecting nutrient intake
- Knowledge and motivation level
- Financial status

CASE APPLICATION FOR THE DENTAL HYGIENIST—cont'd

Nutritional Diagnosis

Several factors are involved with Mrs. Owen's poor nutrient intake: xerostomia; root caries; an ill-fitting prosthesis; frequent intake of hard candy; lack of variety in food; choice of soft, low-nutrient foods; and social isolation.

Nutritional Goals

Mrs. Owen has agreed to improve her overall nutritional status gradually by replacing soft, low-nutrient foods with high-fiber foods and using sugar-free candies and soda to prevent root caries.

Nutritional Implementation

Intervention: Increase intake of calcium-rich foods, such as low-fat milk, yogurt, and cheese.

Rationale: Adequate calcium and vitamin D intakes help to protect the alveolar bone from resorption.

Intervention: Provide education on xerostomia and the effects on the oral cavity and dietary process.

Rationale: An understanding of the cause and effect of xerostomia can help Mrs. Owen make necessary changes.

Intervention: Limit the intake of commercial frozen prepared meals and other processed foods high in sodium. Suggest that when the patient feels like cooking, she could prepare several meals and freeze them in individual portion sizes.

Rationale: An occasional frozen meal is quick and effortless and a better choice than not eating. However, they are expensive and generally need to be supplemented with other foods for adequate nutrients. Because many are high in sodium, an important factor because of Mrs. Owen's hypertension, remind her to read labels and to purchase ones that contain less than 500 mg of sodium per serving.

Intervention: Suggest (1) frequent sips of a nutritious beverage (e.g., milk or juices) or a noncariogenic fluid (e.g., water or diet soda) throughout the day; (2) use of products designed for patients with xerostomia, such as Biotène or Oral Balance; (3) foods containing non-nutritive sweeteners or sugar alcohols (e.g., products containing xylitol); and (4) foods that stimulate saliva flow, such as citrus, tart, or sour foods (e.g., sugar-free lemon drops). Remind the patient of gastrointestinal distress associated with excessive consumption of products containing sugar alcohols.

Rationale: High-nutrient or noncariogenic fluids keep the mouth moist to relieve xerostomia. Products containing xylitol consumed after a meal can hinder demineralization and promote remineralization. Citrus, tart, or sour foods and chewing gum stimulate the flow of saliva.

Intervention: Emphasize the importance of practicing proper oral hygiene techniques, and explain the caries and periodontal disease process.

Rationale: Because it has been shown that dentition status is related to nutritional status, Mrs. Owen would benefit by retaining each natural tooth as long as possible. Xerostomia is also a contributing factor to root caries; however, plaque biofilm must be present for xerostomia to play a role in caries development. Proper daily oral hygiene care would improve her oral status and prevent further complications.

Intervention: Apply topical fluoride in the office, and instruct the patient on self-applied home fluoride treatments.

Rationale: Topical fluoride application reduces caries risk by disrupting destructive bacteria from metabolizing fermentable carbohydrates. Application of fluoride is based on caries risk, not age.

Intervention: Instruct the patient to use a daily antimicrobial rinse for 2 weeks after each treatment.

Rationale: Antimicrobial agents are used as an adjunct to other strategies for caries reduction. Antimicrobial agents effectively control plaque biofilm formation and maturation.[8]

Intervention: Avoid dry, spicy, and some acidic foods; alcohol; caffeine; and tobacco.

Rationale: These choices can worsen xerostomia or irritate the mucosa.

Intervention: Encourage involvement with a local senior group and provide information for food assistance programs for older adults, such as Meals on Wheels.

Rationale: An older adult who lives alone may experience a decreased appetite and lack motivation to prepare appropriate meals. Socializing with others during meals enhances the enjoyment of eating.

Evaluation

Mrs. Owen's mandibular partial denture has been adjusted. The nutrition goals established with the dental hygienist are gradually being met. She has substituted a few pieces of sugar-free candy for the hard candy containing sugar, prepares more meals, and has joined the community senior citizen center. She recently began using home fluoride treatments, completed the antimicrobial rinse, and remains caries-free. She seems to be a much happier individual.

STUDENT READINESS

1. To understand what a patient with xerostomia experiences, eat several saltine crackers with no fluid, and note the dryness of the oral cavity. Imagine this situation indefinitely and its impact on a patient's food intake. Now try a product designed to relieve xerostomia to understand its effect before recommending it to a patient.

2. Discuss at least two changes in the oral cavity that can change a patient's taste sensation. What recommendations can a dental hygienist provide?

3. Prepare an educational program for interdisciplinary healthcare professionals on recognizing changes in the oral cavity affecting nutrient intake and, ultimately, general health. List at least three healthcare professionals who would benefit from this knowledge.

References

1. Story M, Newmark-Sztainer D, French S: Individual and environmental influences on adolescent eating behaviors. J Am Diet Assoc 2002; 102:S40-S51.
2. Grushka M, Epstein J, Gorsky M: Burning mouth syndrome. Am Fam Physician 2002 Feb; 65:615-620.

3. Tilliss TS, Keating JG: Understanding and managing dentin hypersensitivity. J Dent Hyg 2002 Fall; 76:296-310.
4. U.S. Department of Health and Human Services, Centers for Disease Control and Prevention, Oral Health Division: Fact Sheet: Key Findings from NHANES 1999-2002 Surveillance for Dental Caries, Dental Sealants, Tooth Retention, Edentulism and Enamel Fluorosis-United States, 1988-1994 and 1999-2002. Atlanta, GA: Centers for Disease Control and Prevention, 2006.
5. Burt BA, Eklund SA: Dentistry, Dental Practice and the Community, 5th ed. Philadelphia: Saunders, 1999.
6. Moynihan P, Bradbury J: Compromised dental function and nutrition. Nutrition 2001; 17:177-178.
7. Faine MP: Nutritional concerns for the dentally compromised client. In Palmer CA (ed): Diet and Nutrition in Oral Health. Upper Saddle River, NJ: Prentice Hall, 2003, p 238.
8. Barber LR, Wilkins EM: Evidence-based prevention, management, and monitoring of dental caries. J Dent Hyg 2002 Fall; 76:270-275.

Chapter 20

Nutritional Assessment and Counseling for Dental Hygiene Patients

OUTLINE

EVALUATION OF THE PATIENT
Health History
Psychosocial History
Dental History

ASSESSMENT OF NUTRITIONAL STATUS
Clinical Observation
Laboratory Information
Determining Diet History

IDENTIFICATION OF NUTRITIONAL STATUS

FORMATION OF NUTRITION TREATMENT PLAN
Integration and Implementation
Evaluation
Documentation

FACILITATIVE COMMUNICATION SKILLS
Listening
Nonverbal Communication
Questioning

LEARNING OBJECTIVES

Upon completion of this chapter, the student will be able to achieve the following objectives:

- Discuss the importance of a thorough health, social, and dental history in relation to assessment of nutritional status.
- Describe the components needed to assess the nutritional status of a patient.
- Explain the types of diet histories, and determine situations in which each is used effectively.

- Formulate a dietary treatment plan for a dental problem influenced by nutrition.
- Identify the steps and considerations in implementing a dietary treatment plan.
- Describe the steps in a nutritional counseling session.
- Discuss several communication skills the dental hygienist should employ when counseling a patient.

KEY TERMS

Anthropometry
Diet history
Food frequency questionnaire

Goal
24-hour recall

372

1. **T/F** When health and dental histories have been reviewed, the dental hygienist has adequate information to begin the dietary counseling with the patient.
2. **T/F** A clinical oral examination is a very sensitive tool for identifying nutritional deficiencies.
3. **T/F** Using food models when counseling helps the patient to learn how to determine portion sizes quickly and accurately.
4. **T/F** When providing nutritional counseling for a patient, the dental hygienist should change the usual intake as little as possible and reinforce positive practices.
5. **T/F** Results of dietary counseling do not need to be documented or communicated with other dental staff members.

6. **T/F** Providing a standardized low-carbohydrate menu is sufficient for most patients with a high caries rate.
7. **T/F** The dental hygienist should highlight all foods on the food diary that may contribute to increasing the risk for caries.
8. **T/F** When the nutritional counseling session has ended, the patient should have enough information and motivation to make the necessary changes.
9. **T/F** "What type of snacks do you eat?" is an example of an open-ended question.
10. **T/F** Listening involves interpreting the words said, the manner in which they are said, and nonverbal actions directly observed.

Health is a multidimensional concept, encompassing the interaction of many elements. Dissemination of information to a patient does not guarantee that the patient will establish healthier patterns. For example, millions of people start or continue smoking despite innumerable documented health risks. To facilitate positive changes toward a desired health behavior, the healthcare educator must tailor the message to meet the patient's needs, practices, habits, attitudes, beliefs, and values.

The relationship between nutrition and the oral cavity has already been established in this book. As you have learned, signs of a nutrient deficiency, excess, or imbalance are detectable in the mouth. Conversely, the integrity of the oral cavity is a factor in nutrient intake. Through the dental hygiene process of care (assessment, diagnosis, planning, implementation, and evaluation), the dental hygienist is ideally situated to address nutritional status as it relates to oral health.[1] The position of the American Dietetic Association is, "Collaboration between dietetics and dental professionals is recommended for oral health promotion and disease prevention and intervention" (p 1418).[2] Nutrition is essential for general health and dental health. The American Dental Hygienists' Association *Standards for Clinical Dental Hygiene Practice*[1] state one of the dental hygienist's responsibilities is assessment of nutrition history and dietary practices with integration of nutrition counseling into comprehensive dental hygiene care. Poor eating habits are widespread among Americans; nutritional counseling is justifiable for most patients.

A nutritional assessment involves compiling and comparing data about the patient from various sources to provide meaningful evaluation and effective counseling. All steps in the assessment require critical thinking by the dental hygienist. The evaluation tools to be discussed in this chapter include health, social, and dental histories; clinical evaluations; dietary intake evaluation; and biochemical analysis.

EVALUATION OF THE PATIENT

For effective counseling, a comprehensive picture of the patient is essential. If information gathered is incomplete, the treatment plan is distorted and may be ineffective or even detrimental to the patient's overall health. Consider this scenario: a patient with rampant caries is told to substitute sugar-free candy for mints. The patient agrees to try this until she discovers that sugar-free mints cost more money and are unrealistic with her limited income. The patient is unaware of other acceptable alternatives and continues with the mints. This healthcare professional overlooked information essential for making suitable recommendations for the patient.

HEALTH HISTORY

The health history is designed to identify health-related considerations and side effects from medications putting a patient at nutritional risk. The presence of some medical conditions could affect nutritional status by interfering with a patient's ability to chew, digest, absorb, metabolize, or excrete nutrients. Medications (over-the-counter and prescription), herbs, and supplements have numerous side effects and interactions altering eating behaviors or affecting nutritional status or both. A patient taking an antihypertensive medication may experience drug-induced xerostomia and its consequent dental complications. Changes in taste and appetite, increased risk of dental problems, gastrointestinal distress, nausea or vomiting, and xerostomia are just a few drug-induced side effects. Many medications also have drug-nutrient interactions (e.g., prednisone), which may influence nutrient needs.

By reviewing the health history and clarifying statements with the patient, the clinician can discover additional health-related information. Patients may not report valuable information because they (1) perceive it as irrelevant for dental professionals, (2) have forgotten it, (3) are confused by the question, or (4) are apprehensive about their visit to the dental office. Patients frequently neglect to disclose the use of oral contraceptives or antiobesity drugs, which have several dental and nutritional implications. A few minutes of further questioning by the dental hygienist can save hours of time and effort spent trying to treat the complications. A thorough health history provides the dental hygienist with a strong foundation for developing a plan for dietary counseling (Fig. 20-1). In addition, a blood glucose level on a patient with diabetes and a blood pressure measurement can be obtained to augment the assessment.

Screening tools, such as a nutritional assessment questionnaire (see Evolve), are helpful. When a nutritional screening is obtained during the initial steps of the assessment, the dental hygienist can detect warning signs to investigate further.

PSYCHOSOCIAL HISTORY

A social history identifies factors influencing food intake. Personal, environmental, or economic influences can imply nutritional problems (Box 20-1). The dental hygienist obtains much of this information through conversation and further questioning. In addition, by asking a patient to describe a "typical day," the dental hygienist can determine routine activities reflective of the patient's lifestyle. Understanding reasons for food choices provides directions for suggesting dietary modifications.

DENTAL HISTORY

Knowing how patients perceive or value their oral health assists the dental hygienist in developing strategies for counseling. Such information is part of a dental history (Fig. 20-2). Tobacco and alcohol use, fluoride history, and snacking patterns are also important components.

If medical, social, and dental history forms are provided before the appointment, information provided by the patient

is more likely to be thorough and accurate than if the information is completed while the patient is waiting for treatment. The most effective technique is for the dental hygienist or a member of the dental staff to interview the patient. Ultimately, the dental hygienist must review the information for clarification, and question the patient for additional pertinent information.

ASSESSMENT OF NUTRITIONAL STATUS

A thorough assessment provides the dental hygienist with enough information to determine the nutritional status of the patient. An assessment of a healthy patient may identify nutritional aspects that can be improved or "fine tuned" for optimal health. For patients experiencing medical or dental complications, the assessment provides information alerting the dental hygienist to nutritional factors that can impede responses to dental treatment or recovery (e.g., a patient with anorexia nervosa, whose fragile nutritional status would delay recovery after periodontal surgery). During the assessment, the dental hygienist can also identify the level of patient readiness for change to provide appropriate guidelines directed toward modifying behavior. Overall, assessment provides the basis for the dental hygienist's well-informed recommendations or referrals.

CLINICAL OBSERVATION

Clinical observation begins as soon as the patient walks through the door. General appraisal should include posture, gait, mobility, skin tone and color, general weight status, significant loss or gain of weight since previous visit, emotional state, personal hygiene, and physical limitations. Unintentional weight loss can be indicative of numerous disease states or even oral problems.

Extraoral and Intraoral Assessments

Visual inspection during an extraoral and intraoral examination identifies abnormal clinical signs. Table 20-1 lists physical signs and symptoms that may indicate an alteration in nutrition. These findings are not a sensitive tool for determining nutrient deficiencies or excesses because they can mirror non-nutritional complications or the possibility of several nutritional difficulties. For example, cheilosis can be the result of a vitamin B complex, iron, or protein deficiency; excess salivation; constantly licking lips; allergies; yeast or fungal infections; or environmental exposure. Observations are used as an adjunct to supplement other assessment techniques.

Examples of extraoral signs and symptoms for the dental hygienist to document are multiple skin bruises or pallor, excessively dry or easily plucked hair, dry eyes, and cracked or spoon-shaped fingernails. Intraoral inspection of the integrity of soft tissues, status of the periodontium, and presence of plaque biofilm and calculus are examples of valuable indicators of the need for nutritional intervention (Fig. 20-3). Data obtained during an extraoral and intraoral examination

---

Box 20-1	**Social Influences of Food Intake**

Examples of factors to be collected by the dental hygienist to understand further the basis of the patient's eating practices.
- Economic resources
- Food preparation and storage facilities
- Cultural, ethnic, or religious background
- Living or eating alone
- Frequency of dining out
- Responsibility of grocery shopping and food preparation
- Motivation level
- Education level
- Transportation issues
- Physical or mental challenges of an individual
- Occupation
- Work or school status
- Physical activity level

HEALTH HISTORY (HHx)

Patient Name: Last   First   Middle

Gender (circle): F   M   Date of Birth (mm/dd/yy): _____   Patient ID: _____

Address: _____
            Number   Street   Apt   City   State   Zip

Phone: (_____) _____   (_____) _____   (_____) _____
            Home   Cell   Business

Emergency Contact: (_____) _____
                        Phone   Name   Relationship

Y   N   Have you been seen by a physician during the past 12 months?
                For _____
Y   N   Are you taking prescribed or over-the-counter medicine including aspirin, vitamins, or herbal supplements?
Y   N   Have you taken the medication at the prescribed time today?

Condition	Medication/Dose/Time Taken	Condition	Medication/Dose/Time Taken

RETURN VISITS: I verify all of the above information is correct.	**Patient's initials:_____** Date:	**Patient's initials:_____** Date:	**Patient's initials:_____** Date:

Dentist's Name: _____

Address: _____

Phone: (_____) _____   Fax (when applicable): (_____) _____

Physician's Name: _____

Address: _____

Phone: (_____) _____   Fax (when applicable): (_____) _____

Y   N   Have you ever been told by a physician that you have a heart murmur?
                Type _____
Y   N   Have you taken steroids in the last two years?
Y   N   Have you ever taken Fosamax (alendroate), Actonel (risedronate), Aredia (pamidronate), Zometa (zoledronate), Boniva or other
                bisphosphonate medication? If yes, which one? _____
                How did you take the medication?   ____orally   ____ IV   How long? _____
Y   N   Have you ever had surgery, childbirth, hospitalization or serious illness? What/When _____
                _____

Have you ever had any of the following?

Y   N   Antibiotics prior to surgery/dental treatment?
Y   N   Infective endocarditis?
Y   N   Heart trouble (pacemaker/fibrillation/heart murmur/angina)?
Y   N   Mitral valve prolapse?
Y   N   Heart attack?
Y   N   Heart attack within the last 6 months?
Y   N   High or low blood pressure, TIA's or stroke?
Y   N   If a stroke, have you had one within the last 6 months?
Y   N   Rheumatic fever/rheumatic heart disease?
Y   N   Shunt/port/stent?
Y   N   Organ or tissue transplant?
Y   N   Cancer/tumor/growth/radiation therapy/chemotherapy?

Y   N   Prosthetic replacement (joints/heart valve; pins, plates, surgical wires, screws, implants)?
Y   N   Diabetes or family history of?
Y   N   Excessive thirst or urination?
Y   N   Fatigue/night sweats/persistent fever?
Y   N   Vision/Cataracts surgery/Lens Implant?
Y   N   Hearing impairment?
Y   N   Epilepsy/seizures/fainting?
Y   N   Mental or physical impairment?
Y   N   Respiratory disorders/tuberculosis/asthma?
Y   N   Surgery within the last 2 years?
Y   N   Drug/alcohol dependency?

FIGURE 20-1 Health history. (Courtesy of Dental Hygiene Program, University of Cincinnati Raymond Walters College, Cincinnati, OH.)

Have you ever had any of the following? (continued)

Y N Anemia, Sickle Cell Anemia or blood disorder/diseases?
Y N HIV positive/ARC/AIDS?
Y N Jaundice, hepatitis, or liver disease?
Y N Kidney disease/trouble/dialysis?
Y N Chest pain/discomfort?
Y N Shortness of breath/swelling of ankles?
Y N Lost weight without dieting?
Y N Blood transfusion, tattoo and/or tongue piercing?

Y N Injectable drugs/current use of recreational drugs?
Y N Thyroid condition/goiter?
Y N Painful or swollen joints/arthritis/spina bifida?
Y N Sexually transmitted disease?
Y N Serious bleeding or family history of ?
Y N Other _____

Y N Are you or Have you used tobacco products? If yes, what? _____ How long? _____
       Amount?_____Cessation Date _____
Y N Females: Do you use oral, subcutaneous or injectable contraceptives?
Y N Females: Are you pregnant?   Weeks_____ Months _____

Do the following make you ill or are you allergic to: (If the answer is yes, describe the reaction.)

Y N Aspirin or codeine? _____
Y N Local or topical anesthetics (Novocaine/Benzocaine)? _____
Y N Iodine, dyes? _____
Y N PABA (sunscreen)? _____
Y N Latex? _____
Y N Penicillin, sulfa drugs or antibiotics? _____
Y N Any other substances or drugs (e.g. food, clothing, animals, bee stings)? _____
Y N Do you have any additional condition, disease or health information? _____
       _____

ASA Classification _____

Date of last radiographs: BWS _____ FMS _____ Pan _____ Medical _____

Y N **HHX TAKEN BY PHONE?** _____   _____
                              DATE   **STUDENT'S SIGNATURE**

_____   _____
    Blood Pressure   Pulse

Remarks: _____
_____
_____
_____
_____
_____

I hereby authorize that the above information is correct to the best of my knowledge. I hereby authorize any physician, hospital or medical care facility to provide all information on my medical history and treatment to Raymond Walters College Dental Hygiene Clinic. I hereby authorize photocopies of this form to be as valid as the original. I hereby consent to preventive services.

_____   _____
Patient/Parent/Legal Guardian/Medical Power of Attorney's Signature   Date

       To the best of my knowledge, I hereby attest that the above information is current and accurate.

_____   _____
Student's Signature   Date

_____   _____
Faculty (Witness) Signature   Date

Revised 09/08

FIGURE 20-I, cont'd

DENTAL HISTORY (DHx)

Date _____   Patient Name_____

1) Do you have any pain or sensitivity in
   your teeth at this time? If yes, explain.   YES   NO

   _____

   _____

2) What was the approximate date of your last
   dental appointment?   _____
   debriding and polishing? _____

3) If under age 55, did you reside in a fluoridated area from
   birth to age twelve?   DK   YES   NO

4) Do you expect to keep your teeth a lifetime?   YES   NO
   Why/why not? _____

5) What type of dental cleaning aids do you use? Frequency?
   a) toothbrush   _____
   b) toothpaste   _____
   c) dental floss   _____
   d) stimulators   _____
   e) toothpick   _____
   f) irrigator   _____
   g) power toothbrush _____
   h) other   _____

6) Do you brush your tongue?   YES   NO

7) What do you eat and drink between meals?

   _____

   _____

8) Do you have now or have you ever had:
   a) canker sores or cold sores?   YES   NO
   b) bleeding gums?   YES   NO
   c) trench mouth or gum disease?   YES   NO
   d) teeth sensitive to hot, cold or sweet?   YES   NO
   e) pain or soreness about your ears or
       temples?   YES   NO
   f) family hx of gum disease?   YES   NO
   g) orthodontic treatment? (when)   YES   NO

8) (continued) Do you have now or have you ever had:
   h) oral surgery? (when)   YES   NO

   i) dental implants? (when, where)   YES   NO

       _____

       What care instructions were you given? _____

   If yes to any of the above, when and what
   treatment: _____

   _____

   _____

9) Do you ever:
   a) have sinus trouble?   YES   NO
   b) clench or grind your teeth?   YES   NO
   c) have sore muscles or teeth
       upon wakening?   YES   NO
   d) breathe through your mouth?   YES   NO
   e) have difficulty swallowing?   YES   NO
   f) have oral habits (thumb sucking,
       biting nails or foreign objects)?   YES   NO
       when/how often?   _____

10) Do you have full or partial dentures?   Full   Partial   N/A
    a)   Do they fit properly?   YES   NO
    b)   Do you remove them at night?   YES   NO
    c)   Do you wear them regularly?   YES   NO
    d)   How do you care for them? _____

    _____

11) Patient's main concern: What are you most concerned
    about regarding your personal oral health?

    _____

PLAQUE CONTROL RECORD

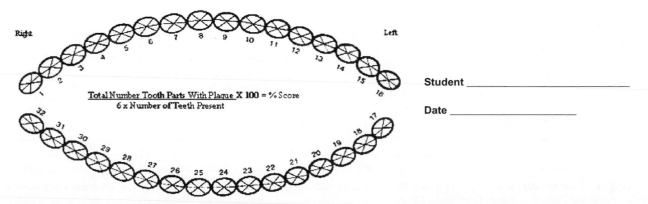

$$\frac{\text{Total Number Tooth Parts With Plaque} \times 100}{6 \times \text{Number of Teeth Present}} = \% \text{ Score}$$

Student _____

Date _____

FIGURE 20-2 Dental history. (Courtesy of Dental Hygiene Program, University of Cincinnati Raymond Walters College, Cincinnati, OH.)

EXTRAORAL & INTRAORAL EXAMINATION

Date of Exam_____   Patient Name: _____

Indicate deviation from normal by placing a check on the line next to the condition or structure.
The lines below or next to each section should be used to describe the deviations. Lines left blank
indicate that the condition or structure is within normal limits.

A. General Appraisal:
    1 _____ Posture, gait
    2 _____ Physical cond. (ht., wt., challenged)
    3 _____ Speech (voice)
    4 _____ Respiration

_____
_____
_____
_____

F. Hard palate:
    1 _____ Hard palate
    2 _____ Incisive papilla
    3 _____ Palatine raphe & rugae
    4 _____ Torus
    5 _____ Maxillary tuberosity

_____
_____
_____

B. Extraoral exam:
    1 _____ Head, Neck & Facial symmetry
    2 _____ Exposed skin
    3 _____ TMJ
    4 _____ Lymph nodes, salivary glands
    5 _____ Facial muscles

_____
_____
_____
_____

G. Soft palate:
    1 _____ Soft palate
    2 _____ Uvula

Pharyngeal area:
    3 _____ Palatine Pillars
    4 _____ Tonsils
    5 _____ Oropharynx

_____
_____

C. Intraoral Exam:
    1 _____ Lips
    2 _____ Vermillion border
    3 _____ Labial commissure
    4 _____ Labial mucosa
    5 _____ Alveolar mucosa
    6 _____ Labial Frenums

_____
_____
_____
_____

H. Tongue:
    1 _____ Papillae
    2 _____ Dorsal surface
    3 _____ Lateral borders
    4 _____ Ventral surface

_____
_____

I. Sublingual area:
    1 _____ Floor of mouth
    2 _____ Lingual frenum
    3 _____ Sublingual folds
    4 _____ Sublingual caruncle

D. Buccal mucosa:
    1 _____ Buccal mucosa
    2 _____ Mucobuccal fold (vestibule)
    3 _____ Parotid papilla
    4 _____ Retromolar area
    5 _____ Pterygomandibular fold

_____
_____
_____

E. Landmarks/Conditions/Other:

_____
_____
_____

J. Alveolar ridge or Alveolus:
    1 _____ Maxillary
    2 _____ Mandibular
    3 _____ Exostosis
    4 _____ Torus

_____
_____

FIGURE 20-3 **A,** Extraoral and intraoral examination. **B,** Periodontal assessment. (**A,** Courtesy of Dental Hygiene Program, University of Cincinnati Raymond Walters College, Cincinnati, OH.)

PERIODONTAL ASSESSMENT FORM   Patient Name_____   Date_____

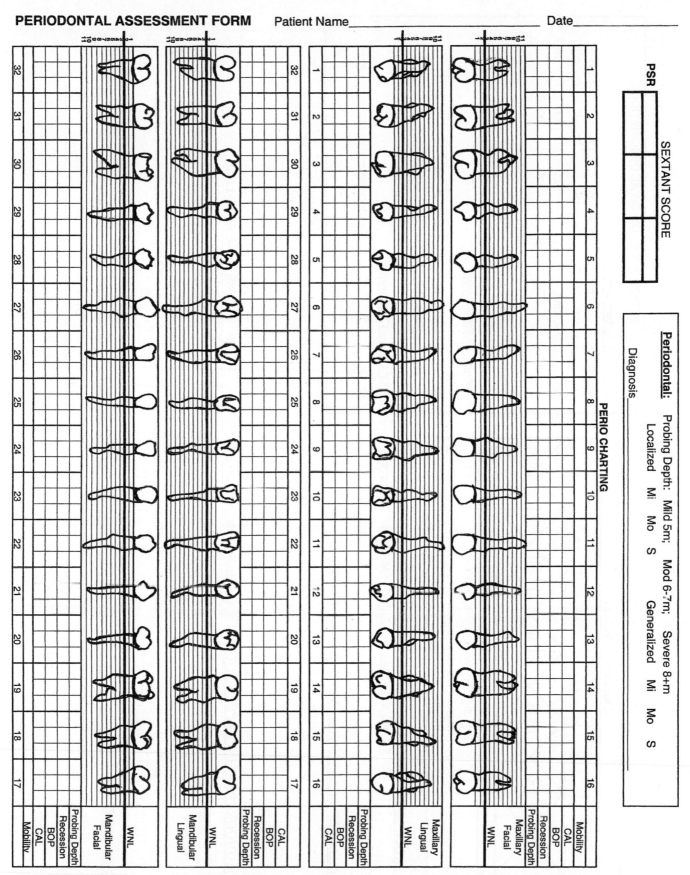

FIGURE 20-3, cont'd **B,** Periodontal assessment. *Continued.*

PERIODONTAL/GINGIVAL DESCRIPTION

Gingival Appearance:

Color: PK	ERY	MAG	PIG	KER	BB
Pap Contour: PT	BLT	CR	EDM	REC	IRR
Marg. Contour: NML	RLD	ENL	GLS	HKER	
Texture:	STP	S	FIB		
Consistency:	FRM	EDM			
Attached Gingiva:	ADQ	INADQ	MGI		

Severity Description:

Gingival:

Localized   Mi Mo S / P M D

Generalized Mi Mo S / P M D

AAP Disease Classification:

I II III **IV** _____

ND V VI VII **VIII** _____

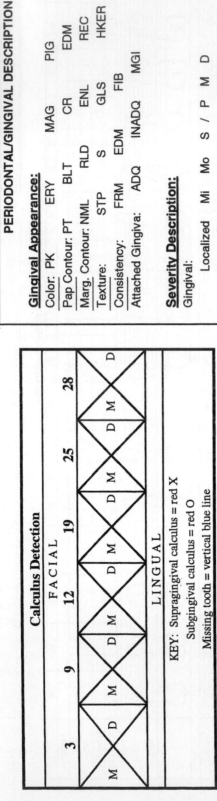

Calculus Detection

FACIAL

| 3 | 9 | 12 | 19 | 25 | 28 |

LINGUAL

KEY: Supragingival calculus = red X

Subgingival calculus = red O

Missing tooth = vertical blue line

CALCULUS: *SUPRAGINGIVAL:* *Light Moderate Heavy*

              SUBGINGIVAL: *Light Moderate Heavy*

CALCULUS CLASSIFICATION: *A B C D E NC*

RADIOGRAPHIC INTERPRETATION:

HORIZONTAL BONE LOSS

Mild   Moderate   Severe

Location: _____

VERTICAL BONE LOSS

Mild   Moderate   Severe

Location: _____

COMMENTS:

_____

_____

_____

FIGURE 20-3, cont'd **B,** Periodontal assessment.

Table 20-1	Nutrition-Related Complications of the Oral Cavity
Nutrient	**Deficiency Symptoms**
Thiamin (B$_1$)	Increased sensitivity and burning sensation of oral mucosa; burning tongue; loss of taste and appetite
Riboflavin (B$_2$)	Angular cheilosis; blue to purple mucosa; glossitis, magenta tongue, enlarged fungiform papillae, atrophy and inflammation of filiform papillae, burning tongue
Niacin (B$_3$)	Glossitis, ulcerations of tongue, atrophy of papillae; cheilosis; thin epithelium; burning of oral mucosa, stomatitis, erythematous marginal and attached gingiva; loss of appetite
Pyridoxine (B$_6$)	Cheilosis; glossitis, atrophy and burning of tongue; stomatitis
Cobalamin (B$_{12}$)	Stomatitis; hemorrhaging; pale to yellow mucosa; glossitis, atrophy and burning of tongue; altered taste; loss of appetite
Folic acid	Glossitis with enlargement of fungiform papillae, ulcerations along edge of tongue; gingivitis; erosion and ulcerations on buccal mucosa, pale mucosa
Biotin	Glossitis; gray mucosa; atrophy of lingual papillae
Vitamin C	Odontoblast atrophy; porotic dentin formation; alterations in pulp; gingival inflammation with easy bleeding, deep red to purple gingiva; ulceration and necrosis; slow wound healing; muscle and joint pain; defects in collagen formation
Vitamin A	Ameloblast atrophy; faulty bone and tooth formation; accelerated periodontal destruction; hypoplasia; xerostomia; cleft lip; keratinization of epithelium; drying and hardening of salivary glands *Toxicity symptoms*: Hypertrophy of bone; cracking and bleeding lips; thinning of epithelium; erythematous gingiva; cheilosis
Vitamin D, calcium, and phosphorus	Failure of bones to heal; mild calcification to enamel hypoplasia; loss of alveolar bone; delayed dentition; increased caries rate; loss of lamina dura around roots of tooth; reduced plasma calcium levels
Vitamin K	Gingival hemorrhaging
Iron	Painful oral cavity; stomatitis; thinned buccal mucosa with ulcerations; pale to gray mucosa, lips, and tongue; angular cheilosis; burning tongue; reddening at lip and margins of tongue; salivary gland dysfunction
Zinc	Thickening of epithelium; thickening of tongue with underlying muscle atrophy; impaired taste
Protein	Smooth, edematous tongue; angular cheilosis; fissures on lower lip; smaller teeth; delayed eruption; salivary gland dysfunction

can supply valuable evidence of a nutritional problem that can be confirmed with other assessment procedures.

Other health professionals, such as registered dietitians, provide a physical assessment that includes the performance of a basic oral examination. A dental hygienist is the professional capable of sharing expertise related to oral health concepts. Educating other health professionals to become competent in oral examinations can lead to identifying potential problems with oral issues and an increase in referrals to dental professionals. Ultimately, the patient benefits from the strategies formulated by an interdisciplinary team.

Anthropometric Evaluation

Anthropometry involves measurements of physical characteristics such as height, weight, and change in weight. Indirectly, an anthropometric evaluation provides an image of body composition and helps to monitor progress of growth of pregnant women, infants, children, and adolescents. This assessment alone is not sensitive enough to determine nutritional status; however, anthropometric measures may be useful in diagnosis.

Although measuring height and weight is unrealistic and inappropriate in most dental environments, it is appropriate to ask the patient his or her height and weight because this information is needed to determine appropriate dosage for

medications and local anesthesia used during dental care. The height and weight information can easily be put into a body mass index (BMI) calculator (available online). The BMI, as described in the *Dietary Guidelines for Americans* (see Chapter 1 or http://www.usda.gov/cnpp), provides the general weight category and associated health risk and is a guide toward measuring nutritional status. However, BMI does not consider variables such as body composition and should not be the only anthropometric measure assessed. In addition, visual inspection assists in detecting unusual leanness, indicating undernutrition, or notable obesity.

Concern arises when weight loss is unintentional. A reduction of 10% of usual weight over 6 months is significant, and a loss of 20% of body weight or greater may indicate depletion of body mass, which may affect the immune response and the patient's ability to heal after invasive dental treatment.

LABORATORY INFORMATION

When available, laboratory tests provide another piece of the puzzle in determining nutritional status. Generally, blood and urine samples supply the most sensitive data. As with other assessment techniques, a laboratory test alone should not be used to diagnose malnutrition because non-nutritional factors also can influence these data. A healthcare provider or registered dietitian generally interprets nutrition-related laboratory tests. Dental hygienists generally do not have access to this information, and it is not commonly used in a dental nutritional assessment.

In a dental environment, laboratory evaluations can include measuring salivary flow, plaque indices, caries risk assessment, determining the number of destructive bacterial cells, testing saliva with pH strips, or monitoring blood glucose. Each of these tests provides invaluable information to be included in the assessment.

Dental Hygiene Considerations

Assessment
- *Physical*: deviations from normal anatomy, particularly of the head and neck areas; diseases or conditions; emotional state; abnormal anthropometric measurements; blood pressure; if accessible or practical, laboratory tests, such as blood glucose values.
- *Dietary*: medications responsible for difficulties in eating; conditions that interfere with obtaining adequate nutrients (e.g., financial status, ability to shop for or prepare food); oral health issues interfering with food intake.

Interventions
- To be an effective nutritional counselor, the dental hygienist must understand eating habits of local cultural, ethnic, or religious groups (see Chapter 15).
- Questioning the patient about mode of transportation and mobility in the community may reveal difficulties in food procurement related to immobility or isolation.
- Have the patient describe past dental experiences to gauge knowledge level, and perception and attitude toward dentistry.
- Information about previous fluoride exposure provides valuable indicators for the assessment. Additional questions include the following: "Were you raised in an area with fluoridated water?" "Did you take fluoride supplements growing up?" "How often did the dentist provide fluoride treatments?" "Were fluoride treatments given at school?" "Have you used fluoridated rinses or gels at home?"
- Observations of the patient's attentiveness, anxiety level, motivation, previous dental treatment, and present oral conditions provide direction when initiating a nutritional treatment plan.
- A simple method to determine a patient's readiness for behavior change is to ask, "On a scale from 1 to 10, how ready are you to substitute 12 oz of milk for 12 oz of soda?" (1 being not ready to change and 10 being ready to change).[3]
- Questions and comments made by the patient reflect existing knowledge and understanding of information presented, and their needs and desires. A dental hygienist should practice active listening skills to gain valuable information needed in the assessment.
- While interviewing, maintain verbal and nonverbal neutrality in response to the patient's statements.

Evaluation
When histories and other information about the patient have been obtained, and the clinical examination has been performed, the dental hygienist should have gained an understanding of the patient's preferences and needs.

Nutritional Directions

Taking the time to gather as much information about the patient as possible results in individualized suggestions by the dental hygienist and greater compliance of the patient. Use of generic health messages and meal plans is ineffective.

DETERMINING DIET HISTORY

To assess the patient's nutritional status further, the evaluation process should include a screening **diet history**, or a review of usual patterns of food intake and the various factors that determine food selection. The overall goal is to determine usual dietary habits so that recommendations are individualized and the diet is modified, while improving the dietary quality. Reviewing intake of the parent, guardian, or caregiver is necessary to understand food choices of a child or adolescent. Questioning may be necessary to clarify information provided. Explain the need for a nutritional assessment before distributing the diet history form. When the form has been completed, additional questioning may be necessary to clarify the information provided. Asking about food preparation, whether foods chosen are nonfat or dietetic, and use of beverages or condiments is common. Also, use of food models, pictures of foods in measured portions, and measuring devices easily and precisely identify the patient's usual serving sizes. Table 20-2 lists appropriate questions the dental hygienist can use to gather accurate information.

The diet history is evaluated according to MyPyramid and the *Dietary Guidelines for Americans* for adequacy and variety of nutrients. An analysis of daily carbohydrate exposures identifies cariogenic potential of the diet. Practical tools used to gain data on dietary intake include the 24-hour recall, food frequency questionnaire, and 3- to 7-day food diary.

Twenty-Four-Hour Recall
The **24-hour recall** (Fig. 20-4; see Fig. 17-7) allows the dental hygienist to collect data on food consumed during a single day. The information is most accurate when interviewing the patient or the parent or guardian of a child and requesting intake from the previous day; this requires little time and is easy to obtain. The patient is generally able to recreate the dietary intake from the preceding day with minimal effort. Snacking patterns and spacing of meals may also be revealed in a 24-hour recall. Another advantage is it allows a general analysis of basic nutrient adequacy, variety, and cariogenicity.

An account of the previous day may not be optimal, however, because that day may not have been a typical day. For example, the patient may have been extremely busy the day before and may have eaten only one meal, instead of the usual three meals and two snacks. Requesting recall of a typical day also may result in unreliable estimates because the patient is more likely to supply information about a "fictitious" day with optimal nutrient intake. It is an option,

Table 20-2 Checklist for Food Records*

Type of Food	Did You Specify
All	Amount eaten? By cup, tablespoon, or teaspoon? By size, giving dimensions (length, width, thickness, or diameter)? By number, for standard-size items? By weight?
Cereals	Size of servings? Brand name? Additions, such as milk, sugar, or fruit? Instant or ready-to-eat type?
Baked goods	Homemade or commercial? From scratch or mix? Topping or frosting? Portion size? Number eaten? Low fat? Low carbohydrate?
Fruits and juices	Cooked, raw, or dried? Peeled? Fresh, frozen, or canned? Sweetened? Size of serving? 100% fruit juice?
Vegetables	Cooked or raw? Fresh, frozen, or canned? Sauces, other additions? Serving size?
Milk products	Percent fat? Made with sweetener? Regular, low fat, or nonfat? Powder or liquid?
Meat, fish, poultry	Type of cut? Oil or water packed? Fat, skin removed? Preparation method? Additions? Cooked weight or dimensions of amount eaten?
Eggs	Added fat? Egg substitutes? Quantity? Preparation method?
Mixed dishes	Homemade or commercial? From scratch or mix? Brand? Major ingredients and proportions? Cooking method?
Soups	Homemade or commercial? Brand? Broth or milk base? Type of milk? Principal ingredients?
Fats and oils	Stick, tub, diet, whipped, liquid, or nonfat margarine? Brand? Major oil? Type of shortening? Homemade or commercial salad dressing? Low kilocalorie or nonfat? Creamy?
Beverages	Brand? Sweetened? Diet? Decaffeinated? Alcohol content? Additions? Amount?
Snacks	Brand? Size, weight, or number eaten?
Restaurant meals	Type? Fast food, ethnic, seafood, steak? How often?
Vitamin-mineral supplements	Type? Reasons? Amount?

From Aronson V: Checklist for food records. In: Guidebook for Nutrition Counselors. Prentice Hall, Englewood Cliffs, NJ, 1990.
*Use this list to help clarify and increase accuracy of a food diary.

MyPyramid Worksheet
Check how you did today and set a goal to aim for tomorrow

Write in Your Choices for Today	Food Group	Tip	Goal Based on a 2000 calorie pattern.	List each food choice in its food group*	Estimate Your Total
	GRAINS	Make at least half your grains whole grains	**6 ounce equivalents** (1 ounce equivalent is about 1 slice bread, 1 cup dry cereal, or ½ cup cooked rice, pasta, or cereal)		ounce equivalents
	VEGETABLES	Try to have vegetables from several subgroups each day	**2 ½ cups** Subgroups: Dark Green, Orange, Starchy, Dry Beans and Peas, Other Veggies		cups
	FRUITS	Make most choices fruit, not juice	**2 cups**		cups
	MILK	Choose fat-free or low fat most often	**3 cups** (1 ½ ounces cheese = 1 cup milk)		cups
	MEAT & BEANS	Choose lean meat and poultry. Vary your choices—more fish, beans peas, nuts, and seeds	**5 ½ ounce equivalents** (1 ounce equivalent is 1 ounce meat, poultry, or fish, 1 egg, 1 T. peanut butter, ½ ounce nuts, or ¼ cup dry beans)		ounce equivalents
	PHYSICAL ACTIVITY	Build more physical activity into your daily routine at home and work.	At least **30 minutes** of moderate to vigorous activity a day, 10 minutes or more at a time.	*Some foods don't fit into any group. These "extras" may be mainly fat or sugar— limit your intake of these.	minutes

How did you do today? ☐ Great   ☐ So-So   ☐ Not so Great

My food goal for tomorrow is: _____

My activity goal for tomorrow is: _____

FIGURE 20-4 MyPyramid food record worksheet for a 2000-calorie intake goal. (From USDA Center for Nutrition Policy and Promotion. Available at www.mypyramid.gov.)

however, for obtaining a typical day's intake when the past 24 hours were atypical. Another limitation is that some patients have difficulty recollecting the previous day's food intake. Take a minute to write down what you ate yesterday to understand how arduous this task can be, and how easy it is to omit snacks and other foods of lesser importance.

Food Frequency Questionnaire

Another dietary evaluation tool is the **food frequency questionnaire**. The purpose of this questionnaire is to determine how often a patient consumes specific foods. A list of foods is provided to the patient with instructions to circle the number of times per day or week the food is chosen (Table 20-3). It requires limited explanation and little time; the patient can fill out the questionnaire while waiting for the appointment. The data gained allow for an analysis of food group consumption and carbohydrate intake.

The food frequency questionnaire is not specific and does not garner enough data to evaluate nutrient content. It also relies on the patient's memory, and the patient can easily improve the choices and supply the healthiest alternatives. A food frequency questionnaire can be used to supplement the 24-hour recall to increase reliability of the information collected. For instance, a patient may have had a glass of milk yesterday; however, the food frequency questionnaire indicates this is unusual. The dental hygienist may not have concentrated on dairy products with only the 24-hour recall, but in combination with the food frequency questionnaire, it becomes a component of the nutritional counseling.

Food Diary

The patient (or parent or guardian) may also be asked to record food and drink consumption for 3 to 7 days, including a weekend day, to evaluate intake. Figure 20-4 is an example of 1 day of a food diary (see Fig. 17-7 for another example). Verbal and written instructions for use of the food diary can be given at the prophylaxis appointment (Box 20-2). For accuracy, the most important point to stress is recording the intake on the actual day of consumption. The patient can return the diary at the recare appointment. Overall, this is

Box 20-2 How to Keep Your Food Record

- Record foods as quickly after eating as possible.
- Record days when not sick or fasting.
- Record all meals and snacks for each day, including one weekend day.
- Estimate portion sizes (e.g., 3 oz fish, 1 cup of cereal, ½ cup of milk, 1 tsp of vegetable oil) as closely as possible.
- Record the food preparation method (e.g., baked, broiled, fried, or grilled).
- Include added sugar, creamer, sauces, gravies, and condiments (e.g., mayonnaise or mustard), with the amount.
- For combination dishes such as casseroles, soups, chili, or pasta, record all the ingredients and the amounts accurately, and the portion eaten.
- Record brand names (e.g., Cheerios or Promise Margarine).
- Enter the time of consumption.
- Include miscellaneous foods, such as mints, gum, and cough drops.

Table 20-3 Food Frequency Questionnaire

Directions: The following questions will help show your (or your child's) normal eating behavior. This information will allow the dental health team to thoroughly evaluate your (or your child's) dental status. Please mark how often you (or your child) ate or drank each of these items in the past week.

Food Item	Never	1 to 3 Times per Month	1 to 3 Times per Week	5 or more Times per Week	1 to 2 Times per Day	3 to 4 Times per Day	5 or more Times per Day
Fruit and juices							
Vegetables, other than starchy choices							
Potatoes and other starchy choices							
Milk and yogurt							
Meat, fish, poultry, eggs							
Cheese							
Cereals (cold and hot)							
Cookies, cake, pies, pastries							
Candy							
Soda							
Diet soda							
Gum							
Sugar-free gum							
Alcohol							

From Thompson FE, Byers TB: Dietary assessment resource manual. J Nutr 1994 Nov; 124(II Suppl):2297S.

the most effective method of obtaining dietary information because the data are more likely to be representative of actual intake. An analysis of nutrient and fermentable carbohydrate intake is more accurate. In addition, the patient becomes actively involved when recording the information and may see obscure eating patterns emerge.

Patient compliance is a deterring factor. Requesting records for too many days may decrease cooperation. The validity of the food diary is threatened by the patient's underestimating food intake by neglecting to record all foods or accurate portion sizes. The patient also may adjust the food diary to reflect optimal eating patterns. By emphasizing this is not a test, but an instrument to use as a guide to evaluate where the patient is and to identify areas for possible modifications to improve overall health and oral health, the dental hygienist can concentrate on applying the data or may be able to dispel myths and misinformation that surface from the food diary. Finally, the food diary represents food consumed only in that period of time and does not always reflect usual intake.

The dental hygienist and other members of the dental team can cooperatively establish the most practical and realistic approach for determining food intake in their setting. Along with other components of assessment, the dental hygienist can generally evaluate the nutritional status of the patient and be knowledgeable about the role of food habits on oral status.

Nutritional Directions

Nutritional analysis of food intake, even if it is computer generated, cannot be used exclusively for diagnosing a deficiency and cannot replace nutritional counseling. Many software programs do not have complete or current data, and they do not consider other factors such as overcooking. Nutrient intakes may not be accurately estimated. Because nutritional analysis provides only an approximation of nutrient content, it should be used only as an assessment tool and a guide in counseling.

IDENTIFICATION OF NUTRITIONAL STATUS

When all of the information is collected, the dental hygienist can begin to identify nutritional status and cariogenicity of the patient's dietary intake and help the patient establish goals. (The cariogenic potential of the diet is described in Chapter 17.) A thorough understanding of the nutrients in each group of MyPyramid helps the dental hygienist to identify nutrients that may be deficient or excessive. A commonly omitted food group is the dairy group, which, if evaluated, would alert the dental hygienist to possible inadequate intake of calcium, vitamin D, protein, and riboflavin. If such inadequacies are found, the dental hygienist could concentrate on helping the patient to find suitable food choices that are appetizing, accessible, and affordable. Preferably, choices to provide these nutrients would be from the dairy group or other food groups, rather than supplements.

Several methods are available to evaluate a dietary intake. A form produced by the Pennsylvania State Nutrition Center provides an interesting and simple approach to evaluating a 24-hour recall of each day of a 3- to 7-day food record (see Fig. 20-4). The foods from the 24-hour recall are transferred to the appropriate food categories with assistance from the patient. It is helpful to have the parent or guardian present when counseling a child or adolescent, while letting the child or adolescent participate as much as possible. The patient easily determines adequacy of intake, and ideas for modifications or substitutions can follow. For a 3- to 7-day food record, the dental hygienist can separate foods into appropriate food groups for each day. The patient can be responsible for 1 day. The number of servings consumed from each group is totaled. Average intakes are determined by dividing the totals by the number of days in the diary, and the averages are compared with MyPyramid. As described in Chapter 17, the patient should be encouraged to circle or highlight each carbohydrate exposure and identify form, frequency, and time eaten (i.e., with a meal or as a snack), to evaluate the cariogenic potential of the diet.

Combination foods can be problematic for the patient because of numerous ingredients and difficulties of assigning different components into appropriate food groups. Each ingredient is considered separately and placed in the appropriate food group with servings. A 1-cup serving of spaghetti

---

Dental Hygiene Considerations

Assessment
- *Physical*: age or status of patient may require a caregiver to provide information.
- *Dietary*: current dietary practices and requirements, adequacy of diet, fermentable carbohydrate intake.

Interventions
- When interviewing a patient for a 24-hour recall, you may want to begin with, "What was the first thing you ate or drank after you got up?" or "What was the first thing you ate or drank yesterday morning?" Do not assume breakfast was eaten. Other questions commonly used are the following: "Do you use gum, mints, antacids, or cough drops?" "Do you eat snacks?" "Tell me what you do to clean your mouth." "What do you usually drink?"
- Allow as much participation by the patient as possible, encouraging the patient to make his or her own decisions and to prescribe his or her own dietary modifications. Active involvement in problem solving is more effective in changing patient habits and making the patient more accountable for his or her actions.

Evaluation
The patient participates in the nutrition assessment process, asking appropriate questions and making statements that reflect understanding.

and meatballs generally is categorized as two bread/starch servings (spaghetti), one meat serving (meatballs), one fat serving (if oil is present in spaghetti sauce or meatballs are fried), and one vegetable serving (tomato sauce).

These types of approaches to determining dietary intake are adequate and practical for most dental patients. The primary goal of a dietary assessment in dentistry is to identify patients with oral concerns related to eating and to improve these habits to prevent dental disease. If a more thorough assessment is required, the patient should be referred to a registered dietitian.

Computer dietary analysis software packages and online programs are available that provide data about dietary intake. (See Relevant Websites on Evolve.) Several packages are specifically designed for the dental office. Nutrients that can be determined include kilocalories, vitamins, minerals, protein, fiber, fat, and cholesterol. The dental team determines which program would meet the needs of the dental environment. Programs vary in complexity, visuals, efficiency, number of food items, and accuracy. A printout of the comparison with the recommended dietary allowances (RDAs), dietary goals, and exchanges provides a useful and "eye-opening" adjunct to the nutritional counseling session.

Use of a computer software program is limited by the cost of the hardware and software and the time factor. Not all software is reliable and accurate. Before relying on the data, randomly compare the nutrient content of several foods to U.S. Department of Agriculture (USDA) nutrient data (http://www.nal.usda.gov/fnic/foodcomp) or the manufacturer's information. Most importantly, use computer feedback to supplement nutrition counseling, not replace it.

FORMATION OF NUTRITION TREATMENT PLAN

After evaluation of data, the results can be shared with the patient and parent or guardian, if appropriate. The dental hygienist and patient can begin to establish an individualized dietary plan and course of action. The patient should be involved in as many processes as possible to improve compliance. When assisting the patient in preparing an altered meal pattern, several strategies need to be considered. As discussed earlier, accommodating factors affecting food intake, whenever possible, are advantageous. The goal is patient adherence so that oral health is improved. Other important considerations are food preferences, habits and behaviors, allergies, and prescribed diets. Compliance is more likely if changes are minimal or deviate as little as possible from the patient's normal pattern of eating. The patient should verify other results indicated by the assessment. For instance, if a patient's intake seems deficient in fruits, further questioning may reveal no fruit was available during the days of recording because of the patient's inability to go to the grocery store. The dental hygienist would interpret this deficiency as atypical, or the situation may occur frequently because of lack of transportation.

INTEGRATION AND IMPLEMENTATION

The purpose of nutritional counseling is to provide accurate information, and motivate and encourage the patient to initiate positive changes in behavior and continue healthful practices. Obtaining knowledge and changing a personal habit requires a patient internalize and accept that modifying a specific behavior is beneficial to himself or herself. A large gap exists between gaining information and applying the information because of difficulties in changing eating patterns. The patient and dental hygienist work together to bridge the gap. Knowledge alone does not determine desired behavior. Providing a sheet with a textbook diet or a list of nutrition "do's and don't's" is unlikely to effect change. These written guidelines are not meaningful because they do not account for each patient's individuality and unique nutritional needs, and for the difficulty in changing established eating patterns. Consider a patient who accurately describes MyPyramid, but continues to omit vegetables. This patient is knowledgeable but does not change behavior; learning is ineffective.

Effective nutritional counseling involves the patient and dental hygienist working together to define the diet/dental problem and formulate solutions. A counseling session in which the dental hygienist points out each negative behavior is not conducive to learning. The dental hygienist's responsibility is to supply accurate information and guide the patient in making healthful decisions toward improving the diet/dental situation. The patient's responsibility is to make changes in food patterns, but the dental hygienist can offer some suggestions.

Setting Goals

Resistance to change, despite knowledge, is a natural response of an individual. Consider the dental health professional who encourages patients to floss, yet he or she does not floss regularly. Box 20-3 presents an exercise to further understanding. Establishing a **goal** is an important aspect of changing behaviors because it sets a concrete standard for change. A meaningful and realistic goal provides the patient with something achievable. The goal chosen should be difficult enough to be challenging, but not so difficult as to seem impossible. Occasionally, behaviors may need to be

Box 20-3	**Exercise to Understand Resistance to Change**

Fold your arms in front of you. Do not glance down to identify which arm rests on top. Quickly unfold your arms and refold them the opposite way. For example, if the right arm was initially on top, it should be under the left arm after the switch.

Note the awkwardness. Does this reflect a change in an established behavior? If even this slight physical change leads to some resistance, think of the implications for more substantial behavioral changes asked of a patient.

Adapted from Newstrom JW, Scannell EE: Games Trainers Play. New York: McGraw-Hill, 1980.

prioritized; a behavior with the most significant impact on oral health is addressed first. Perhaps frequent use of cough drops has led to an increased caries rate. The dental hygienist should emphasize the reason this behavior is detrimental and guide the patient in establishing goals to decrease use of or eliminate cough drops. This guidance may include referring the patient to a healthcare provider to determine what is causing the sore throat or cough, or explaining to the patient why the mouth is so dry.

A goal needs to be measurable or observable. "Eat one vegetable each day" is a very specific goal that can readily be measured. However, "improve oral health" is vague and difficult to observe; this goal should be more specific. Creating goals for multiple behavior changes at one time could be overwhelming. Gradual changes in behavior are more successful and can be accomplished by breaking goals into smaller steps. The dental hygienist can work with the patient to select and develop a realistic goal. When established, the goal should be modified as needs change. For example, "Eat one vegetable every other day" may be more appropriate for someone eating no vegetables at all than "Eat three to five servings of vegetables each day as recommended." The latter example may prove to be too difficult, and the patient may give up. Successful achievement of smaller steps motivates one toward larger changes. When smaller steps are accomplished, the patient can modify the goal to eating one vegetable every day and eventually work toward eating three to five vegetables per day.

Menu Creation

When the patient has a grasp of the dietary need and has direction as to how to accomplish it, he or she should create a realistic menu for a day. Figure 20-5 provides an example of a menu planning record that a dental hygienist can use. The dental hygienist assists the patient in establishing a menu that follows the principles discussed, including nutritionally adequate and noncariogenic situations. It should vary as little as possible from the original intake and include foods the patient likes. Often the patient may suggest an ideal intake, modeling MyPyramid. The dental hygienist can intervene and suggest more practical options to improve long-term compliance. For instance, most individuals know it is unwise to eat frequently at fast food restaurants, but it is unrealistic to instruct patients never to eat there. The dental hygienist can help the patient determine the best food selections available if the patient eats fast food several times each week.

The feedback given by the patient to formulate a menu is one indicator the dental hygienist can use to determine whether learning has occurred. A patient who provides an ideal menu reflects knowledge-based skills, but this is a signal for the dental hygienist to redirect the patient toward more workable modifications.

Follow-up

A follow-up appointment to monitor the patient's progress and to evaluate the care provided can be scheduled sepa-

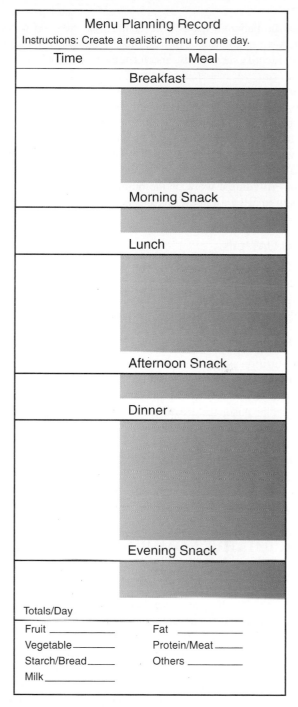

FIGURE 20-5 Menu planning. (A customizable version is available on Evolve.)

rately or in conjunction with another dental appointment. Primary approaches for the dental hygienist include supporting continued change, establishing challenging goals or revising existing goals, and clarifying information. Reviewing a new food record with the patient promotes feedback of progress, particularly when compared with the original. Rather than expressing disappointment over not meeting a goal, the dental hygienist points out the positive behaviors, no matter how small. Praise is more motivating for the patient. Perhaps the initial interventions established did not meet the patient's needs. The dental hygienist can use the follow-up appointment to listen to the patient, reassess the plan, identify new needs, and formulate new goals.

Review

The dental hygienist concludes the session by summarizing the pertinent points and giving the patient a sense of accomplishment and direction after leaving the appointment. A firm commitment toward change may not always occur, but an agreement to think about it can be a successful conclusion. Providing a work phone number and encouraging the patient to call with questions also helps the patient recognize your concern.

EVALUATION

Evaluation is an ongoing process that occurs in all stages of assessment and counseling. The dental hygienist needs to revise the nutritional assessment and counseling continuously, and make appropriate changes as needed.

DOCUMENTATION

The nutrition assessment process must be documented in the treatment record. Because this is a permanent legal document, if it is not recorded, presumably the intervention did not occur. Also, the treatment record serves as a tool for communication with other members of the dental team and other healthcare professionals. At a restorative appointment, the dentist or dental assistant can reinforce the nutrition message initiated by the dental hygienist from the information provided on the treatment record. Documentation should include the dental issues, assessment, plan, and outcomes.

FACILITATIVE COMMUNICATION SKILLS

Intertwined with implementing an effective nutrition care plan are the interpersonal communication skills of the dental hygienist. An atmosphere of sincerity, trust, and empathy should be established to help the patient relax and feel more comfortable in revealing accurate information and be more cooperative in working toward a goal. Good rapport is the foundation; without it, very little is accomplished (Fig. 20-6). Using nonjudgmental and noncritical responses encourages a patient to provide accurate accounts of food intake without the threat of being reprimanded. If a patient's food record reveals donuts and soda for breakfast, it would be judgmental for the dental hygienist to say, "I can't believe you eat that for breakfast!" Instead, a noncommittal verbal and nonverbal acknowledgment of the food, such as, "Is this usual?" would elicit a more accurate reply. Phrases discounting a patient's feelings do not promote the warm and caring atmosphere essential for good rapport. Phrases such as, "You're making a mountain out of a molehill," "Don't be ridiculous," or "It is good, but ...," are guaranteed to inhibit the patient's participation.

LISTENING

Listening to the patient is an important and distinguishing feature of effective communication that the dental hygienist

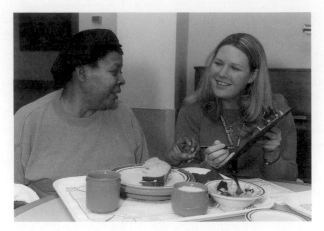

FIGURE 20-6 Counseling. (From Peckenpaugh NJ: Nutrition Essentials and Diet Therapy, 10th ed. Philadelphia: Saunders, 2007.)

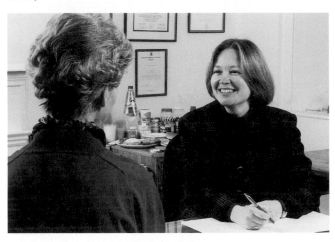

FIGURE 20-7 Listening. (From Mahan LK, Escott-Stump S: Krause's Food and Nutrition Therapy, 12th ed. Philadelphia: Saunders, 2008.)

must practice. Listening involves more than hearing. It includes interpreting what is said, how it is said, and nonverbal actions observed. Active listening is difficult and requires the full attention of the listener (Fig. 20-7). Active listening can actually save time, however, because the dental hygienist gains a better understanding of a situation.

Impediments to active listening include interrupting, preparing a response while the other person is speaking, distracting mannerisms, daydreaming, and finishing the speaker's sentences. Awareness of personal barriers to listening allows the dental hygienist to focus on establishing appropriate alternatives for more effective communication.

To improve listening skills, the dental hygienist can practice being attentive by shutting out external distractions or not interrupting (e.g., decreasing the number of questions asked, not taking the subject in another direction). A patient feels more comfortable and important when he or she is being heard.

NONVERBAL COMMUNICATION

Facial expressions, eye contact, body movements, personal distance, head nodding, and vocal cues are nonverbal behaviors serving to enhance verbal behavior. Positive nonverbal communications increase the effectiveness of the message and create a comfortable atmosphere for the patient. Eye contact is a significant interaction between the dental hygienist and patient. Good eye contact communicates interest, understanding, and warmth, whereas a lack of eye contact or staring can be interpreted as indifference or preoccupation. Eye contact and other nonverbal signals can communicate what cannot be verbalized.

QUESTIONING

Asking open-ended questions encourages the patient to expand on the answers, which can include much more information about food choices than anticipated. "What is your evening routine?" would evoke a more detailed response than a question with a yes or no reply, such as, "Do you snack in the evening?"

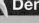

Dental Hygiene Considerations

Assessment
- *Physical*: attitude and interest of patient toward behavior change; nonverbal signs from patient.
- *Dietary*: completed and analyzed dietary intake.

Interventions
- Avoid scheduling nutritional counseling after a long or difficult dental appointment.
- The operatory causes anxiety for many patients; when possible, choose a quiet and private location for nutritional counseling so that the patient feels more relaxed and less apprehensive.

- The room designated for nutritional counseling should be equipped with educational material such as pertinent literature, posters, flannel boards, food packages, food models, and measuring utensils to enhance the learning experience.
- Explain to patient you will be making notes of what is being discussed so that you will not forget important information.
- Resist the temptation to create an ideal diet prescription and solve all nutritional problems for the patient. Help patients to adapt and develop a less than perfect menu plan that is more likely to be followed routinely.
- When appropriate, request that a family member or friend participate with the patient in the counseling session, especially an individual who is responsible for the cooking and food shopping. Assistance is also warranted when a physical or mental impairment interferes with the patient's understanding.

Evaluation
The patient is an active participant, making a change toward food choices and behaviors agreed to in the nutritional counseling session; at the follow-up visit or next recall appointment, there is successful achievement of the first set of goals and advancement to implement other, more difficult suggestions; many questions are asked and comments are made that verify interest and understanding.

Nutritional Directions

Establishing good eating habits is a wise investment toward lifelong positive health and dental status. Prevention, alleviation, or postponing the onset of a disease is possible with good nutrition.

CASE APPLICATION FOR THE DENTAL HYGIENIST

As 70-year-old Mr. B walks into the operatory, it is noted he continues to lose weight and has less energy than at his previous 4-month recare visit. His health history reveals no significant findings except one daily medication to control hypertension. The social history reveals his wife has been deceased for 2 years, and his limited income makes it difficult to purchase the foods he needs. He complains of a loose-fitting maxillary denture and xerostomia.

Nutritional Assessment
- Medical, dental, and social history
- Nutritional assessment questionnaire (see Evolve)
- Extraoral and intraoral examination
- Periodontal evaluation
- Anthropometric evaluation for weight changes
- 3-day food record

Nutritional Diagnosis
Social and oral factors are affecting the desire and ability to obtain adequate nutrients.

Nutritional Goals
The patient will seek support from suggested referrals and begin to improve his caloric intake and variety of food.

Nutritional Implementation
Intervention: Examine the oral cavity for any deviation from normal and the fit of the maxillary denture.
Rationale: Ill-fitting dentures can be a result of weight loss, which can be responsible for creating sore spots. The presence of oral infections can decrease the ability and desire to eat, ultimately affecting nutrition status. Identifying such areas can allow for treatment and education on prevention.
Intervention: Provide instruction for completing a 3-day food record.
Rationale: This component completes the assessment process. Determining typical eating habits and patterns and the variety of foods gives direction to the nutritional counseling. Look for the predominant use of soft foods, highly salted foods, convenience foods, and fermentable carbohydrates; variety; low kilocalories; and number of meals daily.
Intervention: Educate Mr. B regarding basic information about nutrient needs and the relationship between diet and health status.
Rationale: Depression over a spouse's death and dining alone are two factors decreasing an older individual's desire to eat. Referral to a community-based senior citizen program may

CASE APPLICATION FOR THE DENTAL HYGIENIST—cont'd

provide support and companionship needed to improve his desire to eat.

Intervention: Explain to Mr. B frequent consumption of acid-containing beverages (e.g., sodas, citrus juices) can put him at high risk for caries. Due to his xerostomia, the lack of protection by saliva may even allow sugar alcohols to create a cariogenic environment, especially if his remaining teeth have gingival recession.

Rationale: Patients with xerostomia have limited cleansing and buffering capabilities because of reduced quantities of saliva. Even foods that are generally noncariogenic when saliva flow is adequate can be detrimental when saliva flow is diminished. Suggest rinsing with water to dilute the effects of citrus juices or to remove carbohydrates (e.g., rinsing away remnants of crackers or pretzels).

Intervention: Provide positive feedback on any changes, even small ones, that Mr. B makes.

Rationale: An older adult may be more resistant to modifications in well-established habits. Small goals are more realistic. Allow him to make the goals based on the information presented to him. Recognize any change is a sign of effort. A follow-up on his progress is important to establish new goals or modify goals as necessary.

Evaluation

At a return visit, Mr. B's new 24-hour recall reveals adequate caloric intake and improvement in variety of food choices. He has slowly begun to gain back some of his weight. He has sought the support of various local senior citizen groups. His denture has been repaired, and he presents a healthy oral cavity.

STUDENT READINESS

1. Examine your own health, social, and dental histories, and identify health-related factors a dental hygienist would find useful in developing a dietary plan. Interview another student to obtain health, social, and dental histories. What questions were effective in clarifying or obtaining additional pertinent information?

2. Select and explain at least two reasons why a dental hygienist should conduct a nutritional assessment for patients.

3. Describe the components needed for an assessment of a patient's nutritional status, and explain the rationale of each.

4. The following 24-hour recall was obtained by a dental hygienist. What questions need to be asked to get a more accurate estimate of the patient's intake?

    Breakfast: Bagel and cream cheese, coffee

    Lunch: Hamburger, French fries, soda

    Snack: Candy bar

    Dinner: Roast beef, potatoes, salad, corn

5. Explain why the following question asked during a nutritional counseling session is undesirable: "Do you realize omitting fruits and vegetables from your day could lead to a deficiency in vitamins A and C?" Reword the question to enhance effectiveness.

6. Establish a nutrition goal you can realistically apply this week, and have a partner evaluate. Review progress with the partner at the conclusion of the week. Would you do anything differently to increase the likelihood of accomplishing the goal?

CASE STUDY

The dental hygienist has reviewed Jim S's medical, dental, and social histories at the prophylaxis appointment, indicating no significant changes. Jim presents with observable weight gain since the last 6-month recall appointment and three new areas of dental caries. He has no idea why the areas of decay occurred. A 3-day food diary is explained, and a nutritional counseling session is established following his restorative treatment. At the restorative appointment, the patient forgot to bring his completed food diary. The dental hygienist attributed this to a lack of interest. A 24-hour recall is obtained, and the session is conducted in the operatory.

1. Prioritize the diet and dental information that Jim S needs.

2. Explain why and how a nutritional counseling session could be beneficial to Jim.

3. What questions should be asked before and during the counseling session to gain additional information?

4. State several reasons why the counseling session may not be effective to motivate behavior change. How could these situations be modified to enhance motivation?

References

1. American Dental Hygienists' Association: Standards for Clinical Dental Hygiene Practice. Chicago: ADHA, 2008. Available at http://www.adha.org/downloads/adha_standards08.pdf.

2. Touger-Decker R, Mobley CC: Position of the American Dietetic Association: Oral health and nutrition. J Am Diet Assoc 2007; 107:1418-1428.

3. Snetselaar LG: Intervention: Counseling for change. In Mahan LK, Escott-Stump S (eds): Krause's Food, Nutrition and Diet Therapy, 12th ed. Philadelphia: Saunders, 2008, p 489.

Appendix A

Glossary

acceptable macronutrient distribution ranges (AMDRs) a part of the latest dietary reference intakes (DRIs); established for the macronutrients (fat, carbohydrate, protein, and two polyunsaturated fats) to ensure sufficient intakes of essential nutrients while reducing risk of chronic diseases.

accessory organs organs, such as salivary glands, liver, gallbladder, and pancreas, that provide secretions essential for the digestive process.

achlorhydria absence of hydrochloric acid in the stomach, a condition that occurs primarily in older patients.

ad libitum as desired, at will

adenosine triphosphate (ATP) main form of energy used by the cells.

adequate intake (AI) average amount of a nutrient that seems to maintain a defined nutritional state; derived from mean nutrient intakes by groups of healthy people.

adipose tissue body fat.

aldosterone hormone secreted by the adrenal cortex to signal the kidney to retain sodium and water, and excrete potassium and hydrogen ions; ultimately causes edema and high blood pressure.

alimentary canal all the body parts through which food passes, extending from the mouth to the anus.

alopecia hair loss.

α-linolenic acid organic compound found in many vegetable oils.

alveolar process crest of the maxilla and mandible.

ameloblasts tall columnar epithelial cells in the inner layer of the enamel.

amenorrhea absence of menses.

amino acids basic building blocks for proteins.

amorphous having no definite form.

anabolism use of absorbed nutrients to build or synthesize more complex compounds.

anencephaly absence of a major portion of the brain and skull.

aneurysm bulge or ballooning in the wall of an artery. When an aneurysm becomes too large, it may burst and cause dangerous bleeding or death.

anion ion carrying a negative charge as a result of an accumulation of electrons.

anorexia lack or loss of appetite.

anosmia loss of smell.

anthropometric measurements of physical characteristics such as height, weight, and change in weight.

anticariogenic reducing the risk of caries by preventing plaque from recognizing a cariogenic food.

anticoagulant drug or substance that delays or prevents the clotting of blood (e.g., heparin).

antidiuretic hormone (ADH) hormone released by the pituitary gland to act on the kidneys to control urine output.

antigenic having the properties of an antigen (substance that comes in contact with target cells, inducing an immune response or sensitivity).

antioxidant synthetic or natural substance that prevents or delays the damaging effects of a reactive substance seeking an electron.

apatite calcium phosphate complex that forms crystalline salts within the matrix of bone and teeth.

appetite external factors that influence people to seek and eat food even when not hungry.

ataxia gait disorder characterized by uncoordinated muscle movements.

atherosclerosis degenerative disease caused by progressive accumulation of fatty materials on smooth inner walls of arteries of the heart, narrowing the arteries and disrupting blood flow.

atrophic gastritis chronic stomach inflammation with atrophy of the mucous membrane and glands, resulting in diminished hydrochloric acid production.

atrophic gingivitis condition characterized by redness, pain, and wasting of the gingival tissue owing to local and systemic causes.

avidin biotin-binding glycoprotein substance present in raw egg white.

baby bottle tooth decay (BBTD) see *early childhood caries*.

bariatric surgery surgical procedure that promotes weight loss by restricting food intake or interrupting the digestive process to prevent absorption of some kilocalories and nutrients.

basal energy expenditure person's total caloric requirement.

basal metabolic rate energy required for involuntary physiological functions to maintain life, including respiration, circulation, and maintenance of muscle tone and body temperature.

beriberi dietary deficiency of thiamin characterized by neuropathy, diarrhea, weight loss, fatigue, and poor memory.

bile emulsifier that helps in the digestion of fats.

binges periods of overeating.

bioavailability amount of nutrient available to the body based on its absorption.

biological value measure of protein quality, with a higher score for proteins of higher quality.

body mass index (BMI) mathematical calculation using a person's height and weight to determine weight status and to predict health risks that increase at higher levels of overweight and obesity (see p. iv).

bolus mass of food that is swallowed and passed into the stomach.

bradykinesia slowness of movement.

bruxism clenching and grinding of teeth that erodes and diminishes the height of dental crowns.

calcitonin polypeptide hormone regulating the balance of calcium and phosphate in the blood by direct action on bone and kidney. It is secreted by the parathyroid, thyroid, and thymus tissue.

calorie-dense foods term used for food usually high in fats (or fat and sugar) and low in vitamins and minerals and other nutrients. A characteristic of calorie-dense foods is less volume of food is needed to furnish energy requirements.

calorimeter device used to measure kilocalories.

cancellous bone internal bone that appears spongy with little hollows that contain bone marrow.

Candida invasive fungal microorganism.

cariogenic fermentable carbohydrate that causes a reduction of salivary pH to less than 5.5.

cariostatic caries-inhibiting; not metabolized by microorganisms in plaque biofilm.

casein principal protein in cow's milk and chief constituent of cheese.

catabolism breakdown of complex substances into simpler substances.

cation ion carrying a positive charge as a result of a deficiency of electrons.

cheilosis unilateral or bilateral presence of cracks and dry scaling around the vermilion border of lips and corners of the mouth; the skin is scaly with red fissures.

chemotherapy treatment of disease by chemical agents.

cholesterol waxy lipid found in all body cells; found only in animal products.

circumvallate lingual papillae 8 to 10 large and distinctive structures forming a V shape on the posterior end of the anterior two-thirds of the dorsum of the tongue.

cleft lip/palate split where parts of the upper lip or palate fail to grow together.

clinical attachment loss (CAL) loss of periodontal attachment.

coenzyme molecule needed to activate an enzyme.

cofactor element similar to an enzyme in that it is necessary to activate reactions, but the molecule required is a mineral or electrolyte.

collagen basic protein substance of connective tissue helping support body structures such as skin, bones, teeth, and tendons.

complementary foods foods that do not contain adequate amounts of all the essential amino acids, but when eaten together make up for insufficient amounts of specific essential amino acids, so that adequate amounts of all the essential amino acids are available.

complex carbohydrates see *polysaccharides*.

compound lipids triglycerides with at least one of the fatty acids replaced with carbohydrate, phosphate, or nitrogenous compounds.

compressional forces actions in which the pressure attempts to diminish a structure's volume, which usually increases density.

conditionally essential amino acids amino acids that are essential in the diet during certain stages of development or in certain nutritional or disease states.

conjugated linoleic acid (CLA) family of at least 13 isomers (or forms) of linoleic acid, found especially in meats and dairy products.

cortical bone compact external part of the skeleton.

crepitus crackling or grating sound made by a joint, such as the temporomandibular joint.

cretinism stunting of growth often characterized by mental deficits and deaf mutism; a result of inadequate iodine intake during pregnancy.

cruciferous vegetables belonging to the botanical family of plants that includes cabbage and mustard.

daily reference values (DRVs) desirable levels of nutrients considered important for health: total fat, saturated fatty acids, protein, cholesterol, carbohydrate, fiber, and sodium.

daily value (DV) term used on food labels indicating the percentage of the DV provided by a serving to show the amount of nutrients provided as a percentage of established standards. The DV is based on a 2000-kcal diet.

demineralization removal or loss of calcium, phosphate, and other minerals from tooth enamel, causing tooth enamel to dissolve.

dentin hypersensitivity extremely painful feeling of exposed dentin resulting from a stimulus, such as temperature or tactile.

dextrins intermediate products of the digestive enzymes on starch molecules; they are long glucose chains split into shorter ones.

diaphoresis excessive sweating.

diet history detailed dietary record; may include 24-hour recall; food frequency questionnaire; and other information such as weight history, previous diet changes, use of supplements, and food intolerances.

dietary acculturation dietary changes that occur as a result of adapting to food resources of a new location.

dietary fiber several different types of nondigestible carbohydrates and lignin intrinsic and intact in plants.

dietary reference intakes (DRIs) set of nutrient-based reference values that identify amounts of required nutrients for various stages of life.

dipeptide two amino acids together.

diplopia perception of two images of a single object; also known as *double vision*.

disaccharides double sugars (two simple sugars joined together) containing 12 carbon atoms.

docosahexaenoic acid (DHA) omega-3 fatty acid with 22 carbons and 6 double bonds synthesized by the body from linolenic acid; present in fish oils.

dysesthesia condition in which a burning sensation is produced by ordinary stimuli.

dysgeusia persistent, abnormal distortion of taste, including sweet, sour, bitter, salty, or metallic.

dysphagia difficulty in swallowing.

early childhood caries (ECC) early rampant tooth decay associated with inappropriate feeding practices.

edentulous without teeth or lacking some or all teeth.

eicosapentaenoic acid (EPA) omega-3 fatty acid with 20 carbon atoms and 5 double bonds synthesized by the body from linolenic acid; present in fish oils.

emulsification to break up fats into smaller particles by lowering the surface tension.

enamel hypoplasia developmental disturbance of the teeth characterized by defective formation of the enamel matrix.

energy ability or power to do work.

enrichment process of restoring nutrients removed from food during processing.

enteral feedings feeding that delivers liquid food through a tube. It is used for infants and children who have a functioning gastrointestinal tract, but are unable to ingest nutrients orally to meet their metabolic needs.

enteric general term for the intestines.

enzymes complex proteins enabling metabolic reactions to proceed at a faster rate without being exhausted themselves.

epilepsy transient disturbance of brain function that results in episodic impairment or loss of consciousness.

epiphyses growing points at ends of long bones.

erythema marginated redness of the mucous membranes caused by inflammation.

erythropoiesis formation of red blood cells.

esophagitis inflammation of the lower esophagus.

essential amino acids (EAAs) amino acids that must be supplied by the diet.

essential fatty acids (EFAs) fatty acids (linoleic acid and linolenic acid) that must be supplied by the diet.

essential hypertension elevated blood pressure of unknown cause.

estimated average requirement (EAR) amount of a nutrient estimated to meet the needs of half of the healthy individuals in a specific age and gender group.

estimated energy requirement (EER) dietary energy intake that is predicted to maintain energy balance in healthy normal-weight individuals of a defined age, gender, weight, height, and physical activity level consistent with good health.

extracellular fluid (ECF) fluid outside the cells.

fatty acids structural component of fats.

fermentable carbohydrate carbohydrates that can be metabolized by bacteria in plaque biofilm to decrease the pH to a level where demineralization occurs; this includes all sugars and cooked or processed starches.

fibroblasts collagen-forming cells.

fibrotic formation of fibrous tissue of the gingiva and other mucous membranes because of chronic inflammation. The tissue may clinically appear to be healthy, concealing the disease.

filiform papillae smooth threadlike structures, which are covered by a nonkeratinized epithelium, on the anterior two-thirds of the dorsum of the tongue.

flexitarian person who primarily follows a plant-based diet, but occasionally eats small amount of meat, poultry or fish; also known as a *semivegetarian.*

fluid volume deficit (FVD) relatively equal losses of sodium and water in relation to their gains.

fluid volume excess (FVE) relatively equal gains of water and sodium in relation to their losses.

fluorapatite fluoride-containing crystalline substance produced during bone and tooth development; resistant to acid.

fluorosis hypomineralization of enamel.

foliate papillae vertical ridges or grooves scattered along the lateral borders of the tongue.

follicular hyperkeratosis condition characterized by the appearance of cone-shaped, horny, hyperkeratinized, scaly eruptions resulting from blocked pores as a result of vitamin A deficiency.

food fad catch-all term covering all aspects of nutritional nonsense, characterized by exaggerated beliefs about the value of nutrition in health and disease.

food frequency questionnaire checklist of many foods used to determine how often specific foods are consumed.

food insecurity lack of access to enough food to fully meet basic needs at all times.

food jags refusing to eat anything except one food for several days.

food pattern customary way of eating, reflecting a person's ethnic or cultural, social, religious, geographical, economic, and psychological components and family lifestyle.

food quackery promotion of nutrition-related products or services having questionable safety or effectiveness, or both, for the claims made.

fortification process of adding nutrients not present in the natural product or to increase the amount above that in the original product.

full liquid diet nutrients provided in a liquid form when solid food is not tolerated. It can provide a transition between a clear liquid and soft diet.

functional fiber isolated, nondigestible carbohydrates that have beneficial physiological effects in humans.

functional foods foods that contain potentially healthful products, including any modified food or food ingredients providing a health benefit beyond the traditional nutrients it contains.

fungating producing fungus-like growth.

fungiform papillae red, knoblike structures on the tongue scattered throughout the filiform papillae.

gastroesophageal reflux disease (GERD) return of gastric contents into the esophagus, causing a severe burning sensation under the sternum.

gastrostomy establishment of a new opening into the stomach; performed to insert a tube to supply nutrition, foods, or medications directly into the stomach, bypassing the mouth and esophagus.

genome all of the DNA contained in an organism or cell, which includes the chromosomes in the nucleus and the DNA in the mitochondria.

ghrelin peptide hormone secreted in the gastrointestinal tract by exocrine cells.

gingivitis inflammation of the gingival tissue.

glossitis inflammation of the tongue.

glossodynia pain in the tongue.

glossopyrosis pain, burning, itching, and stinging of the tongue with no apparent lesions.

gluconeogenesis synthesis of glucose from noncarbohydrate sources.

gluten protein found mainly in wheat and to a lesser degree in rye, oat, and barley.

glycemic effect amount a carbohydrate increases the blood glucose level.

glycogen carbohydrate storage form of energy in humans.

glycogenesis process by which sugars, including fructose, galactose, sorbitol, and xylitol, are stored as glycogen.

goal achievable aim or target that would be meaningful in changing behaviors by setting a concrete standard for change.

goiter chronic enlargement of the thyroid gland occurring most frequently in areas with low iodine in the soil.

goitrogens naturally occurring substances in foods that interfere with the synthesis of thyroid hormone production; may cause goiter if consumed in large amounts.

gravida pregnant woman; gravida followed by a Roman numeral or preceded by a Latin prefix (e.g., "primi-," "secundi-") designates the number of pregnancies for the woman (e.g., gravida I or primigravida is a woman in her first pregnancy).

gustatory sense of taste.

health claim claim that describes a health relationship between a food, food component, or dietary supplement ingredient and reduced risk of a disease or a health-related condition.

hematopoiesis formation of red blood cells.

heme iron iron provided from animal sources.

hemosiderin storage form of iron in the liver when the amount of iron in the body exceeds storage capacity.

herpetic related to the herpesvirus; ulceration on the tongue or esophagus or both.

hiatal hernia partial protrusion (herniation) of the stomach through the esophageal opening into the chest cavity.

high-energy phosphate compounds instant source of energy for cells; also called *ATP*.

high-quality proteins foods that contain adequate amounts of the nine essential amino acids to maintain nitrogen balance and permit growth.

homeostatic mechanisms body's ability to correct nutritional imbalances, for instance, decreased nutrient intake accompanied by an increase in absorption or efficiency or use.

hormone compound produced and secreted by cells of the body, transported in the blood to another site where it has a specific regulatory function.

hormone replacement therapy (HRT) therapy using medication that contains one or more female hormones, usually estrogen and progestin.

hunger physiological drive to eat.

hydrogenation process in which polyunsaturated vegetable oil is converted to a solid by a commercial process whereby hydrogen is added to the oil; this process increases the proportion of saturated fatty acids, alters the shape of the fatty acid, and creates *trans* fatty acids.

hydrolysis splitting of a large molecule into smaller ones that are water soluble and can be used by cells; the reaction requires water.

hydroxyapatite inorganic component of bones and teeth.

hypercalcemia excessive levels of calcium in the blood.

hypercarotenemia excessive levels of carotene in the blood, characterized by yellowing of the palms of the hands and soles of the feet.

hypergeusia heightened taste acuity.

hyperglycemia elevated blood sugar.

hyperkalemia elevated potassium concentrations in the blood.

hyperlipidemia elevated concentrations of any or all of the serum lipids, especially triglycerides or cholesterol or both.

hypernatremia elevated serum sodium level.

hypertension persistent high arterial blood pressure. Hypertension is considered a risk factor for heart disease, kidney disease, and stroke.

hypervitaminosis A condition resulting from the ingestion of excessive amounts of vitamin A.

hypocalcemia deficient levels of calcium in the blood.

hypodipsia diminished thirst.

hypogeusia loss of taste.

hypoglycemia low blood sugar (less than 70 mg/dL).

hypokalemia low potassium concentrations in the blood.

hyponatremia lowered sodium in the blood.

hypotonic solution having less osmotic pressure than another solution.

iatrogenic adverse condition resulting from treatment (medications, irradiation, surgery) by a healthcare provider.

immune response body's ability to protect itself from the destructive bacteria and infection that are present in the body.

immunocompromised immune response that has been weakened by a disease or pharmacological agent.

immunoglobulins antibodies, the body's main protection from disease.

incontinence inability to control urinary excretion.

indirect calorimetry method to estimate metabolic energy by measuring oxygen consumption, carbon dioxide production, respiratory quotient, and resting energy expenditure as a means to assess and manage a patient's nutrition.

innate inborn.

insulin hormone that lowers blood sugar levels.

interstitial spaces between cells within a tissue or organ.

interstitial fluid fluid located between cells and in body cavities, including the joints, pleura, and gastrointestinal tract.

intracellular fluid (ICF) liquid within cells.

intrinsic factor glycoprotein synthesized by the parietal cells in the stomach; required for vitamin B_{12} absorption.

irradiated foods process of treating food with controlled amounts of ionized radiation for a prescribed period to kill the spoilage-causing and disease-causing bacteria and molds in food.

ischemia inadequate blood flow and lack of oxygen because of constriction or obstruction of arteries.

Kaposi's sarcoma malignant tumor of blood vessel origin that occurs on the skin and oral mucosa.

Kayser-Fleischer ring greenish yellow pigmented ring encircling the cornea; consists of copper deposits in the Descemet membrane.

Keshan disease cardiomyopathy (disease of the heart muscle) resulting from the deficiency of selenium found in women and children, primarily in Keshan, China.

ketoacidosis accumulation of ketone bodies in the blood.

ketones normal products of lipid metabolism in the liver; can be used by muscles for energy if adequate amounts of glucose are available.

ketonuria ketones excreted in the urine as a result of high levels in the blood.

ketosis accumulation of ketone bodies in the blood.

kilocalorie (calorie, Calorie) amount of heat needed to increase the temperature of 1 kg of water 1° C; measurement of the potential energy value of foods and energy within the body, equivalent to 1000 calories; more frequently referred to as calorie.

kwashiorkor nutritional deficiency disease that occurs when adequate kilocalories are available, but protein is inadequate.

lactovegetarian person who consumes only products from plants and dairy products.

large intestine cecum, colon, and rectum.

leukemia generalized malignant disease characterized by distorted proliferation and development of white blood cells.

leukoplakia white, yellow, or gray thickened patches on the mucous membranes of the oral mucosa that cannot be wiped away; appearance may be wrinkled, fissured, nodular, or smooth.

linoleic acid essential fatty acid with 18 carbon atoms and 2 double bonds; also called *omega-6 fatty acid.*

lipids compounds that contain carbon, hydrogen, and oxygen with less oxygen in proportion to hydrogen and carbon than carbohydrates; provide 9 kcal/g.

lipogenesis process of converting glucose to fats.

lipolysis fat breakdown.

lipoprotein compound lipids composed of triglycerides, phospholipids, and cholesterol combined with protein; produced by the body.

long-chain fatty acids fatty acid that contains 12 or more carbon atoms.

longitudinal fissure slits or wrinkles that extend lengthwise on the tongue.

low birth weight (LBW) weighing less than 5½ lb (2500 g) at birth.

lower esophageal sphincter (LES) group of very strong circular muscle fibers located just above the stomach.

low-quality proteins plant proteins that lack one or more essential amino acids or may lack a proper balance of amino acids; also called *incomplete proteins.*

lysosomes intracellular bodies containing hydrolytic enzymes that promote the breakdown of materials taken into the cells.

macrodontia larger than normal teeth.

macronutrients nutrients needed in large amounts by the body to provide energy—carbohydrates, protein, and fats.

macules flat lesion of abnormal color.

manganese madness severe psychotic and neuromuscular symptoms that resemble the symptoms of parkinsonism.

marasmus nutritional deficiency caused by inadequate protein and kilocaloric intake.

masticatory efficiency how well the patient prepares the food for swallowing.

mechanical soft diet regular diet altered in consistency during periods when chewing is difficult. It can provide a transition between a liquid diet and a regular diet.

medium-chain fatty acids fatty acid that has 6 to 10 carbon atoms.

megaloblastic anemia condition in which the red blood cells are extra large in size but fewer in number.

melting point temperature at which a product becomes a liquid.

menopausal gingivostomatitis changes in the oral mucosa that result in a dry, shiny gingiva that bleeds easily. The color can range from an abnormally pale pink to a deep red. This condition is often alleviated with the use of estrogen hormone replacement.

menopause cessation of the menses, which occurs when production of the hormones estrogen and progesterone ceases.

meta-analysis systematic analysis that is applied to separate experiments on a related topic involving pooling the data to provide larger study samples that generate information about statistically significant results from the cumulative research on a topic.

metabolism continuous processes whereby living organisms and cells convert nutrients into energy, body structure, and waste.

microflora microorganisms living in the large intestine.

micronutrients nutrients needed by the body in small amounts (e.g., vitamins and minerals).

microvilli minute cylindrical processes located on the surface of the intestinal cells, greatly increasing their absorptive surface area.

mineralization deposition of inorganic minerals on an organic matrix.

modified barium swallow assessment to measure the physiological and anatomical abnormalities associated with swallowing.

monosaccharides simple sugars containing two to six carbon atoms.

monounsaturated fatty acid (MUFA) fatty acid containing one double bond; found in olive, peanut, and canola oil.

mucositis ulcerations and sores of the mucous membrane in the mouth or throat, usually caused by chemotherapy or radiation.

myelin lipid substance that insulates nerve fibers and affects transmission of nerve impulses.

myxedema severe hypothyroidism.

nanotechnoiogy the ability to measure and detect molecular structures nonometes or smaller, allowing determination of minute amounts of substances in the food supply.

necrosis degeneration and death of cells.

necrotizing ulcerative gingivitis (NUG) oral condition caused by nutritional deficiencies, stress, infection, and depressed immune responses; characterized by erythema and necrosis of the interdental papillae.

neural tube defects (NTD) birth defects of the skull, brain, and spinal cord.

neurotransmitters substance released at the end of a nerve cell when a nerve impulse arrives there, which diffuses across to the next cell to excite or inhibit it.

neutropenia diminished number of neutrophils in the blood; also called *leukopenia* or *agranulocytosis.*

night blindness inability to adapt to bright lights when the eyes are adapted to darkness.

nitrogen balance balance of reactions in which protein substances are broken down and rebuilt.

nocturia excessive urination at night.

noma severe gangrenous process usually manifesting as a small ulcer on the gingiva that becomes necrotic and spreads to the lips, cheek, and tissues covering the jaw; caused by inadequate amounts of protein.

nonessential amino acids (NEAAs) amino acids essential to the body, but are not required in the diet.

nonheme iron iron provided primarily from plant sources and supplements; less efficiently absorbed than heme iron.

non-nutritive sucking sucking on objects that do not provide nutrition (i.e., pacifier, fingers).

nutrient content claim characterizes the level of a nutrient in a food; terms used are "free," "low," "high," and "reduced."

nutrient-dense containing a high percentage of nutrients in relation to the number of kilocalories provided.

nutrient density amount of a specific nutrient of a food relative to the number of kilocalories it provides.

nutrients biochemical substances that can be supplied in adequate amounts only from an outside source, normally from food.

nutrition study of foods and nutrients and their effect on health, growth, and development of the individual.

nutritional deficiency inadequate amounts of a nutrient available to sustain biochemical functions.

nutritional insult deficiency or excessive amounts of specific nutrients.

nutritionist person who has at least a 4-year degree in foods and nutrition and usually works in a public health setting assisting people in the community with diet-related health issues. In most states, this title is legally defined, and nutritionists are licensed or certified.

nystagmus involuntary rapid movement of the eyeball.

obesity excess weight for height, with a BMI above 30.0.

odontoblasts tissue cells that deposit dentin and form the outer surface of dental pulp adjacent to the dentin.

odynophagia pain associated with swallowing.

oils fats that are liquid at room temperature.

olfactory nerves receptors for smell.

omega-3 fatty acid unsaturated fatty acid with its first double bond at the third carbon atom from the methyl end; includes eicosapentaenoic acid and docosahexaenoic acid.

omega-6 fatty acid unsaturated fatty acid with its first double bond at the sixth carbon atom from the methyl end; includes linoleic acid and linolenic acid.

organic foods that meet U.S. Department of Agriculture (USDA) standards and do not contain parts of other slaughtered animals, have not been given growth hormones or antibiotics, and have been allowed outdoors; are not genetically engineered or irradiated; are grown on land that has not been fertilized with sewage sludge or chemical fertilizers or treated with pesticides.

osmoreceptors neurons in the hypothalamus that are stimulated by increased osmolality, enhancing the release of ADH.

osmosis movement of water from an area of lower solute concentration to a higher solute concentration. When solute concentrations in the body are different, water moves across the membrane.

osteoblasts assists in production of collagen; helps in building and reformation of new bone.

osteocalcin vitamin K–dependent, bone-specific protein that is released into blood from the resorbed bone matrix and from the osteoblasts that make it.

osteoclasts resorbed bone in microscopic cavities.

osteodystrophy abnormal bone development, similar to osteomalacia.

osteoid young bone that has not undergone calcification.

osteomalacia softening of bones.

osteonecrosis term used to describe a condition in which the bone dies or undergoes necrosis.

osteoporosis age-related disorder characterized by decreased bone mass, causing bones to be more susceptible to fracture.

osteosclerosis increased bone formation resulting in reduced marrow spaces and increased radiopacity.

overweight excess accumulation of body fat, or a BMI between 25.0 and 29.9.

ovolactovegetarian vegetarian diet supplemented with milk, eggs, and cheese.

ovovegetarian type of vegetarian whose diet consists of foods from plants with the addition of eggs (no meat, poultry, fish, or dairy products).

oxidation process of hydrolyzing triglycerides into two-carbon entities to enter the Krebs cycle for energy production.

pancreatic enzymes enzymes that hydrolyze carbohydrates, protein, and fats.

parasympathetic division of autonomic nervous system.

Parkinson's disease progressive neurological condition characterized by involuntary muscle tremors, muscular weakness, rigidity, stooped posture, and peculiar gait.

parotitis inflammation of the parotid gland.

pathogenic harmful.

pedometer instrument carried by a walker, which measures approximately the distance covered in walking by recording the number of steps.

pellagra deficiency resulting form inadequate intake of niacin, which results in the four D's (diarrhea, dermatitis, dementia, and death).

perimenopause time leading up to menopause, in which the ovaries begin to shut down, making less of certain hormones, such as estrogen and progesterone.

periodontal disease group of infections and lesions affecting tissues that form the attachment apparatus of a tooth or teeth.

periodontitis inflammatory process involving interproximal and marginal areas of two or more adjacent teeth.

periodontium hard and soft tissues that surround and support the teeth: gingiva, alveolar mucosa, cementum, periodontal ligament, and alveolar bone.

peripheral in the extremities, such as the legs and feet.

peristalsis involuntary rhythmic waves of contraction traveling the length of the alimentary tract.

pernicious anemia megaloblastic anemia in which there is a decrease in red blood cells that occurs when the body cannot properly absorb vitamin B_{12} in the gastrointestinal tract.

petechia (*pl.* petechiae) small, pinpoint, round red spot caused by submucous hemorrhage.

phantom taste dysgeusia without identifiable taste stimuli.

phenylketonuria genetic disorder characterized by inability to metabolize the amino acid phenylalanine.

phospholipid fat-related substances that contain phosphorus, fatty acids, and a nitrogen-containing base; constituent of every cell.

photosynthesis compounding or building up of chemical substances under the influence of light; green plants use chlorophyll and energy from sunlight to produce carbohydrates from water and carbon dioxide and to liberate oxygen.

phytochemical plant chemical that can stimulate estrogen function.

pica abnormal consumption of specific food and nonfood substances, such as dirt, clay, starch, or ice; occurs more frequently during pregnancy.

plant sterols essential components of plant membranes that resemble the chemical structure of cholesterol and carry out similar cellular functions in plants. They are naturally present in small quantities in fruits, vegetables, nuts, seeds, legumes, and oils.

plaque biofilm well-organized community of bacteria that is embedded in a slime layer and adheres tenaciously to tooth surfaces, restorations, and prosthetic appliances.

plethora red appearance resulting from an excess of blood.

pocketed foods foods retained in the mouth, especially in the vestibule.

polycythemia sustained increase in the number of red blood cells, which may result in iron-deficiency anemia.

polypeptide several amino acids joined together.

polysaccharides (complex carbohydrates) sugars containing more than 12 carbon atoms.

polyunsaturated fatty acid (PUFA) fatty acid containing two or more double bonds.

postabsorptive state time when digestive and absorptive processes are minimal, not affecting the basal metabolic rate.

ppb parts per billion.

prebiotics nondigestible food ingredients having beneficial effects on the host by stimulating growth or activity of probiotics in the colon.

precursor substance from which another biologically active substance is formed.

preeclampsia development of hypertension as a result of pregnancy or the influence of recent pregnancy. It usually occurs after the 20th week of pregnancy.

premature born before the state of maturity, occurring with a gestational age (length of pregnancy) of less than 37 weeks.

primigravida woman in her first pregnancy.

probiotics products containing live bacteria that aid in restoring and maintaining an intestinal balance of healthful bacteria.

prognathism overgrowth of the mandible.

prostaglandins hormone-like compounds derived from unsaturated fatty acids.

protein digestibility corrected amino acid score (PDCAAs) official assay for evaluating protein quality in humans.

protein-energy malnutrition (PEM) nutritional deficiency condition caused by consistently consuming inadequate amounts of energy and protein.

protein-sparing energy source so that protein can be used for building and repairing (i.e., fats and carbohydrates).

proteolytic enzymes enzymes that function to hydrolyze proteins.

prothrombin first stage in forming an insoluble clot; a deficiency results in impaired blood coagulation.

purging use of laxatives, enemas, emetics, diuretics, or exercise to negate effects of overindulgence.

purpura condition characterized by hemorrhaging into tissues, under the skin, and through the mucous membranes; the three types are petechiae, ecchymoses, and hematomas.

purulent exudates consisting of or containing pus; generally the result of inflammation.

pyogenic producing pus.

radical group of atoms that forms a fundamental constituent of a molecule.

R-binder protein produced by the salivary glands necessary for absorption of vitamin B_{12}.

recommended dietary allowances (RDAs) specific amounts of essential nutrients that adequately meet the known nutrient needs of 97% to 98% of healthy Americans.

reference daily intakes (RDIs) term used on food labels, based on the former RDAs. There are five sets of RDIs, which are designed for special foods for infants, children younger than 4 years, pregnant women, lactating women, and children older than 4 years and adults.

registered dietitian person who has completed a bachelor's degree in foods and nutrition with training in normal and clinical nutrition, food science, and food service management, and advanced training in medical nutrition therapy.

remineralization restoration or return of calcium, phosphates, and other minerals into areas that have been damaged, as by incipient caries, abrasion, or erosion.

remodeling resorption and reformation of bone.

renal failure inability of the kidneys to maintain normal function of excreting toxic waste materials.

renal osteodystrophy changes in bones associated with renal failure.

renin enzyme synthesized in the kidney and released in response to low blood pressure.

residue total amount of fecal solids, including undigested or unabsorbed food, and metabolic (bile pigments) and bacterial products.

resistant starch starch that resists digestive enzyme action and reaches the colon; a starch that is encased in a nondigestible plant seed coat or modified by cooking or processing can be resistant.

retinoic acid form of vitamin A that can be produced by the body and can be made in the laboratory. It is used in combination with other drugs to treat leukemia and to treat acne.

rhodopsin light-sensitive pigment that allows the eye to adjust to changes in light.

rickets condition resulting from vitamin D deficiency, especially in infancy and childhood, resulting in disturbance of normal bone formation.

sarcopenia progressive loss of muscle mass, strength, and function, owing to the aging process.

satiety feeling of fullness.

saturated fatty acid fatty acid that does not contain any double bonds.

scorbutic similar to scurvy.

sealants clear or shaded plastic material that is applied to the occlusal surfaces of permanent teeth.

secretory immunoglobulin antibody present in oral, nasal, intestinal, and other mucosal secretions; provides the first line of defense in the oral cavity.

severe early childhood caries (SECC) see early childhood caries (ECC).

severe sensory neuropathy impairment of the ability to sense touch, vibration, temperature, and pinprick.

short-chain fatty acid fatty acid that contains fewer than six carbon atoms.

signs objective evidence of disease that is perceptible to the clinician.

small intestine duodenum, jejunum, and ileum.

solutes dissolved substances in fluid.

solvent fluid in which substances are dissolved.

sphincter muscles any of the ringlike muscles encircling an opening that is able to contract to close the opening, such as the sphincter pylori between the stomach and the small intestine.

stable nutrients nutrients of which more than 85% is retained during processing and storage.

stannous containing tin.

stomatitis inflammation of the oral mucosa.

Streptococcus mutans bacteria found in dental plaque biofilm.

structural lipids fats that are a component of cell membranes, tooth enamel, and dentin (i.e., phospholipids).

structural polysaccharides see *dietary fiber*.

sugar alcohols formed from or converted to sugar; also called *polyols*.

suppuration discharge or formation of pus.

sympathetic exhibiting a mutual relationship between two organ systems or parts of the body.

symptoms subjective evidence of abnormality as perceived by the client.

synbiotic mixing of probiotics (microorganisms that are similar to beneficial bacteria found in the gut) and prebiotics (nondigestible food ingredients that stimulate growth or activity of beneficial bacteria in the gut).

synergistic effect combined sweeteners yield a sweeter taste than that provided by each sweetener alone.

syrup of ipecac cardiotoxic drug used to induce vomiting after accidental ingestion of a chemical or poison.

systemic condition disease or disorder that affects the whole body.

taste buds receptors for the sense of taste.

temporomandibular disorder (TMD) group of symptoms that cause pain and dysfunction in the head, face, and temporomandibular region.

tensional forces actions in which the pressure stretches or strains the structure.

tetany neuromuscular disorder of uncontrollable muscular cramps and tremors.

thermic effect increase in metabolism that occurs during digestion, absorption, and metabolism of energy-yielding nutrients.

thermogenesis process of heat production in warm-blooded organisms. Thermogenesis occurs when the metabolic rate increases above normal, and is influenced by many factors, including digestion of food and activity.

thiaminase active enzyme found naturally in foods (e.g., raw fish) that inactivates thiamin.

thromboembolism plug or clot in a blood vessel formed by coagulation of blood.

thrombus blood clot.

tinnitus noise in the ears, which sometimes may be heard by others.

tocopherols name given to vitamin E and compounds chemically related to it.

tocotrienols component of vitamin E.

tolerable upper intake level (UL) maximum daily level of nutrient intake that probably would not cause adverse health effects or toxic effects for most individuals in the general population.

total fiber sum of dietary fiber and added fiber.

total parenteral nutrition (TPN) nutrition provided to a patient who cannot use the digestive tract. It is a special liquid food mixture administered into the blood with a needle through a vein.

trabecular bone spongy internal bone.

trans **fatty acid** unsaturated fatty acid that is usually monounsaturated; may be formed during hydrogenation, in which the hydrogen ions rotate so that the hydrogens stick out on opposite sides of the bond.

transferrin serum protein that transports iron in the blood.

triglycerides major form of lipid in the body and in food that is composed of three fatty acids bonded to glycerol, an alcohol.

24-hour recall a method of assessing everything a person has consumed (foods, supplements, and beverages) in a 24-hour period; this may or may not reflect a typical day.

unsaturated fatty acid of or related to an organic compound, especially fatty acids, containing one or more double or triple bonds between carbons.

upper level (UL) see *tolerable upper intake level*.

uremic condition in which too much urea and other nitrous waste is present in the blood.

valves/sphincter muscles circular muscles in the gastrointestinal tract that regulate the flow of bolus between different segments.

varicose veins unnaturally and permanently distended veins.

vegan person who eats only plant foods.

viscous fiber water-soluble fibers, including pectins, gums, psyllium, mucilages, and algal polysaccharides, which are physiologically important for their gel-forming ability.

vitamins general term for numerous related organic, noncaloric substances present in foods in small amounts.

xeroderma dry, rough, scaly skin.

xerophthalmia abnormally dry and thickened surface of the conjunctiva and cornea of the eye.

xerostomia dryness of the mouth resulting from inadequate salivary secretion.

xylitol sugar alcohol used as a sugar substitute. It is considered a nutritive sweetener because it provides four calories per gram, similar to sugar.

Growth Charts

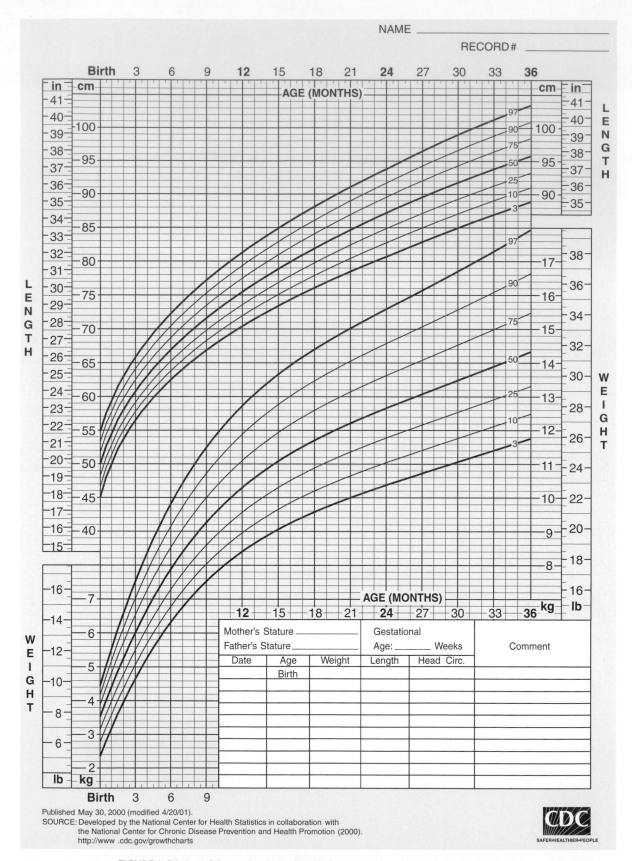

Published May 30, 2000 (modified 4/20/01).
SOURCE: Developed by the National Center for Health Statistics in collaboration with
the National Center for Chronic Disease Prevention and Health Promotion (2000).
http://www.cdc.gov/growthcharts

FIGURE 1 Birth to 36 months: boys length-for-age and weight-for-age percentiles.

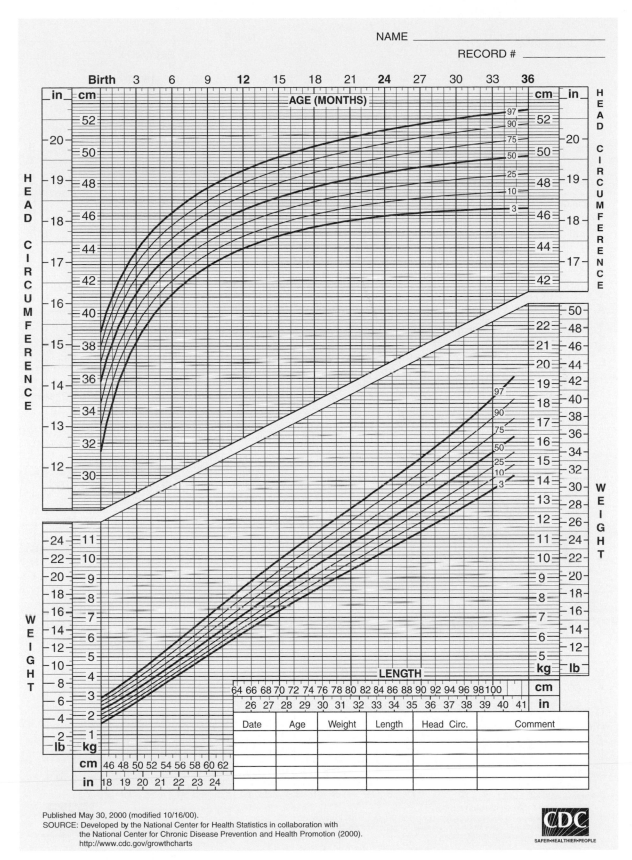

NAME _____

RECORD # _____

FIGURE 2 Birth to 36 months: boys head circumference-for-age and weight-for-length percentiles.

Published May 30, 2000 (modified 10/16/00).
SOURCE: Developed by the National Center for Health Statistics in collaboration with
the National Center for Chronic Disease Prevention and Health Promotion (2000).
http://www.cdc.gov/growthcharts

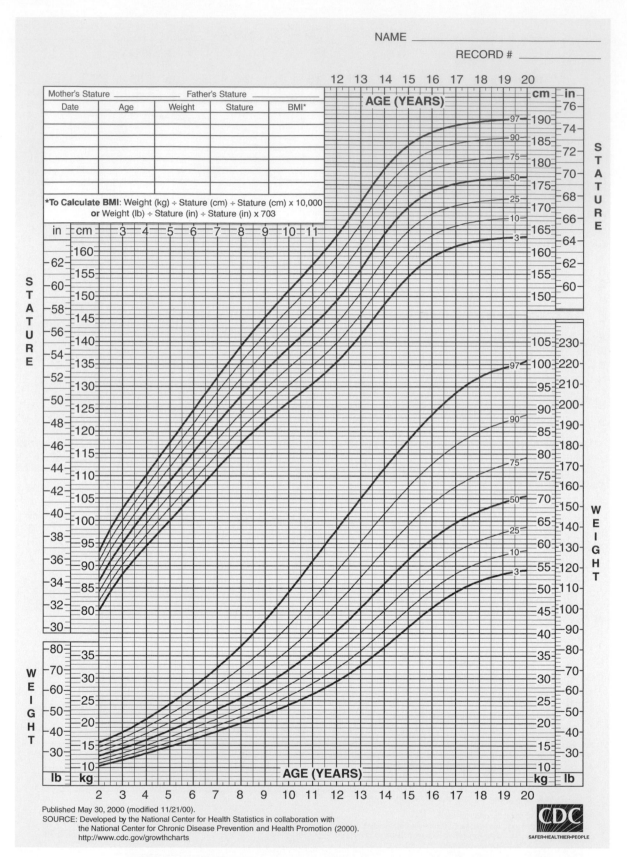

FIGURE 3 2 to 20 years: boys stature-for-age and weight-for-age percentiles.

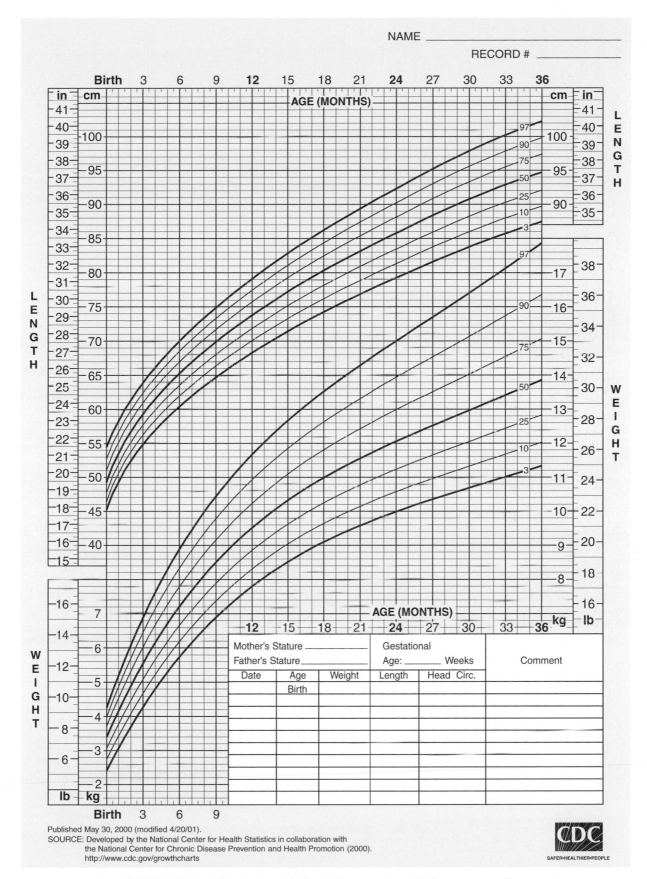

FIGURE 4 Birth to 36 months: girls length-for-age and weight-for-age percentiles.

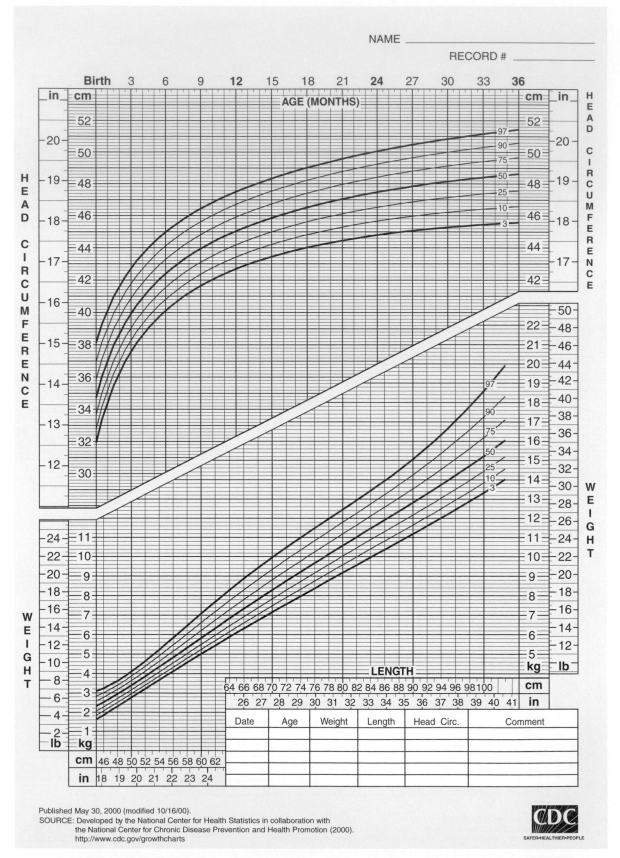

NAME _____

RECORD # _____

Published May 30, 2000 (modified 10/16/00).
SOURCE: Developed by the National Center for Health Statistics in collaboration with
the National Center for Chronic Disease Prevention and Health Promotion (2000).
http://www.cdc.gov/growthcharts

FIGURE 5 Birth to 36 months: girls head circumference-for-age and weight-for-length percentiles.

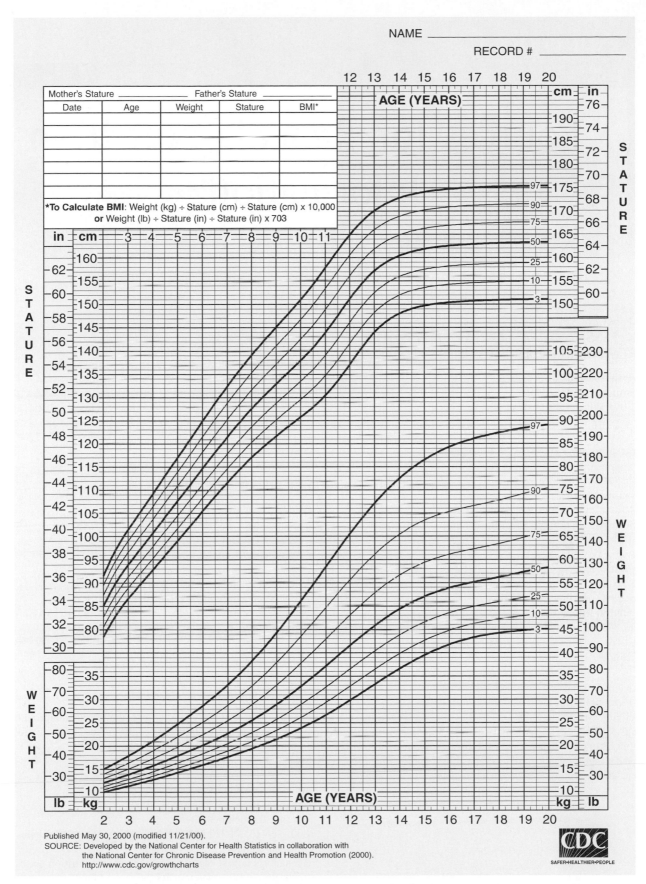

FIGURE 6 2 to 20 years: girls stature-for-age and weight-for-age percentiles.

Appendix C

Sources for Reliable Nutrition Information*

PROFESSIONAL ASSOCIATIONS AND ORGANIZATIONS

American Academy of Pediatrics
141 Northwest Point Blvd.
Elk Grove Village, IL 60007-1098
www.aap.org

American Association for Health Education
1900 Association Dr.
Reston, VA 20191-1598
www.aahperd.org

American Association of Dental Research
1619 Duke St.
Alexandria, VA 22314-3406
www.iadr.com

American Cancer Society
1599 Clifton Rd., N.E.
Atlanta, GA 30329-4251
(800) ACS-2345
www.cancer.org

American Cleft Palate-Craniofacial Association
1504 E. Franklin St., Ste. 102
Chapel Hill, NC 27514-2820
(800) 24-CLEFT
The American Cleft Palate-Craniofacial Association is an international nonprofit medical society of healthcare professionals who treat and perform research on birth defects of the head and face.
www.cleftline.org/default.htm

American Council on Science and Health
1995 Broadway, 2nd Fl.
New York, NY 10023-5860
The American Council on Science and Health, Inc. (ACSH) is a consumer education consortium concerned with issues related to food, nutrition, chemicals, pharmaceuticals, lifestyle, the environment, and health. ACSH is an independent, nonprofit, tax-exempt organization.
www.acsh.org

American Dental Association
211 E. Chicago Ave.
Chicago, IL 60611
www.ada.org
website for patient information:
www.ada.org/prof/resources/topics/index.asp

American Dental Hygienists' Association
444 N. Michigan Ave., Ste. 3400
Chicago, IL 60611
www.adha.org

American Diabetes Association
National Center
1701 N. Beauregard St.
Alexandria, VA 22311
The American Diabetes Association is the leading nonprofit health organization in the United States. It provides diabetes research, information, and advocacy.
www.diabetes.org

American Dietetic Association
120 South Riverside Plaza, Ste. 2000
Chicago, IL 60606-6995
(800) 366-1655 (National Center for Nutrition and Dietetics consumer hotline)
The nation's largest organization of food and nutrition professionals, the American Dietetic Association (ADA) serves the public by promoting optimal nutrition, health, and well-being.
www.eatright.org

---

*Note: Updated and additional Web addresses can be found on this text's Evolve site.

American Heart Association, National Center
7272 Greenville Ave.
Dallas, TX 75231-4596
www.americanheart.org

American Institute for Cancer Research
1759 R St., N.W.
Washington, DC 20009
(800) 843-8114
The American Institute for Cancer Research (AICR) supports research into the role of diet and nutrition in the prevention and treatment of cancer. It also offers a wide range of cancer prevention education programs.
www.aicr.org/site/PageServer

American Medical Association
Department of Foods and Nutrition
515 N. State St.
Chicago, IL 60610
(800) 621-8335
www.ama-assn.org

American Public Health Association
800 I St., N.W.
Washington, DC 20001-3710
The American Public Health Association (APHA) is an association of individuals and organizations working to improve the public's health and to achieve equity in health status for all.
www.apha.org

American Red Cross, National Headquarters
2025 E. St., N.W., 8th Floor
Washington, DC 20006
www.redcross.org

American School Health Association
7263 State Route 43
P.O. Box 708
Kent, OH 44240
www.ashaweb.org

Center for Science in the Public Interest (CSPI)
1875 Connecticut Ave., N.W., Ste. 300
Washington, DC 20009-5728
www.cspinet.org

Food Allergy Network
11781 Lee Jackson Highway, Ste. 160
Fairfax, VA 22033-3309
(800) 929 4040
www.foodallergy.org

Food Research and Action Center
1875 Connecticut Ave., N.W., Ste. 540
Washington, DC 20009
The Food Research and Action Center (FRAC) is a leading national organization working to improve public policies to eradicate hunger and undernutrition in the United States.
www.frac.org

Institute of Medicine
500 Fifth St., N.W.
Washington, DC 20001
www.iom.edu

International Food Information Council
1100 Connecticut Ave. N.W., Ste. 430
Washington, DC 20036
The International Food Information Council (IFIC) communicates science-based information on food safety and nutrition to health and nutrition professionals, educators, journalists, government officials, and others providing information to consumers. The IFIC is supported primarily by the broad-based food, beverage, and agricultural industries.
www.ific.org

International Life Science Institute, North America
Office of Education and Public Affairs
One Thomas Circle, 9th Fl.
Washington, DC 20005
The International Life Science Institute (ILSI) is a nonprofit, worldwide foundation that seeks to improve the well-being of the general public through the pursuit of balanced science. Its goal is to further the understanding of scientific issues relating to nutrition, food safety, toxicology, risk assessment, and the environment by bringing together scientists from academics, government, and industry.
www.ilsina.org

National Association of Nutrition and Aging Services Programs
1612 K St. N.W., Ste. 400
Washington, DC 20006
The National Association of Nutrition and Aging Services Programs (NANASP), a membership organization, supports a broad range of nutrition and related services for community-dwelling older people by training nutrition providers and advocating for older people.
www.nanasp.org

National Cattleman's Beef Association
9110 E. Nichols Ave., Ste. 300
Centennial, CO 80112
www.beef.org

National Council Against Health Fraud, Inc.
119 Foster St.
Peabody, MA 01960
The National Council Against Health Fraud (NCAHF) is a private nonprofit, voluntary health agency that focuses on health misinformation, fraud, and quackery as public health problems.
www.ncahf.org

National Dairy Council
10255 W. Higgins Rd., Ste. 900
Rosemont, IL 60018-5616
The National Dairy Council (NDC), the nutrition marketing arm of Dairy Management, Inc., has been the leader in dairy nutrition research, education, and communication since 1915. The NDC provides timely, scientifically sound nutrition information about fostering a healthier society.
www.nationaldairycouncil.org

National Foundation/March of Dimes
1275 Mamaroneck Ave.
White Plains, NY 10605-5298
www.modimes.org

Nutritional Screening Initiative
1010 Wisconsin Ave., N.W., Ste. 800
Washington, DC 20007
The Nutrition Screening Initiative (NSI) is a broad, multidisciplinary effort led by partner organizations the American Academy of Family Physicians and American Dietetic Association and a diverse coalition of more than 25 national health, aging, and medical organizations. The goal of the NSI is to promote the integration of nutrition screening and intervention into health care for older adults.
www.aafp.org/online/en/home.html

Society for Nutrition Education
7150 Winton Dr., Ste. 300
Indianapolis, IN 46268
www.sne.org

Special Care Dentistry
211 E. Chicago Ave., Ste. 740
Chicago, IL 60611
SCD promotes oral health and well-being for people with special needs.
www.scdonline.org

GOVERNMENTAL ENTITIES

Cancer Information Service
Office of Cancer Communication
NCI/NIH, Bldg. 31, 10A07
31 Center Dr. M5C2580
Bethesda, MD 20892-2580
(800) 4-CANCER
The Cancer Information Service (CIS) is a resource for the latest, most accurate cancer information from the National Cancer Institute (NCI).
cis.nci.nih.gov

Centers for Disease Control and Prevention
U.S. Department of Health and Human Services
1600 Clifton Rd., N.E.
Atlanta, GA 30333
www.cdc.gov

Center for Nutrition Policy and Promotion
3101 Park Center Dr., Rm. 1034
Alexandria, VA 22302-1594
The Center for Nutrition Policy and Promotion (CNPP) works to improve the health and well-being of Americans by developing and promoting dietary guidance that links scientific research to the nutrition needs of consumers. CNPP staff help to define and coordinate nutrition education policy within the U.S. Department of Agriculture (USDA), and to translate nutrition research into information and materials for consumers, policymakers, and professionals in health, education, industry, and media.
www.usda.gov/cnpp

Food, Nutrition, and Consumer Services
Special Nutrition Programs
U.S. Department of Agriculture
3101 Park Center Dr.
Alexandria, VA 22302
The Food, Nutrition, and Consumer Services (FNCS) ensures access to nutritious, healthful diets for all Americans. Through food assistance and nutrition education for consumers, the FNCS encourages consumers to make healthful food choices. Today, rather than simply providing food, the FNCS works to empower consumers with knowledge of the link between diet and health, providing dietary guidance based on research.
www.fns.usda.gov/fncs

Food and Drug Administration
U.S. Department of Health and Human Services
5600 Fishers Lane
Rockville, MD 20857
(888) 463-6332
www.fda.gov

Food and Nutrition Information Center
National Agricultural Library Bldg.
U.S. Department of Agriculture
Beltsville, MD 20705
The Food and Nutrition Information Center (FNIC) website provides a directory to credible, accurate, and practical resources for consumers, nutrition and health professionals, educators, and government personnel. Visitors can find printable format educational materials, government reports, research papers, and more.
www.nal.usda.gov/fnic

Food Nutrition and Consumer Service
Child Nutrition Division
U.S. Department of Agriculture
3101 Park Center Dr., Rm. 1017
Alexandria, VA 22302
www.fns.usda.gov/cnd

National Cancer Institute
U.S. Department of Health and Human Services
9000 Rockville Pike
Bethesda, MD 20892
(800) 4-CANCER
official website: **www.nci.nih.gov**
for the National Cancer Institute's (NCI) 5-a-day program:
www.5aday.gov

National Center for Education in Maternal and Child Health
2115 Wisconsin Ave., N.W., Ste. 601
Washington, DC 20007-2292
The Maternal and Child Health Library provides accurate and timely information on a broad range of topics. Materials include the weekly newsletter *MCH Alert,* resource guides, full text publications, databases, and links to quality Maternal and Child Health sites.
www.mchlibrary.info

The Surgeon General's call to action urges that oral health promotion, disease prevention, and oral health care have a presence in all health policy agendas set at local, state, and national levels. For this to happen, the public, health professionals, and policymakers must educate themselves to understand that oral health is essential to general health and well-being at every stage of life.
www.mchlibrary.info/KnowledgePaths/kp_oralhealth.html

National Institute on Aging
U.S. Department of Health and Human Services
Bldg. 31, Rm. 5C27
31 Center Dr., MSC 2292
Bethesda, MD 20892
www.nia.nih.gov

National Institutes of Health
Information Services
9000 Rockville Pike
Bethesda, MD 20892
The National Institutes of Health (NIH) is the steward of medical and behavioral research for the United States. It is an agency under the U.S. Department of Health and Human Services (USDHHS).
official website: **www.nih.gov**
website for health information: **//health.nih.gov**
Medline plus: **www.nlm.nih.gov/medlineplus**

National Cholesterol Education Program
National Heart, Lung, and Blood Institute C-200
National Institutes of Health
P.O. Box 30105
Bethesda, MD 20824-0105
The goal of the National Cholesterol Education Program (NCEP) is to contribute to reducing illness and death from coronary heart disease (CHD) in the United States by reducing the percentage of Americans with high blood cholesterol. Through educational efforts directed at health professionals and the public, the NCEP aims to raise awareness and understanding about high blood cholesterol as a risk factor for CHD, and the benefits of lowering cholesterol levels as a means of preventing CHD.
www.nhlbi.nih.gov/about/ncep

National Institute of Dental and Craniofacial Research
National Institutes of Health
Bethesda, MD 20892-2190
The mission of the National Institute of Dental and Craniofacial Research (NIDCR) is to promote the general health of the American people by improving their oral, dental, and craniofacial health. Through the conduct and support of research and the training of researchers, the NIDCR aims to promote health, prevent diseases and conditions, and develop new diagnostics and therapeutics.
www.nidr.nih.gov

Office on Women's Health
National Women's Health Information Center
U.S. Department of Health and Human Services
8550 Arlington Blvd., Ste. 300
Fairfax, VA 22031
(800) 994-9662
The Office on Women's Health offers reliable free information for women with special sections for heart disease and pregnancy.
www.4woman.gov

President's Council on Physical Fitness and Sports
Department W
200 Independence Ave., S.W., Room 738-H
Washington, DC 20201-0004
The President's Council on Physical Fitness and Sports (PCPFS) serves as a catalyst to promote, encourage, and motivate Americans of all ages to become physically active and participate in sports.
www.fitness.gov
www.presidentschallenge.org
www.smallstep.gov

U.S. Department of Agriculture
1400 Independence Ave., S.W.
Washington, DC 20250
www.usda.gov

U.S. Department of Health and Human Services
200 Independence Ave., S.W.
Washington, DC 20201
www.dhhs.gov

OTHER WEBSITES

Food Guide Pyramid
The Food and Nutrition Information Center has general information and clip art.
www.nal.usda.gov/fnic/Fpyr/pyramid.html

Dietary Reference Intakes
Dietary Reference Intakes: An Update
ific.org/publications/other/driupdateom.cfm

National Academy of Sciences
www.iom.edu/iom/iomhome.nsf/Pages/FNB+Reports

General Health and Nutrition
Food and Nutrition Information Center
www.nal.usda.gov/fnic/index.html

Healthfinder
Sponsored by the U.S. Department of Health and Human Services (USDHHS), Healthfinder provides health information from "A to Z"—prevention and wellness, diseases and conditions, and alternative medicine—plus medical dictionaries, an encyclopedia, journals, and more.
www.healthfinder.gov

National Health Information Center, U.S. Department of Health and Human Services
Website provides national referral resources.
(800) 336-4797
www.health.gov/nhic

Wellness web homepage
www.wellweb.com
Healthy People 2010 website
www.healthypeople.gov

FOOD LABELING

Food Labeling and Nutrition
www.cfsan.fda.gov/label.html

OBESITY AND DIET

Nutrition and Obesity
www.niddk.nih.gov/health/nutrit/nutrit.htm

BODY WEIGHT

Aim for a Healthy Weight
www.nhlbi.nih.gov/health/public/heart/obesity/lose_wt/index.htm

DIETARY ANALYSIS

Interactive Healthy Eating Index, developed by the U.S. Department of Agriculture's (USDA) Center for Nutrition Policy and Promotion, analyzes daily food intake and provides a Healthy Eating Index (HEI) "score" representing the overall quality of the diet in terms of total fat, saturated fat, cholesterol, sodium, variety, and intake of five food groups.
www.nhlbi.nih.gov/health/public/heart/obesity/lose_wt/index.htm

Fat Calories is not specifically a diet analysis tool, but provides valuable information on the nutritional facts of 10 popular fast food restaurant chains.
www.fatcalories.com

FitDay offers numerous tracking options for users, including food intake, physical activity, and weight and online journaling.
www.fitday.com

Life Clinic allows users to set personalized weight, meal, and nutrition goals.
www.lifeclinic.com

The U.S. Department of Agriculture (USDA) National Nutrient Database for Standard Reference provides data for 6220 foods for 117 nutrients and food components. The data files can be viewed or downloaded for use later on your computer.
www.ars.usda.gov/ba/bhnrc/ndl

DietSite offers a simple diet and recipe analysis program.
dietsite.com

My Nutrition Analysis Tools, developed by faculty from the University of Illinois, has numerous features for analyzing food intake.
nat.uiuc.edu

VEGETARIAN NUTRITION

Food and Nutrition Information Center, U.S. Department of Agriculture (USDA)
fnic.nal.usda.gov/nal_display/index.php?info_center=4&tax_level=1

North American Vegetarian Society
www.navs-online.org

Seventh-day Adventist Dietetic Association
www.sdada.org

Vegetarian Resource Group
www.vrg.org

PHYSICAL ACTIVITY

The President's Council has an interactive website to encourage activity and fitness.
www.presidentschallenge.org
www.fitness.gov

Nutrition and physical activity page from the Centers for Disease Control and Prevention (CDC)
www.cdc.gov/nccdphp/dnpa/physical/index.htm

America on the Move is a website that encourages people to become more active through organized groups and prevent weight gain by increasing activity (steps) slightly and reducing total calories by 100 kcal per day.
www.americaonthemove.org

DIETARY AND HERBAL SUPPLEMENTS

The Federal Trade Commission (FTC) enforces a variety of federal antitrust and consumer protection laws and provides guidance on advertising dietary supplements.
www.ftc.gov/bcp/conline/pubs/buspubs/dietsupp.htm

U.S. Food and Drug Administration (FDA) Center for Food Safety and Applied Nutrition
www.cfsan.fda.gov

FDA warnings regarding certain dietary supplements
www.cfsan.fda.gov/~dms/supplmnt.html

National Institutes of Health Office of Dietary Supplements provides health information, research programs and information, and fact sheets for various dietary supplements.
dietary-supplements.info.nih.gov

Consumer Lab provides consumers and healthcare professionals with results of independent tests of products that affect health and well-being.
www.consumerlab.com

The Council for Responsible Nutrition, a science-based trade association of the dietary supplements industry, reports on vitamin and mineral safety.
www.crnusa.org

About Herbs contains unbiased monographs with citations from the scientific literature that bolster or refute the purported clinical properties of herbs or supplements. This website was created and is maintained by the Integrative Medicine Service at Memorial Sloan-Kettering Cancer Center in New York. The website also explains some of the conditions the agents are used to treat, adverse effects, and potential drug interactions.
www.mskcc.org/aboutherbs

HerbMed, sponsored by Alternative Medicine Foundation, Inc., is an interactive, electronic herbal database providing scientific data underlying the use of herbs for health.
www.herbmed.org

International Bibliographic Information on Dietary Supplements (IBIDS) Database is a database produced by the Office of Dietary Supplements (ODS) at the National Institutes of Health (NIH) and the Food and Nutrition Information Center, National Agricultural Library (USDA) to assist the public, healthcare providers, and researchers in locating credible, scientific literature on dietary supplements.
ods.od.nih.gov/databases/ibids.html

The U.S. Pharmacopeia (USP) helps ensure that consumers receive medicines of the highest possible quality by setting the standards that manufacturers must meet to sell their products in the United States. The USP provides standards for more than 3700 medicines, dietary supplements, and dosage forms. The website provides monographs on selected dietary supplements.
www.usp.org

VERIS Research Information Service is a not-for-profit corporation that strives to provide a responsible source of information on the role of nutrition in health with an emphasis on antioxidants.
www.verisconsulting.com/NewsArticle.aspx?newsArticleId=-32680

Ergogenic Aid/Athletic Supplements
www.geocities.com/HotSprings/Spa/9971/index.html

PREGNANCY AND LACTATION

La Leche League International
www.lalecheleague.org

March of Dimes Birth Defects Foundation
www.modimes.org

National Osteoporosis Foundation
www.nof.org

INFANTS AND CHILD HEALTH

Infant Formula
www.cfsan.fda.gov/~dms/inf-toc.html

Growth charts for infants and children
www.cdc.gov/growthcharts

Bright Futures
brightfutures.org

Exercise and nutrition related to children
www.healthfinder.gov/kids
www.cdc.gov/nccdphp/dnpa

Eat Smart, Play Hard Resources
www.fns.usda.gov/eatsmartplayhard
www.health.state.ny.us/nysdoh/nutrition/resources/pages/ewph.htm

Physician-approved health information about children from before birth through adolescence
kidshealth.org

Maternal and Child Health Library
Oral Health and Children and Adolescents
www.mchlibrary.info/knowledgepaths/kp_oralhealth.html

ACTIVATE is an educational outreach program of the International Food Information Council (IFIC) Foundation, developed in partnership with the American Academy of Family Physicians, American College of Sports Medicine, American Dietetic Association, International Life Sciences Institute Center for Health Promotion, and National Recreation and Park Association. ACTIVATE is committed to promoting healthy family lifestyles to help prevent kids from becoming overweight to reduce their risk of having obesity-related chronic diseases as adults.
www.kidnetic.com

OLDER ADULTS

Administration on Aging
www.aoa.dhhs.gov

Meals on Wheels Association of America
www.mowaa.org

National Aging Information Center, U.S. Administration on Aging
www.aoa.gov/eldfam/nutrition/nutrition/aspx

National Institute on Aging Information Center
www.nih.gov/nia/health/health.htm

Tufts University's Jean Mayer Human Nutrition Research Center on Aging
hnrc.tufts.edu

FOOD SAFETY

Iowa State University Extension's Web-based food safety question and answer service is science-based and peer-reviewed by qualified food safety experts from academics, federal government, associations, and industry.
www.foodsafetyanswers.org

The American Dietetic Association and ConAgra jointly sponsor this site regarding consumer food handling. Recent food safety research surveys indicate consumer food handling practices.
www.homefoodsafety.org

Partnership for Food Safety Education (government, professional, and trade associations) sponsors this site with information for consumers, media, and educators regarding food safety.
www.fightbac.org

U.S. government gateway to food safety information is easy for consumers to use.
www.foodsafety.gov

Center for Food Safety and Applied Nutrition
www.cfsan.fda.gov

Food Safety and Inspection Service
www.fsis.usda.gov/index.htm

FOOD INSECURITY AND HUNGER

American's Second Harvest
www.secondharvest.org

Child and Adult Care Food Program
www.fns.usda.gov/cnd/Care/CACFP/cacfphome.htm

Food Research and Action Center
www.frac.org

The Hunger Site
www.thehungersite.com

Appendix D

Recommended Journals and Newsletters*

American Family Physician; available at www.aafp.org/afp

American Journal of Clinical Nutrition; available at www.ajcn.org (abstracts available; subscription required for access to articles)

American Journal of Dentistry; available at www.amjdent.com (subscription required for access to articles)

American Journal of Public Health; available at www.ajph.org (subscription required for access to articles)

British Dental Journal; available at www.bmj.com

Caries Research; available at content.karger.com

Circulation (publication of the American Heart Association); available at circ.ahajournals.org (abstracts available; subscription required for access to full articles)

Compendium Continuing Education Dentistry; available at http://ce.compendiumlive.com/default.asp

Dairy Council Digest (National Dairy Council); available at www.nationaldairycouncil.org/NationalDairyCouncil/; www.newenglanddairycouncil.org/health/hp-sub-home.html; www.newenglanddairycouncil.org

Dental Update; available at www.dental-update.co.uk

Diabetes; available at www.diabetesjournals.org

Diabetes Forecast; available at www.diabetes.org/diabetesforecast

Dimensions of Dental Hygiene; available at www.dimensionsofdentalhygiene.com

FDA Consumer; available at www.fda.gov/fdac/fdacindex.html

Journal of the American College of Nutrition; available at www.jacn.org (abstracts available; subscription required for access to full articles)

Journal of the American Dental Association; available at http://jada.ada.org

Journal of the American Dietetic Association; available at www.eatright.org. (subscription required for access to articles)

Journal of the American Medical Association; available at www.jama.ama-assn.org

Journal of Contemporary Dental Practice; available at www.thejcdp.com

Journal of Dental Education; available at www.jdentaled.org

Journal of Dental Hygiene; available at www.adha.org

Journal of Dental Research; available at jdr.iadrjournals.org

Journal of Nutrition Education and Behavior; available at www.jneb.org (subscription required for access to articles)

Journal of Pediatrics; available at www.mosby.com/jpeds (abstracts available; subscription required for access to articles)

The Lancet; available at www.thelancet.com (abstracts available; subscription required for access to articles)

Mayo Clinic Health Letter; available at www.newsletters@mayoclinic.com

New England Journal of Medicine; available at http://content.ncjm.org

Nutrition Action Health Letter; available at www.cspinet.org/nah/index.htm

Nutrition and Cancer; available at www.informaworld.com

Nutrition and the MD; available at wwnewsletters.com (subscription required for access to articles)

Nutrition Reviews; available at www.ingentaconnect.com/content/ilsi/nure (subscription required for access to articles)

Pediatrics; available at www.pediatrics.org (abstracts available; subscription required for access to articles)

RDH; available at www.rdhmag.com

School Nutrition; available at www.schoolnutrition.org (subscription required for access to articles)

Supermarket Savvy Newsletter; available at www.supermarketsavvy.com

Today's Dietitian; available at www.todaysdietitian.com (subscription required for access to articles)

Tufts University Health Nutrition Letter; available at www.healthletter.tufts.edu (abstracts available; subscription required for access to articles)

University of California, Berkeley Wellness Letter; available at www.wellnessletter.com

---

*Note: Updated and additional Web addresses can be found on this text's Evolve site.

Appendix E

Comparison of Popular Diets

Diets used for weight loss generally fit into several classifications (Box E-1). Research is seldom conducted on a specific diet, but rather by general macronutrient distribution. Although some particular differences exist between diets (e.g., one diet may emphasize *trans* fatty acids, whereas another may ignore them), much of the research available pertains to all the diets within that classification. For one of each classification of diets, this appendix presents a detailed description with research that has been conducted. References to research studies supporting statements in this paper are listed at the end.

Any diet should be evaluated in terms of its allowing adequate amounts from each of the food groups and adhering to the principles of the *Dietary Guidelines for Americans* to ensure a nutritionally balanced diet without excessive amounts of food components that may contribute to a chronic disease. Kilocalories consumed must be less than the amount the body needs. It is the position of the American Dietetic Association that successful weight management to improve overall health for adults requires a lifelong com-

mitment to healthful lifestyle behaviors emphasizing sustainable and enjoyable eating practices and daily physical activity.

Other diets exist that are based on consumption of one particular food purportedly responsible for the weight loss; these diets are considered "gimmick" diets. No information is presented about these diets because of a lack of research regarding them. Some examples of these diets include the "raw food," "cabbage soup," and "miracle" diets. No food contains a magic ingredient that causes weight loss.

Losing weight is important, but, statistically, losing weight and maintaining that weight loss are more difficult than kicking a heroin or cocaine addiction. In addition to increased activity levels, restricted energy intake must occur in such a manner that the individual is likely to remain compliant and experience satiety. To date, no easy answers are available. Many weight loss approaches have been harmful to health. The goal is to lose weight in ways that make the person healthier rather than cause harm.

Box E-1 | Popular Diets by Classification*

Low Carbohydrate, High Fat†‡
- New Diet Revolution (Dr. Atkins)
- Sugar Busters (Leighton Steward and Associates)
- Protein Power Lifeplan (Michael and Mary Eades)
- The Carbohydrate Addict's Lifespan Program (Richard and Rachael Heller)

High Carbohydrate, Low Fat¶
- Eat More, Weight Less (Ornish)
- Pritikin (Nathan Pritikin)
- Weight Watchers (Weight Watchers)
- Slimfast Meal Replacement (Slimfast)
- An Eating Plan for Healthy Americans (American Heart Association)

Moderate Carbohydrate, Moderate Fat§
- South Beach (Arthur Agatston)
- Zone (Barry Sears)
- Mediterranean (Oldways Preservation and Exchange Trust and Harvard School of Public Health)
- Low Glycemic Diet (Richard Podell)
- DASH (National High Blood Pressure Education Program)
- The McDougall Program for Maximum Weight Loss (John and Mary McDougall)
- Eating Well for Optimum Health (Andrew Weil)
- Dieting for Dummies (Jane Kirby)
- Mayo Clinic Healthy Weight Pyramid (Donald Hensrud)
- Volumetrics (Barbara Rolls and Associates)

*Up-to-date information and lists of current diet trends can also be found on the Evolve site for this text.
†Contain 20% or less of the kilocalories from carbohydrate; 25% to 30% from protein, and 55% to 65% from fat.
‡Generally, these diets are low in vitamins E, A, and B₆; thiamin; folate; calcium; magnesium; iron, zinc; potassium; and dietary fiber. Dietary supplements are usually recommended.
§Contain 40% to 60% of the kilocalories from carbohydrate, 20% to 30% from protein, and 30% or less from fat.
¶Contain approximately 65% of the kilocalories from carbohydrate, 15% to 20% from protein, and 10% to 19% from fat.

Low Carbohydrate, High Fat: *Dr Atkins' New Diet Revolution*	Moderate Carbohydrate, Moderate Fat: *South Beach Diet*	High Carbohydrate, Low Fat: *Eat More, Weigh Less (Ornish Diet)*
Basic Premise	**Basic Premise**	**Basic Premise**
Carbohydrates cause obesity, and sugar causes great swings in insulin levels, which makes excess fat stores. Eliminating or minimizing carbohydrate intake results in weight loss and longevity of life. Minimal carbohydrate intake results in ketosis, "which is simply the most efficient path ever devised for getting you slim," and ketosis "suppresses hunger and lowers appetite."	This diet, which has three phases, teaches an individual how to rely on the right carbohydrates and fats.	As indicated by the name of this diet, a very-high-starch, very-high-fiber diet allows a person to eat a greater volume of food while still losing body fat. Fat is about one-third the usual amount found in the typical American diet. Very small quantities of meat and limited dairy products make this diet semivegetarian. The limited meats allowed are more of a garnish rather than a major component of the meal. Because of the reliance on low-energy dense foods, weight loss is almost a given; weight gain would be practically impossible. The diet recommends whole-grain products, legumes, fruits and vegetables, and minimal amounts of saturated fat and all added fats.
During the *induction* phase, which lasts for only 2 weeks, carbohydrate intake is less than 20 g daily. Liberal combinations of fat and protein, including meat, cheese, eggs, and fats (including saturated fats), are allowed with instructions to "eat until full, not stuffed." This introductory phase is supposed to "kick-start" the body to switch over to using fat for energy.	In phase 1, normal-sized portions of low-fat meats (chicken, turkey, fish, and shellfish) with adequate servings of vegetables, low-fat cheese, eggs, and nuts are allowed in three balanced meals and three snacks daily. Bread, rice, potatoes, pasta, baked goods, ice cream, beer or alcohol, fruit, and sugar are not allowed during this first 2-week period. The body should become acclimated to lack of unhealthy sugars and starches, and "physical cravings that ruled your eating habits will be gone." The dieter is warned against staying on the diet for more than 2 weeks, but the book indicates that many stay on longer because of more rapid weight loss. Amounts are not limited, and the dieter should never feel hungry. Meals should be just enough to satisfy hunger. Weight loss is expected to be 8 to 13 lb over the 2-week period.	Dr. Ornish encourages much more than healthy eating; physical activity and stress reduction are heavily emphasized. He has conducted research on this diet for many years and promoted it for its ability to reduce blood cholesterol levels. He states that sometimes it is "easier for people to make more comprehensive changes in diet and lifestyle because they experience the benefits so quickly and to a much greater degree."
During the *ongoing weight loss (OWL)* phase, 5 g of carbohydrate per week is added, but weight loss continues. The most crucial phase, *pre-maintenance,* begins when dieters have less than 10 lb to lose. Dieters should be accustomed to eating a certain way to prepare for permanent slimness and new healthier lifetime eating habits. The *maintenance* phase warns that the dieter must stick to the diet to some extent for the rest of his or her life to avoid weight rebound. "Your best carbohydrate level is the one you can be happiest on without weight regain."	In phase 2, healthy carbohydrates, some fruit, whole-grain bread and rice, whole-wheat pasta, low-fat milk and yogurt, sweet potatoes, and pinto beans are introduced. This phase lasts until achievement of the target weight. Certain foods are avoided: refined wheat products, cookies, white potatoes and rice, beets, carrots, corn, potatoes, bananas, canned fruit and fruit juices, pineapple, raisins, watermelon, honey, ice cream, and jam.	

Low Carbohydrate, High Fat: *Dr Atkins' New Diet Revolution*

Moderate Carbohydrate, Moderate Fat: *South Beach Diet*

High Carbohydrate, Low Fat: *Eat More, Weigh Less (Ornish Diet)*

Phase 3, the most liberal stage of the diet, is how the individual should eat for life. However, after overindulgences, the first phase may need to be implemented for 1 or 2 weeks. No food list is provided for the third phase.

Facts

The high-protein, low-carbohydrate, high-fat diet produces rapid weight loss (fluid, body fat, reduced loss of lean body mass) more quickly, partially because of increased diuresis and loss of body fat; spares muscle loss; protein is possibly directly related to weight loss related to a metabolic advantage; reduces plasma triglycerides, total cholesterol, and LDL cholesterol levels, and increases HDL cholesterol; enhances glycemic control; increases satiety; increases thermogenesis; and causes ketosis or halitosis (65% of dieters) with an anorectic effect (especially malodorous when combined with periodontitis).

Facts

After the first phase, this diet is rich in vegetables, fruits, whole grains, and lean protein, and it does not omit any major food groups. Eliminating highly processed carbohydrates and simple sugars and limiting the amount of fats, especially saturated fats, is good nutrition.

However, Agatston's book contains many glaring nutrition inaccuracies, contradictions, and claims of scientific evidence that simply are not available yet. The premise that a high-carbohydrate diet causes high blood glucose levels resulting in insulin secretion and hypoglycemia, leading to hunger and cravings, has no scientific basis. It is well established that unless diabetes mellitus is present, blood glucose levels remain remarkably stable. Research has not linked relatively low blood glucose levels to hunger. Although the book says the diet is "distinguished by the absence of calorie counts" or "rules about portion size," recipes clearly indicate how many servings each one contains along with caloric value. Another inconsistency is the fact watermelon is to be avoided because it is full of sugar, but cantaloupe is allowed. (A cup of either contains 14 g of sugar.)

Based on one study using a high-protein, low-fat diet, body weight and fat mass declined more with individuals being more satiated than individuals on the high-carbohydrate diet. Total levels of cholesterol, insulin, and uric acid decreased. A high-protein, low-fat, energy-restricted diet can promote healthful weight loss.

Facts

The diet provides large amounts of fiber and copious amounts of antioxidants and phytochemicals that are effective in reducing blood cholesterol levels. Limitations on milk and meat products may affect the adequacy of essential minerals such as niacin, iron, magnesium, calcium, and phosphorus.

Low Carbohydrate, High Fat: *Dr Atkins' New Diet Revolution*	**Moderate Carbohydrate, Moderate Fat:** *South Beach Diet*	**High Carbohydrate, Low Fat:** *Eat More, Weigh Less (Ornish Diet)*
Nutritional Evaluation Induction phase—1500-1800 kcal, 30% protein, 57% fat, 8% carbohydrate (20 g) OWL phase—1600-1800 kcal, 31% protein, 56% fat, 11% carbohydrate (46 g) Pre-maintenance—1500-1800 kcal, 21% protein, 65% fat, 12% carbohydrate (45 g) This diet is inadequate in many nutrients, especially calcium, magnesium, potassium, thiamin, vitamins D and E, fiber, and phytochemicals because limited amounts of fruits and vegetables and dairy products are consumed; the diet is very high in cholesterol, fat, and saturated fat.	**Nutritional Evaluation** Phase 1—1400-1500 kcal; 33% protein, 54% fat, 13% carbohydrate Phase 2—1500-1600 kcal; 22% protein, 41% fat, 42% carbohydrate Phase 3—1600 to 1800 kcal; 18% protein, 39% fat, 45% carbohydrate	**Nutritional Evaluation** Less than 10% fat, 15%-20% protein, 70%-75% carbohydrate, and 5 mg cholesterol This diet may be deficient in vitamins E and B_{12} and zinc.

Potential Health Implications

Low Carbohydrate, High Fat

Weight loss over the long-term is unproven; weight loss at 1 year is not significantly different from other diets. The diet may also contribute to mood swings and depression resulting from lack of serotonin production, impaired cognitive performance, lack of energy, headaches (54% of dieters), constipation (70% of dieters), hair loss (10%), gout, dehydration and electrolyte abnormalities, and more serious problems such as kidney and heart problems.

Potential Health Implications

Moderate Carbohydrate, Moderate Fat

Long-term weight loss is unproven; phase 1 may contribute to mood swings and depression as a result of lack of serotonin production; it may also contribute to impaired cognitive performance.

Potential Health Implications

High Carbohydrate, Low Fat

This diet promotes weight reduction and reduces harmful total cholesterol and LDL cholesterol levels. A published peer review study found blood flow to the heart improved on a very-low-fat diet and was detrimentally affected by the low-carbohydrate, high-fat diet. One study showed the diet accompanied with lifestyle changes can lead to regression of atherosclerosis, which was sustained for 5 years. Another study found greater reductions in anginal frequency; body weight; body mass index (BMI); blood pressure; and total cholesterol, LDL cholesterol, glucose, and insulin levels than in individuals in a usual-care control group. Total cholesterol levels, weight, LDL cholesterol levels, and insulin levels improved more than on any of the other diets. In most studies using this diet, HDL cholesterol levels remained the same or decreased. HDL cholesterol is generally thought of as "protective" against heart disease. Per Dr. Ornish, "HDL is like a garbage truck that goes around picking up garbage or bad cholesterol. When you don't have as much bad cholesterol, or garbage, you don't need as many garbage trucks."

Low Carbohydrate, High Fat: *Dr Atkins' New Diet Revolution*	Moderate Carbohydrate, Moderate Fat: *South Beach Diet*	High Carbohydrate, Low Fat: *Eat More, Weigh Less (Ornish Diet)*
Recommendation	**Recommendation**	**Recommendation**
This diet is not recommended because of many questions about the effects of high fat intake, and studies indicate people with higher BMIs generally consume a high-fat diet. In favor of the diet, Americans like eating large amounts of protein foods and like the easy-to-follow, no calorie counting/complicated meal plans. Rapid weight loss may contribute to a lower dropout rate. Long-term compliance is poor.	This diet is questionable, especially with all the inconsistencies found in the book, but it is safer than the Atkins diet. Individuals should not stay on phase 1 of the diet longer than 2 weeks, and skipping that phase would be even better. Studies show high-carbohydrate diets are generally more nutritionally adequate, and high-carbohydrate, moderate-fat diets result in the lowest BMIs.	This diet is recommended for patients with diagnosed heart disease who can adapt to a lifestyle with minimal amounts of meat. Extreme changes necessitated by this diet results in very poor long-term compliance.
Patients with health problems such as intestinal, liver, or kidney disease or diabetes mellitus; women who are pregnant or are trying to get pregnant; and adolescents and athletes should consult their physician before starting the low-carbohydrate regimen.	Patients with health problems such as intestinal, liver, or kidney disease or diabetes mellitus; women who are pregnant or are trying to get pregnant; and adolescents and athletes should consult their physician before starting the low-carbohydrate regimen.	

References

Agatston A: The South Beach Diet. New York: Rodale Press, 2003.

Aldana SG, et al: Cardiovascular risk reductions associated with aggressive lifestyle modification and cardiac rehabilitation. Heart Lung 2003 Nov-Dec; 32(6):374-382.

Appel LJ, et al: Effects of protein, monounsaturated fat, and carbohydrate intake on blood pressure and serum lipids: results of the OmniHeart randomized trial. JAMA 2005 Nov 16; 294(19):2455-2464.

Atkins RC: Dr. Atkins' New Diet Revolution. New York: M Evans & Co, 1999.

Batterham RL, et al: Critical role for peptide YY in protein-mediated satiation and body-weight regulation. Cell Metab 2006 Sep; 4(3):223-233.

Bravata DM, et al: Efficacy and safety of low-carbohydrate diets. JAMA 2003 Apr 9; 289(14):1837-1850.

Clifton PM, Keogh JB, Noakes M: Long-term effects of a high protein weight loss diet. Am J Clin Nutr 2008 Jan; 87(12):23-29.

Dansinger ML, et al: One-year effectiveness of the Atkins, Ornish, Weight Watchers, and Zone Diets in decreasing body weight heart disease risk. Presented at the American Heart Association Scientific Sessions, Orlando, November 11, 2003.

Fleming R, Boyd LB: The effect of high-protein diets on coronary blood flow. Angiology 2000 Oct; 51(10):817-826.

Foster GD, et al: A randomized trial of a low-carbohydrate diet for obesity. N Engl J Med 2003 May 22; 348(21):2082-2090.

Gardner CD, et al: Comparison of the Atkins, Zone, Ornish, and LEARN diets for change in weight and related risk factors among overweight premenopausal women: the A to Z Weight Loss Study: a randomized trial [Erratum in JAMA 2007 Jul 11; 298(2):178]. JAMA 2007 Mar 7; 297(9):969-977.

Halton TL, et al: Low-carbohydrate-diet score and the risk of coronary heart disease in women. N Engl J Med 2006 Nov 9; 355(19):1991-2002.

Johnston CS, Tjonn SL, Swan PD: High-protein, low-fat diets are effective for weight loss and favorably alter biomarkers in healthy adults. J Nutr 2004 Mar; 134(3):586-591.

Kennedy ET: Popular diets: correlation to health, nutrition, and obesity. J Am Diet Assoc 2001 Apr; 101(4):411-420.

Layman DK, Baum JI: Dietary protein impact on glycemic control during weight loss. J Nutr 2004 Apr; 134(4):968S-973S.

Levine MJ, Jones JM, Lineback DR: Low-carbohydrate diets: assessing the science and knowledge gaps, summary of an ILSI North American workshop. J Am Diet Assoc 2006 Dec; 106(12):2086-2094.

Luscombe-Marsh ND, et al: Carbohydrate-restricted diets high in either monounsaturated fat or protein are equally effective at promoting fat loss and improving blood lipids. Am J Clin Nutr 2005 Apr; 81(4):762-772.

Maki KC, et al: Effects of a reduced-glycemic-load diet on body weight, body composition, and cardiovascular disease risk markers in overweight and obese adults. Am J Clin Nutr 2007 Mar; 85(3):724-734.

Metcalf N (ed): New diet winners. Consumer Reports 2007 Jun. Available at www.ConsumerReports.org.

Ornish D: Was Dr. Atkins right? J Am Diet Assoc 2004 Apr; 104(4):537-542.

Ornish D, et al: Intensive lifestyle changes for reversal of coronary heart disease. JAMA 1998 Dec 16; 280(23):2001-2007.

Schoeller DA, Buchholz AC: Energetics of obesity and weight control: does diet composition matter? J Am Diet Assoc 2005; 105 (Suppl 1, 5):S24-S28.

Stern L, et al: The effects of low-carbohydrate versus conventional weight loss diets in severely obese adults. Ann Intern Med 2004 May 18; 140(10):778-785.

Weigle DS, et al: A high-protein diet induces sustained reductions in appetite, ad libitum caloric intake, and body weight despite compensatory changes in diurnal plasma leptin and ghrelin concentrations. Am J Clin Nutr 2005 Jul; 82(1):41-48.

Westman EC, et al: Effect of 6-month adherence to a very low carbohydrate program. Am J Med 2002 Jul; 113(1):30-36.

Wing RR, Vazquez JA, Ryan CM: Cognitive effects of ketogenic weight-reducing diets. Int J Obes Relat Metab Disord 1995 Nov; 19(11):811-816.

Wolfe RR: The underappreciated role of muscle in health and disease. Am J Clin Nutr 2006 Sep; 84(3):475-482.

Answers to Nutritional Quotient Questions

CHAPTER 1: OVERVIEW OF HEALTHY EATING HABITS

1. False. No single food contains all the essential nutrients in amounts needed for optimal health.
2. False. Only consumption of added sugars should be reduced. Naturally occurring sugars, especially from milk and fruits, are desirable.
3. True.
4. False. DRIs are a set of categories of nutrient-based reference values that include the estimated average requirements, recommended dietary allowances, adequate intakes, and tolerable upper intake levels intended to be used for planning and assessing diets of healthy Americans and Canadians.
5. True.
6. False. Three to five servings are recommended for vegetables, and two to four servings are recommended for fruit.
7. True.
8. False. Sugar is implicated in dental caries, but not in other major diseases, such as hypertension, cardiovascular disease, or diabetes mellitus.
9. True.
10. False. The nutrients that provide energy are carbohydrates, fats, and proteins.

CHAPTER 2: THE ALIMENTARY CANAL: DIGESTION AND ABSORPTION

1. True.
2. False. This is the hydrolysis of lipids or fat; carbohydrate yields monosaccharides.
3. False. Absorption occurs primarily in the small intestine.
4. False. Long-chain triglycerides enter the lymphatic system; short-chain and medium-chain triglycerides enter the portal circulation.
5. True.
6. False. Most enzymes end in -ase (e.g., lactase); lactose is a sugar found in milk.
7. True.

8. False. Villi are located in the small intestine.
9. True.
10. True.

CHAPTER 3: CARBOHYDRATE: THE EFFICIENT FUEL

1. False. The FDA has labeled raw sugar as unfit for direct use as a food or a food ingredient because of the impurities it contains.
2. True.
3. False. Oral bacteria are unable to metabolize xylitol, which is a calorie-containing sugar alcohol.
4. False. The desire for sweetness is not considered an acquired taste because newborn infants exhibit a preference for it.
5. True.
6. True.
7. False. Excessive caloric intake leads to obesity, whether from carbohydrates, proteins, fats, or alcohol.
8. False. Sucrose is table sugar.
9. False. Many other factors, including consumption of other fermentable carbohydrates, contribute to development of caries.
10. True.

CHAPTER 4: PROTEIN: THE CELLULAR FOUNDATION

1. True.
2. False. The breed of hen determines the color of eggshell, and color is not related to its nutritional value.
3. False. Gelatin does not contain all the EAAs.
4. False. The protein requirement is at least equal to that of a young adult and may be increased.
5. False. Adequate amounts of protein are needed for development of healthy teeth, but increasing protein beyond the RDA would not have any effect on tooth enamel.
6. True.
7. True.

419

8. False. It is a protein-deficiency and kilocalorie-deficiency disorder.
9. False. In addition to foods from plants, dairy products are consumed. Eggs are excluded.
10. True.

CHAPTER 5: LIPIDS: THE CONDENSED ENERGY

1. False. The overall average of fat intake is important; foods, such as margarine and oils, are 100% fat, but can be used safely in the diet.
2. False. As an antioxidant, vitamin E protects the oil to which it is added to some degree; however, in doing so, vitamin E is inactivated, so it cannot be used by the body.
3. True.
4. False. The AMDR for fat is estimated to be 20% to 35% of energy intake for adults.
5. False. Bananas contain a trace of fat; avocados are 88% fat. However, they are both plant products, so they do not contain any cholesterol.
6. False. All fats produce 9 kcal/g.
7. True.
8. False. Even though they are nutritious foods, for most Americans, their use should be limited because of their high fat content.
9. True.
10. True.

CHAPTER 6: USE OF THE ENERGY NUTRIENTS: METABOLISM AND BALANCE

1. True.
2. True.
3. False. BMR stands for basal metabolic rate, which is the amount of energy needed to maintain involuntary physiologic functions.
4. True.
5. True.
6. False. Hunger is the physiological drive to eat, whereas appetite implies a desire for specific types of food.
7. False. Fats are stored by the body for energy, but they must first be converted into a form the body can use. Glycogen stores, which depend on carbohydrate intake, are readily available for energy.
8. True.
9. True.
10. False. Only fats, carbohydrates, proteins, and alcohol provide energy.

CHAPTER 7: VITAMINS REQUIRED FOR CALCIFIED STRUCTURES

1. True.
2. True.
3. True.
4. True.
5. False. Retinol is obtained from animal foods; beta carotene is found in fruits and vegetables.
6. True.

7. True.
8. False. A deficiency of vitamin D causes rickets.
9. False. Vitamin K is essential for blood clotting; vitamin D functions in regulation of blood calcium and phosphorus levels.
10. True.

CHAPTER 8: MINERALS ESSENTIAL FOR CALCIFIED STRUCTURES

1. True.
2. False. Many nutrients work together in building strong healthy bones, including protein, calcium, phosphorus, magnesium, fluoride, and vitamins C and D.
3. True.
4. True.
5. False. Based on the DRIs, teenagers need 1300 mg of calcium. To obtain adequate amounts of calcium, $4\frac{1}{2}$ cups of milk are recommended for teenagers (300 mg calcium/cup $\times$ $4\frac{1}{2}$ = 1350 mg calcium).
6. False. Fluoridation of community water supplies is the most effective method of preventing dental caries.
7. False. Calcium supplements by themselves probably are not beneficial to women older than 30.
8. True.
9. False. Caffeine decreases calcium absorption.
10. False. Bottled waters vary in fluoride content.

CHAPTER 9: NUTRIENTS PRESENT IN CALCIFIED STRUCTURES

1. False. The IOM has established ULs for copper, manganese, and molybdenum, but not for chromium.
2. True.
3. True.
4. False. Alzheimer's disease and aluminum toxicity are two different conditions.
5. True.
6. False. Unrefined foods generally provide more trace minerals.
7. False. Aluminum is cariostatic, especially in combination with fluoride.
8. True.
9. False. Sugar is not a good source of any nutrients except kilocalories; sugar consumption results in increased insulin levels, affecting the chromium requirement.
10. False. Selenium supplements are not recommended because selenium can be toxic.

CHAPTER 10: VITAMINS REQUIRED FOR ORAL SOFT TISSUES AND SALIVARY GLANDS

1. True.
2. False. Vitamin D is called the sunshine vitamin because sun facilitates the body's production of vitamin D; vitamin B_6 is also called pyridoxine, pyridoxal, and pyridoxamine.
3. False. Beriberi is caused by a thiamin deficiency; niacin deficiency causes pellagra.
4. True.

5. False. Flushing and intestinal disturbances are symptoms of niacin toxicity. No toxicity symptoms have been observed for thiamin.
6. True.
7. True.
8. False. Liver, leafy vegetables, legumes, grapefruit, and oranges are rich sources of folate.
9. True.
10. True.

CHAPTER 11: WATER AND MINERALS REQUIRED FOR ORAL SOFT TISSUES AND SALIVARY GLANDS

1. True.
2. True.
3. True.
4. True.
5. False. The IOM has established an AI for total fluid (beverages, water, and food) requirements to be 15 to 16 cups per day for men and 11 to 12 cups per day for women.
6. False. The minimum requirement for sodium is 500 mg per day for adults, but no RDA has been established for sodium.
7. True.
8. False. Potassium is principally within the cells (intracellular).
9. True.
10. False. Oral pallor is a sign of iron-deficiency anemia.

CHAPTER 12: NUTRITIONAL REQUIREMENTS AFFECTING ORAL HEALTH IN WOMEN

1. False. These do not reflect natural instincts for required nutrients.
2. True.
3. False. If the diet is deficient in calcium, the fetal calcium requirements would be met first, but some of the calcium may come from her bones, not from her teeth.
4. False. Although she is "eating for two," normal energy requirements are not doubled. Depending on the prepregnancy weight, approximately 300 calories more than her usual caloric requirement are needed during the second and third trimesters.
5. True.
6. False. Iron and folate are usually the nutrients needing supplementation.
7. True.
8. False. Breast milk is normally thin and is nutritionally adequate.
9. False. The more often an infant nurses, the more milk is produced. Milk production is most active during infant sucking.
10. True.

CHAPTER 13: NUTRITIONAL REQUIREMENTS THROUGH THE LIFE CYCLE AND EATING HABITS AFFECTING ORAL HEALTH

1. True.
2. False. Fluoride supplements are not recommended for infants older than 6 months even though breast milk and artificial breast milk are low in fluoride.

3. False. Solid foods are introduced between 4 and 6 months of age, not at 6 weeks.
4. False. Orange juice is one of the last juices to be introduced because of the high frequency of allergies.
5. True.
6. True.
7. False. Breastfed infants need a supplement of 200 IU vitamin D beginning during the first 2 months to prevent rickets.
8. False. Suckling, as occurs when extracting milk from the breast, encourages maximum development of the genetically defined jaw and chin; breastfed infants are less likely to develop malocclusion.
9. True.
10. False. Toddlers and children need snacks because of their high energy needs; however, wholesome snacks (e.g., cheese cubes, fresh fruit, raw vegetable sticks, milk, or yogurt) that do not promote tooth decay are recommended.

CHAPTER 14: NUTRITIONAL REQUIREMENTS FOR OLDER ADULTS AND EATING HABITS AFFECTING ORAL HEALTH

1. False. Because of changes in nutrient requirements secondary to physiological changes, the IOM has developed DRIs for individuals 51 to 70 years old and older than 70 years.
2. True.
3. True.
4. False. The texture for edentulous patients is determined by their own preferences.
5. False. Dehydration is a frequent occurrence in elderly individuals for many reasons—impaired homeostatic mechanisms, decreased thirst sensation, inability of the kidney to concentrate urine, changes in functional status, side effects of medications, and mobility disorders.
6. True.
7. False. Intake requirement is lower because of menopause.
8. True.
9. False. Although it is highly likely that an elderly individual may benefit from taking a dietary supplement, toxicity or nutrient imbalances may occur. An older individual should consult a healthcare provider before deciding to take a vitamin supplement.
10. False. Physical activity can help ameliorate some chronic health problems, improve physiological well-being, and relieve symptoms of depression and anxiety.

CHAPTER 15: OTHER CONSIDERATIONS AFFECTING NUTRIENT INTAKE

1. True.
2. False. Patterns and attitudes internalized during childhood promote a sense of stability and security for older patients.
3. False. No culture has ever been known to make food choices solely on the basis of nutritional values of food. The factors that seem to predominate in food choices are cultural and economic.
4. False. Only about 10% of the American food dollar is spent on food.
5. False. Fad diets may be physically harmless, but they are usually not based on sound nutritional principles.

6. False. Scientific research to date has not shown any nutritional benefits from the use of organically grown foods.
7. False. Although some food processing is detrimental to the nutritive value of foods, the goal of food processing is to maintain optimum qualities of color, flavor, texture, and nutritive value.
8. True.
9. True.
10. True.

CHAPTER 16: EFFECTS OF SYSTEMIC DISEASE ON NUTRITIONAL STATUS AND ORAL HEALTH

1. True.
2. True.
3. False. Supplements for anemia should not be prescribed without the results of blood testing to determine the type of anemia. High intakes of iron could possibly complicate the situation.
4. False. Because of the various considerations involved in constructing a meal plan and lifestyle changes for a patient with diabetes, the patient must be referred to diabetes specialists.
5. True.
6. True.
7. False. Kaposi's sarcoma is a tumor that occurs frequently in immunocompromised patients.
8. True.
9. False. Although a patient with an eating disorder should be referred to a physician or an eating disorder program, it is the dental hygienist's responsibility to approach the patient with the objective findings.
10. False. Bulimics are generally of normal weight or sometimes above recommended body weight.

CHAPTER 17: NUTRITIONAL ASPECTS OF DENTAL CARIES: CAUSES, PREVENTION, AND TREATMENT

1. False. A combination of diet, host, environment, and saliva are necessary for initiation of dental decay.
2. True.
3. True.
4. True.
5. False. Sugar alcohols are fermented slowly by oral bacteria, and they are noncariogenic. Xylitol is cariostatic because of its ability to inhibit production of *Streptococcus mutans.*
6. False. An acid environment is required to demineralize a tooth; a cariogenic food causes the plaque pH to decrease to less than 5.5. Foods allowing plaque pH to increase to greater than 6 are considered noncariogenic.
7. False. It is the least important factor to consider. Identifying frequency of intake, physical form, and spacing of food within a day or meal would provide a more accurate assessment.
8. True.
9. False. Although the RDAs provide a lot of factual information, they are too overwhelming for most patients. MyPyramid and *Dietary Guidelines for Americans* provide practical and general nutrition information relevant to preventing dental decay and improving overall health.

10. False. Information alone does not guarantee a behavioral change.

CHAPTER 18: NUTRITIONAL ASPECTS OF GINGIVITIS AND PERIODONTAL DISEASE

1. True.
2. False. Indirectly, firm, fibrous foods reduce the amount of bacterial plaque biofilm by stimulating salivary flow, which promotes oral clearance of food and lessens food retention.
3. False. A nutrient deficiency can be a contributing factor to gingivitis, but local irritants (plaque biofilm and calculus) must be present. The inflammation can be exaggerated by a nutrient deficiency, and by reduced resistance and recovery time.
4. True.
5. False. A patient may interpret this advice as condoning ice cream, gelatin, and chicken noodle soup, which would not provide enough nutrients or kilocalories for quick recovery. The dental hygienist should provide a specific list of nutrient-dense foods for the patient to purchase before the periodontal surgery.
6. True.
7. True.
8. True.
9. True.
10. False. If surgery is indicated for a periodontal patient, optimally, the nutritional assessment and counseling should be done before the procedure to increase nutrient reserves that would expedite the recovery period.

CHAPTER 19: NUTRITIONAL ASPECTS OF ALTERATIONS IN THE ORAL CAVITY

1. False. Although root surface caries can be a complication of xerostomia, other causes are possible, such as frequent intake of hard candy. Also, a complete and thorough assessment of the patient is essential. No single factor is adequate to diagnose the presence, extent, or cause of root caries. An inaccurate evaluation can lead to inappropriate recommendations.
2. False. Although xerostomia is a common complaint in an older adult, the changes in saliva in a healthy older individual are minimal. Xerostomia has been strongly associated with multiple factors, such as use of medications, one or more systemic diseases, and radiation, all of which are common to this population.
3. True.
4. False. Root caries appear on the root surface, in areas of gingival recession. This condition is seen more often in older adults who have experienced periodontal disease or toothbrush trauma.
5. True.
6. False. It is important to have nutrient-dense foods available, but in different consistencies. A full liquid diet, progressing to a mechanical soft diet and then to a regular diet would allow the patient to adjust to swallowing, chewing, and biting with the new appliance.
7. True.
8. False. Spongy cancellous bone is the major component of alveolar bone.

9. True.
10. True.

CHAPTER 20: NUTRITIONAL ASSESSMENT AND COUNSELING FOR DENTAL HYGIENE PATIENTS

1. False. Although the health and dental histories provide valuable information, they are not enough to determine the patient's nutritional status. Other evaluation tools include clinical assessment and dietary intake.
2. False. Clinical oral examinations detect physical signs and symptoms of many nutrient deficiencies. However, deficiencies generally do not appear until an advanced state exists. An oral examination should be used as an adjunct in identifying potential nutritional deficiencies.
3. True.
4. True.
5. False. Dietary counseling must be documented and other staff members informed about the nutritional counseling for consistency and reinforcement of the information at future appointments.
6. False. Changing a dietary habit is difficult and requires a meal plan and lifestyle behavior changes tailored to meet the patient's needs. A thorough assessment identifies many factors that should be considered. Active involvement of the patient in establishing a meal pattern enhances compliance.
7. False. The dental hygienist is responsible for providing information and guiding the patient to make healthier decisions. Active participation, problem solving, and decision making allow for greater compliance. The patient should highlight the fermentable carbohydrates.
8. False. Changing food habits is very difficult. The first attempt established by the dental hygienist and patient may not have been successful, and other alternatives may need to be established. Follow-up is an essential component of the nutritional counseling process.
9. True.
10. True.

Index

Page numbers followed by *f*, *t*, and *b* indicate
figures, tables, and boxed material, respectively.

425

Meats
   contributions of, in daily nutrition, 19t
   or meat substitutes
      in MyPyramid Food Guidance System, 18
      recommended, and frequency, 14t
Mechanical soft diet, 357–359, 358b
Medication use, during pregnancy, 229
Mediterranean diet. *See* Popular diets.
Medium-chain fatty acids, 86
Megadoses, of vitamins, 193b–195b
Megaloblastic anemia
   dental hygiene considerations in, 320b
   and folate deficiency, 187
   nutritional directions for, 321b
   oral manifestations in, 319–320
Menopause
   dental hygiene considerations in, 242b
   nutritional directions for, 242b
   nutritional requirements in, 241–244
Mental health disorders, oral manifestations in,
      317t, 332–337
Mental illness, oral manifestations in, 334–337
Menu creation and planning, 387, 387f
Mercury, 171–174
Meta-analysis, 141b–142b
Metabolic disorders, oral manifestations in,
      317t, 324–328
Metabolic pathways, 105, 105f
Metabolism, 105–106, 109–110
   anabolic processes in, 105–107
   catabolic processes in, 105, 107–109
   endocrine effects on, 111
   and energy balance, 113–115
   and energy production, 110
      from alcohol, 108–109
      basal metabolic rate in, 110–111
      from carbohydrates, 106–107, 109
      dental hygiene considerations of, 109b
      key terminology of, 104–105
      from lipids, 108–109
      nutritional directions for, 110b
      from proteins, 107–109
   health application in, 116b–119b
   and patient health
      dental hygiene considerations of, 106b
      nutritional directions for, 106b
   references on, 122
   and role of kidneys, 106
   and role of liver, 106
   and satiety center, 114
Microflora, of large intestine, 44–45, 55
Micronutrients, 6–7
Microvilli, of small intestine, 42
Milk, analysis of fat content of, 95t
Milk and milk product group, in Food Pyramid
      Guidance System, 18
Milk and milk products, 150
   anticariogenic properties of, 345–346, 345f
   for children over two years, 261
   daily consumption of, by Americans, 148
   for infants, 250. *See also* Infant formula(s).
   recommended, and frequency, 14t
Milk consumption, versus soft drink
      consumption, 59, 60f
Milk sugar, 52–53
Mineral electrolytes
   case application in, 222b
   chloride in, 211

Mineral electrolytes *(Continued)*
   health application in, 220b–221b
   insufficiency of, in older adults, 283
   iodine in, 218–223
   iron in, 213–214
   in oral soft tissue physiology, 199, 206. *See
      also specific mineral electrolyte.*
   potassium in, 211–213
   references on, 223–224
   sodium in, 206–210
   terminology of, 199
   zinc in, 216–217
Mineralization, 146
Minerals, 147b, 145–163, 164–174
   and calcified structure physiology, 146. *See
      also* Calcium; Fluoride; Magnesium;
      Phosphorus.
      bone growth in, 146
      case application of, 161b–162b
      health application of, 160b–161b
      key terminology of, 145–146
      references on, 162–163
      tooth formation in, 146–147
   as food additives, 306t–307t
   insufficiency of, in older adults, 281–283
   in pregnancy, recommended dietary
      allowance (RDA) of, 230
   supplemental, for older adults, 284–289
   trace, in calcified structures, 165. *See also*
      Chromium; Copper; Manganese;
      Molybdenum; Selenium; Ultratrace
      elements.
Misinformation, about nutrition, 305–313
   dental hygienist's role in combating,
      309–313
   identifying sources of, 308–309, 309b
Molybdenum, 169
   dental hygiene considerations of, 169b
   hyper-states and hypo-states of, 169
   nutritional directions for, 169b
   nutritional requirements for, 169, 170t
   physiologic roles of, 169
   recommended dietary allowance (RDA) for,
      169, 170t
   sources of, 169
Monosaccharides, 51–53, 51f
   metabolism of, 106–107
Monounsaturated fatty acids (MUFAs), 86–87
   food sources of, 93, 93t
   physiologic actions of, 90t
Mouth. *See* Oral cavity.
Mucositis, 319
My Nutrition Analysis Tools, 410
Myelin synthesis, vitamin B_{12} (cobalamin) in,
      188
MyPyramid Food Guidance System, 7, 13
   for children, 253f, 257
   dental hygiene considerations of, 20b, 348
   discretionary kilocalories group in, 19
   drawbacks of, 14
   following food intake over time on, 15
   food group representation in, 14
   food industry promotion of, 16
   foundation for, 7
   fruits group in, 16–18
   grains group in, 14–20
   in-depth information about food groups in,
      14–15

MyPyramid Food Guidance System
      (Continued)
   and intake comparison to *Dietary Guidelines
      for Americans,* 15
   links to MyPyramid Tracker on, 15
   menu planner on, 15–16
   milk and milk products group in, 18
   nutritional directions for, 20b
   oils group in, 18–19
   for older adults, 282f, 283–289
   personalization of, 15
   physical activity information incorporated in,
      15
   for pregnant and lactating women, 235, 236f.
      See also MyPyramid for Moms.
   professional use of, 16
   protein foods group in, 18
   sample menu plan based on, 10f–11f
   tools of, 14
   vegetables group in, 16
MyPyramid food record worksheet, 383f
MyPyramid for Kids, 253f, 257, 257f
MyPyramid for Moms, 239, 240f
MyPyramid Menu Planner, 15–16
MyPyramid Tracker tool, 15

N

National Academy of Sciences, 409
National Aging Information Center, 411
National Association of Nutrition and Aging
      Services Program, 407
National Cancer Institute, 408
National Cattleman's Beef Association, 407
National Center for Education in Maternal and
      Child Health, 408
National Cholesterol Education Program, 409
National Council Against Health Fraud, 407
National Dairy Council, 407
National Foundation/March of Dimes, 408
National Health Information Center, 410
National Institute of Dental and Craniofacial
      Research, 409
National Institute on Aging, 409
National Institute on Aging Information Center,
      411
National Institutes of Health, 409
   Office of Dietary Supplements, 410
National Nutrient Database for Standard
      Reference, 410
National Osteoporosis Foundation, 411
National Osteoporosis Foundation, vitamin D
      intake recommendations of, 130–131
Natural food products, lack of definition of,
      304
Natural killer cells, and folate, 187
Necrosis, 76–77
Necrotizing ulcerative gingivitis (NUG), 359–
      362, 359f
   bland diets in, 360, 360b
   dental hygiene considerations in, 360b–
      361b
   nutritional and dietary considerations in, 360
   nutritional directions for, 361b
   and protein energy malnutrition, 76–77
Necrotizing ulcerative periodontitis (NUP),
      359–362
Neoplastic disorders, oral manifestations in,
      317t, 330–331, 330f

book 3 HO
book H
book P box 1-1

page 5 box 1-1
page 14
page 346.